Series Editors:
David R. Beukelman, Ph.D.
Joe Reichle, Ph.D.

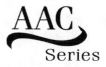

AAC
Series

Communicative Competence
for Individuals Who Use AAC

Also in the Augmentative and
Alternative Communication Series:

*Exemplary Practices for Beginning
Communicators: Implications for AAC*
edited by Joe Reichle, Ph.D.,
David R. Beukelman, Ph.D.,
and Janice C. Light, Ph.D.

*Augmentative and Alternative Communication
for Adults with Acquired Neurologic Disorders*
edited by David R. Beukelman, Ph.D.,
Kathryn M. Yorkston, Ph.D.,
and Joe Reichle, Ph.D.

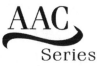

AAC
Series

Communicative Competence for Individuals Who Use AAC

From Research to Effective Practice

edited by

Janice C. Light, Ph.D.
The Pennsylvania State University–University Park

David R. Beukelman, Ph.D.
University of Nebraska–Lincoln

and

Joe Reichle, Ph.D.
University of Minnesota–Twin Cities

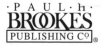

·P·A·U·L·H·
BROOKES
PUBLISHING C°®

Baltimore • London • Sydney

MW

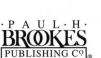

Paul H. Brookes Publishing Co.
Post Office Box 10624
Baltimore, Maryland 21285-0624

www.brookespublishing.com

Typeset by Integrated Publishing Solutions, Grand Rapids, Michigan.
Manufactured in the United States of America by
Versa Press, Inc., East Peoria, Illinois.

Library of Congress Cataloging-in-Publication Data

Communicative competence for individuals who use AAC : from research to effective
    practice / edited by Janice C. Light, David R. Beukelman, and Joe Reichle.
        p.   cm.–(AAC series)
    Includes bibliographical references and index.
    ISBN 1-55766-639-3
    1. Communicative disorders–Treatment. 2. Communicative disorders–Patients–
    Rehabilitation. 3. People with disabilities–Means of communication
    I. Light, Janice C. (Janice Catherine) II. Beukelman, David R., 1943–
    III. Reichle, Joe, 1951– IV. Series.
    RC423.C654 2003
    616.85'506–dc21   2003044305

British Library Cataloguing in Publication data are available from the British Library.

5/21/04

Contents

I Definition of Communicative Competence

II Linguistic Competence

Series Preface

The purpose of the *Augmentative and Alternative Communication Series* is to address advances in the field as they relate to issues experienced across the life span. Each volume is research-based and practical, providing up-to-date and ground-breaking information on recent social, medical, and technical developments. Each chapter is designed to be a detailed account of a specific issue. To help ensure a diverse examination of augmentative and alternative communication (AAC) issues, an editorial advisory board assists in selecting topics, volume editors, and authors. Prominent scholars, representing a range of perspectives, serve on the editorial board so that the most poignant advances in the study of AAC are sure to be explored.

In the broadest sense, the concept of AAC is quite old. Gestural communication and other types of body language have been widely addressed in the literature about communication for hundreds of years. Only recently, though, has the field of AAC emerged as an academic discipline that incorporates graphic, auditory, and gestural modes of communicating. The series concentrates on achieving specific goals. Each volume details the empirical methods used to design AAC systems for both descriptive groups and for individuals. By tracking the advances in methods, current research, practice, and theory, we will also develop a broad and evolutionary definition of this new discipline.

Many reasons for establishing this series exist, but foremost has been the number and diversity of the people who are affected by AAC issues. AAC consumers and their families, speech-language pathologists, occupational therapists, physical therapists, early childhood educators, general and special educators, school psychologists, neurologists, and professionals in rehabilitative medicine and engineering all benefit from research and advancements in the field. Likewise AAC needs are not delineated by specific age parameters; people of all ages who have developmental and acquired disabilities rely on AAC. Appropriate interventions for individuals across a wide range of disabilities and levels of severity must be considered.

Fundamentally, the field of AAC is problem driven. We, the members of the editorial advisory board, and all professionals in the field are dedicated to solving problems in order to improve the lives of people with disabilities. The inability to communicate effectively is devastating. As we chronicle the advances in the field of AAC, we hope to systematically dismantle the barriers that prevent effective communication for all individuals.

Editorial Advisory Board

Volume Preface

> If I could not express myself, I would become like the tree in the forest–the one for which it does not matter if it makes a sound when it comes crashing down, because there is no one around to hear it. Unfortunately there are still a great many silent fallen trees all around us if we stop and look. (Williams, 2000, p. 250).

Approximately 12 of every 1,000 people are unable to meet their daily communication needs through speech. They require augmentative and alternative communication (AAC) (e.g., signs, gestures, communication boards, voice output communication aids). Unless these individuals receive effective AAC interventions and supports, they will not have a "voice"; they will remain silenced. This quotation by Bob Williams underscores how important it is that people receive the necessary interventions and supports to develop the communicative competence essential to communicate effectively with others and participate fully in society. The ability to communicate is at the very center of people's lives, for communication allows people to express their thoughts and feelings, to define who they are, to connect with others in meaningful ways, and to participate in education and work. The development of communicative competence is essential to express needs and wants, share information with others, and develop social closeness with family and friends.

For people with significant communication disabilities who require AAC, the journey to attain communicative competence presents many challenges. The goals are the same whether one communicates using natural speech or AAC: 1) to develop the means, knowledge, judgment, and skills required to communicate effectively; and 2) to ensure the opportunities and supports required to meet a full range of communication objectives, including the expression of needs and wants, social closeness interactions with others, information exchange, and social etiquette routines.

Although these goals are the same, the path to attaining communicative competence is fundamentally different for individuals who use AAC compared with those who use natural speech. The tools of communication and the skills required of the communicator are different. So, too, are the opportunities and the environmental supports available for communication and the barriers that must be overcome. These differences result from the motor, sensory perceptual, cognitive, social, and linguistic capabilities of the individuals who require AAC; the characteristics of the AAC systems; the characteristics of the environment; and the knowledge, attitudes, and interaction skills of communication partners.

This book explores the development of communicative competence by individuals with developmental disabilities who require AAC. Specifically, it discusses the means, knowledge, judgment, skills, and psychosocial attributes required by individuals who use AAC to attain communicative competence as well as the effects of environmental barriers and supports. The book presents interventions to enhance communicative competence and discusses methods to evaluate outcomes of these interventions.

The intent of this volume is to review the current research, to summarize what is known based on this research foundation, and to discuss the implications for effective practice to enhance the communicative competence of individuals who require AAC. The volume also delineates the gaps in current knowledge and understanding and defines priorities for future research. It is written for those with advanced interests in AAC and individuals with developmental disabilities and will be of interest to educational and rehabilitation professionals, students, researchers, and anyone else with an interest in the development of communicative competence by individuals with developmental disabilities who require AAC.

ORGANIZATION OF THE BOOK

This book is divided into six parts: an introductory section; sections on linguistic competence, operational competence, social competence, and strategic competence; and a section on issues related to interventions to enhance communicative competence. Section I: Definition of Communicative Competence provides an overview chapter (Chapter 1) by Janice C. Light that discusses a framework for considering the development of communicative competence by individuals who require AAC, including factors intrinsic to the individual who uses AAC and those extrinsic in the environment. Specifically, Light discusses the knowledge, judgment, and skills required in linguistic, operational, social, and strategic domains; she also considers the effects of various psychosocial factors such as motivation, attitude, confidence, and resilience. Finally, Light considers the communicative demands of the environment and the barriers or supports available that may hinder or facilitate communicative competence.

The next four sections of the book each focus on one of the domains of knowledge, judgment, and skills that are critical to the development of communicative competence by individuals who use AAC: linguistic, operational, social, and strategic domains (Light, 1989).

Section II: Linguistic Competence includes five chapters, each focused on a fundamental issue in the development of linguistic competence by individuals who use AAC, including the development of receptive and expressive skills within the spoken language(s) of the family and community as well as skills in the "language code" of the AAC systems. In Chapter 2, Katherine C. Hustad and Kathy L. Shapley discuss the relationship between natural speech and AAC for various groups of individuals with developmental disabilities and include an examination of speech production capabilities, speech intelligibility, use of speech, communicative effectiveness, and integration of multiple modes of communication including AAC and natural speech.

In Chapter 3, Susan Blockberger and Ann Sutton consider how children with developmental disabilities and extremely limited speech acquire linguistic skills in the language(s) of their community. They also consider how the development of linguistic competence affects learning to use AAC.

In Chapter 4, Beth Mineo Mollica focuses on the language representation component of AAC systems, specifically the visual representation of language through pictures. She examines the many factors that affect an individual's ability to use picture-based representations to communicate, including characteristics of the communicator, characteristics of the representational media, and the nature of the task itself.

In Chapter 5, MaryAnn Romski and Rose A. Sevcik provide a general overview of the role of language input in the development of linguistic and communicative competence and then consider the specific role of input language in AAC interventions. They review the research on the effects of augmented input (i.e., the use of speech plus AAC as input) and provide a conceptual framework for considering these effects. Finally, Romski and Sevcik discuss implications of augmented input for effective practice.

In the final chapter in Section II (Chapter 6), Martine M. Smith and Nicola Clare Grove consider three factors that influence language acquisition and the development of linguistic competence: the structural characteristics of the language, the input provided to the language learner, and the processing of the input by the language learner. Specifically, they consider these factors with reference to the unique experiences of language learners who require AAC where the modalities of input (typically speech) differ from those of output (AAC with or without some speech). These authors consider the clinical and educational implications of this asymmetry between input and output and suggest priorities for research to advance understanding and improve language outcomes.

Section III: Operational Competence encompasses knowledge, judgment, and skills in tool use. Particularly important are skills that lead to the accurate and efficient operation of AAC systems (e.g., skills producing the correct hand shape, movement, and configuration of signs or gestures; skills accessing the aided AAC system). This section includes three chapters that discuss the impact of motor skills (Chapter 7), cognitive skills (Chapter 8), and visual skills (Chapter 9) on the development of operational competence by individuals with developmental disabilities who use AAC.

In Chapter 7, Jutta Treviranus and Vera Roberts discuss motor impairments experienced by various groups of individuals with developmental disabilities who require AAC. These authors consider the impact of motor impairments on skill acquisition as it relates to the operation and use of AAC. According to Treviranus and Roberts, learning to use AAC systems is like learning to play a musical instrument. Like a musician, the individual who uses AAC requires specialized skills, acquired through intense instruction and practice, to control AAC systems effectively. Treviranus and Roberts consider techniques to optimize AAC systems for motor control and operational competence, including factors related to unaided systems as well as those related to aided systems (e.g., the control act, input device, selection method). Finally, they discuss the significant challenges confronted in research and product design. They propose strategies to overcome these challenges and improve the design of AAC systems to enhance functional use.

In Chapter 8, Charity Rowland and Philip D. Schweigert address the relationship between communication skills and cognitive skills for individuals who require AAC. Specifically, they debunk the myth that there are cognitive prerequisites to communication intervention. Rowland and Schweigert then discuss six cognitive factors and consider their relevance to AAC interventions: awareness, communicative intent, world knowledge, memory, symbolic representation, and metacognitive learning.

In addition to motor and cognitive skills, it is also important to consider the impact of vision on the development of operational competence by individuals who require AAC. Most AAC systems use visual symbols whether they are unaided or aided. In Chapter 9, Tracy M. Kovach and Patricia Bothwell Kenyon provide background information on visual impairments often experienced by individuals with developmental disabilities who require AAC. They discuss the impact of these impairments on communication development and consider interventions to enhance visual functioning. Finally, Kovach and Kenyon discuss the design of auditory scanning systems to enhance the communicative competence of individuals with significant speech, motor, and visual impairments.

With the development of linguistic and operational competencies, individuals who require AAC have the tools necessary to communicate; however, they must also develop the skills to use these tools effectively to communicate in social interactions. Section IV: Social Competence explores the sociolinguistic as well as the sociorelational aspects of social competence. Teresa A. Iacono (Chapter 10) reviews the research literature related to the development of sociolinguistic or pragmatic skills by individuals with developmental disabilities and considers the implications for individuals who use AAC across various stages of development. She presents strategies to enhance pragmatic development in light of factors intrinsic to individuals who require AAC and extrinsic in the environment. Iacono also considers gaps in our understanding of pragmatic development and presents directions for future research to address these gaps.

In addition to the development of sociolinguistic or pragmatic skills, it is also important for individuals who use AAC to develop sociorelational competence, which requires knowledge, judgment, and skills in the interpersonal aspects of communication. Janice C. Light, Kara B. Arnold, and Elizabeth A. Clark (Chapter 11) tackle the issue of sociorelational competence, which is an issue that has long been neglected in the AAC field. Light and colleagues review what is known about the development of sociorelational skills by individuals who require AAC and consider implications for effective practice. They also review what is known about the attitudes of others toward individuals who require AAC and consider the influence of attitude barriers and other opportunity barriers on the development of sociorelational competence.

Despite interventions to develop the linguistic, operational, and social competencies of individuals who require AAC, given the significant speech, motor, language, sensory perceptual, and/or cognitive impairments and the environmental barriers experienced by individuals who require AAC, it is inevitable that they will encounter limitations in their linguistic, operational, and social competencies that restrict their communication. In these situations, individuals who require AAC must rely on strategic competence. Section V: Strategic Competence includes a chapter by Pat Mirenda and Karen D. Bopp (Chapter 12) that addresses the temporary and long-term strategies used by individuals who require AAC to overcome operational, linguistic, social, and environmental constraints to attain communicative competence. Despite the critical importance of strategic competence for individuals who require AAC, as of 2003 there has been very little research in this area. As a result, Chapter 12 draws heavily on the personal accounts of individuals who use AAC. Mirenda and Bopp conclude their chapter by identifying key questions and issues for future research to enhance our understanding of the development of strategic competence.

The final section of the book, Section VI: Interventions to Build Communicative Competence, presents a summary discussion of intervention issues. In Chapter 13, Joe Reichle, Mary Jo Cooley Hidecker, Nancy C. Brady, and Nancy Terry provide an overview of the continuum of intervention strategies that can be used to establish communicative symbol use, ranging from those with minimal involvement of an interventionist (e.g., fast mapping) to those with substantial interventionist involvement (e.g., direct instruction). Reichle and colleagues discuss the challenges in designing interventions to develop a full range of communicative acts, to ensure that these skills are well discriminated but highly generalized, and to ensure the use of appropriate modes of communication.

Finally, in Chapter 14, Ralf W. Schlosser discusses approaches to measuring the outcomes of AAC interventions to ensure that they are truly making a positive difference in the lives of individuals with significant communication disabilities, their families, and other facilitators. Schlosser focuses specifically on three potential approaches to outcome measurement: goal attainment scaling, measures of participation, and quality of life measures. He provides descriptions of these approaches, discusses strengths and limitations, and illustrates these measures with applications from the AAC field. The chapters by Reichle and colleagues and by Schlosser provide an important framework for planning, implementing, and evaluating effective AAC interventions to enhance communicative competence.

CONCLUSION

This book is dedicated to the many individuals with developmental disabilities who have significant communication disabilities and require AAC. Their journey to attain communicative competence presents many challenges. As Bob Williams poignantly illustrates in the opening quote to this preface, too many individuals who require AAC have been effectively silenced in their lives due to a lack of appropriate interventions and supports. It is our hope that this book will serve to advance knowledge and practice in the field so that these individuals receive the effective instruction and the supports that they require to attain communicative competence and meet their full potential. It is our belief that all people who require AAC have the fundamental right to an effective "voice" to communicate and that society has a responsibility to ensure that every voice is heard.

REFERENCES

Light, J. (1989). Toward a definition of communicative competence for individuals using augmentative and alternative communication systems. *Augmentative and Alternative Communication, 5,* 137–143.

Williams, B. (2000). More than an exception to the rule. In M. Fried-Oken & H.A. Bersani, Jr. (Eds.), *Speaking up and spelling it out: Personal essays on augmentative and alternative communication* (pp. 245–254). Baltimore: Paul H. Brookes Publishing Co.

About the Editors

Janice C. Light, Ph.D., Professor, Department of Communication Sciences and Disorders, The Pennsylvania State University, 110 Moore Building, University Park, Pennsylvania 16802. Dr. Light is actively involved in research, personnel preparation, and service delivery in the area of augmentative and alternative communication (AAC). Her primary interest has been furthering understanding of the development of communicative competence and self-determination in individuals who use AAC, and she is co-author of the book *Building Communicative Competence with Individuals Who Use Augmentative and Alternative Communication* (1998, Paul H. Brookes Publishing Co.). Dr. Light is the principal investigator on several federally funded research grants to improve outcomes for individuals with significant communication disabilities through the use of AAC. She is also one of the project directors in the Augmentative and Alternative Communication Rehabilitation Engineering Research Center (AAC-RERC), a virtual research consortium funded by the National Institute on Disability and Rehabilitation Research. In 1996, Dr. Light was recognized as the Don Johnston Distinguished Lecturer by the International Society of Augmentative and Alternative Communication for her leadership in the AAC field. In 1999, she received the Dorothy Jones Barnes Outstanding Teaching Award at The Pennsylvania State University. In 2002, Dr. Light received the Evan G. and Helen G. Pattishall Outstanding Research Achievement Award from The Pennsylvania State University in recognition of her dedication to scholarship and her excellence in research.

David R. Beukelman, Ph.D., Professor, Department of Special Education and Communication Disorders, University of Nebraska, 202F Barkley Memorial Center, Post Office Box 830732, Lincoln, Nebraska 68583. Dr. Beukelman is Barkley Professor of Communication Disorders at the University of Nebraska. He is also Director of Research and Education of the Communication Disorders Division, Munroe-Meyer Institute for Genetics and Rehabilitation at the University of Nebraska Medical Center in Omaha, Nebraska, a research partner in the Augmentative and Alternative Communication Rehabilitation Engineering Research Center (AAC-RERC). In addition, Dr. Beukelman is Senior Researcher in the Institute for Rehabilitation Science and Engineering at the Madonna Rehabilitation Hospital in Lincoln, Nebraska. He is co-author with Pat Mirenda of the textbook *Augmentative and Alternative Commu-*

nication: Management of Severe Communication Disorders in Children and Adults, Second Edition (1998, Paul H. Brookes Publishing Co.). Dr. Beukelman also served as editor of the *Augmentative and Alternative Communication* journal for 4 years.

Joe Reichle, Ph.D., Professor, Department of Communication Disorders, University of Minnesota, 164 Pillsbury Drive SE, 115 Shevlin Hall, Minneapolis, Minnesota 55455. Dr. Reichle is responsible for the master's, doctoral, and postdoctoral personnel preparation programs in the area of augmentative and alternative communication (AAC) at the University of Minnesota. Dr. Reichle has worked for 20 years in general and special education programs serving school-age children with moderate to severe disabilities and providing services to families, teachers, therapists, and paraprofessionals. In addition to being interested in communication intervention, Dr. Reichle is a recognized expert in communicative approaches to managing challenging behavior. He has served as a co-principal investigator of model in-service projects and outreach projects, which have been designed to develop technical assistance teams in local school districts to serve children with severe challenging behavior in inclusive classroom environments. Dr. Reichle has published numerous articles about AAC and challenging behavior and, along with Dr. Steven F. Warren, served as series editor of the *Communication and Language Intervention Series* (Paul H. Brookes Publishing Co.). He is also Associate Editor of the *Journal of Speech, Language, and Hearing Research.*

About the Contributors

Kara B. Arnold, MS., Speech-Language Pathologist, Chester County Intermediate Unit, 585 James Hance Court, Exton, Pennsylvania 19341. Ms. Arnold is a graduate of The Pennsylvania State University, where she received bachelor of science and master of science degrees in communication disorders. She is employed by the Chester County Intermediate Unit in Chester County, Pennsylvania, where she works with children in kindergarten through fifth grade who have a variety of communication disorders. Her caseload includes children with cerebral palsy, autism, developmental delays, and Down syndrome who use augmentative and alternative communication.

Susan Blockberger, Ph.D., S-LP(C), Augmentative Communication Consultant, School District #38 (Richmond), Learning Services Department, Gilmore Office, 8380 Elsmore Road, Richmond, British Columbia V7C 2A1, Canada. Dr. Blockberger has worked with individuals with severe communication impairments since 1972. She is the Augmentative Communication Consultant for School District #38 in Richmond, British Columbia, and a clinical assistant professor in the School of Audiology and Speech Sciences, University of British Columbia, Vancouver. She has a longstanding interest in language acquisition by individuals who use augmentative and alternative communication, a topic she explored in her doctoral research.

Karen D. Bopp, M.Sc., S-LP(C), Speech-Language Pathologist and Doctoral Student, Department of Educational Counseling Psychology and Special Education, The University of British Columbia, 2125 Main Mall, Vancouver, British Columbia V6T 1Z4, Canada. Ms. Bopp is a certified speech and language pathologist and is pursuing her doctoral degree at the University of British Columbia. She has worked extensively with children with developmental disabilities and their families. Her primary area of interest is in augmentative and alternative communication intervention techniques for young children with autism spectrum disorders.

Nancy C. Brady, Ph.D., Associate Research Professor, Kansas Mental Retardation and Developmental Disability Research Center, University of Kansas, 1052 Dole Center, Lawrence, Kansas 66045. Dr. Brady conducts research on the acquisition and use of communication systems by individuals with severe disabilities.

Elizabeth A. Clark, M.S., Speech-Language Pathologist, Lower Merion School District, 301 East Montgomery Avenue, Ardmore, Pennsylvania 19003. Ms. Clark earned a bachelor of art degree from the University of Connecticut in 1999 and a master's degree from The Pennsylvania State University in 2001. She currently works as a speech-language pathologist for Lower Merion School District in Pennsylvania.

Nicola Clare Grove, Ph.D., M.Sc., PGCE, Senior Lecturer, Department of Language and Communication Science, Northampton Square, City University, London, EC10HB England. Dr. Grove is a speech-language pathologist who lectures on the training course at City University, London. She specializes in work with people with intellectual impairments and in augmentative and alternative communication. She is currently developing projects around storytelling with adults and children with severe communication difficulties.

Mary Jo Cooley Hidecker, M.A., CCC-A/SLP, Speech-Language Pathologist and Audiologist, Department of Audiology and Speech Sciences, Michigan State University, 378 Communication Arts and Sciences Building, East Lansing, Michigan 48824. Ms. Hidecker's diverse clinical experiences include augmentative and alternative communication (AAC) use by children and adults. As a doctoral student at Michigan State University, her research interests focus on AAC outcomes and family involvement in AAC intervention.

Katherine C. Hustad, Ph.D., CCC-SLP, Assistant Professor, Department of Communication Sciences and Disorders, The Pennsylvania State University, 110 Moore Building, University Park, Pennsylvania 16803. Dr. Hustad's primary areas of interest include the integration of augmentative and alternative communication (AAC) and natural speech, interventions for improving speech intelligibility in individuals with chronic dysarthria, and linguistic variables that influence intelligibility and comprehensibility. As a clinician, Dr. Hustad has worked in a variety of settings with both children and adults. Her clinical work has focused on AAC applications for individuals with neuromotor disorders.

Teresa A. Iacono, M.App.Sc. (Spe. Path.), Ph.D., Senior Research Fellow, Monash University, Centre for Developmental Disability Health Victoria, Suite 202, 3 Chester Street, Oakleigh, Victoria 3166, Australia. As Senior Research Fellow with the Centre for Developmental Disability Health Victoria, Dr. Iacono directs the center's research activities. She also assists in the research work of the Communication Resource Centre in Scope, Victoria. In these roles and throughout her career, Dr. Iacono has focused on people with complex communication needs. Dr. Iacono is the editor of the journal *Augmentative and Alternative Communication.*

Patricia Bothwell Kenyon, M.A., OTR, CHT, Occupational Therapy Specialist, The Children's Hospital, 1056 East 19th Avenue, Denver, Colorado 80218. Ms. Kenyon has been an occupational therapist for more than 30 years. She has worked in the area of assistive technology and cortical visual impairments for 15 years and is part of the Assistive Technology Clinic at The Children's Hospital of Denver, where she specializes in evaluating options for modified access to communication systems.

Tracy M. Kovach, Ph.D., Speech-Language Pathologist, The Children's Hospital, 1056 East 19th Avenue, Denver, Colorado 80218. Dr. Kovach is Coordinator of the Augmentative Communication and Learning Enhancement Program and Satellite Speech-Language Therapy Programs at The Children's Hospital in Denver. She has more than 25 years of experience as a speech-language pathologist working with individuals with severe speech impairments and multiple disabilities. Dr. Kovach has an appointment to the Department of Pediatrics, School of Medicine, University of Colorado Health Sciences Center in Denver and the Department of Speech, Language and Hearing Sciences at the University of Colorado at Boulder, where she regularly teaches graduate-level courses in the area of augmentative and alternative communication. She is active in professional organizations related to this field, such as American Speech-Language-Hearing Association (ASHA) and the United States Society for Augmentative and Alternative Communication (USSAAC), where she has been elected to leadership positions.

Beth Mineo Mollica, Ph.D., Scientist, Center for Applied Science and Engineering, Alfred I. DuPont Hospital for Children, 1600 Rockland Road, Wilmington, Delaware 19803. Dr. Mineo Mollica is Associate Professor in the Department of Linguistics at the University of Delaware and Scientist at the Center for Applied Science and Engineering. She develops and evaluates assistive technology devices and strategies for people with significant disabilities, and her research has focused primarily on language representation issues. As the director of Delaware's statewide assistive technology project, she facilitates improved technology access and utilization for people with disabilities.

Pat Mirenda, Ph.D., Associate Professor, Department of Educational and Counseling Psychology and Special Education, The University of British Columbia, 2125 Main Mall, Vancouver, British Columbia V6T 1Z4, Canada. Through the years, Dr. Mirenda has concentrated on augmentative and alternative communication (AAC) for people with developmental disabilities.

In addition, she has focused on the inclusion of individuals who use AAC in general education classrooms. From 1998 to 2002, Dr. Mirenda was the editor of the journal *Augmentative and Alternative Communication.* She is also co-author of the book *Augmentative and Alternative Communication: Management of Severe Communication Disorders in Children and Adults, Second Edition* (co-authored with David R. Beukelman, 1998, Paul H. Brookes Publishing Co.). Her current research is focused on the impact of early intervention for children with autism spectrum disorders.

Vera Roberts, M.A., Research Officer, Adaptive Technology Resource Centre, University of Toronto, J.P. Robarts Library, First Floor, 130 St. George Street, Toronto, Ontario M5S 3H1, Canada. Ms. Roberts is a usability researcher at the University of Toronto's Adaptive Technology Resource Centre as well as a doctoral candidate at the university's Ontario Institute for Studies in Education. Her research interests include applications of technology for education and for injury prevention as well as inclusive software usability evaluation methods. Ms. Roberts is the former Curriculum Coordinator of the Special Needs Opportunity Windows (SNOW) web site.

MaryAnn Romski, Ph.D., Professor, Department of Communication, Georgia State University, 1 Park Place South, Box 939, Atlanta, Georgia 30303. Dr. Romski is a certified speech-language pathologist. Her research has focused on studying the language acquisition process of children with developmental disabilities who use augmentative communication devices, and she has written more than 50 articles on this topic.

Charity Rowland, Ph.D., Associate Professor of Pediatrics, Oregon Health & Science University, Design to Learn Projects, 1600 SE Ankeny Street, Portland, Oregon 97214. Dr. Rowland has conducted extensive research on communication development and cognitive development in children and adults with severe and multiple disabilities, including deafblindness, severe mental retardation, autism spectrum disorders, and severe orthopedic impairment. She has developed intervention strategies, assessment instruments, and training materials for use with these populations and has published widely. Dr. Rowland is presently Director of the Oregon Health & Science University's Design to Learn Projects in Portland, Oregon.

Ralf W. Schlosser, Ph.D., Associate Professor, Department of Speech-Language Pathology and Audiology, Northeastern University, 151B Forsyth Building, 360 Huntington Avenue, Boston, Massachusetts 02115. Dr. Schlosser holds a doctorate in special education with an emphasis in augmentative and alternative communication from Purdue University. He is a tenured associate professor in the Department of Speech-Language Pathology and Audiology at

Northeastern University in Boston. He is also a Distinguished Switzer Fellow of the National Institute on Disability and Rehabilitation Research (NIDRR) and a fellow of the American Association on Mental Retardation (AAMR).

Philip D. Schweigert, M.Ed., Senior Instructor, Oregon Institute on Disability and Development, Oregon Health & Science University, 3181 SW Sam Jackson Park Road, Portland, Oregon 97201. Mr. Schweigert is a senior instructor with the Oregon Institute on Disability and Development of the Oregon Health & Science University in Portland. He is Project Coordinator for several federally funded research projects developing strategies to enhance the communication and cognitive skills of individuals with severe and multiple disabilities. During the past 25 years, Mr. Schweigert has been involved in numerous research and demonstration efforts and has written and presented extensively. He has also been a classroom teacher and program manager for children with severe disabilities.

Rose A. Sevcik, Ph.D., Associate Professor, Department of Psychology, Georgia State University, 1 Park Place South, Atlanta, Georgia 30303. Dr. Sevcik's research interests include language and communication acquisition and impairments, mental retardation, and reading development and disorders. She has an extensive publication record and has given numerous presentations to national and international audiences.

Kathy L. Shapley, M.A., Doctoral Candidate, Department of Communication Disorders, University of Nebraska–Lincoln, 318K Barkley Memorial Center, Lincoln, Nebraska 68583. Ms. Shapley is a doctoral candidate in communication disorders at the University of Nebraska–Lincoln. Clinically, she has worked in early intervention settings implementing a variety of strategies to improve functional communication. Her research interests are in the area of developmental speech perception.

Martine M. Smith, Ph.D., Lecturer in Speech-Language Pathology, School of Clinical Speech & Language Studies, Trinity College Dublin, 184 Pearse Street, Dublin 2, Ireland. Dr. Smith has worked as a speech and language therapist with individuals with severe congenital speech and physical impairments since the early 1980s. She is currently a lecturer in speech-language pathology in Trinity College Dublin, and she continues her clinical work with individuals who use augmentative and alternative communication. Her particular research interests are the acquisition of language, including written language in individuals using aided communication.

Ann Sutton, Ph.D., Assistant Professor, École d'orthophonie et d'audiologie, Université de Montréal, Pavillon Marguerite d'Youville, 2375 Côte Sainte-Catherine local 3026, Montréal, Québec H3T 1A8, Canada. Dr. Sutton is an assistant professor at the École d'orthophonie et d'audiologie (The School of Speech-Language Pathology and Audiology) at the Université de Montréal. She is Principal Investigator on federally and provincially funded research grants. Her two primary research interests are the structural aspects of language acquisition in augmentative and alternative communication and the acquisition of Canadian French by typically developing children.

Nancy Terry, M.A., CCC-SLP, Speech-Language Pathologist, St. Anthony–New Brighton Public Schools, 3600 Highcrest Road, NE, St. Anthony, Minnesota 55418. Ms. Terry is a speech-language pathologist in St. Anthony–New Brighton School District. She works with students with speech and language disorders and students with mild to moderate mental impairments, autism spectrum disorders, and Down syndrome who use a combination of low and high technology augmentative communication devices.

Jutta Trevarinus, M.A.Spec.Ed., Resource Centre for Academic Technology, University of Toronto, Fourth Floor, 130 St. George Street, Toronto, Ontario M5S 3H1, Canada. Ms. Treviranus directs the Resource Centre for Academic Technology (RCAT) at the University of Toronto. She also established and directs the Adaptive Technology Resource Centre (ATRC), a center of expertise on barrier-free access to information technology. Ms. Treviranus has worked as a researcher and clinician in the area of assistive technology for more than 20 years.

Acknowledgments

This book is dedicated to all of the individuals who use augmentative and alternative communication (AAC) and their families who have shared their experiences and valuable insights with us. These insights have guided our research and informed our practice. We are also grateful to our colleagues and our students who have challenged us by asking important questions and who have shared their time and effort to support our research to find the answers to these questions. We wish to acknowledge the external funding support that we have received to build the AAC programs at our universities, including funding from the United States Department of Education, the National Institute on Disability and Rehabilitation Research, and the Barkley Trust. We are grateful to the Paul H. Brookes Publishing Co. for their support of our efforts to disseminate information and improve practices through the publication of the AAC series and through this volume specifically. Finally, we wish to thank our families, who have provided so much love and encouragement.

I

Definition of Communicative Competence

1

Shattering the Silence

Development of Communicative Competence by Individuals Who Use AAC

Janice C. Light

> The silence of speechlessness is never golden. We all need to communicate and connect with each other—not just in one way, but in as many ways as possible. It is a basic human need, a basic human right. And much more than this, it is a basic human power. (Williams, 2000, p. 248)

As Williams's statement so eloquently illustrates, communication is essential to attaining quality of life. It is a basic human need to connect with others—to touch others' lives and have others touch our lives. It is a basic human right to express ideas, thoughts, and feelings freely. Communication is a basic human power that allows people to articulate their personal, educational, vocational, and social goals and to achieve their full potential. As a person develops communicative competence, he or she meets this human need, realizes this human right, and attains this human power.

Individuals who have significant disabilities that limit their communication with others face considerable challenges in attaining communicative competence. This chapter is about the development of communicative competence by individuals with developmental disabilities who use augmentative and alternative communication (AAC; e.g., manual signs, gestures, communication boards of line drawings, voice output communication aids). Specifically, this chapter proposes a model of communicative competence for individuals who use AAC, extending the work of Light (1989).

"Shattering the silence" is a reference to a quote from Williams (2000). The quote is included at the end of the chapter.

MODEL OF COMMUNICATIVE COMPETENCE

Light (1989) posited that the goals of communicative competence are similar whether one uses natural speech or augmented means to communicate. In broad terms, as Williams (2000) described, these goals include meeting the human need to communicate, realizing the human right to communicate, and exercising the human power that communication provides. What differs between individuals who use natural speech to communicate and those who use AAC is the road traveled to attain communicative competence. For example, speech is a fast, dynamic method of communication. There are numerous models of effective communication via natural speech throughout daily life. Speech is well accepted as a means of communication within society. In contrast, communication via AAC is typically much slower and takes more effort. Often, individuals who use AAC are constrained in the symbols available to them to communicate. They rarely, if ever, see models of competent communicators who use AAC. They may witness social rejection or negative attitudes toward AAC. As a result of these challenges and many others, individuals who use AAC face some unique circumstances in their development of communicative competence.

This chapter proposes a model of communicative competence for individuals who use AAC that builds on the work of Light (1989, 1997a). The model posits that communicative competence is affected by factors intrinsic to the individual who uses AAC as well as environmental factors (see Table 1.1). Relevant intrinsic factors include the knowledge, judgment, and skills that the individual who uses AAC brings to the interaction. These, in turn, are mitigated by psychosocial factors such as motivation, attitude, confidence, and resilience. The knowledge, judgment, and skills of the individual who uses AAC in combination with relevant psychosocial factors define the resources that the individual brings to communicative interactions. Extrinsic factors in the environment define the communicative demands on the individual as well as the external barriers or supports available to the individual in attempting to meet these communication demands. Ultimately, factors intrinsic to the individual who uses AAC and environmental factors will interplay and serve to facilitate or impede the attainment of communicative competence. The following sections discuss in more detail the intrinsic and extrinsic factors that impact the attainment of communicative competence by individuals who use AAC.

FACTORS INTRINSIC TO INDIVIDUALS WHO USE AAC

In 1989, Light argued that the attainment of communicative competence by individuals who use AAC rests on their integration of knowledge, judgment,

Table 1.1. Intrinsic and extrinsic factors that contribute to the attainment of communicative competence by individuals who use AAC

Type of factor	Specific aspects
Intrinsic factors	
Knowledge, judgment, and skills	Linguistic Operational Social Strategic
Psychosocial factors	Motivation Attitude toward AAC Confidence Resilience
Extrinsic factors	
Communication demands	Social roles Interaction goals
Environmental barriers and/or supports	Policy Practice Attitude Knowledge Skill

and skills in several interrelated domains. The acquisition and application of this knowledge, judgment, and skills will be affected by underlying psychosocial factors such as motivation, attitude, confidence, and resilience. These two sets of intrinsic factors are discussed in further detail in the sections that follow.

Knowledge, Judgment, and Skills

The attainment of communicative competence by individuals who use AAC requires a complex interplay of knowledge, judgment, and skills across four domains: linguistic, operational, social, and strategic (Light, 1989). Table 1.2 provides an overview of the four domains and examples of skills within each of these domains that may contribute to the attainment of communicative competence.

Linguistic Domain   Linguistic competence is fundamental to the development of communicative competence. Although some level of communication can be established without linguistic competence, the depth and breadth of this communication will be severely constrained in the absence of symbolic meaning. For example, an individual with minimal linguistic competence may be able to express basic needs and wants via nonsymbolic means (e.g., crying to express discomfort, looking at a glass of water to request a drink), but may be unable to share information with others or communicate more complex ideas, thoughts, and feelings.

Table 1.2. Knowledge, judgment, and skills required to attain communicative competence for individuals who require AAC

Domain	Examples of knowledge, judgment, and skills that may affect communicative competence
Linguistic domain	Develop skills in the native language(s) spoken in the individual's family and social community • Understand the form, content, and use of the spoken language(s) used by others • Develop as many expressive skills (form, content, and use) in the spoken language(s) as appropriate • Code switch between different linguistic codes and cultural values as required Develop skills in the "linguistic codes" of the AAC systems • Develop lexical knowledge of AAC symbols; express concepts via AAC • Develop semantic-syntactic skills using AAC; combine AAC symbols meaningfully to express more complex messages
Operational domain	Produce unaided symbols (e.g., conventional gestures, pantomime, signs) as required. For example, • Plan and produce the required hand shape, position, orientation, and movement to produce manual signs or gestures (e.g., the manual sign for MORE, thumbs-up signal) • Plan, sequence, and produce body movements to act out messages via pantomime (e.g., to communicate swimming or eating) • Look up to communicate yes Operate aided AAC systems accurately and efficiently as required. For example, • Open communication book, turn pages, and point to desired AAC symbol • Use paper and pencil to draw concept • Use row–column scanning or Morse code to access required AAC symbols
Social domain	Develop appropriate sociolinguistic skills • Take obligatory turns; fulfill nonobligatory turns • Initiate topics appropriately • Produce contingent responses to maintain conversations • Add additional comments/questions to develop conversations • Terminate conversations appropriately • Produce a full range of communicative functions appropriately as required (e.g., protest, request information, provide information, request attention) Develop appropriate sociorelational skills • Participate actively in interactions • Be responsive to partners • Demonstrate interest in partners • Put partners at ease • Project a positive self-image • Engage partners in interaction • Maintain a positive rapport with partners

Domain	Examples of knowledge, judgment, and skills that may impact communicative competence
Strategic domain	Use appropriate strategies to bypass limitations in linguistic domain. For example, • Ask partner to write or point to AAC symbols in addition to speaking to bypass limitations in comprehension • Use mementos to bypass vocabulary limitations and establish topic of interaction • Provide clues and ask the partner to "guess" to bypass vocabulary limitations Use appropriate strategies to bypass limitations in operational domain. For example, • Use partner prediction when communicating with alphabet board to enhance rate • Turn on electronic activation feedback beep to signal that message construction is occurring to avoid interruptions from partners Use appropriate strategies to bypass limitations in social domain • Use an introduction strategy to put partners at ease • Teach personal care attendant to always direct conversation back to augmented communicator

From Light, J.C., & Gulens, M. (2000). Rebuilding communicative competence and self-determination. In D.R. Beukelman & J. Reichle (Series Eds.) & D.R. Beukelman, K.M. Yorkston, & J. Reichle (Vol. Eds.), *Augmentative and alternative communication series: Augmentative and alternative communication for adults with acquired neurologic disorders* (p. 148). Baltimore: Paul H. Brookes Publishing Co.; adapted by permission.

Developing linguistic competence is a complicated enterprise for individuals who use AAC. They must develop knowledge, judgment, and skills not only in the native language(s) spoken by their families and broader social community but also in the linguistic codes of the AAC systems they use (Light, 1989).

Skills in the Spoken Language of the Community

Most individuals who use AAC are first exposed to language through the spoken language of their families and, later, of the broader social community. Despite the trend toward early intervention, many individuals with significant communication impairments are not introduced to AAC until they are 3 or 4 years old or even older. As a result, the spoken language of the family and the community may be their only language during the critical early years of development (Light, 1997a, 1997b). This spoken language (or languages) will continue to be the primary means of input throughout these individuals' lives as they attempt to develop communicative competence. Research suggests that communication partners seldom augment their natural speech with AAC: Romski and Sevcik (1996) found that partners who had been trained to use augmented input (i.e., use AAC to augment their natural speech) did so in only 9% of their messages; partners who have not been trained would be expected to use AAC even less frequently. Thus, it is essential that individuals who use AAC develop receptive language skills in the spoken language of the family and broader social community in order to attain communicative competence.

As of 2003, there has been minimal research to investigate the development of receptive language skills by individuals who use AAC (Romski & Sevcik, 1996). Almost all of the research has focused on expressive language capabilities. Sevcik and Romski (2002) referred to language comprehension as the "forgotten partner" in AAC interventions. Yet, the development of communicative competence not only requires skills as a "speaker" in interactions, but also requires skills as a listener. The development of receptive language skills by individuals who use AAC may be particularly challenging for a number of reasons, including the following:

- Individuals who use AAC who have motor or sensory perceptual impairments may be significantly restricted in their access to the environment; as a result, they may have an impoverished experiential base for conceptual and lexical development (Light, 1997b).
- Individuals who use AAC may hear words spoken in their environment but may have limited means to test hypotheses about the meanings of these words (Light, 1997b). They must develop comprehension skills with minimal access to language production.
- Partners may have difficulty determining appropriate levels of language input in interactions with individuals who use AAC; language input may be quantitatively and/or qualitatively different for individuals who use AAC (Light, 1997b; see Chapter 3).
- AAC interventions tend to focus on production to the neglect of comprehension; individuals who use AAC may be asked to produce communication without an adequate foundation of understanding (Sevcik & Romski, 2002).

Future research is urgently required to investigate the development of receptive language skills by individuals who use AAC, including specification of the challenges in this development and delineation of strategies that may facilitate the development of comprehension. (See Chapters 3 and 5 for further discussion of these issues.) Future research is also required to delineate the effects of receptive language skills on AAC acquisition and use (Sevcik & Romski, 2002).

In addition to receptive language skills in the spoken language of the family and community, most individuals who use AAC develop some expressive language skills as well. These may range from a few vocalizations that are understood as signals for specific needs or wants by familiar partners to connected speech that is understood by familiar partners in known contexts but requires augmentation to be understood reliably by unfamiliar partners or in novel contexts. To date, there has been only limited attention given to the development of natural speech by individuals who require AAC and to the impact of AAC on the development, use, and communication effectiveness of natural speech. (See Chapter 2 for further discussion of the effects of AAC on natural speech.)

Diverse Cultural and Linguistic Backgrounds   Society is becoming significantly more diverse. As a result, there are increasing numbers of individuals who require AAC for whom the family cultural background and the first language spoken in the home differ from those of the schools and broader social community. Individuals who use AAC who come from diverse cultural and linguistic backgrounds face additional demands in developing communicative competence because they must learn receptive and expressive skills in the language spoken by their family as well as receptive and expressive skills in the language of the broader social community (e.g., educational system, business community). In addition, they must learn how to switch between the different language codes, dialects, and cultural norms or values of their family and community (Light, 1997b). Furthermore, they must do so with limited access to expressive language in either language. Gus Estrella described the challenges he experienced growing up between two different cultures and languages:

> I felt trapped. I had so much to say to people and so many questions to ask, and yet how could I? They knew I had something to say but couldn't figure out how to get it out of me. I was like a time bomb ready to explode. To add to my dilemma, I was brought up, for the most part, in a bilingual family and Spanish was spoken most of the time. Prior to starting preschool, my family and friends all spoke to me in Spanish. That was all I knew. So you can imagine my reaction when I started going to preschool. I was entering uncharted territories. I was about to be left with total strangers, foreigners! It was doubtful that anybody would know any Spanish, so what was the likelihood of somebody understanding my little signs for when I needed something . . . .These were the concerns that a little boy had to deal with and figure out how to cope with his new surroundings. So to whom could I turn for help and support? Basically, no one as there wasn't anybody who could relate to my situation. (2000, p. 33)

The challenges of bilingualism (or multilingualism) may be magnified when service delivery is culturally insensitive and ignores the family's linguistic and cultural heritage. Lund and Light (2001) conducted a study of the long-term outcomes of seven young men who had used AAC for at least 15 years, including three men who came from diverse cultural and linguistic backgrounds. These three men and their families reported that cultural barriers had negatively affected outcomes. Specifically, they noted the lack of AAC systems that allowed access to two languages and the lack of cultural sensitivity from professionals providing services. Too often, the AAC systems provided reflected the norms and language of the school system and failed to address the cultural values and language of the family, leaving the individual who used AAC isolated from the family and cultural community. The sister of one of the young men explained

> The hardest thing for us has been my parents and the language barrier. They're still not able to read an English word . . . They [the professionals] started introducing him to words, but the thing is my parents didn't understand what the word meant because it was in English—so that was it. (Lund & Light, 2001, p. 77)

Future research is urgently required to determine effective approaches to AAC assessment and intervention that are culturally sensitive and appropriate to meet the needs of individuals who require AAC from diverse cultural and linguistic backgrounds.

Skills in the Linguistic Code of the AAC Systems

In addition to developing receptive and expressive skills in the spoken language(s) of the family and broader social community, individuals who use AAC must also develop skills in the *linguistic codes* of the AAC systems used. For example, individuals must learn how to use AAC symbols to represent meaning and how to combine symbols to express more complex ideas. (See Chapter 4 for further discussion of the development of representational competence.) Sometimes, the AAC symbols used are graphic representations of the oral language(s) spoken by the family or community (e.g., written words or letters of the alphabet combined to produce words through letter by letter spelling); however, often the AAC symbols bear no direct relationship to the oral language(s) spoken by the family and community (e.g., manual signs, conventional gestures, photographs, line drawings, Blissymbols). Thus, the linguistic codes of the AAC system(s) are different than the linguistic codes of the spoken language(s) of the family and community.

The challenge of developing linguistic competence is magnified significantly for individuals who use AAC for at least three reasons:

- There is a distinct asymmetry between the language input received by individuals who use AAC and the language output they can produce.
- Communication via AAC is typically multimodal, combining various linguistic codes (e.g., manual signs, conventional gestures, photographs, and line drawings) to express meaning.
- Many AAC systems are not true languages and lack the phonological, semantic, syntactic, and/or pragmatic features of true languages.

Future research is required to investigate the relationship between the linguistic codes of the spoken languages that provide input and the linguistic codes of the AAC systems and to determine the impact on the development of linguistic competence by individuals with developmental disabilities who use AAC. (See Chapters 3 and 6 for further discussion.)

Operational Domain   Linguistic skills ensure that individuals who use AAC are able to understand and use symbols to communicate their ideas, thoughts, and feelings to others; operational skills are required to access or produce the symbols expressively. Operational skills refer to skills in the technical production and operation of AAC systems. They include the skills to produce the hand (or body) shapes, positions, orientations, and movements required to form unaided symbols (e.g., manual signs, conventional gestures, pantomime) as well as the sequencing of these to produce more complex messages. Operational skills also include the skills required to technically operate aided AAC systems, including light-technology systems (e.g., communication books, alphabet boards) as well as high-technology systems (e.g., electronic communication aids). The latter skills include skills to operate the access techniques (e.g., use single-switch row–column scanning, use Morse code), adjust the volume, correct errors, and so forth.

The development of operational skills is essential to ensure that communication is effective (i.e., gets the message across accurately), efficient (i.e., does so in a reasonable amount of time), and as minimally fatiguing as possible. Operational skills are dependent on the motor, cognitive, linguistic, and sensory perceptual capabilities of the individual. (See Chapter 7 for further discussion of motor issues, Chapter 8 for further discussion of cognitive issues, and Chapter 9 for further discussion of visual issues.)

In a consumer-driven research study, individuals who used AAC and their families reported that current AAC systems impose significant learning demands on consumers, their families, and professionals; they called for concerted research and development to simplify AAC technologies (Racken-sperger, Williams, Krezman, & McNaughton, 2001). Future research is required to investigate the learning demands of AAC technologies and to redesign these systems to reduce what Beukelman (1991) referred to as the "cost" of learning. (See Light & Drager, in press, for further discussion of issues in redesigning AAC systems for young children with developmental disabilities.)

Social Domain   Linguistic and operational skills ensure that individuals who use AAC have the tools required to communicate. Social skills ensure that individuals who require AAC are able to use these tools effectively to communicate with others. Light (1989) proposed that there are two types of social skills required: sociolinguistic skills and sociorelational skills.

Sociolinguistic skills have traditionally been referred to as pragmatic skills. These skills encompass discourse strategies (e.g., turn taking, topic initiation and development, cohesion and coherence of conversation) and communicative functions (e.g., requests for objects or actions, requests for attention, protests, provisions of information, and requests for information). (See Chapter 10 for further discussion of sociolinguistic or pragmatic skills.)

According to Light (1989), the sociorelational domain includes knowledge, judgment, and skills in the interpersonal aspects of communication. Light, Arnold, and Clark (Chapter 11) proposed the following types of sociorelational skills that may further communicative competence: participating actively in interactions, being responsive to partners, demonstrating interest in partners, putting partners at ease, projecting a positive self-image, engaging partners in interactions, and maintaining a positive rapport with partners. AAC interventions have largely neglected these types of sociorelational skills, yet they may be critical to the successful attainment of meaningful social relationships with others and may facilitate communicative interactions generally. (See Chapter 11 for further details.)

Strategic Domain   Because of the significant disabilities experienced by individuals who use AAC and because of the constraints of AAC systems, individuals who use AAC will invariably experience limitations in the development of linguistic, operational, and/or social skills despite intervention. For example, young children who are preliterate and use AAC are dependent on others to provide access to vocabulary within their aided systems and will no doubt encounter situations where they lack the necessary AAC symbols to communicate a desired message due to the vocabulary constraints of their system. Adolescents or young adults who have significant motor impairments and must use single-switch scanning to control their AAC systems will no doubt experience significant limitations in their rate of communication regardless of the amount of training provided. In these cases, individuals who use AAC will require strategies to allow them to minimize limitations in the linguistic, operational, and/or social domains. These strategies may be long term, utilized by individuals who use AAC for many years to support communication, or they may be short term, employed temporarily by individuals who use AAC until further linguistic, operational, and/or social skills are developed. For example, individuals with slow rates of communication may rely on partner prediction as a long-term strategy to enhance the rate of communication with familiar partners. Children who are preliterate who do not have access to a vocabulary item that they require may direct a partner to ask a multiple choice question to guess the item; this may be a temporary strategy to bypass vocabulary limitations used until the child develops sufficient literacy skills to spell novel words.

Given the considerable linguistic, operational, and social constraints experienced by many individuals who use AAC, development of strategic competence is critical. Strategic competence can allow individuals to attain communicative competence in the face of significant linguistic, operational, and/or social impairments (Holland, 1982). Despite the importance of strategic competence to the attainment of communicative competence, as of 2002, issues of strategic competence have largely been neglected by the AAC research community. In contrast, individuals who use AAC have clearly recognized the importance of compensatory strategies; their personal writings document a wide range of strategies used successfully to bypass limitations and facilitate communication. (See Chapter 12 for a review of these strategies.) Future research is required to document linguistic, operational, and social constraints experienced by individuals who use AAC and to determine effective strategies to overcome these constraints.

Integration of Knowledge, Judgment, and Skills Across Domains   Light (1989) proposed that communicative competence requires the integration of knowledge, judgment, and skills across the linguistic, operational, social, and strategic domains. As of 2002, little is known about the specific constellation of skills that are required to attain communicative competence. It is doubtful that researchers will actually identify a list of specific linguistic, operational, social, and strategic skills that are required of all individuals who use AAC to attain communicative competence. Rather, Light (1997a) proposed that different paths may lead to communicative competence for different individuals who use AAC. The specific constellation of linguistic, operational, social, and strategic skills may vary across individuals who use AAC depending on the nature and severity of disability, profiles of strengths and limitations, personality, and so forth.

Table 1.2 presents a summary of some examples of linguistic, operational, social, and strategic skills that may affect the communicative competence of individuals who use AAC. It is important to note that, as of 2002, there is still only limited empirical evidence as to which of these skills actually contribute to improved communicative competence.

Psychosocial Factors that Influence the Attainment of Communicative Competence

Acquisition and application of the knowledge, judgment, and skills required to become a competent communicator will no doubt be influenced by a variety of psychosocial factors including motivation, attitude, confidence, and resilience. (See Table 1.3 for examples of psychosocial factors that may influence the attainment of communicative competence.)

Motivation   Motivation is critically important to the attainment of communicative competence, for individuals who use AAC typically must expend substantial effort to communicate effectively with others. "During each day in the lives of individuals [who use AAC] . . . choices are made regarding when, how, and with whom to engage in social interactions" (Fox & Sohlberg, 2000, p. 8). Without strong motivation to communicate, individuals who use AAC may be overwhelmed by the high-energy demands imposed by AAC

Table 1.3.   Examples of psychosocial factors that may influence the attainment of communicative competence by individuals who use AAC

Psychosocial factor	Definition	Potential impact on communicative competence
Motivation to communicate	Drive to communicate influenced by the belief that the goal (i.e., communication) is important and valued and that it can be attained	Defines the individual's desire or drive to communicate with others in specific situations
Atttitude toward AAC	Ideas about AAC charged with emotion (positive or negative) which predispose use of AAC (or nonuse) in particular social situations	Influences the individual's willingness to use AAC to communicate with others in specific situations
Communicative confidence	Self-assurance based on the individual's belief that he or she will communicate successfully in specific situations	Influences the propensity of the individual to actually act (i.e., communicate) in specific situations
Resilience	Capacity to prevent, minimize, or overcome the damaging effects of adversities; capacity to compensate for problems and recover from failures	Influences the individual's persistence in continuing to communicate in the face of barriers, adversities, and communication failures

and may elect to limit their communication to specific situations and not others (Fox & Sohlberg, 2000).

Motivation is influenced by two factors: 1) the belief that the goal (in this case communication) is important and valued and 2) the belief that it can be attained. According to Bandura (1986), people are most apt to be motivated by activities in which they believe that they are competent and which result in self-satisfaction or a sense of achievement. Estrella wrote the following about the importance of motivation in his life:

> Some might argue that luck had a lot to do with my success and others might say it was the people I knew. Personally I think it's a combination of the two, but there are other factors that can be added to the equation. One is me, personally. It was me that had the dreams and desire of making something of myself. I mean I could have been given the top job in the country, but without that desire of succeeding that job would have been meaningless! (2000, p. 43)

Because individuals who use AAC experience significant challenges in attaining communicative competence, sustaining their motivation to communicate may be at risk.

Attitude   The attitudes of individuals with significant communication disabilities toward AAC will no doubt influence their attainment of communicative competence. If individuals are motivated to communicate but have negative attitudes toward AAC and are therefore unwilling to use AAC in situations where it is required, they may struggle to attain communicative competence. According to Triandis, an attitude is "an idea charged with emotion which predisposes a class of actions to a particular class of social situations" (1971, p. 2). In this case, the individuals' ideas about AAC, overlaid with their emotions about AAC, may predispose individuals with significant communication disabilities to use AAC (or not) when required in social situations. Attitudes may be influenced by the knowledge that individuals have about AAC and their expectations as well as their prior experiences with AAC, including past successes or failures, the reactions of others, and so forth.

To date, there has been minimal research to investigate the attitudes of individuals with significant communication disabilities toward AAC. Culp and Carlisle (1988) reported on a pilot study that investigated the impact of an intensive intervention program involving 11 children with cerebral palsy who used AAC (ages 3–13) and their primary caregivers. Both parents and children demonstrated positive attitudes toward talking or speech as a means of communication regardless of the severity of the child's expressive communication disability. Most of the children also reported positive attitudes toward AAC as a means of communication: 74% strongly agreed with the statement "I like to use my [AAC system]" prior to involvement in the intervention and 100% strongly agreed 3 months after completion of the intervention program. Interestingly, the parents' perceptions of their children's attitudes toward AAC were not as positive as the children's report: Only 36% of parents strongly agreed with the statement "My child likes to use his/her [AAC system]" prior to the intervention program and 42% strongly agreed 3 months postintervention. Furthermore, the parents' own attitudes toward AAC were not as positive as their children's: Only 44% of the parents strongly agreed with the statement "I like my child to use his/her [AAC system]."

Future research is required to investigate the attitudes of consumers toward AAC and to determine factors that contribute to the formation of positive or negative attitudes toward AAC. It seems reasonable to suppose that numerous factors will affect an individual's attitudes toward AAC. Lasker and Bedrosian (2000) proposed the "AAC Acceptance Model" to begin to explain the acceptance (or lack of acceptance) of AAC by adults with acquired disabilities. According to this model, adapted from Scherer's (1993) Matching Person and Technology (MPT) model, three branches of factors interact to determine the individual's acceptance of AAC: person factors (e.g., personality, age, communication status, literacy, technology experience, needs, intervention history), milieu factors (e.g., partners, environment, funding), and technology factors. Future research is required to determine the validity of this model; to investigate the effects of person, milieu, and technology factors on acceptance of AAC by individuals with developmental disabilities; and to explore techniques to change attitudes where appropriate.

Finally, research is required to delineate the relationship between attitudes toward AAC and actual AAC use. The relationship between attitudes and actual behaviors is not well understood. In general, it is assumed that attitudes predispose the individual to act in certain ways (Triandis, 1971). For example, it might be assumed that those with positive attitudes toward AAC might be more apt to devote time and energy to learning to communicate via AAC and might be more willing to use AAC to interact with others than those with more negative attitudes toward AAC; however, human behavior is a complex enterprise, and it seems doubtful that the relationship between attitudes and behaviors is a simple, one-dimensional one. Other factors besides attitudes may influence individuals in their behaviors as well (e.g., motivation, confidence, social norms, peer expectations).

Confidence   While motivation will determine the individual's drive to communicate and attitudes toward AAC may determine the individual's willingness to use AAC to communicate, confidence may influence the individual's actual propensity to act, in this case, to attempt to communicate with others in a given situation. Although there has been only limited consideration of the effect of confidence on communication in the AAC field, there has been considerable discussion of the importance of confidence in the development of communicative competence in the area of second language learning. For example, Rubin (1975) argued that "good" language learners who are likely to attain competence are confident, lack inhibition, and are willing to make mistakes in order to communicate. Savignon also emphasized the importance of self-assuredness in relation to the attainment of communicative competence in a second language:

> It may be that communicative confidence leads to communicative competence. To use the swimming analogy . . . , communicative confidence in language learning may be like learning how to relax with your face under water, to let the water support you. Having once known the sensation of remaining afloat, it is but a matter of time until you learn the strokes that will take you where you want to go. (1983, p. 45)

Attaining communicative competence via AAC, like second language learning, requires individuals to dive into unfamiliar and, in the case of AAC, largely uncharted waters. In fact, the waters of AAC may seem very murky because most individuals who use AAC typically have limited or no access within their daily lives to others who use AAC and who have attained communicative competence. It will require considerable confidence on the part of users. Seeing others who use AAC who have attained communicative competence and successfully achieved educational, vocational, social, and personal goals may play a critical role in building communicative confidence among people who use AAC. Creech explained, "Until we have seen a fluent, interactive, augmented speaker who shares our physical circumstances, there may have been little in our personal experience to indicate that we, ourselves, could someday actually 'talk'" (1995, p. 12).

Second language learners typically find the foundation for communicative confidence in their successful communication experiences as learners in their first language. These learners have successfully attained communicative competence in a first language and can draw on this successful experience in their attempts to communicate in the second language. In contrast, individuals with developmental disabilities who use AAC do not have prior experience as competent communicators that they can draw on to build their confidence as AAC learners. Furthermore, they may face environmental circumstances that impose significant barriers (e.g., situations where partners are unfamiliar, are unskilled in AAC, and/or hold attitudes that are not favorable) (see Extrinsic Environmental Factors that Influence Communicative Competence for further discussion of these potential environmental barriers). The need for communicative confidence to build communicative competence may be even more pivotal in these challenging situations. In order to foster communicative confidence, it will be important for individuals who use AAC to have many diverse communication experiences from an early age. These experiences should be appropriately challenging and should provide the necessary scaffolding to support success.

Resilience   Although confidence may determine the individual's propensity to act, it is resilience that will influence whether the individual perseveres with communication despite many barriers and despite failure when it occurs. Resilience has been defined as the "capacity which allows a person . . . to prevent, minimize, or overcome the damaging effects of adversity" (Grotberg, 1995). Resilience includes the ability to overcome or compensate for problems and the ability to recover from failure. Resilience arises out of people's belief in their own self-efficacy and in their ability to solve problems. Resilience is critical to the well-being of children and adults and may be exceptionally important to individuals who use AAC for they may confront significant problems within their daily lives due to the severity of their disabilities, the limitations of AAC systems, and environmental barriers (D. Beukelman, personal communication, August 5, 2002). The following e-mail message, written by a 15-year-old girl who uses AAC, illustrates the importance of resilience in the face of significant environmental barriers: "The other kids at school still are rude. . . . I mean I don't have any friends in school. They just freak out about my chair. . . . I'm too tired with everyone's reactions. . . . I gave up with my peers" (R. Ehresman, personal communication, 2001).

Resilience is a dynamic factor, affected by the nature of the specific adversity and by the presence of protective factors, including individual resources and environmental supports. Individual protective factors that may support resilience include problem-solving skills, self-esteem, and optimism.

Social or environmental protective factors that may contribute to resilience include support from family (parents and siblings), mentors, teachers, and peers. Research suggests that individuals who have access to clusters of protective factors (personal and social) are more apt to be resilient and to overcome adversity (Gore & Eckenrode, 1996; Rak & Patterson, 1996). People who are resilient are better equipped to overcome the adversities they face and are more apt to develop communicative competence. Those who are not resilient may have difficulty rebounding from adversities, learning from failures, and ultimately developing communicative competence.

To date, there has been minimal attention given to the resilience of individuals who use AAC. Research with other populations of individuals with disabilities (e.g., children with learning disabilities, with chronic illness, or at risk for delinquent behavior) suggests that interventions can be implemented to build resiliency. Typically, these interventions include access to positive supportive role models, encouragement to develop autonomy and accept responsibility, instruction in effective problem-solving strategies, instruction in effective communication, and instruction in the management of feelings.

Light and colleagues (2000) developed, implemented, and evaluated the effectiveness of an Internet-based mentoring program for adolescents and young adults who use AAC; one of the goals of the AAC Mentor Project was to build resiliency. The project involved a web-based leadership-training program for adults who used AAC who had successfully attained personal, educational, vocational, and/or social goals and who were positive role models for adolescents and young adults who used AAC. These individuals completed three web-based instructional modules that provided instruction in effective communication skills (see Chapter 11 for further details), collaborative problem solving, and access to disability-related resources and information. All of the adults who used AAC successfully acquired the targeted skills through the web-based instruction.

Subsequent to the leadership training, the adults were matched with adolescents and young adults who used AAC and served as mentors over a year-long period. The mentors interacted with their protégés via e-mail on a regular basis, providing social support, positive role models, encouragement to build autonomy, and support in problem solving and goal setting. A total of 32 mentor–protégé dyads participated in the project: 96% of the mentors and protégés reported that they were very satisfied with the AAC Mentor Project. The protégés indicated that they 1) found it very beneficial to have the opportunity to talk with someone who really understood, 2) got new ideas for goals in many areas of their lives, and 3) learned how someone else overcame problems and met goals. The protégés used the interactions with their mentors to set goals and solve a wide range of problems including those related to education, employment, personal relationships, family, transportation, independent living, personal care attendants, finances, communication, and technology. Goal attainment data indicated that the protégés made positive progress on 85% of the more than 75 goals that they set.

Results of the AAC Mentor Project highlighted the many problems confronted by individuals who use AAC in their daily lives and the need for effective problem-solving strategies to build resilience. McCarthy and Light (2002) are involved in a follow-up study to develop, implement, and evaluate the effectiveness of Internet-based instruction in problem solving for adolescents who use AAC. Future research is required to further investigate the effectiveness of interventions to build resilience among children and adults who use AAC to ensure that these individuals have the capacity to overcome the damaging effects of adversities within their lives and the ability to recover from their failures.

EXTRINSIC ENVIRONMENTAL FACTORS THAT INFLUENCE COMMUNICATIVE COMPETENCE

Light argued that "communicative competence is a relative, not an absolute, concept" (1989, p. 138). Communicative competence is context dependent (Hymes, 1972). Although all individuals will be affected by environmental factors in their communication, the extent of the impact may be influenced by the communication resources of the individual. Individuals who are beginning communicators and have yet to develop competence in linguistic, operational, social, and strategic domains will rely on environmental supports to a greater extent and therefore will be more affected by environmental factors. For example, Sigafoos and Mirenda (2002) provided a continuum of formats for requesting that ranged from ones that provided maximal partner support and therefore minimized the demands on the individual who uses AAC (e.g., the partner offers a choice by holding out two objects, the person who uses AAC indicates the desired item) to ones that provided no partner support and therefore posed increased communicative demands on the individual who uses AAC (e.g., the individual who uses AAC must secure the partner's attention and indicate the desired item unambiguously). Beginning communicators may demonstrate competence in the former situation, in which there is significant environmental support for communication, but not in the latter. Those individuals with well-developed linguistic, operational, social, and strategic competencies will bring greater resources to the interaction and will rely less on environmental scaffolding to attain competence.

Depending on environmental factors, individuals who use AAC may be competent communicators within some contexts (e.g., communicating basic needs and wants to parents at home) but not in other situations (e.g., as a student participating in group literacy activities within the classroom). A number of contextual factors may affect the communicative competence of individuals who use AAC, including the communication demands of the situation and the environmental barriers or supports available to the individual who uses AAC within the situation (see Table 1.1).

Communication Demands

The communication demands that individuals who use AAC encounter within their daily lives are defined by two sets of factors: the social roles that they fulfill and their interaction goals within these social roles.

Social Roles   Although there has been some discussion of social roles in the AAC literature on adults with acquired neurological disorders (e.g., Fox & Sohlberg, 2000), there has been minimal consideration of the social roles of children and adults with developmental disabilities who use AAC. Social roles determine the communication demands that individuals who use AAC will encounter in their daily lives and define priorities for intervention. Table 1.4 presents some social roles that may be important for individuals with developmental disabilities who use AAC across the life span. This list builds on the work of Super and Nevill (1986) and Fox and Sohlberg (2000), who identified five broad categories of roles that adults perform in their daily lives: student, worker, citizen, homemaker/family member, and leisurite.

Table 1.4 demonstrates the growth and change in social roles across the life span as individuals mature from infancy through the preschool and school-age years to adolescence and adulthood as well as the decline in the number of social roles in late adulthood. After considering the list of potential social roles and reflecting on the lives of individuals with developmental disabilities who use AAC, it is clear that there are many restrictions in the range of social roles that most individuals who use AAC experience as they mature. For example, adolescents and adults who use AAC may typically be cast in the roles of son or daughter, student, and recipient of rehabilitation services. They may have significant difficulty attaining and then fulfilling the roles of friend, significant other (or husband or wife), parent, employee or employer, and citizen due to attitude barriers and societal prejudice, reduced expectations in society, lack of appropriate education and preparation, and other barriers (see Environmental Barriers and Supports Available for further discussion). For example, a young woman who used AAC wrote this e-mail message describing her frustrations with her exclusion from important social roles:

> I would love to find someone to go out with. It bothers me that I don't date anyone . . . I get lonely for friends of my own age . . . To me dating for people with disabilities seems to be a problem. I hope someday things will be to where everyone is treated equal. Is that dreaming too much? (C. Smith, personal communication, 2001)

Table 1.4. Social roles that may be assumed by individuals who use AAC across the life span

Stage in the life span	Social roles
Infancy/toddlerhood	Son or daughter/family member Recipient of services
Preschool age	Son or daughter/family member Preschool student Friend Recipient of services
School age	Son or daughter/family member Student Friend Recipient of services
Adolescence	Son or daughter/family member Student Friend Significant other (girlfriend/boyfriend) Volunteer or worker Participant in community activities Member of community organizations Recipient of services
Young adulthood	Son or daughter/family member Student Friend Significant other/husband or wife Volunteer Employee or worker Citizen Participant in community activities Member of community organizations Recipient of services
Middle adulthood	Son or daughter/caregiver for parents Friend Significant other/husband or wife Mother or father/family member Volunteer Employee or worker Employer Participant in community activities Member of community organizations Citizen Recipient of services
Late adulthood	Friend Significant other/husband or wife Mother or father/family member Volunteer Participant in community activities Member of community organizations Citizen Recipient of services

According to Fox and Sohlberg (2000), accessing a range of social roles and creating a balance among them is critical to well-being. Individuals who assume multiple social roles tend to have increased self-esteem (Crist-Houran, 1996). With limited opportunities available to participate in meaningful social roles, individuals who use AAC may be at risk of not attaining a high quality of life. Significant advocacy may be required by individuals who use AAC, their families, and professionals to ensure that they have access to the breadth of social roles that may be important to them. If AAC interventions are to be consumer responsive and effectively meet the needs of individuals who use AAC, it is critical that the individuals' current social roles be assessed, priorities for participation in a greater range of social roles are identified, barriers to greater participation are determined, and action plans are developed to improve access to social roles that are considered a priority.

Within each of the social roles delineated in Table 1.4, individuals who use AAC are called on to engage in different types of communicative interactions in order to fulfill the designated role. Some social roles involve diverse communication demands. For example, as an employee, an adult who uses AAC may be called on to report to the boss on various job-related issues, interact socially with co-workers at breaks or lunch, direct care on the job through a personal care attendant, and so forth. Other social roles are more limited in the diversity of interactions involved. For example, when interacting as a friend on the weekend, the same adult may just hang out with friends, watching a favorite sports team on television and chatting about the game. As the range of social roles increases, the communication demands faced by the individual who uses AAC increase and greater resources (i.e., knowledge, judgment, and skills) are required to be a competent communicator.

Interaction Goals   Individuals who use AAC may have a variety of interaction goals within their social roles. Light (1988, 1997a) proposed that there are four main goals in communicative interactions: 1) to express needs and wants, 2) to develop social closeness with others, 3) to exchange information with others, and 4) to fulfill social etiquette expectations. The communication demands differ across interactions that are intended to fulfill these different purposes (see Table 1.5). For example, in an interaction where the primary purpose is to regulate the behavior of someone else to obtain a need or want, the primary communication demands are 1) to obtain the attention of the partner and initiate the interaction, 2) to indicate the desired item or action, and 3) to terminate the interaction appropriately. For example, if a school-age child who uses AAC wants to ask for a drink at breakfast, the child must first get her mom's attention and then indicate that she wants a drink. Ideally, she would terminate the interaction by thanking her mother. In some situations, the child may also need to confirm her mother's understanding of the request and provide clarification if required.

Table 1.5. The communicative demands of interactions intended to fulfill the four main communication goals

Type of interaction	Communication goal	Communication demands
Express needs and wants	To regulate the behavior of others to fulfill needs and wants (Light, 1988)	Get partner's attention as required Indicate desired object or action (or indicate rejection of undesired object or action) Use politeness markers as appropriate Terminate interaction
Develop social closeness	To establish and develop personal relationships (Light, 1988)	Identify shared activities/topics that are of mutual interest Initiate interaction through these shared activities/topics Make eye contact and attend to the partner's comments, questions, and actions Provide appropriate listener feedback to the partner (e.g., smile, nod) Identify appropriate opportunities to participate (e.g., following partner's questions, comments, or actions) Fulfill these turn opportunities with appropriate comments, questions, or actions Express positive affect/empathy as appropriate Resolve conflicts appropriately Continue to participate actively throughout the interaction
Exchange information	To obtain information and/or impart information to others (Light, 1988)	Attend to the partner's comments and questions Identify appropriate opportunities to ask questions or share information on topic (e.g., following partner's questions/comments or following a pause in the discussion) Produce a contingent response to the partner's question, or produce an appropriate comment/question using vocabulary available Add additional relevant information to develop the topic Initiate new topics as appropriate Confirm partner's understanding or clarify as required Continue to fulfill these demands throughout the extent of the interaction
Fulfill social etiquette requirements	To conform to social conventions of politeness (Light, 1988)	Identify required opportunities to participate (e.g., greetings) Fulfill these opportunities as required Terminate interaction appropriately

In contrast, in an interaction where the primary purpose is to develop social closeness with peers, the communication demands are very different. In this case, the primary goal is to develop the interpersonal relationship or friendship with the peer. The focus is on the relationship, not on obtaining a desired item or exchanging information. In order to develop the relationship, it is important for the child to participate actively in the interaction and to demonstrate an interest in the peer. In order to do so, the child must

1. Identify shared activities that are of mutual interest
2. Initiate interaction through these shared activities
3. Make eye contact and attend to the peer's comments, questions, and actions
4. Provide appropriate listener feedback to the peer (e.g., smile)
5. Identify appropriate opportunities to participate (e.g., following peer's questions, comments, or actions)
6. Fulfill these turn-taking opportunities with appropriate comments, questions, or actions
7. Express positive affect as appropriate
8. Resolve conflicts appropriately as they arise

In interactions to develop social closeness, the focus is on sustaining the interaction over time in order to develop the interpersonal relationship. Therefore, the child must continue to participate actively in this way throughout a sustained interaction.

If the same child is participating in a small-group literacy activity in a school classroom, the communication demands are again very different. Here, the primary focus is to obtain information from others or to impart information to others. In this type of interaction, the child must

1. Attend to the comments and questions expressed by the teacher and/or peers
2. Identify appropriate opportunities to participate within the small group session (e.g., following the teacher's questions or following a pause in the discussion)
3. Indicate his or her desire to participate appropriately (e.g., raise hand) and wait until called on
4. Produce a contingent response to the teacher's question or produce an appropriate comment/question using the vocabulary available
5. Confirm the teacher's and peers' understanding or clarify as required
6. Continue to fulfill these demands throughout the extent of the literacy activity

Here the focus is on the information communicated and greater linguistic complexity may be required within these interactions.

The demands on the communicator within these interactions differ substantially depending on the goal of the interaction, be it to express a basic need or want, develop social closeness, or exchange information. In order for individuals who use AAC to attain communicative competence, they must have the necessary knowledge, judgment, and skills to achieve different interaction goals within their social roles. Too often, AAC interventions focus on the expression of needs and wants to the neglect of other interaction goals (Light, 1997a). It is critical that intervention prepares individuals who use AAC to participate not only in interactions to express needs and wants, but also in interactions to exchange information and especially interactions to develop social closeness (Light, Parsons, & Drager, 2002; see also Chapter 11).

Environmental Barriers or Supports Available

The communicative competence of individuals who use AAC will be influenced not only by the communication demands of the situation but also by the barriers and supports available within the context. These may serve to either impede the communicative competence of the individual, in the case of barriers, or facilitate the attainment of communicative competence, in the case of supports. Sometimes the supports available may be sufficient to offset the existing environmental barriers and allow the individual to attain communicative competence. At other times, additional intervention may be required to remove existing environmental barriers and/or increase available environmental supports. Careful assessment is required to delineate the environmental barriers and supports and to determine the impact of these barriers and supports on the individual's communication.

Environmental barriers and supports interact dynamically with the individual's skills and capabilities to determine communicative competence. Individuals who use AAC and who have significant impairments in their linguistic, operational, social, and strategic skills may be able to attain communicative competence in specific situations if the right environmental supports are in place. For example, Light, Roberts, DiMarco, and Greiner (1998) presented a case study of a 6-year-old boy with autism who had significant impairments in his receptive language skills that made it difficult for him to follow directions and meet the communication demands in his class, resulting in frustration and challenging behaviors; however, when his teacher and paraprofessional provided augmented input in the form of writing paired with speech, his comprehension significantly improved. With appropriate environmental supports (in this case, the use of augmented input by his teachers), this boy was able to enhance his communicative competence. In contrast, an individual who has well-developed linguistic, operational, social, and strategic skills may find it difficult to attain communicative competence in situations where there are significant environmental barriers to successful communication. For example, a young woman who uses AAC may have difficulty interacting socially and making friends at college, despite her linguistic, operational, social, and strategic competencies, if the other students consistently avoid her due to attitudinal barriers.

Beukelman and Mirenda (1998) proposed that there are potentially five types of barriers that might limit opportunities for communication by individuals who use AAC: policy, practice, attitude, knowledge, and skill. Conversely, there may be supports available in any or all of these five areas that will enhance the communicative competence of individuals who use AAC. Table 1.6 provides an overview of these five areas with examples of potential barriers and potential supports to the attainment of communicative competence in each of these areas.

Policy Barriers and Policy Supports   Policy barriers are limitations to an individual's communication that occur as a result of the "official written laws, standards, or regulations that govern the contexts in which AAC users find themselves" (Beukelman & Mirenda, 1998, p. 222). Conversely, policy supports refer to the official laws, standards, and regulations that facilitate or enhance the individual's opportunities to communicate and participate. In the early years of the AAC field, during what Beukelman and Mirenda (1998) referred to as the "pioneering phase," there were few policy supports available for individuals with disabilities who use AAC. In more recent years, as the field entered what Beukelman and Mirenda referred to as the "public policy phase," important legislation has been passed to facilitate access to communication and participation in society by individuals with disabilities, including those who use AAC. For example, individuals who used AAC identified, in web-based focus-group discussions, the following policy supports to communication and participation:

- Civil rights legislation that provides legal protection from discrimination for people with disabilities (e.g., in the United States, the Americans with Disabilities Act [ADA] of 1990 [PL 101-336])
- Government programs that provide financial assistance for assistive technology
- Programs that provide access to rehabilitation services (McNaughton, Light, & Arnold, 2002; McNaughton, Light, & Groszyk, 2001)

Unfortunately, most of the individuals who participated in the focus group also noted that numerous policy barriers still exist: Some existing legislation and policies are not enforced as they should be; others include eligibility requirements for funding or services that restrict who receives services and for how long. Further legislation and policy change is required to better support access to communication by individuals who use AAC (e.g., increased funding for assistive technology, increased availability of personal care services, guaranteed access to medical insurance, increased availability of reliable

Table 1.6. Potential environmental barriers and supports to the attainment of communicative competence

Environmental factor	Examples of potential barrier	Examples of potential support
Policy	Funding restrictions on AAC systems or services Eligibility requirements that restrict who receives services and for how long	Legislation that supports inclusion of individuals who require AAC Policies that ensure funding of AAC systems Legislation that prohibits discrimination against individuals with disabilities
Practice	Limited use policies in some school districts Inefficiency of service delivery/funding system Lack of trained AAC professionals; limited services	Efficient consumer-responsive service delivery by professionals with expertise in AAC Funding support for assistive technology and services
Attitude	People's reduced expectations for participation by individuals who use AAC People's limited attention to communicative attempts by individuals who require AAC "Talking down" to individuals who use AAC	Advocacy efforts/public education to dispel myths about people with disabilities People's acceptance of individuals who use AAC
Knowledge	Lack of knowledge of AAC systems Lack of knowledge of available AAC services	Knowledge of funding sources, skilled service providers, AAC resources Knowledge of AAC symbols and transmission techniques Understanding of positioning requirements Understanding of vocabulary selection and system development Knowledge of operation and programming of AAC systems Knowledge of daily care and maintenance routines Strategies for troubleshooting and technical support Strategies for integrating AAC into daily use
Skill	Communication partners who do not use appropriate strategies to facilitate interactions with individuals who use AAC (e.g., do not wait for individual to communicate, provide inappropriate language input, chain questions, fail to confirm their understanding)	Communication partners who use interaction strategies that support communication with individuals who use AAC (e.g., wait for individual to communicate, provide appropriate language input, confirm his or her understanding)

accessible transportation, assistive technology loan programs; McNaughton et al., 2001). Concerted advocacy efforts and, in some cases, legal action are required to eliminate restrictive policy barriers and to enhance policy supports available to individuals who use AAC to facilitate their attainment of communicative competence (Beukelman & Mirenda, 1998).

Practice Barriers and Practice Supports   Practice barriers are conventions or procedures within a school, workplace, or social community that limit the communication and participation of individuals who use AAC; these conventions are not written as policy and may in fact contravene established policy or law (Beukelman & Mirenda, 1998). For example, practice barriers may occur when schools limit the use of AAC systems to the classroom, thus restricting the student's access to the assistive technology that is necessary for communication at home and in the broader social community. Practice barriers may occur when there are limitations to the quality of AAC services due to the paucity of trained professionals. Practice barriers may also exist because of what Williams (2000) referred to as "systems inertia," or "the lack of urgency and sustained effort" in the delivery of required AAC services (p. 251). Sometimes practice barriers exist even when the professionals providing services are knowledgeable if they fail to work collaboratively as a team. For example, one parent described the practice barriers that she encountered in service delivery for her son:

> A very negative experience is the lack of collaboration . . . .Each sector of professionals believes they can do it on their own . . . In the early years, we had about 40 people involved with [my son] from physicians to school personnel and they wouldn't talk to each other . . . .There are lots of good skills around the table and lots of good problem solving skills, but because of professional ideology and people not knowing how to work together, the whole process is diminished. (Lund & Light, 2001, p. 104)

When individuals who use AAC encounter practice barriers within their daily lives, advocacy efforts may be required to eliminate these barriers. Beukelman and Mirenda (1998) cautioned that these advocacy efforts will be most effective if they are paired with education to ensure that professionals and others have the knowledge and support required to change their practices. Changing the well-established behavior of professionals requires significant planning and support. The good news is that systems can and do change, as is apparent in the Internet revolution in business and education. The bad news is that effecting system change may be a challenging process. McNaughton (2001) proposed that systems are most apt to change when three factors are in place:

1. There is a relative advantage for the new practices compared to the old.
2. The new practices are compatible with the values of the organization.
3. The new practices are easy to understand and implement.

The AAC field faces challenges on all three of these fronts. As of 2003, there are only limited data documenting the positive outcomes (relative advantages) of AAC interventions; future research is urgently required to document the benefits and relative advantages of AAC interventions from the perspectives of all stakeholders (see Chapter 14 for further discussion of AAC outcomes). Unfortunately, many people within the educational system, business community, and broader social community demonstrate negative attitudes toward individuals with disabilities; these values result in reduced expectations for participation and communication by individuals who use AAC. AAC interventions that emphasize increased communication and participation may be in conflict with underlying system values and beliefs. The following quote from Williams illustrates the conflict:

> Why are so many people consigned to lead lives of needless dependence and silence? Not because we lack the funds, nor because we lack the federal policy mandates needed to gain access to those funds. Rather, many people lead lives of silence because many others still find it difficult to believe that people with speech disabilities like my own have anything to say or contributions to make. (2000, p. 250)

Future research is required to investigate effective practices to change the systemic attitudes within educational, business, and social environments. Finally, AAC technologies and interventions frequently impose significant learning demands on both the user and facilitators (e.g., family, educational staff, co-workers; Light & Drager, in press). Future research is required to improve the design of AAC technologies to ease the learning demands for facilitators and to increase the efficiency and effectiveness of AAC service delivery.

In contrast to practice barriers that limit communication opportunities for individuals who use AAC, practice supports occur when conventions and practices within the family, school, place of employment, and broader social community serve to support access to communication for individuals who use AAC. Practices have improved significantly since the 1980s in the AAC field, providing improved support for individuals who use AAC. Lund and Light (2001) conducted a study of the long-term outcomes for seven young adults who had used AAC for at least 15 years. One of the factors identified by these adults and their parents as a factor that had contributed to positive outcomes was the AAC services they received from competent and knowledgeable professionals. For example, one parent said, "[We've had] some very dedicated augmentative communication professionals that had a vision and then had incredible dedication and commitment to finding how he was going to communicate."

The policy and practice barriers and supports described will influence the opportunities that individuals who use AAC have to develop communicative competence. These policy and practice barriers and supports occur at a "systems" level in society. There are also a variety of environmental barriers and supports that occur at the level of individuals within society; specifically, these include attitude, knowledge, and skill barriers and supports.

Attitude Barriers and Attitude Supports Attitude barriers occur when people hold negative ideas and feelings that predispose them to act in ways that limit the communication opportunities of individuals who require AAC. Attitude barriers can have a devastating effect on opportunities for meaningful social interactions (see Chapter 11 for further discussion). Attitude barriers can also result in inappropriately low expectations and exclusion from educational and vocational opportunities and other services. For example, a parent described the frustration his son who used AAC experienced trying to convince employers that he could assume the role of an employee: "Convincing everyone that he could do a productive job independently was the hardest part" (McNaughton, Light, D'Silva, & Gulla, 2002).

Overcoming attitude barriers such as those described will require concerted intervention. Research suggests that positive attitude change may be effected through provision of information about disability, contact with people with disabilities, education by individuals with disabilities (e.g., use of an introduction strategy by individuals who use AAC), vicarious experience, persuasive messages, and so forth (e.g., Gorenflo & Gorenflo, 1991; Light & Binger, 1998; Rosenbaum, Armstrong, & King, 1986; Shaver, Curtis, & Strong, 1989). See Chapter 11 for further discussion of interventions to change attitudes.

In contrast to attitude barriers, attitude supports occur when people in the community, educational system, and places of employment have positive beliefs and feelings that predispose them to provide opportunities for individuals who use AAC to communicate and participate actively in family, educational, vocational, and community environments. For example, an employer who had hired an individual who used AAC made these comments, illustrating the powerful role that attitude supports can play:

> They [people with disabilities] are often very intelligent people with incredible capabilities that are trapped in a body that doesn't work as well as some of the rest of us. Do not be intimidated by the AAC equipment or the user. Getting to know [the individual who uses AAC] has opened up a whole new world for me. (McNaughton, Light, & Gulla, 2002)

Knowledge Barriers and Knowledge Supports Knowledge barriers occur when people lack information about AAC and AAC services, and thus limit opportunities for communication and participation by individuals who use AAC (Beukelman & Mirenda, 1998). Since the 1980s, the AAC field has seen concerted research to advance knowledge and understanding; there is a growing base of empirical knowledge in the field that can be used as evidence to guide effective practice. Unfortunately, there is typically a gap between the state-of-the-art knowledge in the field and the actual practices of professionals and families.

At least two factors contribute to this gap between state-of-the-art knowledge and actual practices: lack of effective preservice training in AAC for professionals and lack of effective dissemination of information to practicing professionals, consumers, and their families. Surveys of preservice training in AAC for special education teachers and speech language pathologists in the United States found that the majority of the programs did not require any course work in AAC (Koul & Lloyd, 1994; Ratcliff & Beukelman, 1995). As a result, most of the current graduates of these preprofessional programs are ill prepared to meet the complex needs of individuals who use AAC (Simpson, Beukelman, & Bird, 1999). Concerted attention is required to improve AAC preservice training of professionals in order to enhance services and thereby improve outcomes for individuals who use AAC and their families.

The AAC field also needs to devote greater attention and resources to ensuring that knowledge is effectively disseminated to all key stakeholders so that it is readily available and accessible in useable formats. Effective dissemination depends on: identifying key stakeholders; determining the content required by these stakeholders; identifying appropriate, accessible media to reach the intended stakeholders; and utilizing familiar and trusted vehicles for dissemination to each stakeholder group (National Center for the Dissemination of Disability Research [NCDDR], 2001). Application of the NCDDR guidelines in the AAC field will result in more effective information dissemination to all relevant constituency groups and will facilitate the removal of knowledge barriers and the development of knowledge supports for individuals who use AAC. Knowledge supports occur when people have the information about AAC and AAC services that they require.

Skill Barriers and Skill Supports   Skill barriers occur when facilitators (i.e., the significant others in the individual's life) do not implement AAC effectively and do not use appropriate interaction strategies when communicating with individuals who use AAC. For example, skill barriers may occur when communication partners do not pause and allow individuals who use AAC the time they need to communicate (e.g., Light, Collier, & Parnes, 1985) or when partners fail to respond to the communicative attempts of individuals who use AAC (e.g., Houghton, Bronicki, & Guess, 1987). Very often knowledge and skill barriers go hand in hand. Partners do not have knowledge of effective AAC practices and therefore have difficulty implementing AAC effectively. Sometimes, however, people have the necessary knowledge but have difficulty translating this knowledge into effective practice (Beukelman & Mirenda, 1998).

Available research suggests that individuals who use AAC frequently encounter skill barriers that limit their opportunities to participate in daily interactions (e.g., Light et al., 1985; Light, Dattilo, English, Gutierrez, & Hartz, 1992; McNaughton & Light, 1989). Concerted intervention may be required with communication partners to address these skill barriers. Kent-Walsh, McNaughton, and Light (2002) reviewed the research on partner training in AAC and found empirical evidence that, with effective instruction, partners who use AAC can learn to use appropriate interaction strategies to support the communication of individuals who use AAC. The skills that were frequently targeted for intervention with communication partners included 1) increased pause time to allow individuals who use AAC time to communicate, 2) increased responsiveness to the communicative attempts of individuals who use AAC, 3) increased use of open-ended questions (as opposed to yes/no questions), and 4) increased modeling of AAC (Kent-Walsh et al., 2002). Partner training in these strategies resulted in increased participation by individuals who use AAC and greater reciprocity in communicative interactions with trained partners. Of particular note is the fact that partner training was typically an efficient intervention; for example, in the study by Light and colleagues (1992), approximately 4 hours of partner instruction were provided and this instruction resulted in greater opportunities for the individuals who used AAC to participate as well as more reciprocal interactions between the partners and the individuals who used AAC.

As of 2002, there has been limited research to investigate the relative effects of different formats for partner instruction; as a result, there is limited understanding of the essential components of effective instruction for partners of individuals who use AAC. Future research is required to investigate the relative effectiveness and efficiency of different approaches to partner instruction in order to maximize skill supports for individuals who use AAC.

CONCLUSION

It has been argued that the development of communicative competence by individuals with developmental disabilities who use AAC rests on their integration of knowledge, judgment, and skills in four interrelated domains: linguistic, operational, social, and strategic. Linguistic and operational knowledge provide the tools for effective communication; social and strategic knowledge ensure that these tools are put into effective use in communicative interactions with others. The attainment and application of linguistic, operational, social, and strategic competencies will be affected by a variety of psychosocial factors, including the individual's motivation, attitudes, confidence, and resilience. Motivation will define the individual's drive to communicate; attitudes may influence the individual's willingness to use AAC to communicate; confidence will impact the individual's propensity to actually engage in communicative interactions with others; and resilience will influence whether the individual recovers from adversities and failures and perseveres in the journey to develop communicative competence.

As Light (1997a) noted, the attainment of communicative competence by individuals who use AAC is a complex process that requires significant time and effort. Communicative competence is not attained in days or weeks; rather, the growth toward communicative competence takes place during many years of learning and practice. The process of developing communicative competence begins in infancy and continues through childhood and adolescence to adulthood. In many cases, significant intervention with individuals who use AAC will be required to build knowledge, judgment, and skills in the linguistic, operational, social, and strategic domains and to bolster motivation, positive attitudes, communicative confidence, and resilience (see Chapter 13 for further discussion of interventions to build communicative competence).

The integration of linguistic, operational, social, and strategic competencies and positive psychosocial factors (e.g., motivation, attitude, confidence, resilience) provides the individual with the foundations for the development of communicative competence. These intrinsic factors are necessary but not sufficient to assure the realization of communicative competence. The attainment of communicative competence will also be affected by a variety of environmental factors.

Communicative competence is a relative construct that depends not only on the individual who uses AAC but also on environmental demands, barriers, and supports. The individual's linguistic, operational, social, and strategic knowledge, judgment, and skills will interact with his or her motivation, attitude, confidence, and resilience to determine the resources that the individual brings to the interaction. The individual's social roles and interaction goals will define the communicative demands of the interaction—in other words, the standards that must be met in order to attain communicative competence. Communicative competence does not require complete mastery of the art of communication; rather, it requires that the individual successfully meets the communication demands of the interaction (Light, 1989). Policy, practice, attitude, knowledge, and skill barriers may limit opportunities for communication and will determine the challenges that the individual must overcome to attain communicative competence. In contrast, policy, practice, attitude, knowledge, and skill supports will serve as external scaffolding support for the individual who uses AAC and may facilitate the attainment of communicative competence.

Future Research Directions

There is much work that remains to be done if we are to ensure that individuals who use AAC develop communicative competence and thus realize the human need, right, and power of communication. Future research is required:

- To determine the specific knowledge, judgment, and skills in the linguistic, operational, social, and strategic domains that are required by individuals who use AAC to attain communicative competence
- To investigate the interaction of the knowledge, judgment, and skills with personal and environmental factors (e.g., individual personality, cultural values, partners)
- To investigate the efficacy of interventions to support the acquisition of linguistic, operational, social, and strategic knowledge, judgment, and skills, and to determine the effect of these interventions on the communicative competence of individuals who use AAC
- To determine the impacts of various psychosocial factors (e.g., motivation, attitude, confidence, resilience) on the acquisition and demonstration of communicative competence
- To investigate the efficacy of interventions to build motivation, positive attitudes toward AAC, communicative confidence, and resilience and to establish the effect of these interventions on the communicative competence of individuals who use AAC
- To explore the social roles that are priorities for individuals who use AAC at various life stages and to identify barriers to the fulfillment of these roles
- To define the communication demands of these roles and to assess the knowledge, judgment, and skills required of individuals who use AAC to meet these demands
- To determine environmental barriers (e.g., policy, practice, attitude, knowledge, and skill barriers) to the attainment of communicative competence by individuals who require AAC
- To develop, implement, and evaluate the effectiveness of interventions designed to remove environmental barriers
- To determine policy, practice, attitude, knowledge, and/or skill supports that facilitate the attainment of communicative competence by individuals who require AAC and to investigate interventions to build these supports

Fulfilling this ambitious research agenda will increase knowledge and will improve practices to develop the communicative competence of individuals who use AAC. With increased knowledge and improved practices, individuals who use AAC will have greater opportunity and support to develop communicative competence and to attain the human need, the human right, and the human power of communication.

> Having the power to speak one's heart and mind changes the disability equation dramatically. In fact, it is the only thing I know that can take a sledgehammer to the age-old walls of myths and stereotypes and begin to shatter the silence that looms so large in many people's lives. (Williams, 2000, p. 249)

REFERENCES

Americans with Disabilities Act (ADA) of 1990, PL 101-336, 42 U.S.C. §§ 12101 et seq.

Bandura, A. (1986). *Social foundations of thought and action: A social cognitive theory.* Upper Saddle River, NJ: Prentice Hall.

Beukelman, D. (1991). Magic and cost of communicative competence. *Augmentative and Alternative Communication, 7,* 2–10.

Beukelman, D.R., & Mirenda, P. (1998). *Augmentative and alternative communication: Management of severe communication disorders in children and adults* (2nd ed.). Baltimore: Paul H. Brookes Publishing Co.

Creech, R. (1995). Outcomes: Choosing our directions: Our freedom is this field's reason for being. In *Pittsburgh Employment Conference Proceedings of the 3rd annual conference* (pp. 9–12). Pittsburgh: SHOUT Press.

Crist-Houran, M. (1996). Efficacy of volunteerism for role-loss depressions: A complement to Weinstein et al. *Psychological Reports, 79,* 736–738.

Culp, D., & Carlisle, M. (1988). *PACT: Partners in augmentative communication training.* Tucson, AZ: Communication Skill Builders.

Estrella, G. (2000). Confessions of a blabber finger. In M. Fried-Oken & H.A. Bersani, Jr. (Eds.), *Speaking up and spelling it out: Personal essays on augmentative and alternative communication.* (pp. 31–45). Baltimore: Paul H. Brookes Publishing Co.

Fox, L., & Sohlberg, M.M. (2000). Meaningful social roles. In D.R. Beukelman & J. Reichle (Series Eds.) & D.R. Beukelman, K.M. Yorkston, & J. Reichle (Vol. Eds.), *Augmentative and alternative communication series: Augmentative and alternative communication for adults with acquired neurologic disorders* (pp. 3–24). Baltimore: Paul H. Brookes Publishing Co.

Gore, S., & Eckenrode, J. (1996). Context and process in research on risk and resilience. In R.J. Haggerty, L.R. Sherrod, N. Garmezy, & M. Rutter (Eds.), *Stress, risk, and resilience in children and adolescents: Processes, mechanisms, and interventions* (pp. 19–63). New York: Cambridge University Press.

Gorenflo, C.W., & Gorenflo, D.W. (1991). The effects of information and augmentative communication technique on attitudes toward nonspeaking individuals. *Journal of Speech and Hearing Research, 34,* 19–26.

Grotberg, E.H. (1995). *A guide to promoting resilience in children: Strengthening the human spirit.* The International Resilience Project from the Early Childhood Development: Practice and Reflections series, Bernard Van Leer Foundation. Available online at http://resilnet.uiuc.edu/library/grotb95b.html

Holland, A. (1982). Observing functional communication of aphasic adults. *Journal of Speech and Hearing Disorders, 47,* 50–56.

Houghton, J., Bronicki, G.J., & Guess, D. (1987). Opportunities to express preferences and make choices among students with severe disabilities in classroom settings. *Journal of The Association for Persons with Severe Handicaps, 12,* 18–27.

Hymes, D.H. (1972). On communicative competence. In J.B. Pride & J. Holmes (Eds.), *Sociolinguistics* (pp. 269–293). Harmondsworth, UK: Penguin Books.

Kent-Walsh, J., McNaughton, D., & Light, J. (2002). *Facilitator instruction in augmentative and alternative communication: A critical review of the literature.* Manuscript in preparation.

Koul, R.K., & Lloyd, L. (1994). Survey of professional preparation in augmentative and alternative communication (AAC) in speech-language pathology and special education programs. *American Journal of Speech-Language Pathology, 3,* 13–22.

Lasker, J.P., & Bedrosian, J.L. (2000). Acceptance of AAC by adults with acquired disorders. In D.R. Beukelman & J. Reichle (Series Eds.) & D.R. Beukelman, K.M.

Yorkston, & J. Reichle (Vol. Eds.), *Augmentative and alternative communication series: Augmentative and alternative communication for adults with acquired neurologic disorders* (pp. 107–136). Baltimore: Paul H. Brookes Publishing Co.

Light, J. (1988). Interaction involving individuals using augmentative and alternative communication systems: State of the art and future directions for research. *Augmentative and Alternative Communication, 4,* 66–82.

Light, J. (1989). Toward a definition of communicative competence for individuals using augmentative and alternative communication systems. *Augmentative and Alternative Communication, 5,* 137–143.

Light, J. (1997a). "Communication is the essence of human life": Reflections on communicative competence. *Augmentative and Alternative Communication, 13,* 61–70.

Light, J. (1997b). "Let's go star fishing": Reflections on the contexts of language learning for children who use aided AAC. *Augmentative and Alternative Communication, 13,* 158–171.

Light, J.C., & Binger, C. (1998). *Building communicative competence with individuals who use augmentative and alternative communication.* Baltimore: Paul H. Brookes Publishing Co.

Light, J., Collier, B., & Parnes, P. (1985). Communicative interaction between young nonspeaking physically disabled children and their primary caregivers: Part I—Discourse patterns. *Augmentative and Alternative Communication, 1,* 74–83.

Light, J., Dattilo, J., English, J., Gutierrez, L., & Hartz, J. (1992). Instructing facilitators to support the communication of persons using augmentative communication systems. *Journal of Speech and Hearing Research, 35,* 865–875.

Light, J., & Drager, K. (in press). Improving the design of augmentative and alternative communication technologies for young children. *Assistive Technology.*

Light, J.C., & Gulens, M. (2000). Rebuilding communicative competence and self-determination. In D.R. Beukelman & J. Reichle (Series Eds.) & D.R. Beukelman, K.M. Yorkston, & J. Reichle (Vol. Eds.), *Augmentative and alternative communication series: Augmentative and alternative communication for adults with acquired neurologic disorders* (pp. 137–179). Baltimore: Paul H. Brookes Publishing Co.

Light, J., McNaughton, D., Krezman, C., Williams, M., Gulens, M., Currall, J., Galskoy, A., Herman, M., & Cohen, K. (2000, August). *The mentor project: Sharing the knowledge of AAC users.* Mini-seminar presented at the biennial conference of the International Society for Augmentative and Alternative Communication, Washington, DC.

Light, J., Parsons, A., & Drager, K. (2002). "There's more to life than cookies": Developing interactions for social closeness with beginning communicators who require augmentative and alternative communication. In D.R. Beukelman & J. Reichle (Series Eds.) & J. Reichle, D. Beukelman, & J. Light (Vol. Eds.), *Augmentative and alternative communication series: Exemplary practices for beginning communicators: Implications for AAC* (pp. 187–218). Baltimore: Paul H. Brookes Publishing Co.

Light, J., Roberts, B., DiMarco, R., & Greiner, N. (1998). Augmentative and alternative communication to support receptive and expressive communication for people with autism. *Journal of Communication Disorders, 31,* 153–180.

Lund, S., & Light, J. (2001). *Fifteen years later: An investigation of the long-term outcomes of augmentative and alternative communication interventions.* Final grant report submitted to the U.S. Department of Education Office of Special Education Programs. (ERIC Document Reproduction Service No. ED458727)

McCarthy, J., & Light, J. (2002). *Exemplary practices for teaching problem-solving skills via the Internet to students who use augmentative and alternative communication.* Grant proposal funded by the U.S. Department of Education Office of Special Education and Rehabilitation Services.

McNaughton, D. (July, 2001). *Supporting the transfer of research to practice: When do we change and why?* Keynote presentation at the Second Annual Institute on Extending Expertise on Exceptional Learners, State College, PA.

McNaughton, D., & Light, J. (1989). Teaching facilitators to support the communication skills of an adult with severe cognitive disabilities: A case study. *Augmentative and Alternative Communication, 5,* 35–41.

McNaughton, D., Light, J., & Arnold, K. (2002). "Getting your wheel in the door": The full-time employment experiences of individuals with cerebral palsy who use AAC. *Augmentative and Alternative Communication, 18,* 59–76.

McNaughton, D., Light, J., D'Silva, K., & Gulla, S. (2002). *Individuals who use AAC and employment: The views of family members.* Manuscript in preparation.

McNaughton, D., Light, J., & Groszyk, L. (2001). "Don't give up": The employment experiences of individuals with Amyotrophic Lateral Sclerosis who use AAC. *Augmentative and Alternative Communication, 17,* 179–195.

McNaughton, D., Light, J., & Gulla, S. (2002). *"Opening a whole new world": Employer and co-worker perspectives on working with individuals who use augmentative and alternative communication.* Manuscript submitted for publication.

National Center for the Dissemination of Disability Research (NCDDR). (2001). *Developing an effective dissemination plan.* Austin, TX: Southwest Educational Development Laboratory.

Rackensperger, T., Williams, M., Krezman, C., & McNaughton, D. (2001, August). *TECH 2010: How do people learn to use an augmentative communication device?* Presentation at the AAC-RERC State of the Science Conference, Minneapolis, MN.

Rak, C.F., & Patterson, L.E. (1996). Promoting resilience in at-risk children. *Journal of Counseling and Development, 74,* 368–373.

Ratcliff, A., & Beukelman, D. (1995). Preprofessional preparation in augmentative and alternative communication: State-of-the-art report. *Augmentative and Alternative Communication, 11,* 61–73.

Romski, M.A., & Sevcik, R.A. (1996). *Breaking the speech barrier: Language development through augmented means.* Baltimore: Paul H. Brookes Publishing Co.

Rosenbaum, P.L., Armstrong, R., & King, S. (1986). Improving attitudes toward the disabled: A randomized controlled trial of direct contact versus Kids-on-the-Block. *Developmental and Behavioral Pediatrics, 7,* 302–307.

Rubin, J. (1975). What the "good" language learner can teach us. *TESOL Quarterly, 9,* 41–50.

Savignon, S. (1983). *Communicative competence: Theory and classroom practice.* Reading, MA: Addison Wesley Higher Education Group.

Scherer, M.J. (1993). What do we know about women's technology use, avoidance, and abandonment. *Women and Therapy, 14*(3–4), 117–132.

Sevcik, R.A., & Romski, M.A. (2002). The role of language comprehension in establishing early augmented conversations. In D.R. Beukelman & J. Reichle (Series Eds.) & J. Reichle, D.R. Beukelman, & J.C. Light (Vol. Eds.), *Augmentative and alternative communication series: Exemplary practices for beginning communicators: Implications for AAC* (pp. 453–474). Baltimore: Paul H. Brookes Publishing Co.

Shaver, J., Curtis, C., & Strong, C. (1989). The modification of attitudes toward persons with disabilities: Is there a best way? *International Journal of Special Education, 4,* 33–57.

Sigafoos, J., & Mirenda, P. (2002). Strengthening communicative behaviors for gaining access to desired items and activities. In D.R. Beukelman & J. Reichle (Series Eds.) & J. Reichle, D.R. Beukelman, & J.C. Light (Vol. Eds.), *Augmentative and alternative communication series: Exemplary practices for beginning communicators: Implications for AAC* (pp. 123–156). Baltimore: Paul H. Brookes Publishing Co.

Simpson, K., Beukelman, D., & Bird, A. (1999). Survey of school speech and language service provision to students with severe communication impairments in Nebraska. *Augmentative and Alternative Communication, 14,* 212–221.

Super, D.E., & Nevill, D.D. (1986). *The salience inventory.* Palo Alto, CA: Consulting Psychologists Press.

Triandis, H.C. (1971). *Attitudes and attitude change.* New York: John Wiley & Sons.

Williams, B. (2000). More than an exception to the rule. In M. Fried-Oken & H.A. Bersani, Jr. (Eds.), *Speaking up and spelling it out: Personal essays on augmentative and alternative communication* (pp. 245–254). Baltimore: Paul H. Brookes Publishing Co.

II

Linguistic Competence

2

AAC and Natural
Speech in Individuals with
Developmental Disabilities

Katherine C. Hustad and Kathy L. Shapley

Clinicians working with children who have significantly compromised speech production capabilities and subsequent reduced intelligibility are often faced with the question, What will happen to natural speech if an augmentative and alternative communication (AAC) system is implemented? Typically, the extent of the individual's speech production challenges influences the level of concern regarding the impact of AAC intervention on natural speech.

For individuals who experience such severe impairments that they are unable to voluntarily produce sound or can only produce gross undifferentiated vocalizations, the decision to implement AAC intervention to enhance communication effectiveness is usually eagerly endorsed by parents and professionals. The opportunity to allow the individual to communicate with others in order to participate in family life, express his or her wants and needs, further develop language, and develop social relationships usually overwhelms concerns about the impact of AAC on speech development. Due to the severity of the speech impairment, most stakeholders realize that the development of functional speech is likely to be a therapy-intensive process that may not be successful. Typically for such individuals, AAC interventions and natural speech interventions continue simultaneously, at least until it becomes clear that natural speech is not progressing, at which time the focus of communication intervention shifts primarily to AAC.

Others with significant communication impairments are able to speak such that they can be partially understood by very familiar partners. For these individuals, the decision to initiate AAC intervention is somewhat more complex than for those with more severe impairments. For individuals who demonstrate the potential to speak, even though their speech may not be functional to meet all communication needs, concerns that implementation of AAC may result in an arrest in speech development or a reduction in desire to use natural speech are often expressed. However, if AAC intervention is withheld until the course of natural speech development is clear, these children may be forced to learn, participate, and develop their social roles with a communication system that is minimally effective or that requires a caregiver to serve as an interpreter for other family members, peers, teachers, relatives, and so forth.

Finally, some individuals are able to use their disordered speech to meet many of their communication needs with familiar people (i.e., family members) in familiar contexts (i.e., home); however, the ability to meet their communication needs is inconsistent with less familiar communication partners (i.e., peers) and in less predictable contexts (i.e., community settings, school). For these individuals, the decision to initiate AAC intervention is often difficult, with parents and professionals, again, concerned about the impact of AAC on natural speech.

In summary, caregivers of individuals with moderately-severe and severe communication disorders face several options regarding AAC intervention:

1. Allow the individual's communication to remain compromised in all or most situations while waiting for his or her speech to develop through maturation and/or aggressive speech intervention.
2. Provide AAC intervention to enhance communication concurrently with speech intervention.
3. Provide AAC intervention to enhance communication while simultaneously providing less intensive speech intervention or discontinuing speech intervention.

To date, there is little direct empirical evidence that addresses the effect of AAC on natural speech. Consequently, AAC practitioners are unable to provide accurate and satisfactory information to families and other professionals regarding this important concern. In the absence of definitive information, clinicians may be tempted to turn to informal or anecdotal reports such as those provided by Silverman (1995).

Following a review of the literature pertaining to AAC and motivation to use natural speech, Silverman stated,

> Teaching a severely communicatively impaired person to use augmentative communication does not appear to reduce his or her motivation for speech communication—a conclusion supported by more than 100 published and unpublished reports. (1995, p. 34)

Based on this same review of the literature, Silverman claims that using AAC "seems to facilitate speech (i.e., increase verbal output)" in at least 40% of individuals who use AAC (p. 34). On the surface, this information is good news for advocates of AAC; however, it is important to note that Silverman's conclusions were not drawn entirely from published research-based evidence but rather from summary results from a number of sources, some of which were anecdotal and unpublished. In addition, Silverman's review encompassed individuals with aphasia, apraxia, dysarthria, autism, and mental retardation—populations with very different underlying problems.

In an attempt to determine the effect of AAC on natural speech production in individuals with developmental disabilities, Millar, Light, and Schlosser (2000) completed a formal meta-analysis of published literature in which documentation of speech production during and/or following AAC intervention was reported. Ultimately, this meta-analysis included 50 studies that were published between 1975 and 1998. Critical to note is that none of the available research examined the effects of AAC on speech directly. Rather, information about speech was reported secondarily to other research questions. Meta-analysis results showed that across all studies, the majority of individuals demonstrated limited increases or no change in speech use following intervention involving AAC. Again, this would appear to be relatively good news to advocates of AAC; however, quantitative measures associated with speech production including segmental analysis, speech intelligibility, and communication effectiveness when natural speech was employed are unknown. Simply measuring the number of productions or verbal communicative attempts, as was the case in many of the studies examined in Millar and colleagues' meta-analysis, provides a gross estimate of speech use but does not address any changes in quality or accuracy of productions. These are important variables to consider when assessing the impact of AAC on natural speech.

Clearly, the question of how AAC affects natural speech is complex, and the answer is not well understood. In part, this may be because the question is too broad to answer without addressing several, more circumscribed, constituent questions. This chapter provides a conceptual framework for considering the relationship between AAC and natural speech through examination of five components, shown schematically in Figure 2.1, that pertain to natural speech and AAC. These components are

1. Speech production characteristics: What do we know about the underlying speech production problems experienced by targeted populations of individuals with developmental disabilities?
2. Speech intelligibility: Does use of AAC make natural speech more understandable to communication partners?
3. Use of speech: How does AAC affect modes of communication employed?
4. Communication effectiveness: How does AAC affect the individual's ability to communicate effectively?
5. Integrating multiple modes of communication: In what ways can speech and AAC be used together to enhance communication?

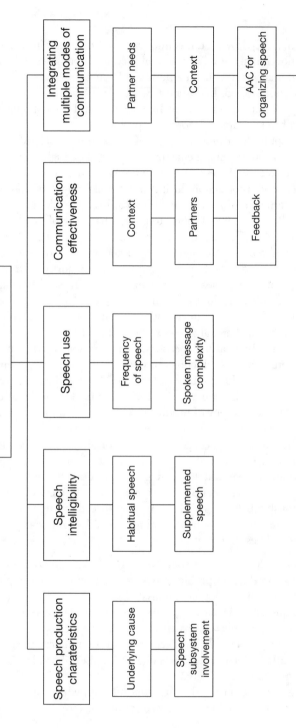

Figure 2.1. Conceptual framework for considering the effects of AAC on natural speech.

This chapter describes what is known about the effects of AAC on natural speech according to each of the five components outlined above and identifies directions for future research. Finally, a case example illustrating consideration of each component is provided.

SPEECH PRODUCTION CHARACTERISTICS

To understand the impact of AAC on speech, it is important to examine specific speech characteristics and their underlying bases, both of which can have important implications for intervention and long-term outcomes. This is particularly true with respect to expectations for changes in speech that might occur with growth and development or with intervention. Three common, yet very different, populations of individuals with developmental disabilities who are frequent candidates for AAC will be addressed in this section. These are individuals with cerebral palsy, Down syndrome, and developmental apraxia of speech (DAS).

Cerebral Palsy

Cerebral palsy is a nonprogressive, neurologically based motor impairment syndrome that is diagnosed in early childhood (Pellegrino & Dormans, 1998). Prevalence estimates of dysarthria associated with cerebral palsy vary between 31% (Wolfe, 1950) and 88% (Achilles, 1955). Speech characteristics observed in those with cerebral palsy are extremely heterogeneous in nature and depend, to a great extent, on underlying pathology—specific muscles and muscle groups that are affected and the physiologic involvement of each. Accordingly, generalizations across individuals, levels of severity, and physiological types are somewhat difficult to draw. Research, although sparse, suggests that speech problems experienced by people with cerebral palsy can affect all speech subsystems—respiration, phonation, resonation, and articulation. Specific effects on each subsystem follow.

In general, respiration is considered the driving force behind the production of speech. It provides the energy source for the phonatory system, which in turn provides the sound source that is filtered by the articulatory and resonatory systems, resulting in the sounds and words of a language (Kent & Read, 1992). Research suggests there are several respiratory problems that may occur in individuals with cerebral palsy, including:

- Respiratory patterns appear to be less flexible than those observed in typically developing children (Hardy, 1964).
- Use of a rapid inhalation and prolonged exhalation pattern of speech breathing employed by speakers without disabilities may be difficult (McDonald, 1987).

- Antagonistic movements of the diaphragm–abdomen and thorax may be more common, resulting in less efficient and reduced inhalatory volume (McDonald, 1987).
- Maintaining consistent subglottal air pressure for speech may be difficult, thus resulting in loudness variation (McDonald, 1987).

Phonatory problems associated with cerebral palsy have received less attention in the research literature; however, McDonald (1987) made the following generalizations:

- Coordinating initiation of phonation with expiration may be difficult.
- Adduction of the vocal folds may be too forceful and regulation of vocal fold tension may be difficult.
- Prevocalizations often result from difficulty with timing the onset of phonation.

Velopharyngeal function in individuals with cerebral palsy has also received little research attention; however, Kent and Netsell (1978) found that individuals with athetoid cerebral palsy tend to have difficulty achieving consistent velopharyngeal closure.

Of all speech subsystems, articulation appears to have received the most attention. Research has demonstrated several different articulatory characteristics of individuals with cerebral palsy. Collective observations across studies are as follows:

- Sounds involving the anterior portion of the tongue tend to be frequently misarticulated (McDonald, 1987; Platt, Andrews, Young, & Quinn, 1980).
- Individuals tend to exhibit a large range of mandibular movements (Kent & Netsell, 1978), including hyperextension (McDonald, 1987).
- Stops, nasals, glides, velars, and bilabials tend to be articulated correctly (Platt, Andrews, Young, & Quinn, 1980).
- Voiceless sounds tend to be misarticulated more frequently than voiced cognates (McDonald, 1987).
- Errors tend to occur more frequently in the word-final than word-initial position (Platt, Andrews, & Howie, 1980; Platt, Andrews, Young, & Quinn, 1980).
- Abnormalities in the timing and range of tongue movements tend to occur (Kent & Netsell, 1978).
- Articulatory transition times tend to be prolonged (Kent & Netsell, 1978).
- Individuals with spasticity and athetosis evidence differing error patterns (Platt, Andrews, & Howie, 1980; Platt, Andrews, Young, & Quinn, 1980).
- Fricatives and affricates are often misarticulated (Platt, Andrews, Young, & Quinn, 1980).

- Vowel productions are often inaccurate (Platt, Andrews, Young, & Quinn, 1980).
- Coarticulation may be problematic (McDonald, 1987).

The constellation, severity, and functional manifestation of subsystem deficits are highly variable among individuals with cerebral palsy. Problems with any one or all of the speech subsystems can result in functional limitations, typically measured by intelligibility and rate of speech (Yorkston, Beukelman, Strand, & Bell, 1999). The relationship among speech subsystems is complex, and problems with a greater number of subsystems do not necessarily constitute greater functional limitations. Some individuals may experience problems primarily with the articulatory system and consequently have profound functional limitations, whereas others may have problems with all of the subsystems and have only mild functional limitations.

Perhaps the most important point regarding speech production in individuals who have cerebral palsy is that the underlying cause is neuromuscular in nature. Consequently, although these individuals may experience some changes in speech with growth, development, and aging, for the most part, problems are static, and gross functional changes without the use of compensatory AAC strategies are not likely.

Down Syndrome

Individuals with Down syndrome present with a unique set of speech production differences relative to those associated with cerebral palsy. Research suggests that 95% of parents of children with Down syndrome sometimes or frequently have difficulty understanding their children's communication attempts (Kumin, 1994). Speech problems appear to be associated with anatomical and neurological differences along with mental retardation. Specific problems include

- Central nervous system structures may differ in size relative to age-matched peers (Florez, 1992; Scott, Becker & Petit, 1983) and consequently may be associated with reduced accuracy, timing, and sequencing of speech movements (Leddy, 1999).
- Larger tongue size in relation to the oral cavity (Arden, Harker, & Kemp, 1972) may affect tongue placement for articulation. Attempts to correct this anatomical difference have included tongue resections, which seem to result in little if any improvement in speech intelligibility (Parsons, Iacono, & Rozner, 1987).
- Abnormal development of the facial bones, including smaller skull (Frostad, Cleall, & Melosky, 1971; Kisling, 1966; Roche, Roche, & Lewis, 1972; Sanger, 1975), may result in a smaller oral cavity.

- Midfacial muscles tend to be poorly differentiated and may result in limited elevation of the upper lip and corners of the mouth for facial expression (Leddy, 1999).
- Hypotonia may make it more difficult for individuals with Down syndrome to control both fine and gross motor movements (Yorkston et al., 1999). Because speech production involves the coordination of many muscles within the four subsystems (i.e., respiration, phonation, resonation, articulation), hypotonia may play a role in decreased speech intelligibility in individuals with Down syndrome.

In addition, problems with articulatory, phonatory, and resonatory subsystems are also characteristic of individuals with Down syndrome (Leddy, 1999). Articulatory problems, in particular, appear to be associated with anatomical and neurological differences outlined previously, as well as a wide range of cognitive abilities. Articulatory characteristics that affect some, but not all, individuals with Down syndrome are as follows:

- Articulation and phonological processing disorder patterns are similar to those of younger children without Down syndrome and include initial cluster reduction, stopping, and final consonant deletion (Bleile & Schwartz, 1984; Iacono, 1998).
- Range and frequency of speech errors seems to be greater for children with Down syndrome than for typically developing children (Parsons & Iacono, 1992)
- Dysarthria or verbal apraxia may influence overall intelligibility (Yorkston et al., 1999) and can compound the effects of an existing phonological processing disorder.
- Tongue thrust patterns may influence both mastication and articulation (Kumin, 1994).

Problems with the phonatory system are most commonly manifest as a hoarse vocal quality (Leddy, 1999). Leddy suggested that anatomical differences, endocrine dysfunction, and an abnormal vocal fold structure may contribute to this percept in the speech of individuals with Down syndrome. Resonatory problems seen in individuals with Down syndrome include hyponasality or hypernasality. Hyponasality may be due to enlarged adenoids or allergies, and hypernasality is often due to flaccid muscle tone (Leddy, 1999).

Finally, fluency disruptions occur in approximately 45%–53% of individuals with Down syndrome (Devenny & Silverman, 1990; Preus, 1990), with dysfluencies tending to be more common among those who have better expressive language skills (Kumin, 1994). Given the wide range of structural and neurological differences, it is not surprising that some researchers believe individuals with Down syndrome have fluency disruptions due to motor-based difficulties, whereas others believe that dysfluencies are linguistically based.

Similar to interventions with individuals with cerebral palsy, AAC interventions do not necessarily have a direct effect on speech production in individuals with Down syndrome. For those with Down syndrome who evidence phonological disorders, particularly children, traditional speech intervention should not be completely abandoned, as there is ample evidence that this type of remediation is effective for other children with phonological disorders (Gierut, 1998); however, generalization of phonological treatment efficacy to individuals with Down syndrome remains largely speculative, and progress is likely to be slow because of cognitive limitations, with changes in speech production that result in functional improvements in spoken communication taking months or even years for some individuals. Consequently, it is important that AAC be implemented for those with reduced intelligibility to enhance functional communication.

Developmental Apraxia of Speech

Developmental apraxia of speech (DAS) is a disorder that is poorly understood and highly controversial in the field of communication disorders (Marion, Sussman, & Marquardt, 1993). "Most definitions of DAS . . . focus on the inability or difficulty with the ability to perform purposeful voluntary movements for speech in the absence of paralysis or weakness of the speech musculature" (Caruso & Strand, 1999, p. 14); however, researchers disagree as to what causes the disorder, with perspectives including motor-level impairment, linguistic deficits, and auditory processing deficits (Strand & Skinner, 1999).

Unlike individuals with cerebral palsy and Down syndrome, those with DAS may seem to be developing typically with the exception of speech production abilities. Although there do not appear to be any anatomical differences, children with DAS may exhibit what some describe as "soft neurological signs," which are characterized by an overall clumsiness or awkwardness, and/or mild sensory aversions to tasks such as brushing their teeth or washing their faces.

Because children with DAS have an outward appearance of being typically developing, their parents and caregivers may resist the implementation of AAC systems and strategies that would make them visibly different to the world around them. Clinical observations suggest that children with DAS sometimes devise their own elaborate signs or gestures to help them communicate. These compensatory strategies may also contribute to parents' resistance to implement AAC. Parents may feel that their child is already using other means to communicate and additional "formal" strategies are not necessary.

The specific speech production characteristics of children with DAS vary among individuals; however, children with DAS generally tend to have particular difficulty with articulation and prosody, which appear to be caused by motor planning deficits. These problems may lead to significantly reduced intelligibility and difficulty with functional communication. Specifically, artic-ulation skills of children with DAS may be characterized by some or all of the following:

- Both consonant and vowel phonemic repertoires are limited (Chappell, 1973; Davis, Jakielski, & Marquardt, 1998; Edwards, 1973).
- Errors are predominantly characterized by omissions, cluster simplifica-tion, and assimilation (Davis et al., 1998; Rosenbek & Wertz, 1972; Smartt, LaLance, Gray, & Hibbert, 1976).
- Vowel errors are numerous, and patterns are sometimes different from children with functional articulation disorders (Crary, 1984; Davis et al., 1998; Rosenbek & Wertz, 1972; Smartt et al., 1976; Yoss & Darley, 1974).
- Articulation errors are not consistent (Davis et al., 1998).
- Children with DAS often rely predominantly on simple syllable shapes, and errors increase on longer units of speech output (Davis et al., 1998).
- Reduced diadochokinetic rates, articulatory groping, and impaired voli-tional oral movements are present (Chappell, 1984; Davis et al., 1998; Rosenbek, Hansen, Baughman, & Lemme, 1974).
- Imitating words and phrases is difficult (Davis et al., 1998).

Prosodic disturbances in children with DAS may include monotony, rate that is too rapid, or rate that is too slow (Davis et al., 1998). Research by Shriberg, Aram, and Kwiatkowski (1997) suggests that inappropriate stress patterns may be a diagnostic marker for DAS. In addition, dysfunctions in speech production may be related to perceptual problems (Shriberg et al., 1997) such as impaired temporal perception of the durational aspects of sounds (Robin, Hall, & Jordan, 1986).

The effect of AAC intervention on speech production in children with DAS is completely unknown and speculation is particularly difficult because of the motor planning problems characteristic of this population. Research with this population is critical to determine the influence of AAC on speech pro-duction. In addition, efficacy research examining the effects of traditional speech-oriented therapy on speech production is also necessary because there is little published empirical evidence.

SPEECH INTELLIGIBILITY

Speech intelligibility is often defined as the degree to which a message pro-duced by a speaker is recovered by a listener (Kent, Weismer, Kent, & Rosen-bek, 1989; Yorkston & Beukelman, 1980; Yorkston, Strand, & Kennedy, 1996). Although the integrity of speech subsystems plays an important role in intelligibility, a direct one-to-one relationship does not exist because a number of other variables, in addition to the integrity of the speech subsystems, contribute to speech intelligibility (Yorkston et al., 1999). These include the listener's ability to apply his or her inherent top–down knowledge of the language and shared context between speaker and listener (Hustad, Beukelman, & Yorkston, 1998).

The ability of parents and other highly familiar caregivers to understand young children, often in spite of compromised intelligibility, illustrates the importance of context and predictability to intelligibility. Parents have shared knowledge regarding such things as the child's experiences, preferences, communication partners, and the general routine of each day. This shared knowledge enables parents to develop expectations for the content of the child's message and, in essence, compensates for the child's reduced intelligibility, enabling an understanding of the intent of the child's message.

In his model of mutuality, Lindblom (1990) discussed the role of two sources of information, signal-dependent and signal-independent information, that contribute to mutual understanding between speaker and listener. Signal-dependent information consists of the speech signal itself, which for many individuals with cerebral palsy, Down syndrome, and DAS is compromised. Lindblom conceptualized signal-dependent information on a continuum ranging from poor to rich, depending on the quality of the acoustic signal produced by the speaker. Signal-independent information consists of knowledge that the listener possesses. Examples include knowledge of the language (i.e., semantics, syntax, morphology, phonology, pragmatics), world knowledge, knowledge of the speaker and the contexts of his or her life, and shared knowledge between speaker and listener (Hustad et al., 1998; Hustad, Jones, & Dailey, in press). Signal-independent information, like signal-dependent information, is also conceptualized on a continuum ranging from poor to rich. According to Lindblom, signal-dependent and signal-independent sources of information are inversely related. If signal-dependent information is compromised (as is the case with individuals who have reduced intelligibility), richer signal-independent information is necessary to compensate so that speaker and listener can achieve mutual understanding. Conversely, when signal-dependent information is rich, little signal-independent information is necessary for speaker and listener to reach mutual understanding because the speech signal is sufficient to carry the communication load.

As children grow older, the signal-independent knowledge specific to the child and all of the contexts of his or her life that communication partners possess may change. Partners may no longer know all of the contexts and situations in a child's life. In addition, as language development proceeds, children may begin to talk about topics and events that are removed in space and time and for which partners do not have shared knowledge or experience. One

AAC intervention that shows promise for increasing intelligibility through enhancement of signal-independent knowledge possessed by listeners is known as speech supplementation (Hustad & Beukelman, 2001; Hustad et al., in press). AAC strategies that can be used to supplement speech include alphabet cues in which the speaker points to the first letter of each word while simultaneously saying the word, topic cues in which the speaker indicates the topic or main idea of a forthcoming message prior to producing it, and combined cues in which both topic and alphabet cues are employed together. A small preliminary body of research suggests that when individuals with reduced intelligibility use these supplemental AAC strategies together with natural speech, intelligibility can be significantly improved, even for those with severe impairments (Beliveau, Hodge, & Hagler, 1995; Beukelman & Yorkston, 1977; Crow & Enderby, 1989; Hustad & Beukelman, 2001; Hustad et al., in press). Although speech supplementation strategies are intended to increase intelligibility by enhancing signal-independent listener knowledge, a byproduct of alphabet supplementation seems to be that speakers reduce their rate of speech and increase word segmentation, thereby modifying production characteristics of speech and making it more intelligible (Beukelman & Yorkston, 1977; Crow & Enderby, 1989; Hustad et al., in press). Consequently, this type of AAC strategy would seem to have a positive effect on both signal-dependent and signal-independent factors. (See Hustad, Morehouse, & Gutmann, 2001, and Hustad & Beukelman, 2000, for detailed discussion of speech supplementation strategies and their implementation.)

Research on the efficacy of speech supplementation strategies has primarily addressed adults with cerebral palsy and other acquired dysarthrias (Beliveau, Hodge, & Hagler, 1995; Beukelman & Yorkston, 1977; Hunter, Pring, & Martin, 1991; Hustad & Beukelman, 2000, 2001; Hustad et al., in press), although preliminary case descriptions suggest that speech supplementation strategies hold promise for children with DAS (Hustad et al., 2001). Additional research is necessary to validate the effectiveness of these strategies with other populations of individuals who have developmental disabilities, including those with Down syndrome.

USE OF SPEECH

One of the obstacles in addressing the impact of AAC on the use of speech is the lack of a consistent operational definition of *speech use*. In the sparse existing literature, this term has been used interchangeably to address the frequency of productions and the complexity of spoken messages. Frequency of productions refers to the number of vocalizations produced and is assessed by counting the number of utterances in a given period of time. Complexity, however, refers to the length and the form of the utterance (consonant–vowel versus consonant–vowel–consonant productions; word-level utterances versus sentence-level utterances).

In general, research examining frequency of speech productions has suggested that availability of AAC does not preclude the use of natural speech and other unaided modes of communication. For example, following implementation of AAC systems and strategies with individuals with mental retardation, Calculator and Dollaghan (1982) found that other, unspecified, modes of communication were used more frequently than AAC systems and strategies for initiating and responding. Similarly, Light, Collier, and Parnes (1985) found that children with severe physical disabilities who used AAC employed vocalizations more frequently than any other communication mode. Further, Beck (1988) reported increases in the frequency of word-level speech productions for children with various developmental disabilities following AAC intervention.

In a study examining the effects of AAC on communication interactions of children with suspected DAS, Cumley (1997) found that AAC did not decrease the frequency of speech use; however, there seemed to be a decrease in the quantity of gestures employed by children who were deemed "high-frequency" users of AAC. Cumley interpreted this as a positive finding because the communication boards employed in this study involved symbols that were more readily understood by a variety of communication partners than gestures.

Less research has focused on changes in the complexity of spoken messages following AAC intervention. However, in a case study, Romski, Sevcik, and Pate (1988) found that complexity of spoken utterances increased from exclusively monosyllabic productions to some bisyllabic productions following intervention emphasizing use of graphic symbols in communicative contexts.

Existing research seems to support the notion that implementation of AAC systems and strategies with individuals who have developmental disabilities does not hinder the use of speech as a mode of communication. Additional research is necessary to further explore the impact of AAC on use of speech. In particular, research should systematically examine individuals with different underlying etiologies, speech impairments of varying severity, different types of AAC systems, and different intervention approaches to further understand the effects of AAC on use of speech.

COMMUNICATION EFFECTIVENESS

Communication effectiveness is a construct that has recently begun to receive increasing attention (Hustad, 2001; Hustad et al., 1998; Yorkston et al., 1999). In general, communication effectiveness refers to the success with which a speaker is perceived to interact, or exchange information, in various communication situations compared with speakers without disabilities of similar age, background, and experience (Hustad et al., 1998). Communication effectiveness is largely a subjective social construct that is measured on the basis of speaker and partner perceptions of success in various communication situations. Yorkston and colleagues (1999) provided an instrument for assessing communication effectiveness in which speakers and partners independently rate success in specific communication contexts using Likert-type rating scales. This type of instrument is useful for systematically determining situations in which the speaker experiences less success, indicating the need for different communication strategies to enhance effectiveness. In addition, the instrument developed by Yorkston and colleagues is useful for determining whether discrepant perceptions between speakers and their communication partners exist. Clinical experience suggests that some individuals may have unrealistic beliefs regarding their own communication effectiveness in different situations and this, in turn, may influence the AAC strategies those individuals choose to employ. For example, those who believe themselves to be effective communicators using speech alone may refuse to use AAC strategies such as alphabet or topic supplementation because they do not see the need. Many of these speakers seem to lack insight into their speech intelligibility challenges and their own behaviors that may propagate reduced communication effectiveness. To some extent, this may be influenced by feedback provided by communication partners.

Skills that seem to be vitally important to effective communication in individuals who use speech that is reduced in intelligibility include the abilities to monitor partners for comprehension, ask partners for feedback, and accept feedback from partners. Conversely, it is critical that communication partners provide honest feedback to speakers with reduced intelligibility, indicating when messages were not fully understood. All too often, listeners of individuals who use speech as a mode of communication are unwilling or uncomfortable indicating that they did not understand the message. As a result, many listeners nod their heads in agreement with the speaker, suggesting that they understand. The consequences of this inaccurate feedback may have far-reaching effects for individuals with speech intelligibility challenges. First, they may fail to develop insight into their intelligibility problems. Second, they may realize that partners did not understand them and come to believe that what they say is not important. Third, they may not learn to look for indicators of comprehension in their communication partners. A quotation from one adult with cerebral palsy illustrates her experiences:

> I know how I feel. I don't like people to say "yeah, yeah" when they really didn't know what I said. I know better than that and I don't like that. I always tell everybody, if you don't know what I said, please just ask me to stop and I will. I will tell you again and again.

It is important to realize that speakers, particularly those who are adolescents and adults, can effect change in their listeners' behavior. Communication, by its very nature, is dyadic. Returning to Lindblom's (1990) model of mutuality, communication or mutual understanding is achieved when the speaker produces a message and the listener processes that message using any and all information available to aid in doing so. When the listener does not have sufficient information to process the message, additional information can be provided by the speaker via AAC strategies. However, the speaker needs to know whether this information is necessary, which can be determined by asking for feedback if it is not provided. It would seem that this type of communication monitoring between speaker and listener should begin early in communication development and continue throughout the life span for individuals who have chronic speech intelligibility challenges. The sooner children learn to identify communication breakdown and acquire tools to repair it, the more effective communication will be.

INTEGRATING MULTIPLE MODES OF COMMUNICATION

The ultimate outcome of any communication intervention should be improvement of the individuals' ability to communicate effectively using any and all means available. For many, this means that both speech and AAC are primary modes of communication, depending on the communication partner and the context. For example, in some situations, exclusive use of AAC may be necessary; however, in other situations, the same person may rely exclusively on speech. Finally, in different situations, this same speaker may benefit from the use of speech supplementation strategies to enhance intelligibility as discussed previously. Often, the mode of communication employed is determined by the communication partner's skill in understanding the message, further illustrating the importance of honest feedback.

Other ways that AAC and speech can be used together include the use of AAC to organize speech. For example, individuals with cognitive disabilities may use low-technology AAC books or boards to structure the content of messages that are then spoken. Finally, AAC can also be used for speech training purposes, serving as a practice partner or a production model. In this type of application, individuals may activate messages stored in a voice output communication device and then repeat those messages using natural speech. The following case example describes a child who benefited from multimodal communication incorporating natural speech, speech supplementation strategies, voice output AAC, and AAC for speech training.

Case Example: Sandy

Sandy was a child with a diagnosis of DAS when she was referred for a speech, language, and AAC assessment at 5 years, 9 months of age. She was just completing kindergarten in a regular education setting and school personnel reported that she was having significant difficulty with communication due to speech intelligibility challenges. Sandy's speech and language intervention to this point had focused primarily on traditional speech-oriented objectives with a strong emphasis on motor planning drill-and-practice activities. Sandy's parents were hesitant to consider AAC options because they felt her speech production was not impaired enough to warrant this. There was also some concern that others weren't "trying hard enough" to understand her. School personnel believed that Sandy's parents did not have a realistic picture of their daughter's communication impairment and her communication needs.

To determine the adequacy of Sandy's speech, quantitative intelligibility measures were collected. This was accomplished through tape recording Sandy's production of a series of structured utterances that were appropriate for her age and language skills. Family members and school personnel were asked to estimate how much of Sandy's speech they thought they typically understood. In addition, they were asked to transcribe the speech sample, writing down each word that they were able to understand. Intelligibility was scored for each listener as the number of words identified correctly divided by the total number of words possible. Results for three family members (mother, father, and a grandparent) showed they estimated that they understood 80%–90% of Sandy's speech. However, transcription intelligibility scores indicated that when signal-dependent information was presented in isolation and family members did not have the full benefit of signal-independent context, quantitative scores ranged from 9% to 35%. For the six school personnel, estimates of intelligibility ranged from 20% to 30% and quantitative measures ranged from approximately 18% to 25%.

These data, displayed graphically in Figure 2.2, illustrate several important points. First, when parents have maximal access to signal-independent information, as they would in a real communication situation, they probably do, in fact, understand 80%–90% of Sandy's messages. Markedly lower estimates of intelligibility by other communication partners who did not have the same comprehensive signal-independent knowledge that her parents have suggest that this signal-independent information is very important for successful communication. Quantitative intelligibility measures of Sandy's speech across school personnel and family reveal that her speech alone is probably not functional when signal-independent information is constrained. In real communication situations, signal-independent information may be limited with unfamiliar communication partners, in situations where the topic or referent is unknown, and in situations where partners do not have shared knowl-

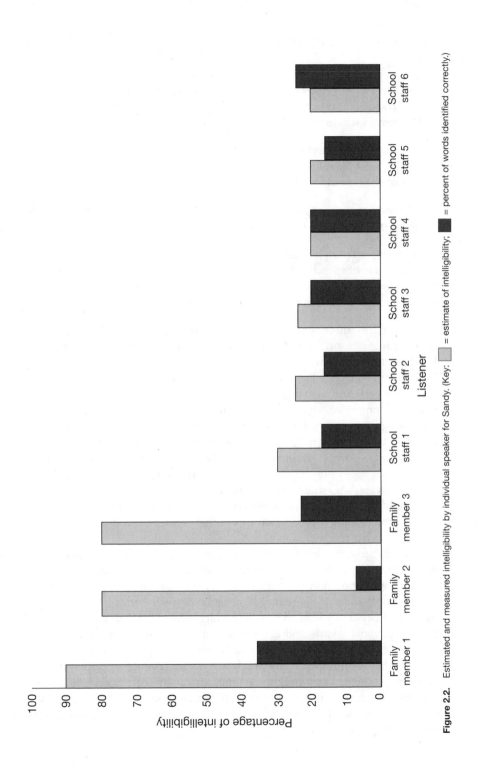

Figure 2.2. Estimated and measured intelligibility by individual speaker for Sandy. (Key: ▢ = estimate of intelligibility; ■ = percent of words identified correctly.)

edge or experience. This is corroborated by responses from a communication effectiveness survey that family and school personnel completed.

In response to the question *In what situations can you understand Sandy's speech best?* answers included the following:

- During routine activities in the classroom
- When the topic is known
- When she is working together with other children on a joint project

In response to the question *In what situations is it hardest to understand Sandy's speech?* answers included the following:

- When no referent is available
- When rate of speech is rapid
- When the general content or topic is unknown
- When there is other noise in the room

Given this information, it seemed very important to provide Sandy with AAC strategies for use when communication partners failed to understand her. Parent education was an important component of intervention for Sandy. When faced with data illustrating the discrepancy between their perception of Sandy's speech and actual performance in decoding her messages without benefit of context, Sandy's family began to see the need for AAC. In addition, comparing intelligibility data from school personnel with their own suggested that difficulty understanding Sandy was probably not associated with failure to try. Sandy's parents continued to advocate for traditional speech therapy; however, they also now agreed to intervention focusing on functional communication via AAC strategies. The suggestion that AAC strategies, in particular use of a voice output communication device, could be used to facilitate speech by providing a production model that Sandy imitated was especially appealing to her parents.

Sandy's intervention focused on use of multiple modes of communication including speech, supplemental AAC strategies, gestures, and voice output communication options. For example, Sandy continued to use speech as her primary mode of communication at home with her family; however, Sandy and her family learned to follow a hierarchy of AAC strategies including use of topic boards and a voice output AAC system for resolution of communication breakdown. At school, Sandy used topic boards in conjunction with her natural speech, and if this was not successful, she employed her voice output device as a backup communication strategy. Speech-language therapy continued to focus on improving speech production as a secondary objective, and use of AAC strategies to enhance functional communication became the primary objective.

SUMMARY

This chapter focused on the relationship between AAC and speech in individuals with developmental disabilities through discussion of five, more circumscribed, issues: underlying speech production variables, effects of AAC on speech intelligibility, effects of AAC on use of speech, communication effectiveness, and the integration of AAC and speech for multimodal communication. Research examining these issues has been somewhat sparse and additional investigation is necessary to fully understand the impact of AAC on each of these speech-related variables. Single-subject and group research designs would both be beneficial in addressing questions identified throughout this chapter so that the effects of AAC on natural speech can be characterized more clearly. Future research is urgently needed to advance understanding in the field and to improve outcomes for individuals with developmental disabilities who have significant speech impairments.

REFERENCES

Achilles, R. (1955). Communication anomalies of individuals with cerebral palsy: I. Analysis of communication processes in 151 cases of cerebral palsy. *Cerebral Palsy Review, 16,* 15–24.

Arden, G.M., Harker, P., & Kemp, F.H. (1972). Tongue size in Down syndrome. *Journal of Mental Deficiency Research, 16,* 160–166.

Beck, A. (1998). Improving natural speech. *Advance for Speech Language Pathologist and Audiologists, 9.*

Beliveau, C., Hodge, M., & Hagler, P. (1995). Effect of supplemental linguistic cues on the intelligibility of severely dysarthric speakers. *Augmentative and Alternative Communication, 11,* 176–186.

Beukelman, D., & Yorkston, K. (1977). A communication system for the severely dysarthric speaker with an intact language system. *Journal of Speech and Hearing Disorders, 42,* 265–270.

Bleile, K., & Schwartz, I. (1984). Three perspectives on the speech of children with Down's syndrome. *Journal of Communication Disorders, 17,* 87–94.

Calculator, S., & Dollaghan, C. (1982). The use of communication boards in a residential setting: An evaluation. *Journal of Speech and Hearing Disorders, 47,* 281–287.

Caruso, A.J., & Strand, E.A. (1999). Motor speech disorders in children: Definitions, background, and a theoretical framework. In A.J. Caruso & E.A. Strand (Eds.), *Clinical management of motor speech disorders in children* (pp. 1–28). New York: Thieme Medical Publishers.

Chappell, G. (1973). Childhood verbal apraxia and its treatment. *Journal of Speech and Hearing Disorders, 38,* 362–368.

Chappell, G. (1984). Developmental verbal dyspraxia: The expectant pattern. *Australian Journal of Human Communication Disorders, 12,* 15–25.

Crary, M.A. (1984). Phonological characteristics of developmental verbal apraxia. *Communication Disorders, 9,* 33–49.

Crow, E., & Enderby, P. (1989). The effects of an alphabet chart on the speaking rate and intelligibility of speakers with dysarthria. In K. Yorkston & D. Beukelman (Eds.), *Recent advances in clinical dysarthria* (pp. 100–108). San Diego: College Hill Press.

Cumley, G. (1997). *Introduction of an augmentative and alternative modality: Effects on the quality and quantity of communication interactions of children with severe phonological disorders.* Unpublished doctoral dissertation, University of Nebraska, Lincoln.

Davis, B.L., Jakielski, K.J., & Marquardt, T.M. (1998). Developmental apraxia of speech: Determiners of differential diagnosis. *Clinical Linguistics and Phonetics, 12,* 25–45.

Devenny, D.A., & Silverman, W.P. (1990). Speech dysfluency and manual specialization in Down's syndrome. *Journal of Mental Deficiency Research, 34,* 253–260.

Edwards, M. (1973). Developmental verbal dyspraxia. *British Journal of Disorders of Communication, 8,* 64–70.

Florez, J. (1992). Neurological abnormalities. In S.M. Pueschel & J.K. Pueschel (Eds.), *Biomedical concerns in persons with Down syndrome* (pp. 159–173). Baltimore: Paul H. Brookes Publishing Co.

Frostad, N.A., Cleall, J.F., & Melosky, L.C. (1971). Craniofacial complex in the trisomy 21 syndrome (Down's syndrome). *Archives of Oral Biology, 16,* 707–722.

Gierut, J.A. (1998). Treatment efficacy: Functional phonological disorders in children. *Journal of Speech, Language, and Hearing Research, 41,* S85–100.

Hardy, J. (1964). Lung function of athetoid and spastic quadriplegic children. *Developmental and Child Neurology, 6,* 378–377

Hunter, L., Pring, T., & Martin, S. (1991). The use of strategies to increase speech intelligibility in cerebral palsy: An experimental evaluation. *British Journal of Disorders of Communication, 26,* 163–174.

Hustad, K.C. (2001). Unfamiliar listeners' evaluation of speech supplementation strategies for improving the effectiveness of severely dysarthric speech. *Augmentative and Alternative Communication, 17,* 213–220.

Hustad, K.C., & Beukelman, D.R. (2000). Integrating AAC strategies with natural speech in adults. In D.R. Beukelman and J. Reichle (Series Eds.) & D.R. Beukelman, K.M. Yorkston, & J. Reichle (Vol. Eds.), *AAC Series: Augmentative and alternative communication for adults with acquired neurologic disorders* (pp. 83–106) Baltimore: Paul H. Brookes Publishing Co.

Hustad, K.C., & Beukelman, D.R. (2001). Effects of linguistic cues and stimulus cohesion on intelligibility of severely dysarthric speech. *Journal of Speech, Language, and Hearing Research, 44,* 407–510.

Hustad, K.C., Beukelman, D.R., & Yorkston, K.M. (1998). Functional outcome assessment in dysarthria. *Seminars in Speech and Language, 19*(3), 291–302.

Hustad, K.C., Jones, T., & Dailey, S. (in press). Implementing speech supplementation strategies: Effects on intelligibility and speech rate of individuals with chronic severe dysarthria. *Journal of Speech, Language, and Hearing Research.*

Hustad, K.C., Morehouse, T.B., & Gutmann, M. (2001). AAC strategies for enhancing the usefulness of natural speech in children with severe intelligibility challenges. In J. Reichle, D. Beukelman, & J. Light (Eds.), *Exemplary practices for beginning communicators: Implications for AAC.* Baltimore: Paul H. Brookes Publishing Co.

Iacono, T.A. (1998). Analysis of the phonological skills of children with Down syndrome from single word and connected speech samples. *International Journal of Disability, Development, and Education, 45*(1), 57–73.

Kent, R., & Netsell, R. (1978). Articulatory abnormalities in athetoid cerebral palsy. *Journal of Speech and Hearing Disorders, 43,* 353–373.

Kent, R.D., & Read, C. (1992). *The acoustic analysis of speech.* San Diego: Singular Press.

Kent, R., Weismer, G., Kent, J., & Rosenbek, J. (1989). Toward phonetic intelligibility testing in dysarthria. *Journal of Speech and Hearing Disorders, 54,* 482–499.

Kisling, E. (1966). *Cranial morphology in Down's syndrome: A comparative roentgenocephalometric study in adult males.* Copenhagen, Denmark: Munksgaard.

Kumin, L. (1994). *Communication skills in children with Down syndrome: A guide for parents.* Bethesda, MD: Woodbine House.

Leddy, M. (1999). The biological bases of speech in people with Down syndrome. In J.F. Miller, M. Leddy, & L.A. Leavitt (Eds.), *Improving the communication of people with Down syndrome* (pp. 61–80). Baltimore: Paul H. Brookes Publishing Co.

Light, J., Collier, B., & Parnes, P. (1985). Communicative interaction between young nonspeaking physically disabled children and their primary caregivers: Part III. Modes of communication. *Augmentative and Alternative Communication, 1,* 125–133.

Lindblom, B. (1990). On the communication process: Speaker–listener interaction and the development of speech. *Augmentative and Alternative Communication, 6,* 220–230.

Marion, M.J., Sussman, H.M., & Marquardt, T.P. (1993). The perception and production of rhyme in normal and developmentally apraxic children. *Journal of Communication Disorders, 26,* 129–160.

McDonald, E.T. (1987). Speech production problems. In E.T. McDonald (Ed.), *Treating cerebral palsy: For clinicians by clinicians* (pp. 171–190). Austin, TX: PRO-ED.

Millar, D., Light, J., & Schlosser, R. (2000). *The impact of AAC on natural speech development: A meta-analysis.* Presentation at the Ninth Biennial Conference of the International Society for Augmentative and Alternative Communication, Washington DC.

Parsons, C., & Iacono, T. (1992). Phonological abilities in individuals with Down syndrome. *Australian Journal of Human Communication Disorders, 20,* 31–46.

Parsons, C.L., Iacono, T.A., & Rozner, L. (1987). Effect of tongue reduction on articulation in children with Down syndrome. *American Journal of Mental Deficiency, 91,* 328–332.

Pellegrino, L., & Dormans, J. (1998). Definitions, etiology, and epidemiology of cerebral palsy. In J. Dormans & L. Pellegrino (Eds.), *Caring for children with cerebral palsy: A team approach* (pp. 3–30). Baltimore: Paul H. Brookes Publishing Co.

Platt, L.J., Andrews, G., & Howie, P.M. (1980). Dysarthria of adult cerebral palsy: II. Phonemic analysis of articulation errors. *Journal of Speech and Hearing Disorders, 23,* 41–55.

Platt, L.J., Andrews, G., Young, M., & Quinn, P.T. (1980). Dysarthria of adult cerebral palsy: I. Intelligibility and articulatory impairment. *Journal of Speech, Language, and Hearing Research, 22,* 28–40.

Preus, A. (1990). Treatment of mentally retarded stutterers. *Journal of Fluency Disorder, 15,* 223–233.

Robin, D.A, Hall, P.K., & Jordan, L.S. (1986, November). *Auditory processing deficits in developmental verbal apraxia.* Paper presented at the Annual Convention of the American Speech-Language-Hearing Association, Detroit, MI.

Roche, A.F., Roche, J.P., & Lewis, A.B. (1972). The cranial base in trisomy 21. *Journal of Mental Deficiency Research, 16,* 7–20.

Romski, M., Sevcik, R., & Pate, J. (1988). Establishment of symbolic communication in persons with severe retardation. *Journal of Speech and Hearing Disorders, 53,* 94–107.

Rosenbek, J., Hansen, R., Baughman, C., & Lemme, M. (1974). Treatment of developmental apraxia of speech: A case study. *Language, Speech and Hearing Services in Schools, 5,* 13–22.

Rosenbek, J.C., & Wertz, R.T. (1972). A review of fifty cases of developmental apraxia of speech. *Language, Speech and Hearing Services in Schools, 5,* 13–22.

Sanger, R.G. (1975). Facial and oral manifestations of Down's syndrome. In R. Koch & F.F. de la Cruz (Eds.), *Down's syndrome (Mongolism): Research, prevention and management* (pp. 32–46). New York: Brunner/Mazel.

Scott, B.S., Becker, L.E., & Petit, T.L. (1983). Neurobiology of Down's syndrome. *Progress in Neurobiology, 21,* 199–237.

Shriberg, L.D., Aram, D.M., & Kwiatkowski, J. (1997). Developmental apraxia of speech: I. Descriptive and theoretical perspectives. *Journal of Speech, Language and Hearing Research, 40,* 273–285.

Silverman, F.H. (1995). *Communication for the speechless* (3rd ed.). Needham Heights, MA: Allyn & Bacon.

Smartt, J., LaLance, L., Gray, J., & Hibbert, P. (1976). Developmental apraxia of speech: A Tennessee Speech and Hearing Association subcommittee report. *Journal of the Tennessee Speech and Hearing Association, 20,* 21–39.

Strand, E.A., & Skinner, A. (1999). Treatment of developmental apraxia of speech: Integral stimulation methods. In Caruso, A.J., & Strand, E.A. (Eds.), *Clinical management of motor speech disorders in children* (pp. 109–148). New York: Thieme Medical Publishers.

Wolfe, W. (1950). A comprehensive evaluation of fifty cases of cerebral palsy. *Journal of Speech and Hearing Disorders, 15,* 234–251.

Yorkston, K., & Beukelman, D. (1980). A clinician-judged technique for quantifying dysarthric speech based on single-word intelligibility. *Journal of Communication Disorders, 13,* 15–31.

Yorkston, K.M., Beukelman, D.R., Strand, E.A., & Bell, K.R. (1999). *Management of motor speech disorders in children and adults.* Austin, TX: PRO-ED.

Yorkston, K., Strand, E., & Kennedy, M. (1996). Comprehensibility of dysarthric speech: Implications for assessment and treatment planning. *American Journal of Speech-Language Pathology, 5,* 55–66.

Yoss, K.A., & Darley, F.L. (1974). Developmental apraxia of speech in children with defective articulation. *Journal of Speech and Hearing Research, 17,* 399–416.

3

Toward Linguistic Competence

Language Experiences and Knowledge of Children with Extremely Limited Speech

Susan Blockberger and Ann Sutton

> Behind the eyes full of life
> Thinking many thoughts
> Thinking if just . . .
> If just these thoughts could become words
> (Dalhoff, 2000)

Light's (1989) influential definition of communicative competence for individuals who use augmentative and alternative communication (AAC) systems proposed that knowledge, judgment, and skills in four domains contribute to communicative competence in individuals who use AAC. One of these four key domains is the *linguistic domain,* which includes comprehension and expression of the spoken language or languages of the community as well as the conveying of language through the medium of the individual's AAC system(s). Although it is possible to communicate without linguistic competence, such communication is limited in both scope and precision of content and is likely to be ineffective with unfamiliar partners. To avoid these significant limitations, people who use AAC must develop knowledge, judgment, and skill in interpreting and producing the linguistic code or codes of their community, and they must also master how language is represented and produced by their AAC systems.

CHILDREN WITH EXTREMELY LIMITED SPEECH

This chapter explores the language experiences and developing linguistic knowledge of children who use AAC or may potentially use AAC, that is, children with extremely limited speech. Like all members of a linguistic community, these children are engaged in the process of learning how to comprehend and formulate words and sentences. This involves learning labels, for example, that the item on the table is called "cup," but it also involves much more. Language acquisition involves acquiring knowledge of *semantics*, that is, words and morphemes (the smallest units of meaning like "un" in unhappy, or "s" in cats), and *syntax*, that is, rules for combining words into sentences. Some examples may illuminate the complexity of the linguistic knowledge that native speakers acquire. Our knowledge of semantics and derivational morphology (morphemes that create new lexical meanings) enables us to understand the meaning and relationship between "tie" and "untie" and to recognize that "undo" is correct, but "unconnect" is not. Our knowledge of syntax and inflectional morphology (syntactically motivated morphemes) allows us to determine who is sad in these sentences: "John noticed the girl on the swing was sad" and "John, noticing the girl on the swing, was sad." It also allows us to recognize that the sentence "John wants to meet the girl in the gazebo" could be interpreted in two different ways. As these examples demonstrate, the linguistic domain is very complex.

Two broad areas of inquiry are addressed in this chapter. The first is how children with extremely limited speech acquire the language or languages of their linguistic community. Which sorts of language acquisition opportunities are available for children with extremely limited speech, and how can the process of language acquisition be facilitated to ensure that every child develops to maximal possible proficiency in this important developmental area? Second, the chapter explores how children's developing linguistic competencies might affect their ease of learning to use an AAC system. Related to this, the chapter speculates on how practitioners might implement systems that "fit" with and take advantage of the child's proclivities and existing language knowledge base as it changes over time. Finally, the chapter discusses directions for future research in the area of language acquisition for children with extremely limited speech.

This discussion is limited to language acquisition in children with extremely limited speech. Although language acquisition is a lifelong endeavor, the bulk of language acquisition, with the possible exception of the area of lexical acquisition, is accomplished in childhood. The early stages of language development are also better researched and described.

Who Are Children with Extremely Limited Speech?

Children with extremely limited speech include individuals with severe speech and physical impairments due to conditions such as cerebral palsy. These children face the double challenge of extreme speech impairments along with motor impairments that significantly affect important functional areas such as independent mobility and play. Also in the extremely limited speech group are children whose speech is extremely limited but whose gross and fine motor abilities are unaffected or mildly affected, as is the case with children with the most severe forms of developmental apraxia of speech. Finally, children with extremely limited speech also include individuals with cognitive impairments who have not developed speech. The term *extremely limited speech*, therefore, includes a wider range of children than does the term *severe speech and physical impairments*, which is commonly used in the AAC literature.

The group of children with extremely limited speech is heterogeneous, a fact that challenges researchers. Nevertheless, these children have several things in common. First and foremost, they are all children. An obvious statement, this fact is worth stating explicitly as a reminder that the large body of information on child development can be fruitfully mined for pertinent information in the quest to understand and describe language development in atypical circumstances. Language development does not proceed at the same pace or in exactly the same way in all children; however, insofar as parameters of human cognitive, social, and physiological architecture constrain the array of possible developmental outcomes, one would expect to see the influence of these factors in both the typical developmental case and in situations where there are differences in some aspects of the child's abilities or circumstances.

Children with extremely limited speech also share characteristics of their early language learning experiences as a result of their inability to produce language in the form of intelligible speech. One striking commonality is that in the earliest language learning years, formal AAC systems are usually not part of the children's expressive repertoires. For a number of reasons, these systems are not usually provided until children are older (often 3, 4, or 5 years old) and well past the age when speaking children have produced their first words. There are several possible reasons for the delay in provision of AAC. Parents may have other more pressing priorities (e.g., stabilizing their child's health) in the earliest years. There may also be reluctance by parents and professionals to introduce AAC because they erroneously see this as abandoning speech development. Parents and professionals may not be aware of AAC options suitable for very young children, and popular AAC systems may not be designed with the skills and abilities of very young children in mind. Without AAC, the ability of the very young child to contribute to conversations is limited. Even once AAC interventions are introduced, the child's linguistic contribution is still limited both by the vocabulary on the system and by the inherent slowness of communicating via AAC compared with natural speech.

The next sections explore commonalties that exist or are thought to exist in the area of spoken language input (i.e., the spoken language addressed to the child) and in language output (i.e., the language produced by the child primarily through AAC). We discuss what theories of language development may predict about the impact of these commonalties, examine what is known about language acquisition by children with extremely limited speech, draw clinical implications, and discuss areas of future research.

LANGUAGE INPUT

Although this discussion is limited to language input as it relates to spoken language, augmented language input is a frequently recommended clinical intervention. Readers are referred to Chapter 5 for a discussion of the role of augmented input.

Children with extremely limited speech, like all children, must discover how language maps onto the world around them. Several researchers have speculated that children with extremely limited speech must map language onto a different and perhaps impoverished base of world knowledge when compared with that of typically developing children, especially when the limited speech is accompanied by motor and/or sensory limitations affecting their ability to explore the environment around them (Light, 1997; Nelson, 1992). For example, children with extremely limited speech and significant motor impairments may not know properties of an object that are not obvious and/or functional properties associated with an object because they have not had an opportunity to explore that object by manipulation.

Regardless of whether children with extremely limited speech are mapping language onto a significantly different knowledge base, there appear to be differences in the language input that they receive relative to that of typically developing children. The fact that children with extremely limited speech have no or limited potential to initiate or contribute in interactions using conventional linguistic forms may affect both the amount and type of linguistic input they are provided.

Some observers believe that children with extremely limited speech receive reduced amounts of linguistic input in their early language experiences (e.g., Calculator, 1997). This conclusion may be based on several observations. Children with disabilities and their caregivers tend to spend proportionally more time in physical care activities than in play (Light & Kelford Smith, 1993). Self-care and physical independence tend to be higher priorities than language-related skills, such as reading and writing, for parents of children with disabilities, but the inverse is true for parents of typically developing children (although communication was a high priority for both parent groups; Light & Kelford Smith, 1993). Furthermore, parents may interact with their children with disabilities in a more directive style than do parents of typically developing children, using increased physical contact and decreased face-to-face communication, even though a responsive rather than directive style has been found to facilitate language development (Girolametto, Weitzman, Wiigs, & Pearce, 1999; Hanzlik, 1990).

The conclusion that children with extremely limited speech receive reduced amounts of linguistic input is called into question by other observations. For example, Cress and associates (2000) argued that parents of children with disabilities tend to engage more frequently in social play than object play and are less directive in that context than in the object play tasks used by Hanzlik (1990). Cress and associates suggested that these parents use directives judiciously to compensate for children's motor limitations when asked to engage in object play tasks, adapting their interaction style to the needs of their children with disabilities. Furthermore, many interaction studies have reported that speaking adults tend to occupy more of the conversational space than do their conversation partners using AAC. In fact, teaching speaking communication partners to provide pauses in order to give the individual using AAC time to respond is a common intervention strategy. In other words, there is a concern that speaking conversation partners talk too much. Although this is clearly a concern from the perspective of providing opportunities for expressive communication, it seems to contradict the notion that children with extremely limited speech receive linguistic input that is quantitatively less than that experienced by typically developing children. The fact that the absolute volume of input that typically developing children receive can vary enormously supports the need to be conservative in drawing conclusions regarding the amount of linguistic input experienced by children with extremely limited speech (Hart & Risley, 1995).

Data on the type of language input provided to children with extremely limited speech is incomplete, but it is believed that there may be qualitative differences compared with input provided to typically developing children. Light, Collier, and Parnes (1985b) examined the communicative functions expressed in conversations between preschool-age children with speech and physical impairments and their primary caregivers. They found that a high proportion of the caregivers' utterances were requests for information. Caregivers often engaged in question–answer routines where the answer was either already known or highly constrained by context. As mentioned, Hanzlik (1990) found that parents of children with cerebral palsy used more directives in an object play task than did parents of typically developing children. In a parental survey conducted by Light and Kelford Smith (1993), caregivers reported that preschoolers with extremely limited speech and physical disabilities spent more time in daily care routines and less time in play and social activities than their peers without disabilities. It follows that the content or topics of conversation are likely to be different—or at least differently distributed—than the content of conversations of peers without physical disabilities. Furthermore, if daily care routines are more likely to involve directives than play or social activities, then the increased amount of time that these activities take may result in an increased proportion of directives.

In classroom environments, Harris (1982) found that teachers' input to children with speech and physical impairments consisted mainly of questions related to physical care, educational questions, or instructions. General interest conversations, passing the time of day, exchange of humor, or anecdotes were described as rare. It is not clear to what extent this type of input is different from that given to speaking children in the same environments (see Cazden, 1988). Harris also noted that the children communicated primarily with adults and only rarely communicated with their peers, although again there were no comparative data for speaking children in the same environments. If children with extremely limited speech do receive proportionately more language input from adults than do speaking children, this might lead to differences in the form and content of that input compared to the input to speaking children.

The literature on typical language development also leads us to predict that the restricted output capabilities of the child with extremely limited speech are likely to have an impact on the nature of the language input. In many cultures (including upper middle class cultures of North America and Europe), adults adjust and simplify their language when speaking to children. It is not entirely clear whether these adjustments are based on the child's language level, cognitive level, or age (see Snow, Perlmann, & Nathan, 1987, for a review of the literature on this topic), and of course usually these three characteristics are highly correlated. These simplifications are felt to facilitate language acquisition and often figure prominently in clinical recommendations to parents of children with language delays (e.g., Manolson, 1985). Caregivers of children with extremely limited speech may have more difficulty in finely tuning their language input to the child's language or cognitive level, given that they do not have the evidence of expressive speech output by which to gauge the child's developmental abilities. Note, however, that there are other cultures (e.g., Samoans, Javanese) in which input is not simplified in this manner, and yet children acquire language within roughly the same time frame as do children in cultures in which input is simplified (Ochs & Schieffelin, 1995). In these cultures, young children are expected to be conversational observers rather than participants and to learn language through other means, such as repeated exposure to unsimplified utterances. Presumably, input to a child with extremely limited speech and to typically developing children would be similar in these cultural milieus.

At least in cultures where input is simplified, language acquisition is facilitated when the topic of that input corresponds to what the child is attending to in that moment. Joint attention refers to instances in which two people are attending to the same object, activity, or topic. The importance of joint attention is highlighted in many accounts of early language development (e.g., Tomasello, 1995). Time spent in joint attention has been found to be positively related to vocabulary acquisition, frequency of communicative utterances, length of conversation, and rate of language development (Kaiser, Hemmeter, & Hester, 1997). Speaking children's comments and questions provide caregivers with illuminating cues about what specifically has captured the child's attention and aid in the establishment of joint attention (Snow, 1984). The child with extremely limited speech may not be able to direct attention to an event or specific object as efficiently, and this limitation may interfere with the establishment of joint attention. As a result, language input to children with extremely limited speech may be less likely to pertain specifically to the aspect of an object or event that has caught their attention. Because of the limited output, there may also be fewer opportunities for adults to provide contingent models and expansions of that output.

Language input to people who use AAC is usually in the form of spoken language. It is rare that the child is given expressive language models in the mode of the AAC system, outside of structured teaching situations (Light, 1997; Romski, Sevcik, & Adamson 1997; von Tetzchner & Jensen, 1996). However, when input does include the graphic modality (i.e., when the partner is modeling use of an aided AAC system employing graphic symbols), the child's attentional resources must be split between the spoken word, the graphic symbol, and the referent rather than between just the spoken word and the referent (Hunt-Berg, 1998).

Role of Language Input in Language Acquisition

It seems likely that children with extremely limited speech experience language input that is quantitatively and qualitatively different than that of their speaking cohorts. Does this affect language acquisition? To address this question, we must examine the role of input in language acquisition. Obviously, input is needed, but how much, when, and what type of input is required or optimal is less clear.

The writings of Clark (1995), Karmiloff-Smith (1992), and Locke (1997) provide examples of theories of language development that include the idea that a threshold of input is required to trigger language analysis and change in the child's linguistic system. Clark (1995) proposed that grammatical acquisition is lexically based and that children learn syntactic characteristics along with lexical items. Once a sufficient number of individual words have been acquired, regularities across items can be analyzed to form grammatical categories and syntactic patterns. All of these theories suggest that there is some level of input needed to trigger language acquisition, but they do not specify how much input is required.

Karmiloff-Smith (1992) proposed a model in which development is viewed as a process driven by the need to establish relationships within and among domains of knowledge. Once a threshold quantity of data from the environment has been stored and represented within a given content domain, the information is redescribed at a higher level of abstraction so that representations are more flexible and more accessible to conscious reflection. This process, called *representational redescription*, is activated by achieving a certain quantity of stored representations at a given level of abstraction. Previously acquired knowledge as well as new information from the environment are available as sources of knowledge acquisition.

Locke (1997) suggested that unanalyzed utterances are stored in memory until storage limitations force analytical mechanisms to identify common patterns within and across utterances.

The developmental timing of input may be important (Elman, 1993). Because of developmental differences in factors such as the child's auditory short-term memory span, the same input may be processed differently at different developmental stages (Newport, 1990). Individuals acquiring language at a later age may bring to the task greater short-term memory storage capacity and greater skills in computational analysis. (Individuals with cognitive impairments acquiring language at a later age may or may not resemble chronologically same-age peers on these parameters.) Paradoxically, these characteristics may actually be disadvantageous for language acquisition because it may be easier to extract form–meaning relationships when the processed input is restricted by short-term memory limitations to shorter strings of data.

Theories also vary by whether they propose that language acquisition occurs *on-line* or *off-line* (Bowerman, 1987). Off-line theories suggest that children compare forms and extract regularities unconsciously even when they are not processing or producing speech. Some input is necessary, but off-line theories place less emphasis on the child's active involvement with language via comprehension or production. On-line theories suggest that children acquire and refine their language base as a result of challenges encountered during language use (either production or comprehension). Blockberger and Johnston (in press) adopted an on-line theoretical stance. They proposed that speaking children learn language through two types of experiences: trying to comprehend input and trying to express themselves through spoken output. Children with extremely limited speech, however, learn language primarily through comprehension. They suggested that early successful comprehension experiences necessitate attention to situational cues and key words. This would encourage identification and acquisition of content words, especially those given emphasis or stress in the input, but comprehension experiences usually do not push a fine-grained analysis of language as do successful production attempts. Following this line of logic, linguistic components not usually crucial to successful comprehension, such as inflectional morphemes, may be more difficult to acquire through comprehension experiences alone.

Lexical acquisition seems most clearly linked to input. Learning specific words, especially content words, depends on having been exposed to them in the environment. Hart and Risley (1995) found that productive vocabularies at age 3 years were approximately $2\frac{1}{2}$ times greater on average for a group of children who were exposed to almost three times as many words on average as a second group of children. It is not known if children with extremely limited speech are exposed to fewer different words than are speaking children, although given the likelihood of restricted experiences and conversational partners, this is a plausible hypothesis.

LANGUAGE OUTPUT

Early Language Output Experiences

The following example is typical of the output experiences of the child with extremely limited speech.[1]

K's first-grade class baked cookies that morning. K approaches the speech-language pathologist and begins a conversation using manual signs:

> K: COOKIE
> SLP: *You made cookies today!*
> K: MOMMY
> SLP: *You're going to give yours to Mommy?*
> K: shakes head no
> SLP: *You're going to show Mommy?*
> K: HOME
> SLP: *You're going to take your cookie home?*
> K: /me/
> SLP: *You and mommy make cookies at home?*
> K: (big smile) nods yes
> SLP: *When did you do that? On the weekend?*
> K: nods yes
> SLP: *You do that almost every weekend, don't you?*
> K: nods yes

A frequently reported conversational phenomenon in dyads involving an individual who uses AAC and a speaking conversational partner is that of co-construction, where the speaking individual expands and elaborates on the message elements provided by the individual who uses AAC (Collins, 1996; Kraat, 1985; Light, Collier & Parnes, 1985a; Soto, 1999; von Tetzchner & Martinsen, 1996). Typically, the person who uses AAC supplies the main

---

[1]In this and all subsequent transcriptions in this chapter, the notational system for the journal *Augmentative and Alternative Communication* is used. That is:
- *Naturally spoken elements are italicized and /phonetic transcriptions are enclosed in forward slashes/*
- *"Words and sentences produced with digitized or synthesized speech are italicized and placed in quotation marks"*
- MANUAL SIGNS are in capital letters
- *GRAPHIC SIGNS* are in capital letters and italicized

content elements, either directly or, if the needed content word is not available, by giving the unaided listener hints or cues. The listener confirms or proposes the content words and expands and elaborates on these components, usually providing the morphosyntactical elements of the message. The resulting message is co-authored over a number of exchanges, although in a sense it represents one conversational turn. The process of co-constructing a message can be arduous, even with a knowledgeable partner. Kraat (1985) gave an example of a co-constructed message—"Can Carl possibly take me home on Saturday with the hospital van?"—that took more than 100 turns and about 20 minutes to accomplish.

Children with extremely limited speech who are attempting to communicate experience many more breakdowns and failures in communication than do children with typically developing speech. Several studies have found that teachers do not respond to most initiation attempts of an individual who uses AAC (Calculator & Dollaghan, 1982; Houghton, Bronicki, & Guess, 1987). Adult responsiveness to communication attempts is similarly an issue for infants and young children, whose communication behaviors may be even more difficult to interpret (Calculator, 1997; Cress et al., 2000). This unfortunate situation has implications for language development, as adult responsiveness to child behavior is known to facilitate language development in the early stages of language development (Yoder, Warren, McCathren, & Leew, 1998). In our experience, and as is illustrated by the following example, the output of an individual who uses AAC, when acknowledged, is often erroneously interpreted as a request when the individual who uses AAC is actually attempting to convey another message.

K's first-grade class baked cookies one morning. K and her speech-language pathologist have just discussed how K and her mom bake cookies together every weekend.

K approaches her teacher and begins a conversation using manual signs:

> K: COOKIE
> Teacher: *No you can't have a cookie right now. We're going to decorate them this afternoon.*
> K: MOMMY
> Teacher: *Mommy will be here at 3:00.*
> Teacher: (to the speech-language pathologist) *She's always asking for her mother!*

Linguistic output produced via AAC systems is often described as telegraphic (e.g., Light et al., 1985a). Despite subject and language elicitation differences, there is a predominance of single-word utterances in the published examples of aided output (Soto, 1997). This could be a modality influence (see Chapter 6), a byproduct of vocabulary limitations, a difficulty with underlying linguistic knowledge, or a conscious strategy for conveying information more quickly given a slow output rate. Conversational partners may also have a hand in creating telegraphic output by jumping in after a single concept has been expressed, thus preventing the individual who uses AAC from communicating longer utterances (Light et al., 1985b). Any or all of these factors may be operating.

It is undeniable that telegraphic output can speed up the conversational exchange with committed and familiar partners. Although telegraphic output may be strategically useful for the timely transmission of information or fulfillment of a conversational turn, there appears to be a cost in social acceptability. When an individual who used AAC communicated in single-word messages (instead of phrases), third party observers judged him to be less involved, less at ease, and less skilled in managing partner attention (Hoag, Bedrosian, Johnson, & Molineux, 1994).

Telegraphic output also places greater interpretative demands on the conversational partner. Correct interpretation of telegraphic utterances often depends on shared knowledge and context. When young speaking children are at the developmental stage where they produce telegraphic utterances, they are usually being cared for by people who have the background knowledge to accurately expand and interpret their utterances. Individuals who use AAC and produce telegraphic speech may attempt to communicate with others who do not share the necessary informational contexts to expand or interpret their utterances accurately. This may partially account for the increased incidence of communicative breakdowns they experience, as the previous example illustrates.

Interestingly, Soto (1999) noted that individuals who use AAC sometimes omit obligatory morphological or syntactic elements even when these are available in their system. Several researchers have also noted that aided output does not necessarily parallel the constituent order of spoken language of the linguistic group (Smith, 1996; Soto, 1999; Sutton & Morford, 1998). For example, Sutton and Morford (1998) found that some children produced object–verb utterances when pointing to Picture Communication Symbols to describe videotaped scenes; they encoded these same scenes in spoken English using a subject–verb–object word order. The atypical order of message elements adds to the challenge of correctly interpreting telegraphic output.

Correct interpretation of a telegraphic utterance may also hinge on a simultaneously occurring transient event (e.g., "no" when carrots are being offered, "doggie" when the neighbor's pet is seen through the window, or "mine" when a sibling has grabbed a toy and is running away with it). Linguistic output via an aided AAC system is characterized by an extremely slow output rate. Whereas conversational speaking rates for natural speakers range from 150 to 250 words per minute, rates for individuals who use AAC are usually less than 15 words per minute. Given this discrepancy, people who use AAC have difficulty producing utterances in a timely fashion, which makes it more likely that they will be misunderstood. Rate limitations also make it difficult for an individual who uses AAC to get and keep the floor in a conversational exchange with a speaking person, which limits conversational opportunities and contributes to a perception of individuals who use AAC as passive communicators.

The aided output of preliterate individuals who use AAC is also characterized by extreme vocabulary limitations. Unless and until they can spell and have an AAC system that affords them that opportunity, people who use aided AAC experience external constraints in their expressive lexicon. The information they can express linguistically is limited by the vocabulary that has been selected by others (usually therapists, teachers, and parents) and included on their device or system. The discrepancy between the expressive lexicon available to a speaking child and that available to an individual who uses AAC is enormous. Consider that a 3-year-old has an expressive vocabulary of about 1,000 words (Mehrabian, 1970). There are very few AAC systems that provide children with access to this many words, and those that do are not likely to be in the possession of 3-year-olds. Even people who use AAC who employ unaided systems, such as manual signs, may experience vocabulary restrictions if (as is often the case) they are interacting with and acquiring their signing skills from others who themselves have very limited knowledge of sign language.

In addition to limitations in the size of the expressive lexicon in the AAC system, there may also be limitations in types of linguistic units under the productive control of the individual who uses AAC. Despite the importance of verbs in constructing multi-word utterances, vocabulary in aided systems is often predominantly nouns, possibly because these are easier to represent graphically. Given the vocabulary size constraints imposed by AAC system design, grammatical morphemes are also less likely to be included—even if they are required by the syntax of the spoken language—particularly if they do not add significantly to the meaning of the utterance.

Because of the limited vocabulary, children are often unable to explore word meanings by labeling and getting feedback on the fit between the word and the presumed referent (Light, 1997). They may also need to rely on overextensions or related concepts to communicate intended meaning (Romski & Sevcik, 1989). It is interesting to speculate about the impact of iconic graphic symbols on the likelihood that symbols will be overextended. Iconicity seems to facilitate symbol learning, but does iconicity constrain the symbol referent, either in the mind of the individual who uses AAC or in the mind of the person receiving the message? This question has yet to be explored.

Soto (1999) noted several metalinguistic strategies that have been employed by people who use AAC to compensate for lack of vocabulary (see also

Chapter 12). These include semantic bypasses (CAR for bus), substitution of a phonologically similar item for unavailable vocabulary (LONG MORE for lawn mower), and use of word modification markers (e.g., using the symbol for OPPOSITE or SIMILAR TO in conjunction with another symbol). Children also use other modalities, such as facial expression, vocalizations, word approximations, or body posture, to convey information. The multiple modalities (i.e., graphic symbols, gestures, speech) may have a complementary relationship where each contributes different information to the message, or a supplementary relationship where one mode contributes information and the other mode modulates or colors that information.

Many aided AAC systems include messages in the form of phrases or sentences, often represented by a single graphic symbol. Most voice output communication aids allow for whole phrases or sentences to be pre-stored into the device as single units. If the individual who uses AAC is preliterate, these messages must be pre-stored by someone else, again usually a caregiver, therapist, or teacher. When the individual who uses AAC then retrieves that phrase or sentence in a conversation, production of these messages has not required language formulation processes that would have been required had the individual who uses AAC selected and combined the morphemes and constructed the phrase or sentence independently.

As discussed previously, the AAC interventions, which provide the tools to produce language, are usually introduced later than spoken language would typically emerge. At the point in time where children with extremely limited speech are provided productive language opportunities through the provision of an AAC system, they bring different sets of skills, linguistic knowledge, and proclivities to the process of acquiring expressive language. In addition, the production experience via the AAC system draws on a different, though overlapping, set of skills than those required by speech. For example, when using an AAC system with graphic symbols, visual-perceptual and visual-motor skills are needed to identify and locate the symbols in the system. The child must also be able to grasp the representational relationship between the graphic symbol and the referent and may need to become conversant with conventions of graphic symbols, such as action lines or thought balloons. (See Chapter 4 for further discussion of representational competence.)

Once a speaking child has mastered production of a word's phonological form, the motor act of producing that word becomes largely automatic. Individuals who use AAC, however, often must devote conscious attentional resources to the process of locating and producing language via their systems. Children who use aided AAC systems must cope with frequent changes in the procedure for producing a linguistic form or structure. The location of a symbol (and hence the motor actions to select it) may change from display to display within one AAC system, or from system to system if the individual who uses AAC employs different systems in various situations. Changes in AAC systems over time may involve adding, reorganizing, or deleting symbols on a display, or even switching to different symbol systems or vocabulary storage approaches (e.g., changing from Picture Communication Symbols to Minspeak). When these changes occur, individuals who use AAC must learn a different procedure for producing a previously mastered linguistic form. In this situation, any automaticity that the individual who uses AAC had previously developed in the expression of that form becomes a liability as the user must suppress previously established motor patterns in order to learn the new procedure for producing the form on the new system.

Individuals who use aided AAC, especially those with mobility impairments, may not be able to independently access their AAC systems, relying on others to get the system, turn it on, or to hook up switches for access. Most people who use AAC are unable to communicate via their aided systems in certain conditions (e.g., in the bathtub) or when in certain positions (e.g., when lying down). It is especially unlikely that people who use AAC and require assistance to access their AAC systems will have opportunities to use their systems for overt practice when alone. As a result, individuals who use aided AAC may have limited or no opportunities for the type of solitary language play and rehearsal in which many speaking children engage.

Role of Language Production in Language Acquisition

The question of the role of language production in the acquisition of language is confused by the fact that researchers often use production measures as the yardstick for acquisition; however, several people have speculated on the role of language production experiences, or at least certain types of production experiences, in promoting language acquisition.

It has been proposed that language production attempts motivate language development and change. Bates (1993) suggested that production experiences may encourage children to attend to details in the linguistic input so that they can later produce the forms. Others have suggested that children's efforts to express ideas draws attention to and strengthens their understanding of the relationships between language form and content (Bloom, 1994; Golinkoff & Hirsh-Pasek, 1995). Clark (1982) suggested a socialization motivation for language development. She suggested that language development often seems to occur not because of a failure to communicate, but because children wish their productions to sound more like the language models they are emulating.

Language or speech production has also been characterized as a venue for both practice and analysis of language. Paul appeared to be suggesting this when she proposed that transitions in language development are "modulated by speech" (1997, p. 142). Paul identified three transitions where speech or language production appeared to be important. These are the transitions 1) from illocutionary to locutionary communication, marked by the emergence of first words; 2) from semantics to syntax, marked by the emergence of word combinations; and 3) from phonology to metaphonology, marked by emergence of phonological analysis skills. Typical children produce language for other than communication purposes. For example, many children engage in *crib talk*, talking to themselves while alone in their rooms. Kuczaj (1983) suggested that one purpose of this solitary language play is to contribute to language mastery by enabling children to reauditorize and analyse linguistic data and to explore language segmentation and distributional characteristics.

If production opportunities are important for the acquisition of language, children with extremely limited speech may be at a significant disadvantage because their language production opportunities are both more limited and qualitatively different from speaking children's. Children may have more difficulty mastering linguistic forms that are not under their productive control. Researchers have speculated that limited opportunities to combine and recombine words as units may influence the child's ability to segment into appropriate word boundaries (Nelson, 1992). Furthermore, there may be a critical mass of vocabulary required to initiate grammatical analysis processes and use of word combinations, and small vocabulary displays may not provide enough vocabulary to trigger this analysis (Sutton, 1999).

WHAT PEOPLE WHO USE
AAC KNOW ABOUT LANGUAGE

> [Not knowing] how to use the English language properly . . . was an added layer of disability for me in my elementary years. (Warren, 1999)

Given the information, known or presumed, about the language input and output opportunities of children with extremely limited speech, one might expect to see differences or difficulties in language acquisition in this group. This is often the case, yet some children do not experience differences or difficulties.

Clinicians and researchers interested in language development issues for children using AAC immediately confront the challenge of how to assess language components in appropriate ways. The assessment methods and strategies used have a direct impact on the data obtained and consequently on the judgments made regarding linguistic knowledge attributed to the individual. For example, an individual who uses AAC and whose output is telegraphic may fare poorly in a language assessment based on analysis of a spontaneous language sample, one of the most popular language assessment methods. Assessment of that same individual who uses AAC using instruments that reduce the motor demands and time pressure may reveal more linguistic competence than was evident in the spontaneous language sample.

For individuals using AAC systems, difficulties in assessing knowledge of syntax and morphology based on language production are readily acknowledged in the literature (e.g., Beukelman & Mirenda, 1998; Blockberger & Johnston, in press; Nelson, 1992). Clinicians and researchers are therefore cautious when interpreting graphic symbol utterances in terms of morphological and/or syntactic skill related to the spoken language of the environment. When compared to spoken communication, AAC message construction involves visually mediated versus verbal-auditory output and additional cognitive effort (Light, Lindsay, Parnes, & Siegel, 1990; Smith, 1996; von Tetzchner, 2000). Furthermore, restricted available vocabulary may lead to the use of compensatory strategies to communicate words and concepts not represented on the AAC display (Soto, 1999). Participation of the communication partner in the message construction process of an individual who uses AAC may also influence the utterance forms produced. Thus, utterance forms produced in the graphic modality may differ from those of spoken language, and it is not clear exactly how specific AAC utterance forms and spoken language structures are related.

Uncertainty about the relationship between graphic modality output and knowledge of the spoken language leads us to consider comprehension tasks for assessing acquisition of morphology, syntax, and vocabulary. Several standardized comprehension tests exist, such as the Test of Auditory Comprehension of Language–Revised (TACL–R; Carrow-Woolfolk, 1985) and the Peabody Picture Vocabulary Test–III (PPVT–III; Dunn & Dunn, 1997). These tests and other similar measures have been used with children with extremely limited speech. Unfortunately, this approach may also be problematic. Motor difficulties may reduce ease of responding on tasks such as toy manipulation and picture pointing, even when all response choices can be demonstrated. Modifications of response options of standardized tests to reduce motor demands may change the task in ways that influence interpretation of the test results. For example, separating pictured response options may require the individual to scan the pictures one by one rather than being able to see them all at the same time. The additional memory component, not part of the original design, increases the cognitive load of the task; as a result, it is inappropriate to interpret the results as if the test had been administered in the standard fashion. Similarly, reducing the number of response options (e.g., by presenting two rather than four pictures per trial) changes the nature of the decision required in order to respond and increases the possibility of correct responding by chance. These concerns apply in addition to more general issues of use of tests in assessing a population not included in the standardization of the test.

One strategy that seems productive in dealing with issues of assessment task design is to obtain converging evidence from performance on tasks with different physical and cognitive demands that target the same linguistic elements. For example, Blockberger and Johnston (in press) used three assessment tasks targeting acquisition of inflectional morphology (e.g., past tense "–ed") by children with extremely limited speech. The tasks—a picture selection task, a grammaticality judgment task, and a written output task—presented different degrees of physical and cognitive demands and tapped into slightly different aspects of acquisition. The picture selection task required the child to be able to scan and process visual images and perform the motor actions necessary to select a picture from an array of three. In comparison, the motor demands of the grammaticality judgment task were minimal, and no visual stimuli or picture interpretation skills were involved, but the metalinguistic demands of this task were relatively high. The structured output task, which involved producing single words to "fill in the blanks" in a story, had relatively high motor demands and required some literacy skills. If only one of these tasks had been used, it could be argued that any difficulties seen were related to the task demands as opposed to difficulties in the acquisition of the inflectional morphemes. The researchers were more confident in concluding that children with extremely limited speech had difficulty in the acquisition of this aspect of language because the children had difficulty with all three tasks and each of these tasks required different skills but tapped knowledge of inflectional morphemes.

Appropriateness of assessment contexts also requires consideration. Situations that appear relatively similar to those used with speaking children may not necessarily present equivalent response options to the child using AAC. For example, Sutton and Gallagher (1995) discussed analysis adjustments needed in order to compare the performance in equivalent contexts for a child using AAC and a speaking child (i.e., following similar types of turns by the conversation partners rather than across all turns). This adjustment was made because the conversational turns produced by the partner of the participant using AAC included few of a turn type that was frequently used by the partners of the speaking participants (i.e., single-utterance turns). Furthermore, the responses of the participant using AAC and those of the speaking participants were compared in a reduced data set because the participant using AAC did not have access to all of the possible response types available to the speaking participants. Thus, comparisons were made only in an equivalent context and for response types that were equally available to all participants. With these adjustments, the performance of the participant using AAC was equivalent to that of the speaking participants even though in the original analysis her performance appeared considerably reduced.

The increasing number of public speeches and published writing by individuals using AAC eloquently demonstrates that limited expressive speech and the need for AAC do not preclude learning to control highly sophisticated linguistic skills (e.g., Fried-Oken & Bersani, 2000; Hohn, 1997; Williams, 1996; Williams & Krezman, 2000). Whether these skills are acquired through typical language acquisition processes, learned through effort, or a combination of these strategies has not been addressed in the literature. Nonetheless, the development of language skills remains a major concern for many individuals using AAC and their intervenors. Language difficulties, if identified, could be related to extremely limited speech and the consequent differences in language acquisition experiences. Language difficulties could also be concomitant with impairments that result in extremely limited speech—for example, cognitive impairment or neurological impairments such as seizures—which place these children at greater risk for language problems regardless of the special circumstances associated with extremely limited speech. Thus, children with extremely limited speech may experience difficulties with language development due to factors orthogonal to having extremely limited speech, as a result of extremely limited speech, or due to a combination of both types of influences. The following sections examine what is known about acquisition of three areas of language—morphology, syntax, and lexicon—for children with extremely limited speech.

Morphology

Morphology is the area of language that seems most vulnerable to breakdown. Many clinical populations experience morphological difficulties (e.g., individuals with specific language impairments, individuals with aphasia). It would not be surprising, therefore, to observe morphological difficulties in children with extremely limited speech, for whom language learning poses multiple obstacles. The few studies of morphological knowledge among individuals using AAC have dealt with inflectional morphology only; derivational morphology has not been addressed thus far. Existing data indicate the presence of morphological difficulties or differences relative to the morphological skills of natural speakers. For example, in reviewing research findings related to language production by people who use AAC, Soto (1999) noted that AAC utterances tend to contain few morphological elements of the environmental spoken language, even when these are available on the AAC display. The observation that available morphological elements are not used consistently could be taken to indicate that morphology may be an area of difficulty. There is also, however, evidence to suggest that this conclusion does not apply to all individuals with extremely limited speech who use AAC. It is clear that this is an area where research is needed.

Kelford Smith, Thurston, Light, Parnes, and O'Keefe (1989) observed morphological errors in some writing samples produced independently by six young adults who used AAC, ages 13–22 years. Although all participants expressed some morphological elements correctly in at least 85% of obligatory contexts, four of the six participants had lower correct response frequencies for at least one morphological element. One participant produced frequent morphological errors (e.g., only 55% of noun endings, 44% of prepositions, and 60% of copulas were correctly produced). All participants noted significant time commitment for writing, reflecting the increased physical demands and cognitive load of writing tasks for them. Despite these findings suggesting difficulties with English morphology, Kelford Smith and colleagues' data also revealed several high levels of morphological competency among their participants. For example, two participants produced all morphological elements with better than 95% and 87% accuracy, respectively, and a third participant demonstrated a similarly high success rate (94% correct or better) for all but one of the morphological elements analyzed (noun endings). Furthermore, participants who experienced difficulty with some morphological elements produced others correctly most of the time (e.g., greater than 80%–90% accuracy).

Blockberger and Johnston (2001) found that children with extremely limited speech exhibited difficulty in the acquisition of inflectional morphemes compared to two groups of children with similar receptive vocabulary levels: a group of typically developing children and a group of children similar in chronological age to the extremely limited speech group but with delayed language development (an "atypical speaking group"). All participants had reasonable comprehension of content vocabulary, obtaining age-equivalent scores between 4.0 and 8.11 on the Peabody Picture Vocabulary Test–Revised (PPVT–R; Dunn & Dunn, 1981). Children in the extremely limited speech group had a mean chronological age of 9.3 and mean PPVT–R age-equivalent score of 6.1. Children in the atypical speaking group had a mean chronological age of 9.4 and a mean PPVT–R age-equivalent score of 6.2. Children in the extremely limited speech group did more poorly on three tasks probing acquisition of inflectional morphology: a comprehension task involving picture selection, a grammaticality judgment task, and a structured written output task employing a fill-in-the-blank procedure. Unlike most children in the other two groups, children in the extremely limited speech group tended to omit morphemes in the obligatory contexts presented in the written output task. On the picture selection task, they attended to the lexical information in the target sentence but ignored the information provided by the inflectional morpheme. Finally, they were unable to judge the grammatical correctness of utterances where the presence or absence of inflectional morphemes was manipulated.

Johnston and Redmond (1999) used a grammaticality judgment task to explore whether three youths with extremely limited speech were aware of tense and agreement marking rules in English. The two participants with developmental disabilities had difficulty detecting tense marking errors, but the participant with a postlingual acquired disability did not. All three participants were sensitive to agreement errors and "–ing" omissions.

Sutton and Gallagher (1993) targeted a single morphological process, affixation (e.g., "play" + "–ed" = "played"). They adapted an affixation process within the access method (a four-digit eye gaze code) used by two adult participants who communicated with AAC for their daily communication. Within their AAC systems, past tense was indicated by encoding (by eye gaze) a four-digit code for the verb (e.g., "play") along with a separate four-digit code for "past." Participants were shown that the new affixation strategy could be used to mark past tense. They were then asked to encode the past tense of both regular and irregular English verbs (e.g., "walk"–"walked"; "run"–"ran"). Whether the affixation strategy was used for both types of verbs could be taken to indicate the participants' awareness of regular versus irregular past tense marking in English. This is a distinction that is acquired fairly early in typical spoken language development, although regularization errors (i.e., using the "–ed" ending on irregular verbs) continue into middle childhood (Marcus et al., 1992). Mature speakers typically have mastered the regular/irregular distinction. One participant in Sutton and Gallagher's study easily mastered the affixation strategy, using it consistently to mark past tense on regular verbs (i.e., equivalent to "–ed") while maintaining her previous strategy for irregular verbs (i.e., "past" plus verb). The fact that she treated regular and irregular verbs differently without instruction suggested that she was aware of the distinction between them even though they could not be encoded distinctively within her AAC system. The second participant also easily learned and applied the new affixation strategy but did not discriminate between regular and irregular verbs: He applied the strategy to encode past tense for both types of verbs. Thus, the results of this study can be interpreted as evidence both of competence (the first participant) and of difficulty (the second participant) in the area of morphology.

Other observations support the notion that morphological difficulties are not necessarily part of the language profile of individuals with extremely limited speech who use AAC. For example, the published writings of some individuals show proficiency and/or mastery of morphosyntactic forms and structures in their writing despite limited or no opportunities to produce them while their language skills were developing (e.g., Fried-Oken & Bersani, 2000; Hohn, 1997; Williams & Krezman, 2000). Anecdotal reports and case studies of children with extremely limited speech who subsequently develop connected speech also suggest that their earlier limited production experience did not preclude the development of competence in morphology. For example, once the child studied by Sutton and Dench (1998) developed connected speech, his language skills, including morphology, advanced more rapidly than would be predicted based solely on the amount of his productive experience with spoken language.

In summary, there is some evidence to suggest that children with extremely limited speech are likely to face challenges in the acquisition of inflectional morphology, although this is not inevitable. Research to date has focused on bound inflectional morphemes (i.e., word endings that fulfill a grammatical role). Acquisition of derivational morphology (i.e., those morphemes that modify meaning) has not been examined.

Syntax

From a structural perspective, language production by individuals using graphic-symbol AAC systems is often characterized as reduced when compared to spoken language structure. Soto (1999) summarized research and descriptive findings in this regard and noted the following structural commonalties across studies: a predominance of single-word utterances and simple declarative clause structures; the use of constituent orders different from those of the spoken language of the environment; and the use of mode combinations within a single message (e.g., graphic, gestural, and vocal). These observations suggest there are important differences between language structures produced using speech and using AAC systems. Although it is possible that these differences reflect differences in syntactic knowledge, there is increasing evidence that the visual-graphic modality of AAC communication may influence utterance structures used and that the patterns seen in language production using AAC systems are a consequence, at least in part, of modality-specific factors as yet not fully understood.

Evidence for a modality effect has been found in several studies of AAC production by speaking participants. Smith (1996) found that five typically developing preschoolers produced mostly single symbol sequences to describe pictures. Similarly, Sutton and Morford (1998) found that children in kindergarten were most likely to use a single picture (usually representing the verb) when using a picture display to describe a video clip even though they produced full subject–verb–object sentences when doing the same task using spoken English. Older children (i.e., in second, fourth, and sixth grades) were increasingly likely to follow English subject–verb–object word order in their picture pointing sentences. When they did not, however, the utterances tended to follow the order object–verb, which contrasts with English constituent order. The findings of constituent order differences when using AAC cannot be attributed to differences in syntactic knowledge because all participants in these studies exhibited typical spoken language development.

Nakamura, Newell, Alm, and Waller (1998) similarly observed frequent use of single-picture or two-picture pointing utterances (contained in the category they called "Other") by both English-speaking and Japanese-speaking adults, even though they used appropriate and complete sentences when speaking. Participants were asked to respond to questions about a story using speech and using a picture-based dynamic AAC display with a main menu containing pictured links to "subject," "verb," and "object" pages. When participants did produce three-constituent utterances, they tended to follow the standard word order of their language (subject–verb–object in English; subject–object–verb in Japanese). English-speaking participants did so regardless of the left-to-right arrangement of the main page pictures (i.e., subject–verb–object or subject–object–verb) but Japanese participants produced the two types of orders with different frequencies depending on the main page arrangement (subject–verb–object orders more frequently using the subject–verb–object arrangement than the subject–object–verb arrangement). When grammatical particles were made available on the main page of the AAC display in a separate experimental condition for Japanese speakers, these participants were more likely to produce a three-constituent utterance and follow Japanese word order (subject–object–verb) than in the condition when the particles were not available. The findings of frequent single-picture and two-picture utterances are consistent with earlier studies (Smith, 1996; Sutton & Morford, 1998). The findings also suggest that the word order patterns of the participants' spoken language play a role in constituent orders produced using AAC systems. Furthermore, they suggest that the availability of morphological markings may influence constituent order of AAC utterances.

Differences in constituent orders using AAC and speech have also been observed for complex as well as single clause utterances (Sutton, Gallagher, Morford, & Shahnaz, 2000). Adult speakers of English were asked to construct complex sentences using a picture–symbol display containing only content words. Because of the absence of grammatical markers (e.g., the relative pronoun "who," verb inflections), constituent ordering was the only strategy available to mark relationships among the constituents. Participants modified the spoken constituent order to encode the relationships among the constituents explicitly by their proximity in the utterance. For example, for the sentence "The girl who pushes the clown wears a hat," the participants encoded WEAR HAT directly following GIRL in order to make the link between them clear (GIRL WEAR HAT PUSH CLOWN), even though they were not in close proximity in the spoken sentence. In contrast, for the sentence "The girl pushes the clown who wears a hat," participants encoded WEAR HAT following CLOWN. This ordering linked the hat with clown, not with the girl (GIRL PUSH CLOWN WEAR HAT).

Taken together, these studies suggest that the reductions and order modifications observed in utterances produced by individuals who use AAC are related at least in part to visual-graphic modality factors (e.g., Soto, 1999). The use of structures in AAC output that do not conform to the spoken language model cannot be taken as a reflection of limited syntactic competence. Whether modality factors can explain all of the reductions and modifications in utterance structures that have been reported in the literature remains an open question. In addition, variables related to AAC communication other than modality, for example, communication efficiency, may influence utterance structures in ways that have not yet been explored.

Although there are difficulties in interpreting AAC language production as an indication of syntactic knowledge, there is some evidence to suggest that extremely limited speech and the need for AAC do not necessarily hinder development of syntactic knowledge. For example, Kraat (1991) and Sutton and Dench (1998) reported case studies of children who made rapid transitions from AAC use to speech that was more complex and well formed than would be predicted based on the time during which the children had full access to speech production for expression. The children (ages 4 and 7) studied by Kraat rapidly acquired spoken language after using communication boards and were described as producing "complete and relatively complex grammatical structures" when speaking, although output via the AAC system at the time of transition was much less complex. The child reported by Sutton and Dench first produced connected speech (i.e., spontaneous two- to four-word utterances) at about 5 years of age. At age 8;6 (i.e., 3;6 years after the onset of connected speech), this youngster's syntactic development had progressed at a faster rate than usual over the 3;6 year period following the emergence of connected speech. Cases such as these suggest that the children's language experiences provided by their language comprehension and by their AAC systems, including residual natural speech communication, prior to the onset of connected speech were adequate to support the development of syntactic competence without extensive production experience.

The notion that production of syntax may develop quickly once the tools become available is supported by accounts (reported primarily anecdotally) of rapid skill acquisition following minimal teaching of structures or major expansion of the AAC system. For example, Harris, Doyle, and Haaf (1996) found that their 5-year-old participant with developmental verbal apraxia learned to produce three- and four-picture utterances in a structured book-reading context although his pre-intervention utterances were typically single items (words, pictures, or gestures). Furthermore, the participant began to use at least some two-picture utterances as soon as he was required to do so within the intervention setting, and this use steadily increased. When three-picture and then four-picture utterances were required, the participant produced them consistently from the first trial. Thus, the participant demonstrated the ability to produce longer utterances even though he did not typically do so.

In contrast, Kelford Smith and colleagues (1989) observed mixed results related to syntax in their study of written communication, described previously. The six participants were adolescents and young adults who used Blissymbolics for face-to-face communication, and who produced written text using computers. These individuals demonstrated a variety of sentence structures in their writing, although with varying levels of accuracy. For example, all participants produced complex sentence structures with at least 80% accuracy but compound sentence structures varied across participants from 8% to 100% correct. Two participants demonstrated high levels of accuracy on simple, compound, and complex sentence types (at least 91% and 100%, respectively). These data can be interpreted to suggest that communication experiences using AAC supported the learning of literacy and the development of competence in English syntax for some of the participants. As the authors note, it is not clear from the study what variables may have distinguished the participants who were successful from those who were not.

Given the known difficulties in assessing syntax through language production using AAC and in interpreting production data in terms of structural knowledge, it is not surprising to observe that limited information is provided regarding the syntactic production skills of participants in research studies; however, the paucity of comprehension studies is somewhat surprising. Despite the interpretive concerns noted previously, comprehension has potential as an accessible assessment format that may more accurately reflect the individuals' knowledge of language than does their production, especially when assessment strategies and tasks are designed to target specific language structures (e.g., Blockberger & Johnston, 2001, for morphology). For example, Udwin and Yule (1990) observed variable comprehension performance among children who were being taught Blissymbols. All of the 20 children in their study, age 3;6–9;8 years, obtained expressive scores on the Reynell Developmental Language Scales that were uniformly below the level expected for the chronological age (i.e., 90% fell below the 24-month level). The children's comprehension scores, in contrast, tended to be somewhat higher. Ninety percent of the comprehension scores were above the 3-year level, including 10% of the children whose comprehension scores were above the 6-year level.

In general, descriptions of participants in studies of language-related issues tend to include insufficient information for evaluating knowledge of syntax. Researchers rarely report comprehension data or evaluate comprehension systematically for their study participants, perhaps in order to avoid making inappropriate judgments regarding language skills. A review of 19 studies of language-related topics where people who use AAC were participants in the *Augmentative and Alternative Communication* journal since the mid-1990s revealed several patterns of reporting language comprehension of participants. In eight studies, standard scores or age equivalents based on standardized tests were used. In two studies, judgments of normal language comprehension were made based on participants' records, without specifying the measures on which the judgments were made. Frequencies of correct responses on an informal task were given without further interpretation in three studies. In one study, group means of performance were provided for a comprehension measure, even though individual data were presented for other characteristics (e.g., diagnosis, schooling, communication system), and one study also reported teacher ratings of students' communication skills. No information regarding language comprehension was included in four studies. In contrast to these generalizations, the study by Harris, Doyle, and Haaf (1996) included both vocabulary and sentence-level comprehension measures and, in addition, provided a (brief) qualitative analysis of error performance related to sentence structure types for the participant in their case study.

Researchers are encouraged to include both quantitative and qualitative information regarding comprehension of vocabulary and syntax in general, as well as more specifically for the tasks to be used in their study. Researchers and clinicians are also encouraged to continue to develop comprehension tasks that elicit equivalent information when performed with a variety of response modes. These tasks will allow us to characterize more accurately the language comprehension skills of children who need AAC.

Lexical Acquisition

There has been speculation that children with extremely limited speech and physical limitations would have an impoverished knowledge base, and that this would lead to difficulty in lexical acquisition; however, this proposal has not to our knowledge been directly investigated. In this area, as in the areas of morphology and syntax, production data are of limited value in determining the presence or absence of difficulties, particularly for preliterate individuals whose productive vocabulary is circumscribed by what is available on their systems. The use of metalinguistic strategies (see Soto, 1999, and Chapter 12)— such as circumlocutions, the exploitation of homophonous relationships, or combining symbols with markers for OPPOSITE OF or SOUNDS LIKE— indicates that, at least some of the time, people who use AAC have probably acquired vocabulary but lack the means to express it directly via their AAC systems.

Because of the obvious problems with inferring vocabulary knowledge from production data in children with extremely limited speech, comprehension data would be of interest. Although vocabulary acquisition has not been the focus of the research, standardized vocabulary comprehension measures such as the PPVT–R are often reported and used as a marker for general language level, as mentioned previously. If we are to look to standardized assessments to determine if vocabulary acquisition is proceeding as expected in children with extremely limited speech, one question is, "What is the appropriate benchmark comparison to be made?" One possible approach would be to compare vocabulary comprehension levels to performance levels on measures of nonverbal or general intelligence. The caveats applied to the use of standardized language measures with this population also apply to the use of standardized intelligence measures; nevertheless, this information is a starting point for considering lexical acquisition in children with extremely limited speech.

Several studies addressing other issues in individuals with extremely limited speech have reported data on participants' single-word vocabulary comprehension levels along with measures of nonverbal cognition or general intelligence. Berninger and Gans (1986) presented language profiles of three individuals with average intellectual abilities and extremely limited speech. Percentile ranks on the PPVT–R for these participants were 26th percentile, 77th percentile, and 1st percentile. The latter score was obtained by a 16-year-old participant with a severe hearing loss that was undetected until he was 8 years old, a factor that undoubtedly had an impact on his acquisition of language.

Smith (1990) studied predictors of literacy for 10 children with cerebral palsy and extremely limited speech who had nonverbal intellectual abilities within the average range. As part of her study, several standardized language measures were given to the participants. Six of these children scored below average on the TACL–R, and eight scored below average on the British Picture Vocabulary Scales.

Bishop, Brown, and Robson (1990) found evidence of vocabulary comprehension impairments in a group of individuals with extremely limited speech and suggested an interesting explanation. They compared adolescent anarthric and dysarthric participants to individuals in the control group matched on chronological age and nonverbal ability as measure by the Raven's Matrices. Compared to the matched controls, both the anarthric and disarthric groups showed evidence of comprehension impairments on a test of vocabulary comprehension (i.e., the British Picture Vocabulary Scales). The anarthric participants were also found to have difficulties on a phoneme discrimination task involving same–different judgments for monosyllabic nonwords. They did not have more difficulty on a phoneme discrimination task for word judgments, where participants were shown a picture, told the label, and asked if the examiner had said it correctly. Bishop and colleagues attributed the poor performance on the same–different judgment task to weak memory for novel phonological strings, related to the role of articulatory recoding in memory for unfamiliar words. They proposed that this deficit could account for both the poor performance on the same–different judgment task and for difficulties in vocabulary acquisition.

Although it is not known whether vocabulary acquisition is particularly impaired as a result of extremely limited speech, many individuals with extremely limited speech have impaired vocabulary comprehension relative to chronological age expectations. Vocabulary comprehension is an important variable in predicting rate of acquisition of graphic symbol comprehension and use. In a longitudinal study of a group of youths with moderate or severe mental retardation, comprehension of speech appeared to be a predictor of rate of progress in System for Augmenting Language, an intervention program in which use of a speech-output communication device with graphic symbols representing a relevant lexicon is taught by modeling its use in natural communicative exchanges (Romski & Sevcik, 1996). With one exception, participants with very poor speech comprehension skills (as measured by PPVT–R and Assessing Children's Language Comprehension) went on to demonstrate "modest" patterns of achievement. In contrast, eight of the nine participants who subsequently demonstrated "advanced" patterns of achievement began the study with better comprehension of spoken language than the modest achievers, as indicated by their performance on these two tests. Romski and Sevcik proposed that the "advanced achievers who comprehended speech readily extracted the critical visual information from the environment, paired it with their extant spoken language knowledge, processed it, and comprehended and produced symbolic communications" (1996, p. 177). In contrast, "Participants with limited comprehension abilities segmented the visual component of the signal, developed a set of visually based symbol experiences, processed the visual information, and comprehended and then produced symbol communications" (Romski & Sevcik, 1996, p. 177).

Even minimal levels of vocabulary comprehension may facilitate acquisition of basic matching skills that may lead to further symbol acquisition for AAC systems. Franklin, Mirenda, and Phillips (1996) evaluated symbol assessment protocols with participants (ages 7–21 years) with severe cognitive impairments, functioning between 24 and 36 months developmental ages. Participants who were able to identify 10 of 12 pretest objects when named were significantly more successful on object–object and object–photograph matching tasks than participants who were able to identify fewer than 7 of 12 pretest objects. (The tasks were among five symbol assessment protocols previously found to be equivalent for typically developing children.) The differences among the performance of the two participant groups could not be attributed to differences in severity of impairment or in level of expressive communication, which was minimal for both groups (not more than a few expressive words or signs).

Of course, saying that comprehension is a predictor for rate of acquisition of an AAC system is not the same as saying that it is a prerequisite. On the contrary, the fact that the "modest achievers" in Romski and Sevcik's (1996) study were apparently able to acquire symbolic communication through a different and visually mediated route (despite years of failure in the acquisition of symbolic communication in the form of speech) would argue against comprehension of spoken language as a prerequisite for the introduction of visually mediated symbols such as graphic symbols or manual signs.

Interestingly, one aspect of the "advanced achievement" profile of the participants in Romski and Sevcik's (1996) study was the ability to fast map (i.e., to quickly acquire an initial partial understanding of new vocabulary with limited exposures). When presented with a novel item (x) along with al-ready-known items and a request to find x, children who fast map will select the unknown item. Seven of the nine advanced achievers in Romski and Sevcik's study showed the ability to fast map novel vocabulary. Furthermore, participants who could fast map retained comprehension of novel words for up to 15 days and generalized their knowledge to production (Romski, Sevcik, Robinson, Mervis, & Bertrand, 1995). Instructional paradigms adapted from the research literature on fast mapping have been used with individuals with extremely limited speech and moderate to severe mental retardation to teach comprehension of spoken vocabulary and recognition of printed words (Wilkinson & Albert, 2001; Wilkinson & Green, 1998). These studies have re-vealed that for some individuals, small methodological differences in how the novel items are presented can affect success.

It is intriguing to speculate about the relationship between the ability to fast map and the impact of limited life experiences. If an individual who uses AAC is a competent fast mapper, it may be less likely that experiential limita-tions would result in an impoverished lexicon, because even very limited ex-posures may result in lexical learning. Furthermore, if there are "holes" in the individual's lexicon related to lack of experience, these would be fairly easy to remediate; however, if the individual who uses AAC is not fast mapping, much more extensive, focused, and systematic instruction may be necessary for the individual to acquire new vocabulary. Individuals who can fast map in some circumstances, but whose ability to do so is affected by other factors such as short-term memory limitations, may also require more—and more carefully controlled—experiences for lexical acquisition to occur.

THE "LINGUISTIC FIT": SOME AAC DESIGN ISSUES

> I just couldn't relate to communicating in numbers; my mind doesn't translate numbers into words. (Staehely, 2000, talking about trying to use a communication device in which words and phrases were stored under numeric codes)

It is good clinical practice to fit the AAC system to the skills and abilities of the child. This is obvious for factors such as visual ability or motor skills, but it is perhaps less obvious that the system should also fit the child's linguistic and conceptual knowledge and skills. Light and Drager (2000) have pointed out that AAC systems are designed by adults and may reflect the conceptual models of adults without disabilities. For a system to be a good fit for a child, the operational demands should involve linguistic or conceptual knowledge within that child's capabilities, and the system should give the child productive control of the linguistic elements the child needs to move forward in language development. There are at least three areas of AAC system design where an appreciation of language development will help us design systems that are a better "fit" for the child. These are the areas of vocabulary selection, representation, and organization.

Vocabulary Selection

One of the first challenges when introducing an AAC system to a child is to decide which vocabulary to include in the system. Given that language acquisition in a wide number of populations follows a similar developmental sequence, it makes sense to look to typical development for guidance on what order to introduce language concepts, forms, and structures. The early vocabularies of typically developing children tend to be comprised predominantly of nouns, specifically object labels (see Blockberger, 1995, for a review). Other words common in first vocabularies are relational words encoding concepts such as recurrence, disappearance, success, or failure (Gopnik & Meltzoff, 1986). Characteristics of first lexicons in typically developing children can be used to guide vocabulary choices for the child with extremely limited speech if the AAC system is provided at about the stage where spoken words would emerge. When expanding an AAC system, either by adding new vocabulary to the system or by teaching the child to retrieve vocabulary in a system with a large pre-stored lexicon, decisions about what forms and structures to be introduced next can be at least partially guided by developmental sequences. Composite lists of vocabulary from children at various ages can also be used when selecting vocabulary (e.g., Fried-Oken & More, 1992). Typical development is not the only source of guidance for vocabulary selection decisions, of course. The reader is referred to Gerber and Kraat (1992) for an excellent discussion and some clinical examples of the thoughtful use of a developmental model of language acquisition with children using AAC.

Vocabulary Representation

A second challenge concerns how the vocabulary should be represented graphically. Graphic symbol sets commonly used in AAC systems (e.g., Picture Communication Symbols, Dynasyms, Blissymbols) were designed by adults and reflect an adult view of word meaning and how to portray that meaning graphically. Many graphic symbols use metaphorical devices and conventions such as thought balloons, action lines, or question marks to convey meaning. Adults sometimes fail to appreciate that children must learn the "language" of graphic symbols and that conventions, such as action lines to portray movement, are not fully appreciated until age 8 or later (Friedman & Stevenson,

1980; Gross et al., 1991). Cultural conventions, such as representing *music* with musical notation, *idea* with a light bulb in a thought balloon, or *good* with a person sporting a halo, must be learned and are not transparent to very young children. (See Chapter 4 for further discussion of the issues surrounding vocabulary representation.)

Support for a gradual development of the ability to interpret graphic symbol conventions is found in a study by Mineo Mollica, Peischl, and Pennington (1998). They found that typically developing 3-, 4-, and 5-year-old children, when asked to select verbs depicted a variety of ways, were most accurate when selecting from video clips, followed by animated line drawings, then static line drawings. Whether the line drawings had visual cues, such as action lines, did not affect the 3-year-olds' performance, but the inclusion of these visual cues did improve accuracy for the 4- and 5-year-olds. This study also provides some support for the use of animated graphic symbols to depict actions, although the authors cautioned that the animated line drawings used in their study are more lifelike than the animated symbols used in many commercial devices.

Lund, Millar, Herman, Hinds, and Light (1998) addressed the question of whether the graphic symbol systems reflect the way children think and what they know about linguistic concepts by exploring how children represented concepts graphically. Four- to seven-year-old children were asked to draw pictures of early emerging language concepts such as *big, eat, all gone,* and *what's that.* The resulting pictures were rich in context and often portrayed personal experiences and familiar individuals. There were similarities across children in how these concepts were portrayed, but there were differences between the children's drawings and the way that commercial AAC symbol sets portray these concepts. Although further research is necessary, it seems likely that graphic symbol systems that are more iconic can be designed for young children.

Vocabulary Organization

The third challenge concerns how to organize vocabulary on aided AAC systems with large vocabularies. This may involve organizing vocabulary on multiple pages in a communication book, on multiple screens in a communication device with dynamic displays, or using an iconic encoding scheme such as Minspeak in a communication device. To minimize the operational demands of using the AAC system, clinicians must organize dynamic displays or multi-page communication so that both the grouping of symbols onto pages and placement of the symbols within those pages is most intuitive for young children. Noting that many first words tend to be used only in context-specific circumstances, Blockberger (1995) suggested that for individuals who use AAC in the earliest stages of language acquisition, vocabulary should be organized schematically by situation or activity. Nelson (1992) noted that there is a shift in typical children's word associations in a free-recall task, from syntactical associations (go–home) to categorical associations (go–stop), at about age 7 and predicted that younger children may do better with grammatical rather than categorical organization patterns.

Light, Drager, and their colleagues at Penn State University explored this issue in a series of studies that compared how well typical 2-, 3-, 4-, and 5-year-olds learned several organizational schemes for AAC systems (Light, Drager, Curran, et al., 2000; Light, Drager, McCarthy, et al., 2000; Light, Drager, Millar, et al., 2000; Light, Drager, Pitkin, et al., 2000). Three organizational systems were explored: a taxonomic grid organization, a schematic grid organization, and a schematic scene organization. In the taxonomic grid organization condition, symbols were presented in a grid and grouped in taxonomic categories (e.g., a "people" page, a "things" page). In the schematic grid organization condition, symbols were presented in a grid and grouped according to situations or activities (e.g., a "going to the party" page, an "eating cake" page). The schematic scene organization presented the symbols actually embedded in scenes (e.g., a scene of children eating birthday cake in a kitchen). After 3–4 hours of instruction over several days, approximately half of the 2-year-olds and virtually all of the 3-, 4-, and 5-year-olds were able to locate some symbols. Children improved in performance as age increased. There was no difference between the organizational systems, except for the 2-year-olds, who performed best with the schematic scene. Again, more research is required to determine how to organize vocabulary within the AAC system so that children may retrieve it most easily.

In Minspeak or in similar systems, the challenge of access to a large vocabulary is handled differently. A relatively small set of icons, chosen for their ability to be richly associated with a large number of linguistic and conceptual elements, are displayed on an AAC device. Words or phrases are stored under icon sequences and retrieved by the people who use AAC selecting the icons in the correct sequence. In popular commercial applications of this approach, such as some versions of the Unity application program, the rationales for the selected icons in a given sequence seem to draw on a college-educated American adult's world knowledge and metalinguistic abilities. For example, sequences for be verb forms (be, is, are, am) include a honey bee, exploiting the homophonous relationship between bee and be. The rationales for these types of associations will likely be beyond the grasp of very young children, and thus, this type of system may represent a relatively poor fit between a typically developing young child's linguistic knowledge and the AAC system demands. Perhaps future incarnations of this system will be modified so that younger children easily understand more of the icon sequence rationales. In the meantime, children who do not have the metalinguistic skills to appreciate the rationales for icon selection can nevertheless learn the icon sequences, either by rote methods (i.e., developing an automatic motor memory for the sequence) or by some alternative "customized" mnemonic strategy. Furthermore, the icon sequences can spark the discussion and teaching of many linguistic concepts, and this may be quite advantageous to the individual who uses AAC. Finally, the disadvantage to the young child engendered by high cognitive and metalinguistic demands of systems may be offset if the systems are powerful ones that afford the individual who uses AAC productive control of linguistic forms and structures.

CLINICAL IMPLICATIONS

> Dig in, get the support of both the school and the social services agencies, get the devices funded, and make us work our little tails off until we master enough language to become competent communicators. (Estrella, 2000)

Up to this point, the chapter has discussed differences between the early language experiences and knowledge of children with extremely limited speech and speaking children. The next step is to determine which differences have clinical significance and, if they do, to intervene. Understanding the factors that lead to clinically significant differences helps to determine what forms the intervention should take. For example, we may decide that the predominance of single-word utterances in aided output is clinically significant. The intervention to avoid or remediate this output characteristic will differ depending on whether we think it represents a conscious strategy to speed up communication, an unconscious modality influence, or a failure to have acquired the linguistic structures in question.

Whether an identified or hypothesized difference should be addressed in clinical interventions depends on many considerations. Some identified differences may not be clinically significant, as clinical significance and statistical significance are not synonymous. In some instances, it may be possible to show statistically significant differences between groups where that difference has no functional impact and is therefore clinically irrelevant. AAC is, of course, a clinically grounded field, so attention must be focused on those differences that are clinically significant. When clinically significant differences are identified, contributing factors must be explored, particularly those factors that could be manipulated through intervention practices. Furthermore, because it is obviously better to avoid problems than to wait until problems occur and must be dealt with, it would help to be able to influence the language acquisition environment so that clinically significant differences do not develop. Finally, practitioners provide services in a condition of uncertainty. We do not fully understand the variables and all the relationships between these variables that lead some individuals who use AAC to the development of linguistic competence and others to experience difficulties in the acquisition of language. We make clinical decisions based on best guesses, knowing that some things we do or suggest may eventually be shown to be unnecessary or ineffective. Furthermore, our suggestions and intervention plans must mesh with the other priorities and time demands experienced by children with extremely limited speech, their families, and caregivers.

With these caveats in mind, how then might practitioners help children with extremely limited speech acquire linguistic competence? Intervention should begin early, with infant and preschool programs and parent information aimed at encouraging caregivers to assist their children in exploring the environment to expand their knowledge base. Such exploration could be encouraged both on a small level (e.g., by assisting the child in exploring the properties of objects) and on a broader level (e.g., by increasing the types of experiences the child has opportunities to participate in). Particularly for children with mobility impairments, facilitation of the exploration of the physical environment may be very important in establishing a rich base of world knowledge on which to map language.

Early intervention could also assist parents in providing rich language input to their children that is connected to and builds on their child's current focus of attention and has proportionately more comments and fewer directives. Because children with physical impairments may give more subtle cues about the focus of their attention, it may be appropriate to sensitize caregivers to attend to signs of their child's attention and interest (Cress et al., 2000). Given that daily care activities (e.g., feeding, dressing) take a proportionately large chunk of the child's day, practitioners need to explore with caregivers easily achievable ways that rich language input can be incorporated into these activities.

A major focus for early intervention is to build a relationship of trust and partnership with parents. From within such a relationship, it is possible to raise the concept of introducing AAC at an earlier developmental stage. In our experience, AAC is a difficult concept for parents to understand and accept at first and must be presented with sensitivity and acknowledgment of parents' questions and fears, both spoken and unspoken. It is particularly important to address the question of whether the provision of AAC may impede acquisition of speech. There is a lot of anecdotal evidence and a small number of scientifically defensible studies that support the clinical belief that provision of AAC does not impede—and if anything may slightly enhance—speech development, although perhaps not to a clinically significant extent (Millar, Light, & Schlosser, 2000). Some parents may be persuaded by the professional literature. Others may be more convinced by testimonials from other parents, or by meeting children similar to their child who use AAC. Most parents need time to adjust to the idea that their child will be, at least temporarily, a non-traditional communicator.

No one approach to the concept of early introduction of AAC is persuasive for all parents. One approach is to design an N of 1 trial and to enter into an agreement with parents on decision rules for whether AAC will be continued or discontinued (i.e., We agree that AAC will be discontinued if vocal–verbal communication attempts decrease by 10%). Another approach is to negotiate the proportion of time spent on various goals, including those involving AAC systems. Yet another approach is focusing on only one AAC intervention in one activity, demonstrating the utility and value of AAC in that particular situation, and using that success to advocate for expansion of the AAC system.

The design challenges for earliest symbolic AAC systems are often not fully appreciated. The ideal would be to provide systems that give maximum productive control of linguistic structures but that are compatible with the conceptual, perceptual, and motor skills of the child right now, thus reducing the amount of effort the child must expend to master the operational demands of the system. Great care should be taken to ensure that the early aided systems are, as much as possible, contiguous with later systems. That way, as the child's abilities and needs expand, the system can expand and the child will only need to do the minimum amount of unlearning and relearning. It is desirable, therefore, for the clinician to have a reasonable idea of what the more fully developed AAC system will look like in the future as he or she designs or introduces the first aided system.

If language production attempts are important for acquisition of morphology and syntax, every effort must be made to provide the individual who uses AAC with opportunities for language production. It will be necessary to provide multiple systems to allow individuals who use AAC to communicate more often and in more situations because no one system is usable in every situation. Whenever possible, design consistency between and among systems should be maintained to reduce operational demands and to allow the individual to achieve automaticity in production. Finally, creating opportunities for output involves more than the situation and the AAC system. Communication partners must be trained to increase their pause time and slow down conversational exchanges to allow the individual who uses AAC to participate given their much slower output rate.

The issue of pre-stored phrases and sentences on AAC systems is somewhat problematic. From the standpoint of conversational expediency and success, it makes sense to have some phrases or sentences pre-stored, especially if the individual uses a very slow access technique such as scanning. But from the standpoint of fostering language acquisition, this tactic is probably not optimal because the ability to break down and analyze the components of the pre-stored phrase is not in the control of the individual who uses AAC. The answer may lie in continuing to provide pre-stored phrases or sentences for certain functional situations but also ensuring that the individual has the opportunity and AAC tools to segment and construct the linguistic forms in other situations. Such an approach was taken by Harris, Doyle, and Haaf (1996), who described an intervention program based on a reciprocal reading procedure that was used to teach a young child to segment syntactic constituents. They pointed out that their goal was not to replace the child's single constituent messages in conversation, but rather "to provide options for more sophisticated, versatile linguistic communication in selected situations" (p. 240).

Another focus of intervention at almost all stages would be to teach parents and other communication partners to model AAC use in appropriate contexts. Refer to Chapter 5 for further discussion of the role and importance of augmented input in assisting individuals to decode language and learn how to express language via the AAC system.

Output characteristics common to many people who use AAC, such as telegraphic utterances, omission of obligatory syntactic morphology, and deviations from word order rules, carry a social liability and may also result in less effective communication, especially with less familiar partners. This fact may suggest a need for intervention, although the possible benefits of more grammatically complete and correct output must be carefully weighed against the cost in terms of the longer time it will take to produce that utterance. Many people who use AAC choose to produce telegraphic output in most communication situations, but it is important that people who use AAC can produce grammatically acceptable output when the situation demands it.

If this area is to be targeted in intervention, the first step is to make sure that the AAC system allows for linguistically acceptable output. The second step is to assess whether, for this individual, failure to produce a linguistic form or structure is a result of speed and efficiency issues, an output modality influence with underlying linguistic knowledge, or a failure to have acquired the underlying linguistic knowledge. Modality influences complicate the assessment picture, and alternative ways to probe acquisition of a linguistic form or structure should be adopted. These include using comprehension probes such as a picture selection tasks; asking the people who use AAC to act something out or to follow directions; asking the individual to make grammaticality judgments; or analyzing written output, especially text produced in situations with reduced time pressure.

If assessment probes have revealed underlying difficulties with the linguistic form or structure in question, specific therapy targeting that form or structure may need to be undertaken. This might involve increasing opportunities for production, and/or comprehension experiences that highlight the linguistic element in question, or with older individuals, overtly teaching grammatical rules. Lund and Light (1999) presented two case studies demonstrat-

ing effective intervention with adults who use AAC targeting specific morphosyntactical forms and structures. Their intervention involved explanations of the targeted forms as well as opportunities to make grammaticality
judgments and to correct errors when these were presented; however, if assessment probes reveal that the telegraphic communicator can manipulate the
linguistic form or structure but typically does not, intervention may focus on
helping the user decide when telegraphic and elaborated utterances are appropriate (e.g., in particular contexts, with certain conversation partners), similar to the sociolinguistic notion of switching between dialects or registers of
the same language. People who are skillful at using AAC appear to vary the
form of their utterances depending on the listener. Morningstar (1981) observed that Blissymbol users constructed more elaborated utterances with listeners who had no experience in AAC than with experienced listeners, as if
they were switching between a formal and informal register.

FUTURE RESEARCH

> Bottom line: Users and facilitators told us that . . . The traditional
> emphasis of AAC research, i.e., technique and symbol set selection,
> is important. But, more important is finding new and better ways
> to teach the social use of language–the application of appropriate
> communication and interaction behaviours to key life experi-
> ences. (O'Keefe, Kozak, Fronda, & Durkacz, 2001, reporting on the
> results of focus-group discussions on research priorities in AAC)

In preparing this chapter, we were struck by two observations: First, there are
many fairly important aspects of language input, output, and language knowledge where we found clinical observations and speculations but small amounts
of data. For example, there is speculation on characteristics of the language
input for children with extremely limited speech but very few studies on the
topic. Second, there were questions for which we found no information, not
even clinical observations. When preparing the sections on morphology and
syntax, we wondered about the language instruction experiences of adults
who use AAC and show good mastery of grammatical morphology and syntax. Did these individuals acquire their impressive level of mastery through
the course of natural exposure to language, or did they receive specific instruction? If so, what type of instruction did they receive, when, and how
much? More generally, what intrinsic and/or extrinsic factors differentiate
people who use AAC and do develop a good grasp of language from those
who do not? We could not find the answers to these questions.

Clearly, more research is needed on a host of topics within this area. Observational research is needed to further explore how extremely limited speech and AAC interventions affect the language environment of the child, particularly in the developmental stages where syntactical forms and structures are usually being mastered. Longitudinal research is needed to explore relationships between AAC interventions and language acquisition, such as the impact of output capabilities and experiences on the acquisition of specific language forms and structures. There are many questions yet to be explored about the role of productive experience in the acquisition of language. Questions include, Does productive experience via AAC facilitate acquisition of language of the child's linguistic community? Is productive experience more important for some aspects of language than others (e.g., aspects of language that are not typically critical for successful comprehension)? If productive experience is important, what aspects of production are important? Is it the practice in segmentation and combination of linguistic units? Is it the feedback from voice output? If it is the latter, does partner reauditorization of the message components fulfill the same role as synthetic voice output?

Because of the challenges in interpretation of productive data, complicated as it is by factors including the influence of the output modality, studies employing comprehension measures as dependent variables would seem to be a fruitful avenue to explore the course of language development in the child with extremely limited speech. This research could also add information to the developmental course of language comprehension in typical children, as well as contributing to the development of assessment probes targeting specific features of interest while controlling factors such as motoric demands.

There are also many questions around clinical decisions that beg for further investigation. For example, because vocabulary limitations are a known challenge associated with aided AAC systems and strategies such as using a SOUNDS LIKE symbol or an OPPOSITE OF symbol have been successfully employed by some people who use AAC to circumvent vocabulary limitations, it would be of great interest to explore when and how children with extremely limited speech acquire the metalinguistic skills to use these vocabulary-expanding strategies. The research examining typical children's abilities to learn various AAC systems' vocabulary organization schemas is interesting, but these types of studies also need to be applied to children with extremely limited speech, who may be entering into this task with different profiles of skills and knowledge.

Research regarding language development in children with extremely limited speech and individuals who use AAC has the potential to illuminate questions about typical language acquisition. This research could help clarify the roles of variables that are typically difficult to investigate separately when studying typically developing children—for example, the role of language production in language acquisition; the relationship of language development to language input and general world experience; the potential power of language comprehension experiences in driving language acquisition; and the relationships among language input, language comprehension, and language production. This research could also help practitioners understand the power and the limits of language acquisition processes and the variety of routes that can be used to acquire language competence. For example, most typically developing children master the bulk of the grammar of their language by about age 6 years. If children and adolescents using AAC tend not to demonstrate grammatical mastery until later, this may suggest that competencies not acquired through typical processes during early childhood can in fact be mastered through other cognitive learning strategies. Thus, answers to research questions generated by considering children with extremely limited speech using AAC may make significant contributions to knowledge of the acquisition process for all language learners.

Whether clinically oriented or theoretically driven, research for children with extremely limited speech and individuals who use AAC has the same ultimate goal. Research can show us the most effective and efficient ways to employ the time, effort, and monetary resources of individuals who use AAC, their families, and intervenors in order to insure that each and every individual with extremely limited speech achieves the highest possible potential in the important area of language acquisition. And that, after all, is the point.

> If just these thoughts could become words
> Words flowing as a stream out of my mouth
> Waves of big words that would fill the room
> Would fill the streets and squares
> Could be heard upstairs and downstairs
> Outside and inside
> (Dalhoff, 2000)

REFERENCES

Bates, E. (1993). Comprehension and production in early language development. *Monographs of the Society for Research in Child Development, 58* (Serial No. 233), 222–242.

Berninger, V., & Gans, B. (1986). Language profiles in nonspeaking individuals of normal intelligence with severe cerebral palsy. *Augmentative and Alternative Communication, 2,* 45–50.

Beukelman, D.R., & Mirenda, P. (1998). *Augmentative and alternative communication: Management of severe communication disorders in children and adults* (2nd ed.). Baltimore: Paul H. Brookes Publishing Co.

Bishop, D., Brown, B., & Robson, J. (1990). The relationship between phoneme discrimination, speech production and language comprehension in cerebral-palsied individuals. *Journal of Speech and Hearing Disorders, 52,* 156–173.

Blockberger, S. (1995). AAC intervention and early conceptual and lexical development. *Journal of Speech-Language Pathology and Audiology, 19,* 221–232.

Blockberger, S., & Johnston, J. (in press). Grammatical morphology acquisition by children with extremely limited speech. *Augmentative and Alternative Communication.*

Bloom, L. (1994). Meaning and expression. In W.F. Overton & D. Palermo (Eds.), *The nature and ontogenesis of meaning* (pp. 215–235). Mahwah, NJ: Lawrence Erlbaum Associates.

Bowerman, M. (1987). Commentary: Mechanisms of language acquisition. In B. MacWhinney (Ed.), *Mechanisms of language acquisition* (pp. 443–466). Mahwah, NJ: Lawrence Erlbaum Associates.

Calculator, S. (1997). Fostering early language acquisition and AAC use: Exploring reciprocal influences between children and their environments. *Augmentative and Alternative Communication, 13,* 149–157.

Calculator, S., & Dollaghan, C. (1982). The use of communication boards in a residential setting: An evaluation. *Journal of Speech and Hearing Disorders, 47,* 281–287.

Carrow-Woolfolk, E. (1985). *Test of Auditory Comprehension for Language–Revised (TACL–R).* Allen, TX: DLM Teaching Resources.

Cazden, C. (1988). *Classroom discourse.* Portsmouth, NH: Heinemann.

Clark, E. (1982). Language change during language acquisition. In M. Lamb & A. Brown (Eds.), *Advances in child development* (pp. 173–197). Mahwah, NJ: Lawrence Erlbaum Associates.

Clark, E. (1995). Language acquisition: The lexicon and syntax. In J. Miller & P. Eimas (Eds.), *Speech, language and communication: Handbook of perception and cognition* (2nd ed., Vol. 11, pp. 303–337). San Diego: Academic Press.

Collins, S. (1996). Referring expressions in conversations between aided and natural speakers. In S. von Tetzchner & M. Jensen, (Eds.), *Augmentative and alternative communication: European perspectives* (pp. 89–100). San Diego: Whurr Publishers.

Cress, C., Linke, M., Moskal, L., Benal, A., Anderson, V., & LaMontagne, J. (2000, November). *Play and parent interaction in young children with physical impairments.* Paper presented at the conference of the American Speech-Language-Hearing Association, Washington, DC.

Dalhoff, F. (2000). The cry. In M. Williams & C. Krezman (Eds.), *Beneath the surface: Creative expressions of augmented communicators* (p. 83). Toronto: International Society for Augmentative and Alternative Communication (ISAAC) Press.

Dunn, L.M. & Dunn, L.M. (1981). *Peabody Picture Vocabulary Test–Revised.* Circle Pines, MN: American Guidance Service.

Dunn, L.M. & Dunn, L.M. (1997). *Peabody Picture Vocabulary Test–III.* Circle Pines, MN: American Guidance Service.

Elman, J. (1993). Learning and development in neural networks: The importance of starting small. *Cognition, 48,* 71–99.

Estrella, G. (2000). Confessions of a blabber finger. In M. Fried-Oken & H.A. Bersani, Jr., (Eds.), *Speaking up and spelling it out: Personal essays on augmentative and alternative communication* (pp. 31–45). Baltimore: Paul H. Brookes Publishing Co.

Franklin, K., Mirenda, P., & Phillips, G. (1996). Comparisons of five symbol assessment protocols with nondisabled preschoolers and learners with severe intellectual disabilities. *Augmentative and Alternative Communication, 12,* 63–77.

Friedman, S., & Stevenson, M. (1980). Perception of movement in pictures. In M. Hagen (Ed.), *Alberti's window: The projective model of pictorial information* (pp. 225–255). San Diego: Academic Press.

Fried-Oken, M., & Bersani, H.A., Jr. (2000). *Speaking up and spelling it out: Personal essays on augmentative and alternative communication*. Baltimore: Paul H. Brookes Publishing Co.

Fried-Oken, M., & More, L. (1992). An initial vocabulary for nonspeaking preschool children based on developmental and environmental language sources. *Augmentative and Alternative Communication, 8*, 41–56.

Gerber, S., & Kraat, A. (1992). Use of a developmental model of language acquisition: Applications to children using AAC systems. *Augmentative and Alternative Communication, 8*, 19–32.

Girolametto, L., Weitzman, E., Wiigs, M., & Pearce, P. (1999). The relationship between maternal language measures and language development in toddlers with expressive vocabulary delays. *American Journal of Speech-Language Pathology, 8*, 364–374.

Golinkoff, R., & Hirsh-Pasek, K. (1995). Reinterpreting children's sentence comprehension: Toward a new framework. In P. Fletcher & B. MacWhinney (Eds.), *The handbook of child language* (pp. 430–461). Malden, MA: Blackwell Publishers.

Gopnik, A., & Meltzoff, A.N. (1986). Words, plans, things and locations: Interactions between semantic and cognitive development in the one-word stage. In S. Kuczaj & M. Barrett (Eds.), *The development of word meaning* (pp. 199–223). New York: Springer-Verlag.

Gross, D., Soken, N., Rosengren, K., Pick, A., Pillow, B., & Melendez, P. (1991). Children's understanding of action lines and the static representation of speed of locomotion. *Child Development, 62*, 1124–1141.

Hanzlik, J. (1990). Nonverbal interaction patterns of mothers and their infants with cerebral palsy. *Education and Training in Mental Retardation, 25*, 333–343.

Harris, D. (1982). Communicative interaction processes involving nonvocal physically handicapped children. *Topics in Language Disorders, 2*, 21–37.

Harris, L., Doyle, E., & Haaf, R. (1996). Language treatment approach for users of AAC: Experimental single-subject investigation. *Augmentative and Alternative Communication, 12*, 230–243.

Hart, B., & Risley, T.R. (1995). *Meaningful differences in the everyday experience of young American children*. Baltimore: Paul H. Brookes Publishing Co.

Hoag, L., Bedrosian, J., Johnson, D., & Molineux, B. (1994). Variables affecting perceptions of social aspects of the communicative competence of an adult AAC user. *Augmentative and Alternative Communication, 10*, 129–137.

Hohn, R. (1997). *More than a watchmaker*. Vista, CA: Author.

Houghton, J., Bronicki, G., & Guess, D. (1987). Opportunities to express preferences and make choices among students with severe disabilities in classroom settings. *Journal of The Association for Persons with Severe Handicaps, 12*, 18–27.

Hunt-Berg, M. (1998, August). *Children's use of pointing cues in aided language intervention*. Paper presented at the Eighth Biennial Conference of the International Society for Augmentative and Alternative Communication (ISAAC), Dublin, Ireland.

Johnston, S., & Redmond, S. (1999, November). *Grammaticality judgments of children with severe speech and physical impairments*. Poster session presented at the annual meeting of the American Speech-Language-Hearing Association (ASHA), Seattle.

Kaiser, A., Hemmeter, L., & Hester, P. (1997). The facilitative effects of input on children's language development: Contributions from studies of enhanced milieu teaching. In L. Adamson & M.A. Romski (Eds.), *Communication and language acquisition: Discoveries from atypical development*. Baltimore: Paul H. Brookes Publishing Co.

Karmiloff-Smith, A. (1992). *Beyond modularity: A developmental perspective on cognitive science*. London: MIT Press.

Kelford Smith, A., Thurston, S., Light, J., Parnes, P., & O'Keefe, B. (1989). The form and use of written communication produced by physically disabled individuals using microcomputers. *Augmentative and Alternative Communication, 5*, 115–124.

Kraat, A. (1985). *Communication interaction between aided and natural speakers: A state of the art report.* Toronto: Canadian Rehabilitation Council for the Disabled.

Kraat, A. (1991). Methodological issues in the study of language development among children using aided language: Reactant paper 1. In J. Bordin & E. Björck-Åkesson (Eds.), *Methodological issues in research in augmentative and alternative communication* (pp. 118–123). Vällingby: The Swedish Handicap Institute.

Kuczaj, S. (1983). *Crib speech and language play.* New York: Springer-Verlag.

Light, J. (1989). Toward a definition of communicative competence for individuals using augmentative and alternative communication systems. *Augmentative and Alternative Communication, 5,* 137–144.

Light, J. (1997). "Let's go star fishing": Reflections on the contexts of language learning for children who use aided AAC. *Augmentative and Alternative Communication, 15,* 13–24.

Light, J., Collier, B., & Parnes, P. (1985a). Communicative interaction between young nonspeaking physically disabled children and their primary caregivers: Part 1– Discourse patterns. *Augmentative and Alternative Communication, 1,* 74–83.

Light, J., Collier, B., & Parnes, P. (1985b). Communicative interaction between young nonspeaking physically disabled children and their primary caregivers: Part II– Communicative function. *Augmentative and Alternative Communication, 1,* 98–107.

Light, J., & Drager, K. (August, 2000). *Improving the design of AAC technologies for young children.* Paper presented at the Ninth Biennial Conference of the International Society for Augmentative and Alternative Communication (ISAAC), Washington, DC.

Light, J., Drager, K., Curran, J., Fallon, K., & Zuskin, L. (2000, August). *Performance of typically developing 2-year-olds on AAC technologies.* Poster presented at the Tenth Biennial Conference of the International Society for Augmentative and Alternative Communication, Washington, DC.

Light, J., Drager, K., McCarthy, J., Mellott, S., Rhoads, S., & Ward, M. (2000, August). *Performance of typically developing 5-year-olds on AAC technologies.* Poster presented at the Tenth Biennial Conference of the International Society for Augmentative and Alternative Communication, Washington, DC.

Light, J., Drager, K., Millar, D., Parsons, A., & Parrish, C. (2000, August). *Performance of typically developing 4-year-olds on AAC technologies.* Poster presented at the Tenth Biennial Conference of the International Society for Augmentative and Alternative Communication, Washington, DC.

Light, J., Drager, K., Pitkin, L., Larsson, B., & Stopper, G., (2000, August). *Performance of typically developing 3-year-olds on AAC technologies.* Poster presented at the Tenth Biennial Conference of the International Society for Augmentative and Alternative Communication, Washington, DC.

Light, J., & Kelford Smith, A. (1993). Home literacy experiences of preschoolers who use AAC systems and of their nondisabled peers. *Augmentative and Alternative Communication, 9,* 10–25.

Light, J., Lindsay, P., Parnes, P., & Siegel, L. (1990). The effects of message encoding techniques on recall by literate adults using AAC systems. *Augmentative and Alternative Communication, 6,* 184–201.

Locke, J. (1997). A theory of neurolinguistic development. *Brain and Language, 58,* 265–326.

Lund, S., & Light, J. (1999). *The effectiveness of grammar instruction for individuals who use AAC.* Paper presented at the annual meeting of the American Speech-Language-Hearing Association (ASHA), Seattle.

Lund, S., Millar, D., Herman, M., Hinds, A., & Light, J. (1998, November). *Children's representations of early emerging concepts: Implications for AAC.* Poster presented at the Annual Conference of the American Speech-Language-Hearing Association, San Antonio, TX.

Manolson, H. (1985). *It takes two to talk: A Hanen early language parent guidebook*. Available from Hanen Early Language Resource Centre, 4–126, 252 Bloor Street West, Toronto, Ontario, Canada.

Marcus, G., Pinker, S., Ullman, M., Hollander, M., Rosen, J., & Xu, F. (1992). Overregularization in language acquisition. *Monographs of the Society for Research in Child Development, 57* (Serial No. 228).

Mehrabian, A. (1970). Measures of vocabulary and grammatical skills for children up to age six. *Developmental Psychology, 2*(3), 439–446.

Millar, D., Light, J., & Schlosser, R. (2000). *The impact of AAC on natural speech development: A meta-analysis*. Paper presented at the Ninth Biennial Conference of the International Society for Augmentative and Alternative Communication (ISAAC), Washington, DC.

Mineo Mollica, B., Peischl, D., & Pennington, C. (1998). *Animation: Does it add to the representation of action words?* Paper presented at the Eighth Biennial Conference of the International Society for Augmentative and Alternative Communication (ISAAC), Washington, DC.

Morningstar, D. (1981). *Blissymbol communication: Comparison of interaction with naive versus experienced listeners*. Unpublished manuscript, University of Toronto.

Nakamura, K., Newell, A.F., Alm, N., & Waller, A.C. (1998). How do members of different language communities compose sentences with a picture-based communication system?: A cross-cultural study of picture-based sentences constructed by English and Japanese speakers. *Augmentative and Alternative Communication, 14,* 71–80.

Nelson, N. (1992). Performance is the prize: Language competence and performance among AAC users. *Augmentative and Alternative Communication, 8,* 3–18.

Newport, E. (1990). Maturational constraints on language learning. *Cognitive Science, 14,* 11–28.

Ochs, E., & Schieffelin, B. (1995). The impact of language socialization on grammatical development. In P. Fletcher & B. MacWhinney (Eds.), *The handbook of child language* (pp. 73–94). Malden, MA: Blackwell Publishers.

O'Keefe, B., Kozak, N., Fronda, S., & Durkacz, A. (2001, August). *Consumer research priorities in augmentative and alternative communication: Phase two*. Paper given at the Canadian Association of Speech-Language Pathologists and Audiologists meeting, Montreal.

Paul, R. (1997). Facilitating transition in language development for children using AAC. *Augmentative and Alternative Communication, 13,* 141–148.

Romski, M.A., & Sevcik, R. (1989). An analysis of visual-graphic symbol meanings for two nonspeaking adults with severe mental retardation. *Augmentative and Alternative Communication, 5,* 109–114.

Romski, M.A., & Sevcik, R.A. (1996). *Breaking the speech barrier: Language development through augmented means*. Baltimore: Paul H. Brookes Publishing Co.

Romski, M.A., Sevcik, R., & Adamson, L. (1997). Framework for studying how children with developmental disabilities develop language through augmented means. *Augmentative and Alternative Communication, 13,* 172–178.

Romski, M.A., Sevcik, R., Robinson, B., Mervis, C., & Bertrand, J. (1995). Mapping the meanings of novel visual symbols by youth with moderate or severe mental retardation. *American Journal on Mental Retardation, 100,* 391–402.

Smith, M. (1990). Reading achievement in nonspeaking children: A comparative study [Abstract]. *Augmentative and Alternative Communication, 6,* 132.

Smith, M. (1996). The medium or the message: A study of speaking children using communication boards. In S. von Tetzchner & M.H. Jensen (Eds.), *Augmentative and alternative communication: European perspectives* (pp. 119–136). San Diego: Whurr Publishers.

Snow, C. (1984). Parent–child interaction and the development of communicative ability. In R. Schiefelbusch & J. Pickar (Eds.), *The acquisition of communicative competence* (pp. 71–107). Baltimore: University Park Press.

Snow, C., Perlmann, R., & Nathan, D. (1987). Why routines are different: Toward a multiple-factors model of the relation between input and language acquisition. In K. Nelson (Ed.), *Children's language* (Vol. 6, pp. 65–97). Mahwah, NJ: Lawrence Erlbaum Associates.

Soto, G. (1997). Multi-unit utterances and syntax in graphic symbol communication. In E. Björck-Åkesson & P. Lindsay (Eds.), *Communication . . . naturally: Theoretical and methodological issues in augmentative and alternative communication* (pp. 26–32). Västerås, Sweden: Mälardalen University Press.

Soto, G. (1999). Understanding the impact of graphic sign use on the message structure. In F. Loncke, J. Clibbens, H. Arvidson, & L. Lloyd (Eds.), *Augmentative and alternative communication: New directions in research and practice*. San Diego: Whurr Publishers.

Staehely, J. (2000). Prologue: The communication dance. In M. Fried-Oken & H.A. Bersani (Eds.), *Speaking up and spelling it out: Personal essays on augmentative and alternative communication* (pp. 1–12). Baltimore: Paul H. Brookes Publishing Co.

Sutton, A. (1999). Language learning experiences and grammatical acquisition. In F. Loncke, J. Clibbens, H. Arvidson, & L. Lloyd (Eds.), *Augmentative and alternative communication: New directions in research and practice* (pp. 49–61). San Diego: Whurr Publishers.

Sutton, A., & Dench, C. (1998). Connected speech development in a child with limited language production experience. *Journal of Speech-Language Pathology and Audiology, 22,* 133–140.

Sutton, A., & Gallagher, T. (1993). Verb class distinctions and AAC language-encoding limitations. *Journal of Speech and Hearing Research, 36,* 1216–1226.

Sutton, A., & Gallagher, T. (1995). Comprehension assessment of a child using an AAC system. *American Journal of Speech-Language Pathology, 4*(3), 60–68.

Sutton, A., Gallagher, T., Morford, J., & Shahnaz, N. (2000). Constituent order patterns and syntactic distinctions in relative clause sentences produced using AAC systems. *Applied Psycholinguistics, 21,* 473–486.

Sutton, A., & Morford, J. (1998). Constituent order in picture pointing sequences produced by speaking children using AAC. *Applied Psycholinguistics, 19,* 526–536.

Tomasello, M. (1995). Pragmatic contexts for early verb learning. In M. Tomasello & W. Merriman (Eds.), *Beyond names for things: Young children's acquisition of verbs* (pp. 115–146). Mahwah, NJ: Lawrence Erlbaum Associates.

Udwin, O., & Yule, W. (1990). Augmentative communication systems taught to cerebral palsied children—a longitudinal study: I. The acquisition of signs and symbols, and syntactic aspects of their use over time. *British Journal of Disorders of Communication, 25,* 195–309.

von Tetzchner, S. (2000). *Introduction to augmentative and alternative communication* (2nd ed.). San Diego: Whurr Publishers.

von Tetzchner, S., & Jensen, M. (1996). Introduction. In S. von Tetzchner & M. Jensen (Eds), *Augmentative and alternative communication: European perspectives* (pp. 1–18). San Diego: Whurr Publishers.

von Tetzchner, S., & Martinsen, J. (1996). Words and strategies: Conversations with young children who use aided language. In S. von Tetzchner & M. Jensen (Eds.), *Augmentative and alternative communication: European perspectives* (pp. 65–88). San Diego: Whurr Publishers.

Warren, F. (1999). *The power of language.* Paper presented at the annual conference of the American Speech-Language-Hearing Association (ASHA), Seattle.

Wilkinson, K., & Albert, A. (2001). Adaptations of fast mapping for vocabulary intervention with augmented language users. *Augmentative and Alternative Communication, 17,* 120–132.

Wilkinson, K., & Green, G. (1998). Implications of fast mapping for vocabulary expansion in individuals with mental retardation. *Augmentative and Alternative Communication, 14,* 162–170.

Williams, M. (1996, August). *The myth of the machine, or how do you give a speech when you've hardly said a word all your life.* Words+ lecture presented at the Seventh Biennial Conference of the International Society for Augmentative and Alternative Communication, Vancouver, Canada.

Williams, M., & Krezman, C. (2000). *Beneath the surface: Creative expressions of augmented communicators.* Toronto: International Society for Augmentative and Alternative Communication.

Yoder, P.J., Warren, S.F., McCathren, R., & Leew, S.V. (1998). Does adult responsivity to child behavior facilitate communication development? In S.F. Warren & J. Reichle (Series Eds.) & A.M. Wetherby, S.F. Warren, & J. Reichle (Vol. Eds.), *Communication and language intervention series: Vol. 7. Transitions in prelinguistic communication* (pp. 39–58). Baltimore: Paul H. Brookes Publishing Co.

4

Representational Competence

Beth Mineo Mollica

For many individuals, speech and orthography simply are not viable currencies for communicative exchange. Very young children, those with developmentally based cognitive disabilities (e.g., mental retardation, autism), those with limited literacy, and those with cognitive impairments resulting from acquired brain injury often are dependent on picture-based representations to convey their communicative intentions.

Pictures may also be important as cognitive scaffolds, providing prompts, cues, or instructions (e.g., picture-based recipes, daily activity schedules) for individuals with cognitive disabilities who can speak (Lignugaris/Kraft, McCuller, Exum, & Salzberg, 1988; Stephenson & Linfoot, 1996). Given the widespread utilization of pictures, it is critical to understand the benefits and challenges associated with picture-based communication in order to maximize the communicative competence of those who rely on pictures as a means for understanding and expressing language.

This chapter focuses on the *language representation* component of AAC systems, which does not refer to the items or notions selected for inclusion in a communication system but rather to the form in which those selections are presented to the user. The visual mode is the most typical for alternate language representations used by augmented communicators, in which language units are accessed via two-dimensional forms such as photographs, pictures, or written words. But language representations can also take the form of gestures, signs, or items that are distinguished from one another on the basis of touch. Although this chapter addresses several language representation issues that are mode-independent, its focus is on the representation of language in the visual domain, with a primary emphasis on pictures.

Research for this chapter was supported in part by Grant No. H133G990115 from the National Institute on Disability and Rehabilitation Research, U.S. Department of Education. The author appreciates the contributions of Jennifer Wandras, research assistant, and thanks Janice C. Light, David R. Beukelman, and Joe Reichle for their insights and encouragement.

The pervasiveness of pictures in our culture—billboards, television, movies, books, consumer product packaging—may lead to the assumption that pictures are the least common denominator when it comes to information transfer. Pictures are regarded as universal, language-independent, and remarkably similar to the realities that they serve to represent (Beilin, 1983). The implications of this assumption lead to the conclusion that pictures are inherently simple and that symbol comprehension can be taken for granted (DeLoache, Miller, & Rosengren, 1997; Rowland & Schweigert, 2000). As this chapter demonstrates, the use of pictures in cognitive and communicative contexts evolves to the point of being automatic in adults, yet the developmental process that results in such automatic recognition is remarkably complex and vulnerable to disruption from myriad factors.

The AAC field lacks definitive guidance about how to maximize language learning and use through pictures. The absence of a comprehensive and systematic examination of picture-based language representation in the AAC literature or elsewhere precludes the emergence of evidence-based justifications for selection of particular types of representations in particular circumstances. Although there are numerous studies examining aspects of picture-based language representation and others that reveal interesting picture-related phenomena as unintended byproducts, it is difficult to link them in any cohesive manner owing to vast differences in theoretical perspectives motivating the research, subject characteristics, and experimental variables (Levie, 1987). Different terminology is often used to refer to the same phenomenon across disciplines, such as cognitive and developmental psychology, applied behavior analysis, and AAC, which further complicates the assimilation of knowledge into a comprehensive account of picture-based language representation (Wilkinson, Dube, & McIlvane, 1998).

This chapter draws on numerous perspectives in its examination of language representation issues in AAC. It examines many of the factors that affect an individual's ability to use picture-based language representations as a means for demonstrating linguistic competence. It will provide evidence that picture-based language performance is influenced by characteristics of the communicator, characteristics of the representational media, and characteristics of the language task itself. With enhanced understanding of how these factors interact, the reader will recognize how linguistic competence can be maximized through representational competence and how linguistic performance can be impeded through the imposition of representational constraints.

SYMBOLIC BEHAVIOR IS THE GOAL

DeLoache (1995) defined a *symbol* as some entity that someone intends to stand for something other than itself. Any two-dimensional representation can serve in a symbolic capacity, although other things—such as objects, miniature objects, and pieces of objects—can serve as symbols if they are intended to stand for something other than themselves. Bates described *symbolic behavior* as

> The comprehension or use, inside or outside communicative situations, of a relationship between a sign and its referent such that the sign is treated as belonging to and/or substitutable for its referent in a variety of contexts: at the same time the user is aware that the sign is separable from its referent, that is, not the same thing. (1979, p. 43)

As beauty is in the eye of the beholder, so is representational power in the eye (and mind) of the potential symbol user. Symbolic behavior is not an all-or-nothing proposition; it develops in accord with an individual's cognitive and linguistic abilities.

DeLoache and her colleagues, who have studied representational behavior among typically developing youngsters for many years, have identified some benchmarks associated with the developmental process that eventually culminates in the acquisition of flexible symbolic behavior. The first of these is the achievement of *representational insight,* which is the recognition of some type of relationship between a symbol and its referent, albeit not necessarily a symbolic one (Uttal, Schreiber, & DeLoache, 1995). Achievement of representational insight can be facilitated by perceptual similarity between the symbol and the referent, by previous experience with other symbolic relationships, and by instruction regarding the relationship between the symbol and the referent (DeLoache, DeMendoza, & Anderson, 1999; Gross et al., 1991; Uttal et al., 1995). Achievement of representational insight is stimulus and situation specific and may be influenced by a single factor or an interaction among factors (DeLoache, 2000; DeLoache et al., 1999).

Although achievement of representational insight heralds the recognition of some relationship between symbol and referent, it is not of sufficient strength and stability to warrant designation as *dual representation,* which marks an individual's transition into true symbolic behavior. Dual representation is achieved when an individual becomes capable of seeing a picture as an object unto itself at the same time that it also stands for a referent (DeLoache, 1991, 1995, 2000). Sigel (1978) characterized this as the "dual reality" of pictures, in that they can have concrete characteristics and abstract functions simultaneously and can function as surrogates for their referents (Levie, 1987). This is an interesting phenomenon, for, in its fullest instantiation, the referent and the representation share meanings but do not allow for the same behaviors (Sidman, 1994; Sigel, 1978). A child may know that a candy bar is delicious, but he also knows that the photo of the candy bar shares none of the real item's delectable qualities. Liben (1999) referred to this distinction as *attribute differentiation.* Some individuals have considerable difficulty achieving dual representation, particularly when the symbol is an interesting or appealing object in its own right.

One final concept of importance in establishing the context for the remainder of this chapter is *symbolic sensitivity*. Another term coined by DeLoache and her colleagues, symbolic sensitivity refers to the individual's general readiness to look for a symbolic relationship between entities (DeLoache et al., 1999). Such readiness emerges when individuals have had sufficient exposure to symbolic relationships that they begin to recognize other symbolic opportunities in their environment (DeLoache, 1995). For example, children who have learned to point to the picture of a milk carton to request a drink may take advantage of other food-related pictures to expand their requesting repertoire at mealtime.

Multiple Factors Influence Representational Ability

The central premise of this chapter is that factors from multiple domains—individual, representational, and linguistic—and the interactions among them influence the extent to which an individual is able to use picture-based representations of language. These factors are either intrinsic or extrinsic to the individual (Romski, Sevcik, & Adamson, 1997). Intrinsic factors are those related to the biological or behavioral profiles of the individual and may include such elements as age, sensory abilities, cognitive skills, communication and language abilities, neurological and neuromotor status, and motivation. Extrinsic factors would include characteristics of the environment (e.g., partners, environments, nature of AAC method and/or tool), instructional methods, characteristics and arrangement of the language representations, and characteristics of the language task. Table 4.1 presents a variety of intrinsic and extrinsic factors that influence picture-based language representation abilities; items in italics are elaborated in this chapter. Our discussion begins with an examination of a critical factor with both intrinsic and extrinsic implications—the nature of the language task itself.

Table 4.1. Intrinsic and extrinsic factors influencing representational competence

Intrinsic factors	Extrinsic factors
Motivation	*Characteristics of language task*
Neurological status	*Characteristics of language representations*
Age	*Array characteristics*
Sensory abilities	*Instructional methods*
Cognitive skills	Environmental characteristics
Communication/ language abilities	
World experience	

EXTRINSIC FACTORS

Linguistic Task Complexity

Despite the salience and transparency of pictures for adults with intact linguistic abilities, picture-based language representation actually belongs on a continuum of complexity. Although most people probably do not remember when they learned to understand pictures, there is no question that pictorial comprehension is an acquired skill (DeLoache et al., 1999; Sigel, 1978).

Developmental Continuum   There is a widespread belief that picture-based operations are second nature to children. Using ingenious methods based on infants' preferential looking patterns, researchers in the 1970s and 1980s demonstrated that infants in the first half-year of life could make connections between people and real objects and their two-dimensional counterparts (Barrera & Maurer, 1981; DeLoache, Strauss, & Maynard, 1979; Rose, 1977; Slater, Rose, & Morison, 1984). These findings led the research community to conclude that babies were capable of equating pictures with their real-life counterparts, suggesting an inherent simplicity in pictures that distinguished them from more complex linguistic stimuli such as spoken and written words. An alternative interpretation, however, is that the babies were not demonstrating sophisticated picture understanding; rather, their recognition of perceptual similarities was mistaken for comprehension (DeLoache & Burns, 1994; Mineo, 1990; Mineo Mollica, 1997; Sigel, 1978).

Although the mere recognition of perceptual similarities among stimuli should not be mistaken for conceptual knowledge, the language development literature suggests that children in the first 6 months of life often exploit perceptual similarity to try to make sense of the world around them (Blockberger, 1995; Stephenson & Linfoot, 1996). They begin to cluster the objects and actions they encounter according to perceptual similarities, yielding the rudiments of early lexical categories (Behl-Chadha, 1996; Bulthoff, Edelman, & Tarr, 1995; Mervis, 1987; Tversky & Hemenway, 1984). For example, through observation and exploration, children encounter spherical objects that can be propelled rapidly across a surface. They begin to anticipate that spherical objects will behave in a characteristic manner. These *image schemas* are then mapped onto words (in this case, "ball") that children observe others uttering when the particular objects or events are present (Golinkoff, Hirsh-Pasek, Mervis, Frawley, & Parillo, 1995; Johnson, 1987).

Language researchers have accumulated considerable evidence that children are active language learners, using their perceptual knowledge and their rudimentary linguistic knowledge to organize new words they encounter. For example, if children hear their mother utter an unknown word in the presence of a never-before-seen object, they assume that the new word refers to the new object (Golinkoff, Mervis, & Hirsh-Pasek, 1994). If, however, the unknown word is spoken in the presence of an object for which children already have a word, they assume that the new word refers to an attribute or a component of the object, or to the action in which the object is involved, because at this early point in lexical development children operate under the assumption that referents cannot have more than one name (Au & Glusman, 1990; Golinkoff, Jacquet, Hirsh-Pasek, & Nandakumar, 1996; Markman, 1989). The rules governing the quick uptake of new words, referred to as *fast mapping,* become increasingly sophisticated as children's experience and linguistic capabilities broaden (Wilkinson, Dube, & McIlvane 1996, 1998; Wilkinson & Tager-Flusberg, 1998).

Clearly, young children will have maximum advantage for language learning if they have 1) an intact perceptual system allowing observation of similarities in form and function among the many objects and actions encountered, 2) a rich environment offering a never-ending supply of stimuli to experience, and 3) people in the environment who engage their attention and who supply labels for the objects and events they witness. As children's symbolic sophistication grows, they become less and less reliant on perceptual characteristics and surface similarity to make associations among items and to assign new stimuli to lexical categories (DeLoache, Kolstad, & Anderson, 1991). Rather, they rely on relational reasoning to refine both their conceptual knowledge and their lexicons (Gentner, 1988).

Children (and adults) who demonstrate some understanding of language appear to have an advantage in language learning and use—even in other language modes—over those who do not demonstrate such comprehension. I witnessed a remarkable example of intentions mapping to one language form and then another in my older daughter, Lauren. I introduced a small set of signs, selected for their social-regulatory power, to Lauren when she was only 6 months old. The signs for MORE and FINISHED were initially implemented exclusively at mealtime, a situation in which I tended to use their spoken counterparts frequently. I first modeled the signs, pairing the movements with the spoken word, as I narrated the relevant junctures in the meal event. I then began to physically guide her through the production of the signs, although I was able to fade this level of guidance rapidly as she began using the signs independently and appropriately within the week. I have no doubt that her rapid learning was due to the fact that she already had the desire to express these intentions (as a way of controlling my behavior!), and I simply had given her the means to express those intentions. As her articulatory mechanics became more refined, she began pairing spoken approximations of "more" and "finished" with the signs at about 8 months of age. As she became more reliant on speech, the signs underwent a transformation, reducing in salience gradually until they were no more than brief flickers of finger movement. By the time she was 1 year old, the hand movements were eliminated from her productions altogether.

In a much more controlled undertaking, Goodwyn, Acredolo, and Brown (2000) taught 11-month-olds to use symbolic gestures. They reported that the receptive and expressive language scores among the children who participated in the intervention group far exceeded those of a control group. Goodwyn and her colleagues attributed the children's success to the fact that the gestures provided them with a linguistic scaffold, enabling them to learn about the symbolic function and about the objects, events, and conditions in the world around them without waiting until speech afforded them this ability:

> Misconceptions are corrected, concepts are honed, and everything is set for the verbal equivalent to slip right in as a label when it does become available. Without symbolic gestures, much of this conceptual work would be delayed, thus slowing down the whole language learning enterprise. (p. 110)

This notion of linguistic scaffolding applies equally well to picture-based language representation. When young children with disabilities are precluded from using speech as their primary means of communication, they should be given an alternative means of exploring and expressing language. Pictures can provide children with opportunities to map their real-world knowledge onto a representational form that—unlike speech—they can manage and master. Yet, as many researchers and clinicians know, the extent to which children will be able to use pictures in this way will depend on their linguistic foundation. Children (and older individuals) who evidence at least some comprehension of spoken language tend to be more successful with a picture-based language system than individuals who have little or no documented language comprehension skills (Carr, Wilkinson, Blackman, & McIlvane, 2000; Franklin, Mirenda, & Phillips, 1996; Romski & Sevcik, 1992, 1993a; Rowland & Schweigert, 2000; Sevcik & Romski, 1986, 1997). Comprehension of spoken language is evidence that individuals have achieved symbolic functioning, which in turn enables them to recast existing conceptual and linguistic understanding onto new language forms, namely pictures (Sevcik, Romski, & Wilkinson, 1991).

This is not to suggest that the introduction of picture-based representations should wait until an individual has demonstrated language comprehension. To the contrary, picture-based language representations can be a very effective means by which to demonstrate the power and teach the functions of language. In doing so, however, one must keep in mind the perils of "input/output asymmetry," in which the modality of instruction (speech) is different from the modality of the targeted language behaviors (picture selection) (Smith & Grove, 1996; see also Chapter 6). As a consequence, learners are provided with no direct model to emulate. The alternative approach, referred to as augmented input or aided language stimulation, is to provide learners with multimodal input, speaking the referent word while simultaneously indicating the associated representation on a communication display (Goossens', 1989; Hunt-Berg, 1996; Light, 1997; Romski & Sevcik, 1996).

Learners whose symbolic capabilities are relatively unsophisticated are likely to rely on perceptual similarity to link a referent with a representation. As linguistic sophistication increases, individuals become better equipped to accommodate the perceptual shortcuts that many types of picture-based representations demand (e.g., seeing something colorful represented in shades of gray, seeing a three-dimensional object in two dimensions, seeing something large occupying a 1-inch square space). These and other challenges posed by aspects of the representations themselves are explored in greater detail later in the chapter.

Linguistic Task Complexity Continuum   Picture-related tasks fall along a continuum of complexity, with some operations requiring essentially no linguistic ability and others requiring much more flexible receptive and expressive skill (Mineo, 1990). The research literature rarely acknowledges the full spectrum of possible picture–referent relations, resulting in speculation about the place of discrete picture-based operations along the complexity continuum (DeLoache & Burns, 1994). My early attempts to define a linguistic task complexity continuum differentiated among recognition, comprehension, and use tasks (Mineo, 1990). *Recognition tasks* were ones requiring only that individuals recognize the similarity between two stimuli (e.g., match a photograph of a dog to a line drawing of that dog). Further along the continuum were *comprehension tasks*, which required individuals to understand (in a conceptual or linguistic sense) a picture-based representation (e.g., associate the notion of "dog" or the receptive label "dog" with the photograph of the dog). *Use tasks* were ones in which information was extracted from a picture to direct action (e.g., place a toy dog on a block in imitation of a picture) or using a picture as a means of expression (e.g., select the picture for "dog" to indicate a choice among various stuffed animals).

The continuum described in Table 4.2 offers further refinement of the original tripartite segmentation. The recognition tasks on the linguistic task complexity continuum require no linguistic ability for successful completion. The least complex of the recognition tasks are ones that can be mastered based on the recognition of perceptual similarity alone, often referred to as identity matching tasks. In identity matching, individuals are required to match a sample to an identical counterpart, often selecting that counterpart from an array of several choices. An identity task—matching an object to an identical object, or a color photograph to an identical color photograph—relies on feature equivalence and is not in and of itself representational (Ittelson, 1996; McIlvane, Dube, Green, & Serna, 1992). Recognition does not imply or require understanding (Sigel, 1978).

Table 4.2. Tasks on the linguistic task complexity continuum

Nature of task	Specific task	Task description
Recognition—associating representation with referent on basis of perceptual similarity	Perceptual identity match	Match of identical stimuli (e.g., matching two identical photographs of a dog)
	Delayed perceptual identity match	Match of identical stimuli with time delay imposed between presentation of sample and presentation of match choices
	Perceptual nonidentity match	Match of nonidentical stimuli that retain some common perceptual characteristics (e.g., matching color photograph of dog to black-and-white line drawing of dog)
Comprehension—associating representation with a concept or label	Conceptual nonidentity match	Match of nonidentical stimuli on the basis of conceptual relationship (e.g., selecting photo of dog in response to spoken word "dog")
	Delayed perceptual nonidentity match	Time-delayed match of nonidentical stimuli on the basis of a perceptual similarity (delay increases task difficulty by forcing reliance on conceptual or linguistic information as a bridge from initial presentation of sample to eventual selection from the match array)
	Delayed conceptual nonidentity match	Time-delayed match of nonidentity stimuli on the basis of a conceptual relationship
	Propositional match	Match indicating comprehension at a complexity level beyond match-to-sample (e.g., selecting the photo of a dog in response to "Find the one that is furry and barks")
Use—using representation as a guide to action or as a means of expression	Label	Selection of representation to name an entity (e.g., select picture of dog in response to "What is this?")
	Direct action	Extraction of information from picture for use as a guide to action (e.g., arrange stuffed animals according to arrangement in photograph)
	Expression (literal)	Language production constrained by a 1:1 relationship between picture and referent
	Expression (categorical)	Language production with a single picture used to refer to multiple referents
	Expression (extensive)	Language production with pictures used as semantic links to referents not represented in the available choices

Farther along the complexity continuum are nonidentity matches, in which individuals are required to match items that are not perceptually equivalent. In their less complex instantiations, these might include matching an object to a photograph of the object or a photograph of an object to a line drawing of the object. These are still essentially perceptually based tasks, as individuals can use features of the stimuli that remain constant from sample to match—such as shape or color—as a cue. The task becomes more complex as the perceptual similarity between the sample and the match diminishes. For example, consider the nonidentity match represented by the presentation of an actual pretzel (the traditional twisted variety) and a photograph of a pretzel nugget. Note that one cannot rely solely on shape similarity as the basis for selecting the match, although there are some subtle perceptual similarities such as color and texture between the real pretzel and the photograph. However, if both the real object and the representation are recognized as pretzels, the matching task is an easy one, and the perceptual differences between them become irrelevant.

Another variable with potential to affect matching performance is the introduction of delay between the presentation of the sample and the selection of the match. Brady and McLean (1998) demonstrated that the insertion of a delay had a negative impact on individuals with mental retardation, more so in the nonidentity matching task than in the identity matching task. In their experimental protocol, the complexity of the matching task was increased in two ways. In their "delayed matching" conditions, they presented a sample for the participants' visual inspection, removed the sample from sight, and imposed a delay prior to offering the match array to the participants. This variation is important because of its similarity to real-world contexts in which picture-based language representations are used. It is usually only in highly structured, instructional contexts that individuals have all the real-world items and events that they might wish to select in their immediate view when they are asked to indicate a choice among them via pictures. For example, at snack time, a classroom assistant might say, "Do you want the goldfish or the gummies or the pretzels?" without offering samples of each for the children's consideration. In order to generate a response, children must attach a meaning to each of the snack terms, identify the means to indicate each using a picture array, and make a selection from the available choices. Without the samples immediately in front of them, children can neither indicate the items directly by gaze or point, nor can they rely on the perceptual similarity between real snack items and their representations to facilitate discrimination among pictures and selection of the desired choice.

As suggested previously, nonidentity matches can intrude far into the conceptual realm. Matching a picture of an airplane to those of other conveyances or matching a picture of a pencil to the spoken stimulus "pencil" are also forms of nonidentity matching. These matches cannot be accomplished on the basis of perceptual similarity, however, because they require instead conceptual/linguistic knowledge for correct performance.

Bear in mind that demonstrated ability to perform nonidentity matches does not always imply comprehension in its fullest sense (Blockberger, 1995; Sigel, 1978; Stephenson & Linfoot, 1996). Oviatt (1980, 1982) drew a distinction between recognitory comprehension and symbolic comprehension. In the former, individuals recognize that a word or picture may be associated with a specific referent, whereas in the latter, individuals evidence a more complete and flexible understanding of the expanse and boundaries of that association. Thus, simply pointing a picture in response to a spoken word would be evidence of recognitory comprehension, yet would not be sufficient evidence for determination of symbolic comprehension. Wilkinson and McIlvane (2001) characterized this more advanced type of comprehension as *decontextualization* and consider individuals to have attained this level of linguistic functioning when an array of behaviors with generative characteristics is observed (e.g., if the target word is applied to a variety of exemplars, used with different listeners, and used in the absence of the exemplar). An even more sophisticated variation of decontextualized comprehension is represented by the last point within the comprehension segment of the continuum. At this performance level, individuals are able to demonstrate comprehension on the basis of conceptual propositions, that is, with information about the referent rather than a direct reference to it.

The preceding discussion emphasizes that language comprehension, rather than being a unitary phenomenon, is a construct embracing both simple and complex behaviors. In much the same way, there are degrees of sophistication in expressive language as well. These are associated both with the complexity of the underlying communicative proposition and with the complexity of the surface form of the message. The distinction between the final point in the comprehension segment and the first one in the use segment—the provision of labels—is a blurry one. With speaking individuals, this distinction is explicit. In a receptive task such as the one in the Peabody Picture Vocabulary Test–Revised (Dunn & Dunn, 1981), individuals hear a word and point to its associated picture. In an expressive task, such as that in the Expressive One-Word Picture Vocabulary Test–Revised (Gardner, 1990), individuals see a picture and speak the associated word. With individuals who rely on pictures to communicate, however, the behavioral topography is identical for receptive and expressive responses. Although a response demonstrating receptive language (pointing to the picture of the sandwich in response to "Show me the sandwich") is identical (i.e., it has the same behavioral topography) to that used spontaneously to request a sandwich, the ability to produce the latter cannot be assumed from the ability to produce the former.

The second point in the use segment—the ability to use pictures as a source of information—is closely related to comprehension as well (DeLoache

& Burns, 1994). This ability requires individuals to identify and extract relevant information from pictures and use the information as a guide for their own action. Several studies suggest that this seemingly straightforward task poses surprising challenges for typically developing children as well as individuals with cognitive limitations. Studies by Klapper and Birch (1969); Kose, Beilin, and O'Connor (1983); and House, Hanley, and Magid (1980) all demonstrated that participants evidenced considerable difficulty in executing actions when the instructions were provided to them in pictorial form. For example, Kose and colleagues required children ages 3–6 years to imitate poses depicted by live models, photographs of live models, and drawings of the models. Although there were some age-related differences evidenced in imitation of the live model, these differences became much more pronounced in the experimental conditions utilizing two-dimensional representations. Three-year-olds performed much more poorly than 5- and 6-year-olds with both photographic and line-drawn models. In fact, the children found it easier to describe the pictures using spoken words than to use pictured information as a guide to their own actions, suggesting that they found the nature of the task to be particularly challenging. These results also demonstrate that the representational form in which the prompts to action were given influenced the outcomes. This notion will be elaborated in a later section addressing interactions among key intrinsic and extrinsic factors.

The final three points on the linguistic task complexity continuum relate to expressive language in a more traditional sense. In the realm of AAC, as in spoken language, the selection of a language unit (word or picture) could reflect a host of intentions, ranging from literal to categorical to extensive. In a literal production, a single symbol represents a single referent: a child talks about his dog using the picture of a dog on his communication display and does not use that picture to refer to any other canine than the one that sleeps in his bed every night. A categorical production demonstrates greater flexibility in symbol use in that a single symbol may be used for a number of referents: a child uses the dog symbol in reference to all dogs in the neighborhood, to Blue and Lassie of television fame, and to the Dalmatians in the storybook. In an extensive production, a single symbol is used to suggest referents outside the typical semantic boundaries of the symbol, but for which the child has no other means of representation. The picture's meaning is extended, sometimes through some very creative associations, with the intention of leading the communication partner to a different referent. As an example, the picture of the dog might be used to talk about the hyena observed on a zoo trip or to talk about the visit of the fire truck to the school (via a dog–Dalmatian association). Individuals who use pictures in this way may be demonstrating conceptual associations as well as a metalinguistic awareness of how to lead one's communication partner to a shared referent through a series of deliberate clues using the tools at hand (e.g., pictures, facial expression, vocalization, eye gaze).

One final consideration in the expressive realm of the linguistic continuum pertains to the functions for which pictures are used. Use of a picture for one communicative function should not be taken as evidence that the picture will be used to express the full range of communicative functions. For example, individuals often demonstrate the ability to use pictures to label objects but not as requests or comments (Raghavendra & Fristoe, 1995; Reichle & Yoder, 1985). Similarly, the nature of the referent (e.g., object, action, descriptor) may also affect both recognizability and ease of learning of picture-based language representations (Mizuko, 1987; Mizuko & Reichle, 1989).

In clinical settings, one often hears that an individual "has" a picture-based language representation (e.g., "Oh, yes, Ben has the symbol for *open*"). Where on the continuum is "having" represented? More often than not, it is assumed that an individual "has" a symbol if it is selected from an array in response to a request such as "Show me *open*." If this behavior is placed on the continuum, it is clear that association of a symbol with a referent or label (devoid of situational context) is a much more primitive skill than being able to select *open* in response to a variety of situations or to select *open* to tell people to open the door, open the box of candy, and open their eyes. It is much more appropriate to conclude that individuals "have" a symbol when they demonstrate flexibility with it all along the continuum of linguistic complexity.

Research studies examining picture-based language representation issues tend to focus on a narrow segment of the continuum. Exceptions to this would be those researchers who probe for comprehension of words or pictures prior to exploring other picture-based operations such as matching or requesting. Surprisingly, a large proportion of researchers, at least in the AAC field, fail to secure their subjects' place on the continuum prior to exploring their prowess in activities at other points along the spectrum.

Representational Complexity

Another factor that exerts considerable influence over picture-based language performance, particularly among those with nascent skill in this domain, is the nature of the representations themselves. In the preceding section on linguistic factors, the role of perceptual similarity was mentioned as a potentially facilitative factor in the achievement of representational insight (i.e., noticing some similarity between the representation and the referent). Unlike the linguistic factors, however, the representational factors do not lend themselves neatly or handily to placement along a continuum of complexity because different representational factors are facilitative for different people. As discussed later in the section on intrinsic factors, the perceptual feature of color will not facilitate representational performance if the individual's neurological status precludes discrimination of one color from another. Although the field has tended toward definition of an immutable representational hierarchy, trending from highly realistic representations to abstract ones, this approach is ill-advised (Mineo Mollica, 1997, 2002; Mineo Mollica & Peischl, 1997; Mirenda, 1985).

The notion of a hierarchy, in and of itself, is not the problem; indeed, it is very likely that certain representational features are much more facilitative of correct performance than others. Rather, it is the notion of an immutable, one-size-fits-all ordering of these factors that lacks empirical justification. It would be far more appropriate to conceive of person-specific hierarchies—defined on the basis of a thorough evaluation of an individual's linguistic and representational abilities—and to refer to higher-order representations and lower-order representations in the context of individual profiles (Franklin et al., 1996). A higher-order symbol is one "that is more abstract (i.e., less iconic), dynamic, and cognitively demanding relative to the other type(s) of symbol(s) being discussed" (Franklin et al., p. 65). Thus, *complexity* becomes a relative term, defined for each individual based on demonstrated performance.

Although the notion of a representational hierarchy is critical to understanding representational competence, the relative placement of representational features along the hierarchy will vary across individuals. Given the interrelationships among so many variables, however, it is often hard to identify those elements on which successful performance relies (Stephenson & Linfoot, 1996). Thus, the only valid method for determining the relative contribution of various representational features is to conduct a series of probes to reveal the conditions under which performance is facilitated and, conversely, those under which performance breaks down (Mineo Mollica, 2002).

A host of representational factors may affect performance. The one that has received the greatest attention in the AAC literature is *iconicity* (Fuller, Lloyd, & Schlosser, 1997; Mizuko & Reichle, 1989), which refers to the degree to which the representation resembles the referent and, thus, enables to perceiver to equate it with the referent. Iconicity, however, is a multidimensional phenomenon, and can be influenced by such representational elements as shape, color, size, and complexity/fidelity.

The literature on human visual perception indicates that the process of object recognition relies more heavily on shape than on any other perceptual feature (e.g., Biederman, 1987; Biederman & Ju, 1988; Davidoff & Ostergaard, 1988; Johnson, 1995). Typical adults do not find color information to be very important to object recognition (Cave, Bost, & Cobb, 1996; Seamon et al., 1997), although they turn to color as a cue or to disambiguate structurally similar forms (Johnson, 1992; Price & Humphreys, 1989). There is evidence, however, that the primacy of shape is a developmental phenomenon. Several researchers have documented a transition from early reliance on color in the preschool years to predominant reliance on form by adolescence (Pick, 1983;

Suchman & Trabasso, 1966; Tomikawa & Dodd, 1980; Zeaman & Stanley, 1983). An enduring preference for color over shape, however, is observed in many individuals with brain damage (Goldstein & Oakley, 1986; Grewal, Haward, & Davies, 1987; Huang & Borter, 1987; Meador, 1984). Evidence shows the facilitatory influence of color on the speed of picture naming, on performance on standardized intelligence tests, and on segmentation of areas within a display (Barrow, Holbert, & Rastatter, 2000; Davidoff, 1991; Husband & Hayden, 1996; Wickens & Andre, 1990).

Fuller and colleagues (1997) also cite size as a relevant dimension. Theios and Amrhein (1989) found that smaller visual stimuli took longer to name than their larger counterparts, and Mineo Mollica (2002) found that the nonidentity matching performance of two individuals with significant cognitive and communicative limitations dropped off markedly when the matching task required the individuals to contend with a size transformation (i.e., full-size to miniature or miniature to full-size).

Although stimulus complexity is often mentioned as an important representational factor, there is no operational definition for this variable and no acceptable metric by which to measure it (Capozzi & Mineo, 1983; Fuller et al., 1997; Levie, 1987; Sigel, 1978). Biederman (1987) suggested that complexity relates to the number of parts comprising an object; Fuller and colleagues (1997) expanded this research to include semantic elements as well as perceptual elements. Snodgrass and Corwin (1988) suggested that it could be measured by the number of pixels in a computerized image, and several researchers apparently believe that complexity is a "you know it when you see it" type of phenomenon, as they based complexity on participant ratings. Capozzi and Mineo (1983) and Silverman (1995) implicated the relationship of the figure to the background as a contributory factor. A somewhat related construct is that of *concreteness* or *fidelity*, which refers to the degree of perceptual distance between the representation and the referent; in this conception, a photograph would be a more high-fidelity rendering of an object than a line drawing, because it retains more of the cues to depth and texture (Mineo, Peischl, Demasco, Gray, & Bender, 1995; Uttal, Scudder, & DeLoache, 1997).

Other factors suspected to influence representational complexity include the cultural relevance or familiarity of the representations and the viewing perspective reflected in the representation (Beukelman & Mirenda, 1998; Huer, 2000; Sigel, 1978). A canonical perspective—that is, the preferred point from which to view the object—maximizes salient information relative to key components and the relationships among them and to relevant surface and depth cues (Johnson, Paivio, & Clark, 1996). A merry-go-round would be more readily identified from the viewpoint of an onlooker standing 10 feet away than from the viewpoint of a helicopter pilot far above the fairground.

As mentioned previously, perceptual similarities between representation and referent may make it easier for some individuals to forge links between them (DeLoache et al., 1991; Gentner & Ratterman, 1991; Marzolf & DeLoache, 1994). In some cases, however, a representation's perceptual salience may actually hinder its utilization in a symbolic capacity. Children's inefficient extraction of information from photographic representations has been blamed on the photograph's overabundance of perceptual information. Johnson (1992) observed that young children performed less efficiently with colored photographs than black-and-white line drawings in an object discrimination task, leading her to speculate that the processing of the richer visual detail in photographs slowed children's performance. In other words, it was easier for children to extract relevant information from line drawings because the rendering of such drawings stripped away extraneous photographic details that only served to slow children down.

Similarly, representations that are too perceptually anchored to their referents lock the user into literal use of the representation and hinder the use of those representations categorically or extensively. Sevcik and colleagues (1991) have conducted longitudinal research in which they facilitated language learning, as well as language expression, among individuals with significant cognitive impairments using a language representation system in which symbols were highly abstract and bore absolutely no similarity to their referents. Although the time required for initial acquisition of the representations was often lengthy, the research team did not have to worry about perceptual similarity inhibiting generalization to other exemplars.

In addition, the use of real objects as representations may pose a significant challenge to the achievement of dual representation. The salience of the object—the perceptual realities only available in three dimensions, as well as the appeal of the object as a manipulable—may inhibit its use as a symbol (Brady & McLean, 1998; DeLoache, Pierroutsakos, Uttal, Rosengren, & Gottlieb, 1998; Mirenda & Locke, 1989).

Array Characteristics

The size and structure of the array (the collection of potential choices available to the individual) contribute to the level of task difficulty in two important ways. First, the task becomes more complex as the array size increases (Davidoff, 1991; Estes & Taylor, 1966; Mandler & McDonough, 1993; Mizuko, Reichle, Ratcliff, & Esser, 1994). Many studies conducted with young children and individuals with disabilities use array sizes of only two or three choices, increasing the probability that participants will select the correct answer and keeping distractors to a minimum number.

Second, several studies have revealed decremented performance when the sample item is of a lower order than the items in the array (Brady & Saunders, 1991; Daehler, Lonardo, & Bukatko, 1979; Franklin et al., 1996; Mineo Mollica, 2002). This is presumably because individuals are challenged by having to discriminate among several exemplars of a representational level they find to be difficult in order to select a match for the sample. Without question, the variability across studies—in terms of task requirements, subject characteristics, representations used, array size, and relative high-order/low-order position of sample and match arrays—precludes straightforward comparison of results.

Instruction

Another extrinsic factor that influences representational ability is that of instruction. The nature, content, and intensity of instruction all have considerable bearing on learning outcomes. While it is beyond the scope of this chapter to address the details of the various instructional paradigms used to teach symbol matching, comprehension, and use, there are several considerations related to instruction that will be highlighted briefly.

First, the primary focus of instruction is language learning and use, not picture learning and use. Picture-based representations are just the outward and visible manifestation of an individual's facility with language. Therefore, instruction aimed at increasing the breadth and robustness of underlying language behaviors is likely also to influence the manner in which the individual can evidence these behaviors through pictures (Johnson et al., 1996; Liben, 1999). It is dangerous, however, to assume that learners will detect new symbol–referent relations effortlessly and without support, regardless of how transparent those relations might appear to those with mature language abilities (DeLoache, 1989; DeLoache, Miller, & Rosengren, 1997; Marzolf & DeLoache, 1994). There are several strategies that may help to bring the representation/referent relationship to the fore:

1. Highlight the salient relationships (many of them related to perceptual features) that are important to typical learners. For example, emphasize similarities in shape by visibly enhancing the important borders and calling attention to those held constant across forms.
2. Avoid teaching rote association behavior (Wilkinson & McIlvane, 2001); instead, emphasize the relationship between the representation and numerous appropriate exemplars (unless, of course, the picture is intended for use as a literal representation only).
3. Capitalize on multiple modalities. When teaching a new representation, associate it with a variety of forms of the referent, such as spoken words, objects, or other representations of the same object or concept (Liben & Downs, 1991). Demonstrate selection of the item from the communication display as a direct model of desired behavior (Hunt-Berg, 1996). Exploit the voice output capabilities of the communication device to reinforce the meaning of the representation (Brady, 2000; Schlosser, Belfiore, Nigam, Blischak, & Hetzroni, 1995).

4. Plan to provide numerous opportunities for learning and practice (Romski & Sevcik, 1993b; Rowland & Schweigert, 2000).
5. Make the representational connection explicit (DeLoache & Burns, 1994; Johnson et al., 1996; Uttal et al., 1997). Explain the relationship between the referent and the representation. Describe why a particular representation was chosen to stand for a particular concept.
6. Make the representational process explicit (Beilin & Pearlman, 1991). Use a Polaroid camera to show how a photograph is derived from an object. Demonstrate shrinking a two-dimensional stimulus on a copy machine. Trace a line drawing from a photograph, then color it in, emphasizing the selection of colors similar to those of the referent.
7. If introducing picture-based language representations for the first time, try to identify words that the individual knows receptively. Use these as the foundation on which to map the new picture-related behavior. Experience with easy symbolic relationships begets facility with the more difficult ones (Bluestein & Acredolo, 1979; Liben, Moore, & Golbeck, 1982; Marzolf & DeLoache, 1994; Mineo & Goldstein, 1990).
8. Do not stop instruction when an individual evidences matching or receptive identification skills. Create opportunities for training requesting, commenting, and other language functions in natural and motivating contexts (Kozleski, 1991; Sigafoos, Doss, & Reichle, 1989).

INTRINSIC FACTORS

Motivation

A discussion of instructional variables would be incomplete without mention of motivation as a key intrinsic element. Teachers can maximize a learner's motivation by building instruction around things and events that the learner finds enjoyable (Rowland & Schweigert, 2000). Reichle (1991) reported that an individual learned an abstract symbol for candy more rapidly than a highly guessable gesture for water. One family with whom I worked was frustrated by the school's insistence that their son was "too low functioning" to evidence symbolic behavior. They knew otherwise, based in part on the youngster's animated response to paraphernalia displaying the logos of his favorite fast-food restaurants. On one particularly telling occasion, the father and son drove past a Taco Bell. The son used contact gestures to convey that he wanted to stop for a bite to eat. When his dad failed to pull into the restaurant parking lot, the youngster began rooting furiously through material that had accumulated on the floor of the car. Out of the debris, he pulled a Taco Bell napkin and excitedly gestured from the logo to his father. The intent and the dual representation were unmistakable. We encouraged the educators to reconsider their training targets before they concluded that instruction would be a waste of time.

Of course, one should not presume what another person will find appealing. The use of preference probes facilitates data-based decision-making in this regard (Rowland & Schweigert, 2000). Care should be taken to avoid the trap of believing that only objects—treats and toys and the like—have inherent appeal. Language items such as "more" and "Look at this!" put tremendous power in the hands of augmented communicators (Gerber & Kraat, 1992; Wilkinson, Romksi, & Sevcik, 1994). Social-regulatory terms may also add to the clarity, range, and flexibility of communications (Adamson, Romski, Deffebach, & Sevcik, 1992).

Neurological Functioning

The system that supports perception and interpretation of visual information is extraordinarily complex. It is beyond the scope of this chapter to offer an exhaustive review of the literature in this regard, yet several key points will be emphasized because of their relevance to later discussions. For a more comprehensive overview, the reader is referred to the Kosslyn and Osherson (1995) volume on visual cognition and to Schwartz (1999) for the clinical perspective on normal and disordered vision. (See also Chapter 9.)

The human visual perceptual system functions to parse, or segment, incoming visual stimuli, and then to identify the nature of that incoming information. Although there is still considerable debate regarding the point in the process at which perception occurs, there is evidence that an intact visual system separates incoming stimuli into two primary streams: one contains information related to perceptual attributes such as shape and color, and the other contains information about motion that guides actions directed at objects (Goodale, 1995; Shapley, 1990; Spelke, Gutheil, & Van de Walle, 1995). Reference to these pathways as the "what" and "where" systems is generally accurate yet simplistic, as there is considerable interconnection and overlap among the two pathways (Parkin, 1996). Information from the retina travels along the optic nerve, continues past the optic chiasm to the dorsal lateral geniculate nucleus (at which point the division into the two distinct systems is quite apparent), and then is routed to the striate cortex and on to higher cortical areas. Approximately 20 distinct areas have been identified as having a role in higher-level cortical processing, including color perception and form (Tanaka, Saito, Fukada, & Moriya, 1991; Zeki, 1993). Rao and colleagues have speculated that integration of the various components of visual input is coordinated in the prefrontal cortex (Rao, Rainer, & Miller, 1997).

This information is relevant to the discussion of picture-based language representations because the functional use of pictures presumes intact perceptual skills. When individuals have sustained an insult to the central nervous system of such magnitude that motor and/or linguistic functioning is insufficient to support speech, it is quite possible that one or more aspects of the visual system also have been affected (Damasio, 1985; Padula, 2000; Troscianko, 1987). If the developing visual system does not receive normal input within the first year of life, typical perceptual development will be precluded (Schwartz, 1999). Unfortunately, many visual anomalies remain undetected or are not detected until the child has entered school. By then, the critical developmental period is long past, and attempts at correction via standard means such as patching are likely to be futile (Spelke et al., 1995). Practitioners must be sure that individuals are capable of perceiving the representations. In some cases, the thin lines characteristic of so many commercially available symbol systems would elude detection. Similarly, disruptions in color vision—experienced by approximately 4.5% of the general population— would preclude the use of color as a facilitative perceptual cue to picture identification (Pokorny, Smith, Verriest, & Pinckers, 1979). Disruption at the higher levels of cortical function may interfere with the coordination of incoming visual stimuli into a coherent percept, with the further identification and labeling of the image, or with the association of the image to a word or a concept that supports the completion of a linguistic act.

INTERACTIONS AMONG KEY FACTORS

The previous sections have emphasized several key factors that influence the development and demonstration of picture-based language capabilities: the linguistic loading of the task, the perceptual and linguistic capabilities of the individual, and features of the representations themselves. Although any of these alone may exert an influence on performance, they may also interact in complex ways that often lead researchers and clinicians to unfounded conclusions about an augmented communicator's representational language capabilities.

The remainder of this section is devoted to the manner in which representational variables and linguistic task variables may influence behavior. Figure 4.1 places the two continua in opposition, allowing construction of a graph individualized to the profile of a particular user. Along one axis are the representational levels in descending order from high-order (more difficult) representations to low-order representations; recall that the relative difficulty of these is determined on an individual basis, not in terms of a preordained hierarchy. The opposing axis represents points along the linguistic complexity continuum. This representational strategy was designed to enable isolation of the focal task and representational variables in a research study or a clinical intervention.

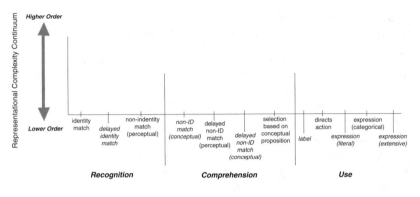

Figure 4.1. Format for presentation of representational complexity/linguistic task complexity interaction. The vertical axis shows the representational levels in descending order from higher-order (more difficult) representations to lower-order (less difficult) representations. The horizontal axis represents the linguistic complexity continuum, from simple identity match (recognition) to extensive expression of the symbol (use).

Knowledge about the full spectrum of representational competence and the factors that influence it is, at best, piecemeal. This graphical strategy for documenting representational performance is suggested as a way that the field might place the outcomes of numerous studies into a common framework. Studies addressing these issues vary enormously in terms of participant characteristics (e.g., age, world experience, developmental status, language competence), the characteristics of the representations involved (e.g., size, color, fidelity), and the nature of the task in which the participant is expected to engage using representations (e.g., recognition versus understanding versus use). A mechanism allowing researchers and clinicians to document representational performance in a consistent manner will help assemble fragmented research and clinical outcomes into a cohesive knowledge base.

In the pages that follow, two studies revealing an interaction between linguistic task variables and representational variables are highlighted. The graphic depiction of their findings will enable the reader to consider performance in the context of both the representations used and the nature of the language tasks. Be aware that this method of representing research outcomes is intended to highlight the relationship between representational complexity and linguistic task complexity. It does not lend itself to representation of actual performance levels relative to specific tasks (e.g., percentage correct); rather, it enables illustration of the relative difficulty of tasks—defined by the representational level used and the linguistic complexity of the task in which they are used.

Study 1: Representational
Incompetence Obscures Language Competence

My colleagues and I examined the influence of representational type on language performance (Mineo Mollica, Peischl, & Pennington, 2002). Evidence from several previous studies had indicated that representations for verbs were not identified as readily as those for nouns (Mizuko, 1987; Mizuko & Reichle, 1989; Raghavendra & Fristoe, 1995), and some have speculated that this is due to the inability of static representations to convey the dynamism of action referents. In light of the emergence of AAC devices capable of animating action representations, we sought to document the effect of movement on the comprehension of graphic representations of action words.

The research required typically developing 3-, 4-, and 5-year-olds to select the representation—from an array of four—that matched a spoken prompt. A trial within any of the four conditions involved the presentation of four picture-based selection options to the child (see Figure 4.2) while issuing the prompt "Show me [action label]." The experimental conditions related to the representational level of the stimuli (see Table 4.3).

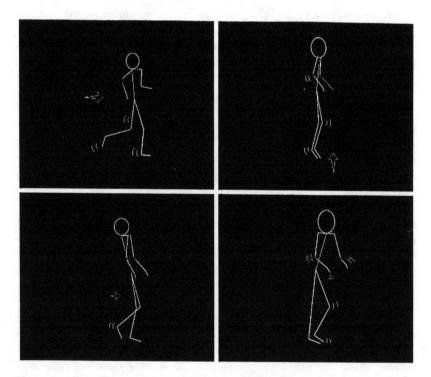

Figure 4.2. "Static with Cues" Trial. *Source:* Mineo Mollica, Peischl, & Pennington, 2002.

Table 4.3. Experimental tasks—Mineo Mollica, Peischl, and Pennington (2002)

Match-to-sample tasks		
Sample	Match	Continuum location
Spoken word	Video	Conceptual nonidentity match
Spoken word	Animation	Conceptual nonidentity match
Spoken word	Static with cues	Conceptual nonidentity match
Spoken word	Static	Conceptual nonidentity match

Source: Mineo Mollica, Peischl, and Pennington (2002)

The *static* level involved a single frame depicting an action in midmotion. In the *static with cues* level, representations identical to those in the static condition were enhanced with pictorial cues such as directional arrows or repeating lines (see Figure 4.2). The *video* level involved black-and-white video clips of an adult engaging in the target actions. The *animation* level showed a moving stick figure engaging in the target actions. The four representational levels all had the same origin: the movement of a human engaging in the target actions. The movements were captured on video as well as recorded in a gait lab; the animated figures were derived from the gait lab data. A single frame of each animation sequence was selected as most representative of each action, and this frame served as the basis for the static and static with cues representations. Children completed 24 trials in each of the four conditions.

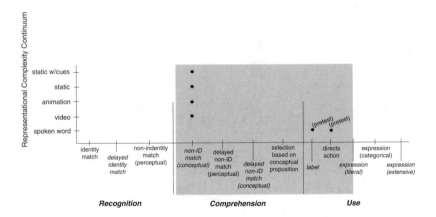

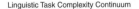

Figure 4.3. Research outcomes for 3-year-olds. The vertical axis shows the representational levels in descending order from high-order (more difficult) representations to low-order (less difficult) representations. The horizontal axis represents the linguistic complexity continuum, from simple identity match (recognition) to extensive expression of the symbol (use). Points represent the highest level linguistic complexity reached in the representational trials. The shaded area indicates the range of the results. (*Source:* Mineo Mollica et al., 2002.)

A condition of participation was that the children had demonstrated understanding of each action word used as a stimulus in the computer-based protocol either receptively (the child performed the requested action) or expressively (the child named the action demonstrated by the examiner). The spectrum of tasks in which the children engaged is summarized in Table 4.3.

The results are depicted in Figures 4.3 and 4.4. The representational complexity dimension is ordered from high- to low-order (most to least difficult). For example, the 3-year-olds found the static with cues level most difficult and the video level least difficult. The ordering of representational levels was very similar for the 4- and 5-year-olds. Although the performance patterns were similar, the raw data revealed a developmental trend, with an increase in overall accuracy of responding with age. Figures 4.3 and 4.4 effectively illustrate a somewhat surprising representational complexity/linguistic task interaction. Regardless of age, the children performed without errors on the pretest task involving higher-order linguistic behaviors found in the expressive region of the continuum. They failed to demonstrate similar performance, however, when pictures were involved in the task, even when the task was a presumably simpler receptive identification activity. Thus, the introduction of picture stimuli, and/or the need to select a match from an array of four choices, interfered with children's ability to demonstrate language proficiency that pretesting had revealed to be within their repertoires. The fact

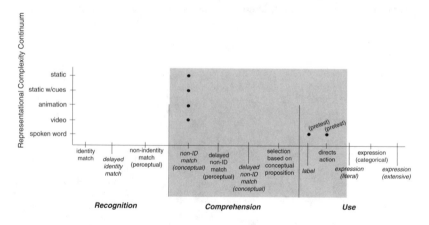

Linguistic Task Complexity Continuum

Figure 4.4.   Research outcomes for 4- to 5-year-olds. The vertical axis shows the representational levels in descending order from high-order (more difficult) representations to low-order (less difficult) representations. The horizontal axis represents points along the linguistic complexity continuum, from simple identity match (recognition) to extensive expression of the symbol (use). Points represent the highest level linguistic complexity reached in the representational trials. The shaded area indicates the range of the results. (*Source:* Mineo Mollica et al., 2002.)

that performance also varied by type of representation suggests an inequality among picture-based language representations, with some more facilitative of correct performance than others. The outcomes of this study serve as a reminder that one should not infer abilities in a visual-graphic mode based on concomitant performance in an auditory-verbal mode. The introduction of picture-based language representations clearly interfered with the demonstration of linguistic knowledge, even among typically developing children.

Study 2: An Intriguing Manipulation of Array Characteristics

Franklin and her colleagues (1996) explored an aspect of assessment and intervention that is often taken for granted—the structure of the task used to determine whether an individual can match stimuli. Matching performance is regarded by many as a critical foundation for development of more sophisticated representational skills, and Franklin and her colleagues attempted to determine if performance would vary as a function of task design. To this end, they engaged three participant groups in five different matching activities. The first group was comprised of typically developing preschool children with a mean age of 35 months. The second and third groups were comprised of individuals with severe intellectual disabilities. These two groups were distinguished from one another by receptive language performance level; the verbal label comprehension group demonstrated understanding of at least 10 of 12 common object labels, whereas the no verbal label comprehension group labeled 7 or fewer of the 12 items correctly.

The matching tasks involved objects, color photographs, and spoken words. Most of the trials required the participant to complete a nonidentity match, although variations on identity matching were also included. The five symbol assessment protocols included in this study are presented in Table 4.4. Also included in the table are three additional match-to-sample activities.

Table 4.4. Experimental tasks—Franklin, Mirenda, and Phillips (1996)

Match-to-sample tasks		
Sample	Match	Continuum location
Object (S)*	Objects (A)*	Perceptual identity match
Objects (S)*	Object (A)*	Perceptual identity match
Spoken word*	Objects (S)*	Conceptual nonidentity match
Photograph (S)	Objects (A)	Perceptual nonidentity match
Photographs (S)	Object (A)	Perceptual nonidentity match
Object (S)	Photographs (A)	Perceptual nonidentity match
Objects (S)	Photograph (A)	Perceptual nonidentity match
Spoken word	Photographs (S)	Conceptual nonidentity match

Source: Franklin, Mirenda, and Phillips (1996).
*pretest or grouping activities

Two of these were used as a pretest; the third evaluated the participants' receptive knowledge of object labels in order to divide those with severe disabilities into the verbal label comprehension and no verbal label comprehension groups. Close inspection of Table 4.4 reveals a key element of the study. Note the systematic variation in the structure of the matching tasks. Both the nature and the positioning of the stimuli are varied in order to determine the extent to which a particular arrangement will influence correct performance.

For example, the design enabled these researchers to evaluate whether a participant found it more difficult to 1) select a picture from an array of four pictures in front of him or her and match it to an object in front of the assessor, or 2) match the single picture in front of him or her to one of four objects in front of the assessor (see Figure 4.5). In all of the matches involving photographs and objects, the items in the "sample" column were those placed closest to the subject (S), and the items in the "match" column were those placed closest to the assessor (A).

To language sophisticates—which in this case includes the typically developing preschool children with whom Franklin and her colleagues interacted—the two tasks illustrated in Figure 4.5 are not discernibly different and are both very easy. In fact, the preschool participants demonstrated very accurate performance on all five symbol assessment protocols. Those with less linguistic sophistication, however, demonstrated markedly different performance across the various experimental tasks. Figures 4.6 and 4.7 illustrate the performance of the participants with severe intellectual disabilities, with the first one representing the performance of the verbal label comprehension

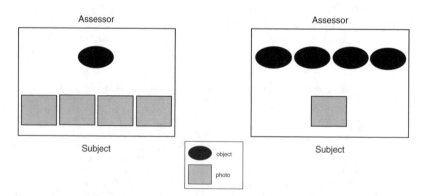

Figure 4.5. Two scenarios for presenting objects to the subject. Participants were asked to either 1) select a picture from an array of four pictures in front of him or her and match it to an object in front of the assessor, or 2) match the single picture in front of him or her to one of four objects in front of the assessor. (From Franklin, K., Mirenda, P., & Phillips, G. [1996]. Comparison of five symbol assessment protocols with nondisabled preschoolers and learners with severe intellectual disabilities. *Augmentative and Alternative Communication, 12,* 63–77; adapted by permission from Taylor & Francis Ltd, http://www.tandf.co.uk/journals)

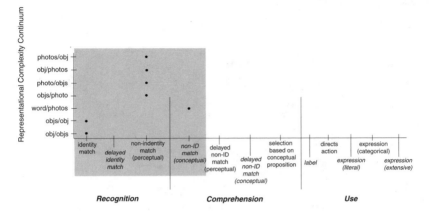

Figure 4.6. Research outcomes for the verbal label comprehension group. The vertical axis shows the representational levels in descending order from high-order (more difficult) representations to low-order (less difficult) representations. The horizontal axis represents the linguistic complexity continuum, from simple identity match (recognition) to extensive expression of the symbol (use). Points represent the highest level linguistic complexity reached in the representational trials. The shaded area indicates the range of the results. (*Source*: Franklin, Mirenda, & Phillips, 1996)

group and the second one representing the performance of the no verbal label comprehension group. Keep in mind that the ordering along the representational complexity continuum reflects the performance of the target group, with those representational levels found to be most difficult in the higher-order positions.

As the inclusion criteria imply, both participant groups performed adequately on the identity matches involving objects; however, both groups were less accurate on the trials in which they had to select from an array of multiple objects in front of them in order to match a single object in front of the assessor. In regard to the trials involving object and photograph stimuli, performance across the two groups revealed an identical trend: multiple-photograph-to-single-object matching was most difficult, and multiple-objects-to-single-photograph was least difficult. The assessment protocols involving multiple photograph arrays were more difficult than those involving multiple object arrays, regardless of whether the arrays were those from which the subject selected or those placed near the assessor. Overall, however, those in the verbal label comprehension group performed more accurately on the assessment protocols involving objects and photographs than did those in the no verbal label comprehension group. The other notable difference between the two groups related to performance on the spoken-word-to-photograph task. It is not surprising that those participants who demonstrated comprehension of

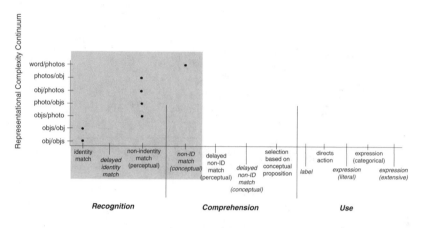

Figure 4.7. Research outcomes for the no verbal label comprehension group. The vertical axis shows the representational levels in descending order from high-order (more difficult) representations to low-order (less difficult) representations. The horizontal axis represents points along the linguistic complexity continuum, from recognition (simple identity match) to full use of the symbol (extensive expression). Points represent the highest level linguistic complexity reached in the representational trials. The shaded area indicates the range of the results. (*Source*: Franklin, Mirenda, & Phillips, 1996)

the names of the pictured objects performed more accurately on this task. What may be surprising to some is that these subjects generally were more accurate in the conceptual nonidentity task involving a spoken-word-to-photograph match than in the theoretically simpler tasks in which matching could be completed on the basis of perceptual characteristics alone.

This finding raises similar questions to those of the Mineo Mollica and colleagues (2002) study. Clearly, some characteristic of the task interfered with participants' ability to demonstrate what they knew. Franklin and her colleagues suggest that object arrays offer multiple salient perceptual cues (e.g., size, color, shape, brightness) that are not equally present in their photographic counterparts, implying that photographs pose greater challenges than objects. Task complexity increases as array size increases, suggesting a compounding of complexity as both array size and representational complexity increase.

The investigators concluded that the protocols investigated in this study did not appear to be "equivalent methods for determining the level of symbolic functioning" (Franklin et al., 1996, p. 75). They suggest that assessments should include multiple combinations and permutations of symbol relationships in order to identify a particular individual's representational strengths. They also note that "AAC systems by their very nature incorporate the use of higher order symbol arrays of varying sizes" (p. 75), and thus may be imposing unintended confounds into attempts to facilitate language learning and use via augmented means.

Variations on the Theme

There are many other fascinating studies that illustrate the reciprocal influence of representational complexity and linguistic task complexity on language performance. The impressive body of research undertaken by DeLoache and her colleagues demonstrated the influence of representational complexity, task instructions, and subject characteristics (particularly age) on children's ability to use scale models as representations of larger spaces. Sorce (1980) deftly revealed how typically developing preschoolers who demonstrate facility with conceptually based matching appear to revert to reliance on perceptual characteristics when the representational level of the research stimuli becomes more complex. Brady and McLean (1998) demonstrated that the insertion of a delay between stimulus presentation and participant response markedly increased task difficulty. Mirenda and Locke (1989) also implicated task characteristics and representational complexity in their study of match-to-sample performance among individuals with severe communication limitations.

These studies alert us to the peril in making assumptions about the inherent simplicity of pictures. All picture-based language representations are not created equal, and the degree to which an individual is able to understand and use pictures will depend on the nature of the picture as well as the nature of the language task. An ability to match a representation to an object should not imply an ability to use that same representation to express an intention. Rather, clinicians must deconstruct scenarios in which pictures are intended as the medium of communicative exchange to be clear about the explicit nature of the task and the impact of the representational form on successful accomplishment of that task.

The strategy for documenting this relationship introduced in Figure 4.1 may be useful to clinicians as a means for graphically representing these task/ representation relationships. This means of plotting performance relative to task complexity and representational complexity also serves as a reminder of the sometimes fine–but nonetheless significant–distinctions among points along the linguistic task complexity continuum. For example, the impact of a time delay on correct responding may seem academic or trivial. Yet, Brady and McLean (1998) demonstrated that the delay variable adds a significant cognitive load to tasks that their participants completed with relative ease in trials without delays. In light of the fact that many daily interactions using AAC devices are, in essence, delayed nonidentity matching tasks, these findings suggest that one should not assume the ability to perform such tasks from demonstrations of more elementary nonidentity matching tasks (e.g., pointing to a picture of a book when shown a real book).

INFORMING THE CLINICAL PERSPECTIVE

Adults with intact language capabilities, who typically process pictured information automatically, tend to regard pictures as a simple, straightforward alternative for representing meaning. There are times, however, when even linguistically competent adults are challenged by pictured information, as in the case of visual illusions or intentionally ambiguous pictures. When confronted with visual anomalies, people become much more deliberate in their processing, using prior experience with similar phenomena, their world knowledge, and their linguistic and cognitive skills to bring order to visual chaos. Very young children and those with significant cognitive challenges cannot rely on the same wealth of resources when confronted with picture-based language representations. Their perceptual apparatus may not be as finely tuned, they may have had few prior interactions with pictures, and, most important, they do not have a sophisticated language system on which they can depend to serve as a bridge between pictures and meaning.

If pictures are to be used as a language representation system, it is imperative that interventionists understand the potential consequences of the decisions they make regarding the types of representations that will be used, the number of representations that will be presented simultaneously, and the arrangement of the representations. It is also critical that interventionists understand that picture matching ability implies neither picture understanding nor the ability to use pictures for expressive communication. Assessment of picture-based language representation skills should probe a variety of representational types at points all along the linguistic task complexity continuum, and instructional paradigms should reflect a sensitivity to the individual's current level of functioning as well as a logical relationship to anticipated communicative outcomes.

FUTURE RESEARCH DIRECTIONS

The field would benefit tremendously from research that further clarifies the relationships among representational types, linguistic tasks, and user characteristics. For example, little is known about how to facilitate representational development. With typically developing youngsters, pictures are an interesting adjunct to language. They function as illustrations and as objects of contemplation, and children are exposed to pictures incidentally through joint book reading activities, television, and interaction with the environment. With children at risk for significant communication limitations, however, pictures may be much more than an embellishment or an adjunct to language; they may become a central conduit for language learning and use. It may be that children whose exposure to pictures is more deliberate and systematic—

with the pictures serving a central communicative function—will demonstrate more rapidly developing picture-related skills or will demonstrate a functional utilization of pictures not typical among speaking children. Investigators need to understand much more about the influence of aided language stimulation/augmented input on the development of picture-based language behaviors and whether certain types of pictures facilitate more efficient learning. They need to learn more about how to influence the environment (both physical environment and caregiver behaviors) to maximize the positive impact of pictures on the development of communication skills.

The field also needs additional research exploring the use of picture-based language representations for various communicative functions. Studies to date have tended to focus on a narrow segment of the linguistic task complexity continuum, preventing investigators from examining the relationship between, for example, picture-based skills in the receptive and expressive domains. Research of this nature would not only inform assessment and instructional practices; it would also expand general knowledge about the relationship between receptive and expressive language. An important pursuit in this regard is the examination of the impact of various elicitation strategies on demonstration of language skill; for example, do "yes/no," matching, and expressive tasks elicit similar responses, and do these responses vary with the representational level of the stimuli?

Investigators also need to examine the implications of the fact that when a person is communicating via pictures, receptive and expressive responses have the same behavioral topography (i.e., selecting, in some manner, a choice from an array). Does this facilitate more rapid development of expressive communication? Despite the similarities in the overt behavior, do children still demonstrate comprehension before they are able to use the same response expressively? There is also considerable need for research that explores whether there are certain performance patterns or representational preferences associated with particular participant or task characteristics. For example, do very young children or those with significant cognitive limitations evidence better performance when color is the most salient perceptual linkage between referent and representation? Are there instances in which intervention should begin with highly abstract representations rather than perceptually similar ones? Are certain types of referents represented more effectively by generic representations rather than ones with highly similar perceptual characteristics? Does the presence of certain visual anomalies summarily preclude the use of certain types of representations?

A growing body of data relative to representational competence will allow a better understanding of the inherent complexity in picture-based language representation arising from factors related to the learner's extant perceptual, cognitive, and linguistic abilities; the nature of the representations utilized; and the nature of the task undertaken via those representations. More will be known about the emergence of early language skills and how they can be either enhanced or hindered by choices related to the language representations themselves or the manner in which they are taught and used. Such knowledge will enable researchers and clinicians to design interventions—responsive to individual skills and needs—that expand the individual's communicative repertoire in the short term and serve as a scaffold on which increasingly sophisticated communication skills can be anchored.

REFERENCES

Adamson, L.B., Romski, M.A., Deffebach, K., & Sevcik, R.A. (1992). Symbol vocabulary and the focus of conversations: Augmenting language development for youth with mental retardation. *Journal of Speech and Hearing Research, 35,* 1333–1343.

Au, T.K., & Glusman, M. (1990). The principle of mutual exclusivity in word learning: To honor or not to honor? *Child Development, 61,* 1474–1490.

Barrera, M.E., & Maurer, D. (1981). Recognition of mother's photographed face by the three-month-old infant. *Child Development, 52,* 714–716.

Barrow, I.M., Holbert, D., & Rastatter, M.P. (2000). Effect of color on developmental pictured-vocabulary naming of 4-, 6-, and 8-year-old children. *American Journal of Speech-Language Pathology, 9,* 310–318.

Bates, E. (1979). *The emergence of symbols: Cognition and communication in infancy.* San Diego: Academic Press.

Behl-Chadha, G. (1996). Basic-level and superordinate-like categorical representations in early infancy. *Cognition, 60,* 105–141.

Beilin, H. (1983). Development of photogenic comprehension. *Art Education, 36,* 28–33.

Beilin, H., & Pearlman, E.G. (1991). Children's iconic realism: Object versus property realism. In H.W. Reese (Ed.), *Advances in child development and behavior* (Vol. 23, pp. 73–111). San Diego: Academic Press.

Beukelman, D.R., & Mirenda. P. (1998). *Augmentative and alternative communication: Management of severe communication disorders in children and adults* (2nd ed.). Baltimore: Paul H. Brookes Publishing Co.

Biederman, I. (1987). Recognition-by-components: A theory of human image understanding. *Psychological Review, 94,* 115–145.

Biederman, I., & Ju, G. (1988). Surface versus edge-based determinants of visual recognition. *Cognitive Psychology, 20,* 38–64.

Blockberger, S. (1995). AAC intervention and early conceptual and lexical development. *Journal of Speech-Language Pathology and Audiology, 19,* 221–232.

Bluestein, N., & Acredolo, L. (1979). Developmental changes in map-reading skills. *Child Development, 50,* 691–697.

Brady, N.C. (2000). Improved comprehension of object names following voice output communication aid use: Two case studies. *Augmentative and Alternative Communication, 16,* 197–204.

Brady, N.C., & McLean, L.K. (1998). Simultaneous and delayed matching to sample in gesture users and speakers with mental retardation. *Research in Developmental Disabilities, 19,* 409–421.

Brady, N.C., & Saunders, K.J. (1991). Considerations in the effective teaching of object-to-symbol matching. *Augmentative and Alternative Communication, 7,* 112–116.

Bulthoff, H.H., Edelman, S.Y, & Tarr, M.J. (1995). How are three dimensional objects represented in the brain? *Cerebral Cortex, 5,* 247–260.

Capozzi, M., & Mineo, B. (1983). Nonspeech language and communication systems. In A. Holland (Ed.), *Language disorders in children* (pp. 173–209). San Diego: College-Hill Press.

Carr, D., Wilkinson, K.M., Blackman, D., & McIlvane, W.J. (2000). Equivalence classes in individuals with minimal verbal repertoires. *Journal of the Experimental Analysis of Behavior, 74,* 101–114.

Cave, C.B., Bost, P.R., & Cobb, R.E. (1996). Effects of color and pattern on implicit and explicit picture memory. *Journal of Experimental Psychology: Learning, Memory, and Cognition, 22,* 639–653.

Daehler, M.W., Lonardo, R., & Bukatko, D. (1979). Matching and equivalence judgements in very young children. *Child Development, 50,* 170–179.

Damasio, A.R. (1985). Disorders of complex visual processing: Agnosias, achromatopsia, Balents syndrome, and related difficulties of orientation and construction. In M.M. Mesulum (Ed.), *Principles of behavioral neurology* (pp. 259–288). Philadelphia: F.A. Davis Co.

Davidoff, J.B. (1991). *Cognition through color.* Cambridge: MIT Press.

Davidoff, J.B., & Ostergaard, A.L. (1988). The role of colour in categorical judgments. *Quarterly Journal of Experimental Psychology, 40A,* 533–544.

DeLoache, J.S. (1989). The development of representation in young children. In H.W. Reese (Ed.), *Advances in child development and behavior* (Vol. 22, pp. 1–39). San Diego: Academic Press.

DeLoache, J. (1991). Symbolic functioning in very young children: Understanding of pictures and models. *Child Development, 62,* 736–752.

DeLoache, J.S. (1995). Early symbolic understanding and use. In D. Medin (Ed.), *The psychology of learning and motivation* (Vol. 33, pp. 65–114). San Diego: Academic Press.

DeLoache, J.S. (2000). Dual representation and young children's use of scale models. *Child Development, 71,* 329–338.

DeLoache, J.S., & Burns, N.M. (1994). Early understanding of the representational function of pictures. *Cognition, 52,* 83–110.

DeLoache, J.S., DeMendoza, O.A.P., & Anderson, K.M. (1999). Multiple factors in early symbol use: Instructions, similarity, and age in understanding a symbol-referent relation. *Cognitive Development, 14,* 299–312.

DeLoache, J.S., Kolstad, D.V., & Anderson, K.M. (1991). Physical similarity and young children's understanding of scale models. *Child Development, 62,* 111–126.

DeLoache, J.S., Miller, K.F., & Rosengren, K. (1997). The credible shrinking room: Very young children's performance in symbolic and non-symbolic tasks. *Psychological Science, 8,* 308–313.

DeLoache, J.S., Pierroutsakos, S., Uttal, D.H., Rosengren, K., & Gottlieb, A. (1998). Grasping the nature of pictures. *Psychological Science, 9,* 205–210.

DeLoache, J., Strauss, M., & Maynard, J. (1979). Picture perception in infancy. *Infant Behavior and Development, 2,* 77–89.

Dunn, L.M., & Dunn, L.M. (1981). *Peabody Picture Vocabulary Test–Revised: Manual for Forms L and M.* Circle Pines, MN: American Guidance Service.

Estes, W., & Taylor, H. (1966). Visual detection in relation to display size and redundancy of critical elements. *Perception & Psychophysics, 1,* 9–16.

Franklin, K., Mirenda, P., & Phillips, G. (1996). Comparison of five symbol assessment protocols with nondisabled preschoolers and learners with severe intellectual disabilities. *Augmentative and Alternative Communication, 12,* 63–77.

Fuller, D.R., Lloyd, L.L., & Schlosser, R.W. (1997). What do we know about graphic AAC symbols, and what do we still need to know about them? In E. Björck-

Åkesson & P. Lindsay (Eds.), *Communication . . . naturally: Theoretical and methodological issues in augmentative and alternative communication. Proceedings of the Fourth ISAAC Research Symposium* (pp. 113–125). Västerås, Sweden: Mälardalen University Press.

Gardner, M.F. (1990). *Expressive One-Word Picture Vocabulary Test–Revised.* Austin, TX: PRO-ED.

Gentner, D. (1988). Metaphor as structure mapping: The relational shift. *Child Development, 59,* 47–59.

Gentner, D., & Ratterman, M.J. (1991). Language and the career of similarity. In S. Gelman & J. Byrnes (Eds.), *Perspectives on language and thought: Interrelations in development* (pp. 225–277). London: Cambridge University Press.

Gerber, S., & Kraat, A. (1992). Use of a developmental model of language acquisition: Applications to children using AAC systems. *Augmentative and Alternative Communication, 8,* 19–32.

Goldstein, L.H., & Oakley, D.A. (1986). Color versus orientation discrimination in severely brain-damaged and normal adults. *Cortex, 22,* 261–266.

Golinkoff, R.M., Hirsh-Pasek, K., Mervis, C.B., Frawley, W.B., & Parillo, M.B. (1995). Lexical principles can be extended to the acquisition of verbs. In M. Tomasello & W.E. Merriman (Eds.), *Beyond names for things: Young children's acquisition of verbs* (pp. 185–221). Mahwah, NJ: Lawrence Erlbaum Associates.

Golinkoff, R.M., Jacquet, R., Hirsh-Pasek, K., & Nandakumar, R. (1996). Lexical principles underlie verb learning. *Child Development, 67,* 3101–3110.

Golinkoff, R.M., Mervis, C.B., & Hirsh-Pasek, K. (1994). Early object labels: The case for lexical principles. *Journal of Child Language, 21,* 125–155.

Goodale, M.A. (1995). The cortical organization of visual perception and visuomotor control. In S.M. Kosslyn & D.N. Osherson (Eds.), *Visual cognition* (pp. 167–214). Cambridge: MIT Press.

Goodwyn, S.W., Acredolo, L.P., & Brown, C.A. (2000). Impact of symbolic gesturing on early language development. *Journal of Nonverbal Behavior, 24,* 81–103.

Goossens', C. (1989). Aided communication intervention before assessment: A case study of a child with cerebral palsy. *Augmentative and Alternative Communication, 5,* 14–26.

Grewal, B.S., Haward, L.R., & Davies, I.R. (1987). The role of color discriminability in the Weigl test. *IRCS Medical Science: Psychology and Psychiatry, 14,* 693–694.

Gross, D., Soken, N., Rosengren, K.S., Pick, A.D., Pillow, B.H., & Melendez, P. (1991). Children's understanding of action lines and the static representation of speech of locomotion. *Child Development, 62,* 1124–1141.

House, B.J., Hanley, M.J., & Magid, D.F. (1980). Logographic reading by TMR adults. *American Journal of Mental Deficiency, 85,* 161–170.

Huang, I., & Borter, S.J. (1987). The color isolation effect in free recall by adults with Down's syndrome. *American Journal of Mental Deficiency, 92,* 115–118.

Huer, M.B., (2000). Examining perceptions of graphic symbols across cultures: Preliminary study of the impact of culture/ethnicity. *Augmentative and Alternative Communication, 16,* 180–185.

Hunt-Berg, M. (1996). *Learning graphic symbols: The role of visual cues in interaction.* Doctoral dissertation, University of Nebraska, Lincoln.

Husband, T.H., & Hayden, D.C. (1996). Effects of the addition of color to assessment instruments. *Journal of Psychoeducational Assessment, 14,* 147–151.

Ittelson, W.H. (1996). Visual perception of markings. *Psychonomic Bulletin and Review, 3,* 171–187.

Johnson, C.J. (1992). Cognitive components of naming in children: Effects of referential uncertainty and stimulus realism. *Journal of Experimental Child Psychology, 53,* 24–44.

Johnson, C.J. (1995). Effects of color on children's naming of pictures. *Perceptual and Motor Skills, 80,* 1091–1101.

Johnson, C.J., Paivio, A., & Clark, J.A. (1996). Cognitive components of picture naming. *Psychological Bulletin, 120,* 113–139.

Johnson, M. (1987). *The body in the mind: The bodily basis of meaning, imagination, and reasoning.* Chicago: University of Chicago Press.

Klapper, Z.S., & Birch, H.G. (1969). Perceptual and action equivalence to objects and photographs in children. *Perceptual and Motor Skills, 29,* 763–771.

Kose, G., Beilin, H., & O'Connor, J. (1983). Children's comprehension of actions depicted in photographs. *Developmental Psychology, 19,* 636–643.

Kosslyn, S.M., & Osherson, D.N. (Eds.). (1995). *Visual cognition.* Cambridge: MIT Press.

Kozleski, E.B. (1991). Expectant delay procedure for teaching requests. *Augmentative and Alternative Communication, 7,* 11–19.

Levie, W.H. (1987). Research on pictures: A guide to the literature. In D.M. Willows & H.A. Houghton (Eds.), *The psychology of illustration: Vol. 1. Basic research* (pp. 1–50). New York: Springer-Verlag.

Liben, L.S. (1999). Developing an understanding of external spatial representations. In S.E. Irving (Ed.), *Development of mental representation: Theories and applications* (pp. 297–321). Mahwah, NJ: Lawrence Erlbaum Associates.

Liben, L.S., & Downs, R.M. (1991). The role of graphic representations in understanding the world. In R.M. Downs & L.S. Liben (Eds.), *Visions of aesthetics, the environment, and development: The legacy of Joachim F. Wohlwill* (pp. 139–180). Mahwah, NJ: Lawrence Erlbaum Associates.

Liben, L.S., Moore, M.L., & Golbeck, S.L. (1982). Preschoolers' knowledge of their classroom environment: Evidence from small-scale and life-size spatial tasks. *Child Development, 53,* 1275–1284.

Light, J. (1997). "Let's go star fishing": Reflections on the contexts of language learning for children who use aided AAC. *Augmentative and Alternative Communication, 13,* 158–171.

Lignugaris/Kraft, B., McCuller, G.L., Exum, M., & Salzberg, C.L. (1988). A review of research on picture reading skills of developmentally disabled individuals. *Journal of Special Education, 2,* 297–329.

Mandler, J.M., & McDonough, L. (1993). Concept formation in infancy. *Cognitive Development, 8,* 291–318.

Markman, E.M. (1989). *Categorization and naming in children.* Cambridge: MIT Press.

Marzolf, D.P., & DeLoache, J.S. (1994). Transfer in young children's understanding of spatial representations. *Child Development, 65,* 1–15.

McIlvane, W.J., Dube, W.V., Green, G., & Serna, R.W. (1992). Programming conceptual and communication skill development: A methodological stimulus class analysis. In S.F. Warren & J. Reichle (Series Eds.) & A.P. Kaiser & D.B. Gray (Vol. Eds.), *Communication and language intervention series: Vol. 2. Enhancing children's communication: Research foundations for intervention* (pp. 242–285). Baltimore: Paul H. Brookes Publishing Co.

Meador, D.E. (1984). Effects of color on visual discrimination of geometric symbols by severely and profoundly mentally retarded individuals. *American Journal of Mental Deficiency, 89,* 275–286.

Mervis, C.B. (1987). Child-basic object categories and early lexical development. In U. Neisser (Ed.), *Concepts and conceptual development: Ecological and intellectual factors in categorization* (pp. 201–233). Cambridge: Cambridge University Press.

Mineo, B. (1990, November). *Picture-based language representation: Implications for AAC and beyond.* Paper presented at the American Speech-Language-Hearing Association Convention, Seattle.

Mineo, B., & Goldstein, H. (1990). Generalized learning of receptive and expressive action-object responses by language-delayed preschoolers. *Journal of Speech and Hearing Disorders, 55,* 665–678.

Mineo, B., Peischl, D., Demasco, P., Gray, J., & Bender, R. (1995). *Assessing picture-related skills using Lascaux: Proceedings of the RESNA 1995 annual conference* (pp. 142–144). Arlington, VA: RESNA Press.

Mineo Mollica, B. (1997, November). Representing the way to language learning and expression. *ASHA SID 12 (AAC) Newsletter.* Rockville, MD: American Speech-Language-Hearing Association.

Mineo Mollica, B. (2002). *Pictorial representation: An analysis of the abilities of two young adults with severe mental retardation.* Manuscript in preparation.

Mineo Mollica, B., & Peischl, D. (1997, August). *Selecting picture-based language representations for AAC.* Paper presented at the United States Society for Augmentative and Alternative Communication Conference, Baltimore.

Mineo Mollica, B., Peischl, D., & Pennington, C. (2002). *Moving targets: Effect of animation on identification of actions.* Manuscript in preparation.

Mirenda, P. (1985). Designing pictorial communication systems for physically able-bodied students with severe handicaps. *Augmentative and Alternative Communication, 1,* 58–64.

Mirenda, P., & Locke, P.A. (1989). A comparison of symbol transparency in nonspeaking persons with intellectual disabilities. *Journal of Speech and Hearing Disorders, 54,* 131–140.

Mizuko, M. (1987). Transparency and ease of learning of symbols represented by Blissymbols, PCS, and Picsyms. *Augmentative and Alternative Communication, 3,* 129–136.

Mizuko, M., & Reichle, J. (1989). Transparency and recall of symbols among intellectually handicapped adults. *Journal of Speech and Hearing Disorders, 54,* 627–633.

Mizuko, M., Reichle, J., Ratcliff, A., & Esser, J. (1994). Effects of selection techniques and array sizes on short-term visual memory. *Augmentative and Alternative Communication, 10,* 237–244.

Oviatt, S.L. (1980). The emerging ability to comprehend language: An experimental approach. *Child Development, 51,* 97–106.

Oviatt, S.L. (1982). Inferring what words mean: Early development in infants' comprehension of common object names. *Child Development, 53,* 274–277.

Padula, W.V. (2000). *Neuro-optometric rehabilitation* (3rd ed.). Santa Ana, CA: Optometric Extension Program Foundation.

Parkin, A.J. (1996). *Explorations in cognitive neuropsychology.* Cambridge, MA: Blackwell Publishers.

Pick, H.L. (1983). Some issues on the relation between perceptual and cognitive development. In T.J. Tighe & B.E. Shepp (Eds.), *Perception, cognition, and development: Interactional analysis* (pp. 293–306). Mahwah, NJ: Lawrence Erlbaum Associates.

Pokorny, J., Smith, V.C., Verriest, G., & Pinckers, A.J.L.G. (1979). *Congenital and acquired color vision defects.* New York: Grune and Stratton.

Price, C.J., & Humphreys, G.W. (1989). The effects of surface detail on object categorization and naming. *Quarterly Journal of Experimental Psychology, 41A,* 797–828.

Raghavendra, P., & Fristoe, M. (1995). "No shoes; they walked away?": Effects of enhancement on learning and using Blissymbols by normal three year old children. *Journal of Speech and Hearing Research, 38,* 174–188.

Rao, S.C., Rainer, G., & Miller, W.J. (1997). Integration of what and where in the primate prefrontal cortex. *Science, 276,* 821–824.

Reichle, J. (1991). Defining the decisions involved in designing and implementing augmentative and alternative communication systems. In J. Reichle, J. York, &

J. Sigafoos (Eds.), *Implementing augmentative and alternative communication: Strategies for learners with severe disabilities* (pp. 39–60). Baltimore: Paul H. Brookes Publishing Co.

Reichle, J., & Yoder, D.E. (1985). Communication board use in severely handicapped learners. *Language, Speech, and Hearing Services in Schools, 16,* 146–157.

Romski, M.A, & Sevcik, R.A. (1992). Developing augmented language in children with severe mental retardation. In S. Warren & J. Reichle (Vol. & Series Eds.), *Communication and language intervention series: Vol. 1. Causes and effects of communication and language intervention* (pp. 113–130). Baltimore: Paul H. Brookes Publishing Co.

Romski, M.A., & Sevcik, R.A. (1993a). Language comprehension: Considerations for augmentative and alternative communication. *Augmentative and Alternative Communication, 9,* 281–285.

Romski, M.A, & Sevcik, R.A. (1993b). Language learning through augmented means. In S.F. Warren & J. Reichle (Series Eds.) & A.P. Kaiser & D.B. Grey (Eds.), *Communication and language intervention series: Vol. 2. Enhancing children's communication: Research foundations for intervention* (pp. 85–104). Baltimore: Paul H. Brookes Publishing Co.

Romski, M.A., & Sevcik, R.A. (1996). *Breaking the speech barrier: Language development through augmented means.* Baltimore: Paul H. Brookes Publishing Co.

Romski, M.A., Sevcik, R.A., & Adamson, L.B. (1997). Framework for studying how children with developmental disabilities develop language through augmented means. *Augmentative and Alternative Communication, 13,* 172–178.

Rose, S.A. (1977). Infants' transfer of response between two-dimensional and three-dimensional stimuli. *Child Development, 48,* 1086–1091.

Rowland, C., & Schweigert, P. (2000). Tangible symbols, tangible outcomes. *Augmentative and Alternative Communication, 16,* 61–78.

Schlosser, R.W., Belfiore, P.J., Nigam, R., Blischak, D., & Hetzroni, O. (1995). The effects of speech output technology in the learning of graphic symbols. *Journal of Applied Behavior Analysis, 28,* 537–549.

Schwartz, S.H. (1999). *Visual perception: A clinical orientation.* Stamford, CT: Appleton & Lange.

Seamon, J.G., Ganor-Sterm, D., Crowley, M.J., Wilson, S.M., Weber, W.J., O'Rourke, C.M., & Mahoney, J.K. (1997). A mere exposure effect for transformed three-dimensional objects: Effect of reflection, size, or color changes on affect and recognition. *Memory and Cognition, 25,* 367–374.

Sevcik, R.A., & Romski, M.A. (1986). Representational matching skills of persons with severe retardation. *Augmentative and Alternative Communication, 2,* 160–164.

Sevcik, R.A., & Romski, M.A. (1997). Comprehension and language acquisition: Evidence from youth with severe cognitive disabilities. In L.B. Adamson & M.A. Romski (Eds.), *Communication and language acquisition: Discoveries from atypical development* (pp. 187–202). Baltimore: Paul H. Brookes Publishing Co.

Sevcik, R.A., Romski, M.A., & Wilkinson, K. (1991). Roles of graphic symbols in the language acquisition process for persons with severe cognitive disabilities. *Augmentative and Alternative Communication, 7,* 161–170.

Shapley, R. (1990). Visual sensitivity and parallel retinocortical pathways. *Annual Review of Psychology, 41,* 635–658.

Sidman, M. (1994). *Equivalence relations: A research story.* Boston: Authors Cooperative.

Sigafoos, J., Doss, S., & Reichle, J. (1989). Developing mand and tact repertoires in persons with severe developmental disabilities using graphic symbols. *Research in Developmental Disabilities, 10,* 183–200.

Sigel, I.E. (1978). The development of pictorial comprehension. In B.S. Rhandhawa & W.E. Coffman (Eds.), *Visual learning, thinking and communication* (pp. 95–106). San Diego: Academic Press.

Silverman, F. (1995). *Communication for the speechless* (3rd ed.). Needham Heights, MA: Allyn & Bacon.

Slater, A., Rose, D., & Morison (1984). New-born infants' perception of similarities and differences between two- and three-dimensional stimuli. *British Journal of Developmental Psychology, 2,* 287–294.

Smith, M., & Grove, N. (1996). Input/output asymmetries–implications for language development in AAC. *Proceedings of the Seventh Biennial Conference of the International Society for Augmentative and Alternative Communication* (pp. 194–195). Vancouver, British Columbia: International Society for Augmentative and Alternative Communication.

Snodgrass, J.G., & Corwin, J. (1988). Perceptual identification thresholds for 150 fragmented pictures from the Snodgrass and Vanderwart picture set. *Perceptual and Motor Skills, 67,* 3–36.

Sorce, J. (1980). The role of operative knowledge in picture comprehension. *Journal of Genetic Psychology, 136,* 173–183.

Spelke, E.S., Gutheil, G., & Van de Walle, G. (1995). The development of object perception. In S.M. Kosslyn & D.N. Osherson (Eds.), *Visual cognition* (pp. 297–330). Cambridge: MIT Press.

Stephenson, J., & Linfoot, K. (1996). Pictures as communication symbols for students with severe intellectual disability. *Augmentative and Alternative Communication, 12,* 244–255.

Suchman, R.G., & Trabasso, T. (1966). Color and form preference in young children. *Journal of Experimental Child Psychology, 3,* 177–187.

Tanaka, K., Saito, H., Fukada, Y., & Moriya, M. (1991). Coding visual images of objects in the inferotemporal cortex of the macaque monkey. *Journal of Neurophysiology, 66,* 170–189.

Theios, J., & Amrhein, P.C. (1989). Theoretical analysis of the cognitive processing of lexical and pictorial stimuli: Reading, naming, and visual and conceptual comparisons. *Psychological Review, 96,* 5–24.

Tomikawa, S.A., & Dodd, D.H. (1980). Early word meanings: Perceptually or functionally based? *Child Development, 51,* 1103–1109.

Troscianko, T. (1987). Color vision: Brain mechanisms. In R.L. Gregory (Ed.), *The Oxford companion to the mind* (pp. 150–152). Oxford: Oxford University Press.

Tversky, B., & Hemenway, K. (1984). Objects, parts, and categories. *Journal of Experimental Psychology: General, 113,* 169–193.

Uttal, D., Schreiber, J.C., & DeLoache, J.S. (1995). Waiting to use a symbol: The effects of delay on children's use of models. *Child Development, 66,* 1875–1891.

Uttal, D.J., Scudder, K.V., & DeLoache, J.S. (1997). Manipulatives as symbols: A new perspective on the use of concrete objects to teach mathematics. *Journal of Applied Developmental Psychology, 18,* 37–54.

Wickens, C.D., & Andre, A.D. (1990). Proximity, compatability and information display: Effects of color, space, and objectness on information integration. *Human Factors, 32,* 61–71.

Wilkinson, K.M., Dube, W.V., & McIlvane, W.J. (1996). A crossdisciplinary perspective on studies of rapid word mapping in psycholinguistics and behavior analysis. *Developmental Review, 16,* 125–148.

Wilkinson, K.M., Dube, W.V., & McIlvane, W.J. (1998). Fast mapping and exclusion (emergent matching) in developmental language, behavior analysis, and animal cognition research. *The Psychological Record, 48,* 407–422.

Wilkinson, K.M., & McIlvane, W.J. (2001). Methods for studying symbolic behavior and category formation: Contributions of stimulus equivalence research. *Developmental Review, 21,* 355–374.

Wilkinson, K.M., Romski, M.A., & Sevcik, R.A. (1994). Emergence of visual-graphic symbol combinations by youth with moderate or severe mental retardation. *Journal of Speech and Hearing Research, 37,* 883–895.

Wilkinson, K.M., & Tager-Flusberg, H. (1998). Applications of a lexical principles framework for studying categorization and word learning in different populations. In S. Soraci & W.J. McIlvane (Eds.), *Perspectives on fundamental processes in intellectual functioning* (pp. 243–264). Stamford, CT: Ablex Publishers.

Zeaman, D., & Stanley, P. (1983). Stimulus preferences as structural features. In T.J. Tighe & B.E. Shepp (Eds.), *Perception, cognition, and development: Interactional analysis* (pp. 103–128). Mahwah, NJ: Lawrence Erlbaum Associates.

Zeki, S.M. (1993). *A vision of the brain.* Oxford, England: Blackwell Scientific.

5

Augmented Input

Enhancing Communication Development

MaryAnn Romski and Rose A. Sevcik

Typically developing children begin the communication development process by being exposed to spoken language input from their caregivers for almost a full year before they begin to produce their own spoken communications. Children and adults who use augmentative and alternative communication (AAC) often do not gain this type of linguistic input with AAC. Yoder and Kraat (1983) argued that there is a lack of communication models in the environment about how to effectively use AAC systems. Thus, children and adults are often asked to communicate with an AAC system that they have not observed employed for communication by another person. The focus of this chapter is on the role that augmented forms of communication input may play in the communication development of children and adults who use AAC systems. The chapter begins with an overview of the role of language input in development, followed by definitions of augmented input used in the AAC field, a framework by which to consider AAC input, and the evidence on augmented input in the literature. Finally, we close by suggesting some directions for research and clinical practice implications.

ROLE OF LANGUAGE INPUT IN DEVELOPMENT

The concept of augmented communication input has its roots in two literatures: the development of language and communication in young children and the concept of total communication discussed and debated in the literature on childhood deafness. In the literature on typical language develop-

The preparation of this chapter was funded by the National Institutes of Health Grant Nos. DC-03766 and DC-03799.

147

ment, language input, or *motherese* as it has been called, is defined as the adult's use of simplified language directed to the young child. The features of motherese include talking about objects, actions, and events in the here and now, short utterances that often omit functor words, exaggerated stress, and variable pitch (Berko-Gleason, 2001). The reasons that the adult's language is simplified has to do with the immaturity of the child's language system. Thus, the adult uses "motherese" to focus the child's attention on the language that is being addressed to him or her.

Since the 1970s, Bruner (1975) and his colleagues have argued that adult input (i.e., motherese) plays an important role in child language development. From birth onward, children are exposed to their native language day in and day out. Much of this input language is naturally matched to the child's level of speech comprehension by the partners. Even though the specific role spoken language input plays in the language development of typically developing children is still under debate, it is clear that language is learned in social, interactive contexts and language input from partners is a natural part of the communicative exchange. Typically developing children are spoken to by their caregivers and others and receive a substantial amount of communicative input prior to speaking themselves (Gallaway & Richards, 1994).

The role of spoken language input, or motherese, has received considerable attention in the literatures on the language development and intervention of children with developmental language disorders who speak (e.g., Conti-Ramsden, 1994; Fey, 1986; Paul, 1995). Warren and Yoder (1997) argued that input matters for these children. The rate and quality of the communication input that children receive is critically important to their development. This literature has focused its attention on assessing potential differences between typically developing children and children with disabilities with the goal of developing intervention strategies that may enhance language development (e.g., Cardoso-Martins & Mervis, 1984; Conti-Ramsden, 1994). Some of these studies have identified aspects of the language environment that differ between children with and without disabilities including adult directiveness and parent social responsivity (Yoder, Warren, McCathren, & Leew, 1998). Interactions between parents and children with language disorders are often different from those between parents and typically developing children because the children encounter difficulty communicating wants and needs. Parents then employ a directive style to compensate for the child's communication difficulties. Responsiveness to a child's communication attempts has been shown to correlate with faster acquisition of vocabulary.

With respect to children with all types of language disorders, enhancing input might have a facilitative effect on language and communication development. Two types of enhancement have been studied in the literature. The first is the addition of the visual mode to the auditory mode. The literature on childhood deafness referred to the term *total communication* as an intervention approach that incorporates both sign and spoken languages as language input (Kretschmer & Kretschmer, 1978). The theoretical rationale for the use of total communication is that children who cannot hear the spoken word need to have access to a visual form of the message in order to develop receptive and expressive language and communication skills. This type of enhancement is clearly one part of AAC intervention. The second type of enhancement comes from the literature on child language disorders including childhood deafness (Gallaway & Woll, 1994). It is linguistically specific (e.g., short sentences, saying verbs before demonstrating actions) and is used as part of language intervention strategies.

Together these literatures provide clear evidence that language input does affect the rate and quality of language development for both typically and atypically developing children (Hart & Risley, 1995). Because language input can be enhanced to facilitate language development, it seems particularly important to consider the role of input language with respect to AAC interventions.

DEFINITIONS OF
AUGMENTED COMMUNICATION INPUT

In the AAC literature, there have been at least two variations on the use of adult communicative input that encompass both types of enhancement and are used as part of broader language intervention approaches. The enhanced input to which children and adults who use AAC systems are typically exposed has been termed *aided language stimulation* (Goossens' & Crain, 1986) or *augmented communicative input* (Romski & Sevcik, 1988).

Goossens' and Crain (1986) defined aided language stimulation as, in many ways, analogous to the total communication and simultaneous communication approaches that appear in the manual sign language intervention literature. When providing aided language stimulation, primary and secondary facilitators (parent, teacher, and/or clinician) use activity-specific aided language stimulation boards throughout daily routines to point out key picture symbols on a communication display. These techniques are employed in conjunction with other ongoing verbal language stimulation. The type of display format or the selection techniques used by the child is irrelevant to the facilitator's use of the technique as noted by Goossens' (1989). Engineering the environment, including developing overlays and selecting vocabulary specific to daily activities, are critical components. One goal of aided language stimulation is that of nurturing the receptive understanding of speech and symbols (Goossens', Jennings, & Kinahan, 2000). Goossens' and her colleagues argue that it is essential to establish receptive language in order to obtain expressive language. Table 5.1 provides an example of aided language stimulation.

Table 5.1.   Example of aided language stimulation

Martha (M) is the facilitator, and George (G) is an adolescent with cerebral palsy who uses an eye-gaze display. They are baking cookies together. Martha points to each capitalized symbol on George's display while talking.

M: Let's get the COOKIE MIX and the BOWL. I'll put the COOKIE MIX IN the BOWL. [uses a sabotage routine by putting the box in the bowl without opening it, thus providing a contextual cue to elicit George's use of the symbol OPEN]

G: [laughs but does not eye gaze to OPEN]

M: Uh-oh! I guess I did something wrong here! I wonder what the problem is? [pauses for 5 seconds to give George time to look at the OPEN symbol (indirect verbal cue)]

G: [vocalizes agreement that something is wrong but does not look at the symbol]

M: [uses a search light cue by scanning her small flashlight across all the symbols on George's display, and then pauses for another 5 seconds]

G: [watches but does not respond]

M: I forgot to do something with the cookie mix box. [direct verbal cue and 5-second pause]

G: [still does not look at the OPEN symbol]

M: [provides a momentary light cue by flashing her light directly on the OPEN symbol for 2–3 seconds]

G: [still does not respond]

M: [provides a constant flashing light cue by shining her light directly on the OPEN symbol until George looks at it to select it]

G: [looks at the OPEN symbol]

M: Oh! Right! I need to OPEN the COOKIE MIX before I PUT it IN the BOWL! Thank you, George! [opens box]

From Beukelman, D.R., & Mirenda, P. (1998). *Augmentative and alternative communication: Management of severe communication disorders in children and adults* (2nd ed., p. 352). Baltimore: Paul H. Brookes Publishing Co.; reprinted by permission.

Romski and Sevcik (1988) defined augmented communication input as one of five components of the System for Augmenting Language (SAL). In SAL, intervention takes place within naturally occurring events in homes, classrooms, and community settings and mandates an integral role in the overall instructional process for the participant's partners. The augmented input component was characterized as the incoming communication or language from the individual's communicative partner that includes speech and is supplemented by AAC symbols, the speech output produced by the AAC device when the symbol is activated, and the environmental context. Communicative partners are encouraged to integrate the use of the devices into their own spoken language communications. In the example, "Jane, let's GO read a BOOK," *go* and *book* are symbols touched on the AAC board or device, produced by the device's speech output (synthetic or digitized), and emphasized verbally by the individual's partner. This communicative model permits each partner to incorporate the device's use more simply into his or her specific communicative interactions as shown in the two examples in Table 5.2.

To ensure that primary communicative partners (e.g., parents, teachers) understand and are comfortable with their roles using SAL, they are explicitly taught to use the device to provide augmented input. This instruction can in-

Table 5.2.   Two samples of partner augmented input

Sample 1
M   Eat your {HOT DOG}.
B   {HOT DOG}.
M   {NAPKIN}.
M   It's on the other side of the plate.
B   XX {points to napkin}.
M   Yeah.

Sample 2
T   Then you get one cracker.
T   One cracker off the plate {PLATE}.
=   In the above utterance, the teacher interrupted herself as she said plate.
P   Plate
T   Sherrie, do you have {NAPKIN}?
=   P Shows T her napkin.
T   OK.
T   Kevin, what do you want to drink today?
K   XX.
T   OK, bring your {GLASS} and your {PLATE}.

From Romski, M.A., & Sevcik, R.A. (1996). *Breaking the speech barrier: Language development through augmented means* (p. 67). Baltimore: Paul H. Brookes Publishing Co.; reprinted by permission.

Note: Transcripts are in Systematic Analysis of Language Transcripts (SALT; Miller & Chapman, 1985) format. Codes are from the Communication Coding Scheme (CCS).

{ } = symbol use; = = comment; XX = unintelligible vocalization; M = mother; T = teacher; K, B, = participants; P = peer.

clude a series of instructional meetings prior to the child's introduction to the device. These meetings serve several functions for the partners, who receive instruction in the physical operation of the speech-output communication device and view videotapes depicting interactions with the devices to illustrate examples of augmented input communicative use. Partners also may engage in role-playing activities to ensure that they are comfortable providing augmented communication input. During the ongoing intervention, the partners' use of augmented communication input is monitored by the clinician and coaching is implemented during the intervention to encourage input from the communicative partners (e.g., teachers, caregivers, siblings).

The rationale for the inclusion of an augmented input component is that the individuals need a model of how to employ the device during daily activities (Romski & Sevcik, 1996). The visual and auditory input provided by the partners may also permit participants to extract previously unobtainable spoken words from the language-learning environment. Speech comprehension can develop even when the individual is not speaking and thus can be a link between the auditory and visual symbol modalities (Sevcik & Romski, 1997, 2002; Sevcik, Romski, & Adamson, 2001).

In summary, these two interventions share many commonalities. They highlight the role of the partner in communication interaction with the individual who uses AAC. They also target the importance of comprehension to the language development process.

CONCEPTUAL FRAMEWORK FOR AUGMENTED INPUT INTERVENTIONS

Augmented input interventions include three interrelated components: the partners, the child or adult who uses AAC, and the broader social community in which the person who uses AAC and partners interact. The partner and the individual who uses AAC interact in social conversations that occur in the broader social context. The scope of the relationships is illustrated in Figure 5.1.

Partners

Partners can be familiar or unfamiliar and can include caregivers, siblings, friends, teachers, and others. Familiar partners interact with the individual who uses AAC on a regular and consistent basis and support the individual in his or her communications. Light and Binger (1998) refer to these familiar partners as facilitators. Unfamiliar partners are those who interact with the individual who uses AAC on an intermittent basis and who often have little prior knowledge of the individual's communication skills and style.

Because augmented input interventions focus on communication in natural settings, a broader concept of partner is fundamental to the communicative process. Partners play two rather obvious roles in the communication exchange: They are speakers providing communicative input to the youth and listeners who then respond to the youth's communications. By virtue of the visual component, the ways in which the partner communicates with the participant are modified. An instructional focus that encompasses partners must then include considerations of both their speaker and listener roles. Additionally, some emphasis needs to be placed on instruction directed towards the partner's physical operation of the speech-output communication device itself. Using this framework for partners, focused attention on instruction for the partner is essential if the intervention strategy is to succeed. This partner instruction must be directed towards adult learning strategies and encompass a broad range of activities over the course of the intervention in order to succeed.

People Who Use AAC

Who is the person who uses AAC who can benefit from enhanced input? By using a theoretical framework grounded in language development, the primary group of individuals who use AAC with whom augmented input would

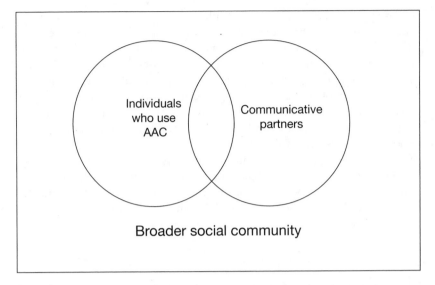

Figure 5.1.   Interrelated components of augmented language intentions.

be employed is children or adults who are just beginning to develop communication skills. Because typically developing children move through the early stages of development so quickly, it is also difficult to specify what role augmented input can play in later stages of language development. In our experience, it can serve to provide models for the development of semantic relations and word order though there is no empirical evidence beyond single words/symbols. It is important to note, however, that the concept of augmented input has also been employed with adults who have severe aphasia. Garrett and Beukelman (1992) categorized the various communication skills of adults with severe aphasia. They described one type of communicator with severe aphasia as the "augmented-input communicator." These were individuals who encountered particular difficulty comprehending spoken language, especially when the language was complex or the conversational focus shifted. Furthermore, Garrett and Beukelman suggested that partners should provide augmented input to supplement the speech of augmented-input communicators through gestures, visual symbols, and written language.

What role does augmented input serve for the individual who uses AAC? Romski and Sevcik (1996) argued that partner-augmented input serves several functions for the child or adult. First, it provides a model for how the AAC device can be used, in what contexts, and for what purposes. When augmented input is employed by the participant's communicative partners, the pairing of the visual symbol with the synthetic or digitized speech output may permit the individual who uses AAC to extract previously unobtainable spoken words from the language learning environment. The specific way in which the symbols are produced and paired with synthetic or digitized speech segments the critical word/symbol from the natural stream of speech (e.g., "Let's see your BIKE") and may facilitate the matching of the symbol or word with its physical referent. This then facilitates the person who uses AAC's comprehension of individual spoken words and/or visual-graphic symbols by highlighting the individual symbol–word relationships. Second, it has the potential to reinforce the effectiveness of using the AAC system; when a partner incorporates the use of the device in successful communicative exchanges, it provides the individual who uses AAC with real-world experiences that illustrate the meaning of symbols and the varied functions they serve. The individual who uses AAC then experiences the potential utility and power of the system. Finally and perhaps most importantly, partner-augmented input makes an implicit statement to the individual who uses AAC and the broader community that the AAC device provides an acceptable vehicle for communicating.

Broader Social Community

The broader social community is the context in which the communications of partners and people who use AAC are embedded. Very little is known about how the use of augmented communication input influences the perceptions and attitudes held by the community as a whole and by unfamiliar partners about the competence of an individual who uses AAC. Use of augmented input may also teach the broader social community about how to communicate with individuals who use AAC through observational learning. Romski and Sevcik reported an exchange that illustrates the potential for partner-augmented input to influence perception.

> One day, a peer tutor was communicating with TF when a friend of the peer tutor joined them. The friend started talking to the peer tutor but ignored TF. The peer tutor said, "This is the way we talk," pointing to the SAL. His friend responded by saying he did not know how to use it. The peer tutor quickly said, "It's easy. You touch it, and it talks for you. TF will show you." The conversation then continued, with all three using the SAL to talk. (1996, pp. 100–101)

We have only begun to consider the broader impact of using AAC on the social community. In the long term, it has the potential to change attitudes and beliefs about AAC communicators.

EVIDENCE ABOUT THE ROLE OF AUGMENTED COMMUNICATION INPUT

There is only modest evidence about the role of augmented communication input. Table 5.3 provides a summary of five investigations directed toward

Table 5.3. Studies about aided language stimulation/augmented communicative input

Study	Type	Participants	Intervention	Findings
Goossens' (1989)	Case study	6-year-old girl with cerebral palsy	7 months of aided language stimulation	Frequent interactive symbol use; emergence of functional speech
Sevcik et al. (1995)	Descriptive report from longitudinal study	13 school-age youth with moderate or severe cognitive impairments and their parents and teachers	System for Augmenting Language (SAL), including augmented input across beginning, middle, and end of a school year	Small percentage of partner's input contained symbol input; more symbol input to beginning SAL achievers than advanced achievers
Peterson et al. (1995)	Case study	7- and 9-year-old boys with autism	One year of intervention with three different communicative inputs	Augmented input facilitated both boys' performance
Romski et al. (1999)	Pilot case study	34-month-old toddler with developmental delays and his mother	10-week parent training intervention focused on augmented input	Increase in speech comprehension skills; emergence of symbol productions
Romski et al. (2001)	Longitudinal study; randomized assignment to one of three interventions	60 toddlers (24–36 months) and their primary caregivers	12-week parent training intervention (augmented input intervention, augmented output intervention, or no augmentation)	Ongoing

AAC and language input. The focus of all of these studies has been on the outcomes for the person who uses AAC rather than the partner or the broader community.

Goossens' (1989) first reported on the successful use of aided language stimulation intervention with a 6-year-old girl with cerebral palsy. Seven months of aided language stimulation seemed to foster frequent interactive symbol use, and functional speech emerged as well.

As part of a longitudinal study of augmented language learning by youth with moderate or severe cognitive disabilities described previously, Romski and Sevcik (1996) used SAL as the intervention approach. One important component of SAL was that the investigators instructed the participants' adult partners (primarily parents and teachers) to serve as a model of AAC use by supplementing their spoken communicative input to the youth with visual-graphic symbols from their speech-output communication system. Sevcik, Romski, Watkins, and Deffebach (1995) then examined the quantity and quality of the symbol input employed by the partners of these 13 youth at three points across one school year (i.e., beginning, middle, and end). They reported that only a small percentage (mean = 9.6%, SD = 6.99) of the partners' overall spoken communicative utterances directed to the youth contained symbol input. The sophistication of the young people's speech comprehension skills, however, differentially affected the amount of AAC symbol input they received from their adult partners. Partners used more AAC symbol input with the beginning SAL achievers who had poor speech comprehension skills (mean = 12.8%) than with the advanced SAL achievers who demonstrated comprehension skills at or greater than 24 months of age (mean = 7.7%). Symbols embedded in the spoken utterances of the adults were significantly more likely to occur in the final position of an utterance than in either the beginning or middle position of the utterance regardless of the youth's achievement pattern. Not surprisingly, school partners (most often teachers) were more directive in their use of augmented input than home partners (most often parents) whose communications were evenly divided between directive and facilitative. The other important result of this study was that home and school adult partners with relatively modest amounts of instruction in how to provide SAL input were quite skilled in presenting the augmented input in a salient and facilitative manner to the youth.

Peterson, Bondy, Vincent, and Finnegan (1995) assessed the effects of interventions in three communicative input modalities on the task performance and frequency of target behaviors of two boys with autism and challenging behaviors (7 and 9 years of age). The three different communicative inputs were spoken language input alone, pictorial or gestural communicative input alone, and augmented input (pictorial or gestural input plus spoken input). They reported that spoken input alone did not facilitate performance as well as the augmented input for either child. In fact, they suggested that spoken input alone may actually increase challenging behaviors.

More recently, Romski, Sevcik, Adamson, Browning, Williams, and Colbert (1999) completed a pilot study to examine the effects of an augmented input intervention focused on teaching a parent to use the strategy with a 34-month-old toddler with disabilities including partial trisomy 13, cerebral palsy, and significant developmental delay. This boy had speech comprehension skills assessed at about 15 months on the Sequenced Inventory of Communication Development–Revised (SICD–R; Hedrick, Prather, & Tobin, 1984). His expressive communication skills on the SICD–R were 6 months, and he had some undifferentiated vocalizations and a laugh that was not employed communicatively. He did not comprehend the meanings for any of the visual-graphic symbols to be taught (e.g., MORE, ALL DONE, BOOK, SNACK, DRINK, BUBBLES, JACK-IN-THE-BOX).

A 10-week intervention protocol was implemented in a structured environment focused on teaching the parent to provide augmented communication input using visual-graphic symbols and a speech-output communication device to her child. There were two 30-minute sessions per week for a total of 20 sessions. The intervention increased his symbol and speech comprehension skills for the target vocabulary items from 0 to 10 words across a 10-week period. After 6 weeks, there was also a steady increase in his spontaneous use of symbols to communicate messages. Initially, his symbol productions appeared random and resembled "babbling." As these random productions decreased, intentional communicative symbol productions increased. There was no comparable change in spoken language production skills over the course of the intervention period. His mother spontaneously reported that she appreciated the intervention approach because it did not place demands on her to make her child use the communication device. This input strategy permitted the parent to be successful regardless of the child's response. That is, the child did not have to perform a specific action in order for the parent to think the child is implementing the intervention strategy (Romski, Sevcik, & Forrest, 2001).

This pilot study provided preliminary evidence that augmented communication input may serve at least three distinct functions. First, it may yield increased symbol and sometimes speech comprehension skills. Second, it may provide an intervention that is comfortable for parents and partners to implement, and third, it may facilitate productive communicative use of symbols. Because it was only a pilot study with one participant, it could not rule out the role of the young child's natural development on the outcome. Additional studies of augmented input interventions are needed to evaluate the effects of utilizing AAC input as an intervention strategy for AAC communicators.

Romski, Sevcik, and Adamson are assessing the relative effects of this augmented input intervention strategy described previously in comparison to two other early communication interventions, one focused on augmented communication output and the other focused on communication interaction with no augmentation. In this ongoing longitudinal study, a total of 60 toddlers with disabilities (24–36 months) are being recruited and randomly assigned to one of these three interventions. The child and his or her parent (primary caregiver) participate in a 12-week parent-implemented intervention protocol and then are followed at 3-, 6-, and 12-month postintervention intervals. The intervention protocol for all three interventions is focused on teaching the parent to use specific communication strategies at home during daily routines. Each 30-minute intervention session includes three 10-minute routines around play, book reading, and snack. Parents first observe the child and an interventionist prior to implementing the interaction themselves with coaching from the interventionist. In this context, we expect to be able to articulate the effects of the augmented input intervention approach for young children with severe communication disabilities. To date, participant recruitment and data collection are underway with approximately 30 participants at one of the three study phases.

In summary, there has been, at best, a modest amount of research on the role of augmented input in the communication development process. The research has focused almost exclusively on the gains made by individuals who use AAC themselves. With the exception of Sevcik and colleagues' (1995) description of the linguistic aspects of the partner's input, there has been little attention directed towards the partner or the broader social community.

FUTURE RESEARCH DIRECTIONS

As the previous discussion suggests, the evaluation of augmented communication input or aided language stimulation as an AAC intervention strategy is in its early stages. Aided language stimulation has been used in clinical practice since the late 1980s without experimental examination of its outcomes (Beukelman & Mirenda, 1998). Augmented input has been employed as part of SAL in research studies on the effects of AAC intervention for individuals with severe developmental and communication disorders. It has not, however, been evaluated in comparison to other strategies. Future research studies must address issues related to SAL's effects on the individual who uses AAC, the role of the partner, and its broader social effects.

There are a number of methodological challenges to studying the effects of augmented communication input on the communication development of individuals using AAC for communication. Perhaps the most striking challenge in studying this augmented language intervention strategy is how to isolate the effects of the input on the individual's communication development. Oftentimes, input is provided in concert with an encouragement of symbol production, and it is difficult to separate the effects of the input alone. In order to do so, the input provided must be operationally defined.

A focus on augmented input requires that researchers rethink how they measure change during beginning AAC interventions. Measurement must include assessments of both the visual and auditory components of the inputs. In SAL, for example, visual symbol input is always paired with auditory speech-output from the communication device. Aided language stimulation does not stress the use of a speech-output communication device but highlights the visual-graphic symbol. What differences are there between using a speech-output communication device versus using a conversation board without speech output? What input is the individual focused on—the visual input, the auditory input, or a combination of both? Measurement tools must be developed that permit investigators to determine the relative effects of different aspects of the input.

Another aspect of augmented input that provides a challenge for investigators is the role of the partner. Partners vary in how they provide augmented input and/or aided language stimulation. How does the communication style of the partner affect the provision of augmented input? In turn, how does the person who uses AAC utilize the input provided? It is also important for investigation to focus some attention on partner instructional strategies including, for example, how well partners implement the strategies and how much generalization there is across settings.

Is augmented input an effective language intervention strategy? Is it better than other intervention approaches and for whom? The precise roles input can play in developing comprehension and production of AAC systems by a range of individuals who use AAC must be specified. Intervention studies that specify the exact effects of augmented input on AAC learning and use are needed. Perhaps most essential are investigations that focus on the role augmented input can play in beginning AAC use because input plays its most critical role during the earliest stages of development. Later, after a new vocabulary is established, does it still play a role in the development of vocabulary and semantic relations?

What is the breadth of application for this intervention? Very little is known about the groups of people who use AAC who can benefit from augmented input interventions. It appears that beginning communicators with a range of etiologies are the primary focus for this type of intervention. Mirenda and Erickson (2000) suggested that children with autism who engage in challenging behaviors may benefit when spoken language is enhanced with the visual modality. It would be important, however, to document the range of individuals who use AAC for whom this intervention is successful or not successful. Finally, does gender or culture affect its implementation?

PRACTICE IMPLICATIONS

With respect to practice implications, there are at least three important considerations for clinicians. The first implication is a philosophical one. Beginning AAC interventions do not have to initially demand symbol production from the individual. This change in focus requires that the clinician communicate information and materials to the individual's partners in a different way. One reason for the almost exclusive focus on production is that the outcome—symbol production—is visible and readily documented. A focus on input suggests that the outcome may be less visible. Thus, the clinician must convey the importance of establishing comprehension as a foundation for productive symbol use. Second, a focus on augmented input requires that researchers rethink how they measure change and document outcomes during beginning AAC interventions. For example, Romski and Sevcik (1996) reported that if they had only measured production, 4 of the 13 participants they studied would have not shown change using the speech-output communication device they were given to communicate because their learning occurred more slowly and, initially, in a different domain (comprehension rather than production) than the remaining nine participants. If an individual has limited speech comprehension skills, augmented language interventions may first need to incorporate a comprehension and input focus before placing demands on the individual to produce symbols. Third, clinicians must support the role partners play in the development of AAC communication skills. From the onset of intervention, this support may come in the form of specific direct instruction and coaching about how to structure language and communication input to the individual who uses AACs. Without this type of targeted support, it is unlikely that augmented input interventions will be successful.

In sum, augmented communication input is an under-utilized component of AAC intervention. It can serve to facilitate communicative competence by expanding symbol and speech comprehension skills, which provide a foundation for symbol production. In turn, it may also facilitate the production of symbols in the beginning communicator.

REFERENCES

Berko-Gleason, J. (2001). *The development of language*. Needham Heights, MA: Allyn & Bacon.

Beukelman, D.R., & Mirenda, P. (1998). *Augmentative and alternative communication: Management of severe communication disorders in children and adults* (2nd ed.). Baltimore: Paul H. Brookes Publishing Co.

Bruner, J. (1975). The ontogenesis of speech acts. *Journal of Child Language, 2,* 1–19.

Cardoso-Martins, C., & Mervis, C. (1984). Maternal speech to prelinguistic children with Down Syndrome. *American Journal on Mental Deficiency, 89,* 451–458.

Conti-Ramsden, G. (1994). Language interaction with atypical language learners. In C. Gallaway & B. Richards (Eds.), *Input and interaction in language acquisition* (pp. 181–196). Oxford: Cambridge University Press.

Fey, M. (1986). *Language intervention with young children*. San Diego: College-Hill Press.

Gallaway, C., & Richards, B.J. (1994). *Input and interaction in language acquisition.* New York: Cambridge University Press.

Gallaway, C., & Woll, B. (1994). Interaction and childhood deafness. In C. Gallaway & B. Richards (Eds.), *Input and interaction in language acquisition* (pp. 197–218). Oxford: Cambridge University Press.

Garrett, K., & Beukelman, D. (1992). Augmentative communication approaches for persons with severe aphasia. In K. Yorkston (Ed.), *Augmentative communication in a medical setting* (pp. 245–338). Tucson, AZ: Communication Skill Builders.

Goossens', C. (1989). Aided communication intervention before assessment: A case study of a child with cerebral palsy. *Augmentative and Alternative Communication, 5,* 14–26.

Goossens', C., & Crain, S. (1986). *Augmentative communication intervention resource.* Wauconda, IL: Don Johnston.

Goossens', C., Jennings, D., & Kinahan, D. (2000, August). *Facilitating strategies for group activities in engineered AAC classrooms.* Preconference workshop presented at the Ninth Biennial Conference of the International Society for Augmentative and Alternative Communication, Washington, DC.

Hart, B., & Risley, T.R. (1995). *Meaningful differences in the everyday experience of young American children.* Baltimore: Paul H. Brookes Publishing Co.

Hedrick, D., Prather, E., & Tobin, A. (1984). *Sequenced Inventory of Communication Development.* Los Angeles: Western Psychological Services.

Kretschmer, R., & Kretschmer, L. (1978). *Perspectives in audiology series: Language development and intervention with the hearing impaired.* Baltimore: University Park Press.

Light, J.C., & Binger, C. (1998). *Building communicative competence with individuals who use augmentative and alternative communication.* Baltimore: Paul H. Brookes Publishing Co.

Miller, J., & Chapman, R. (1985). *Systematic Analysis of Language Transcripts (SALT)* [Computer software]. Madison: University of Wisconsin.

Mirenda, P., & Erickson, K.A. (2000). Augmentative communication and literacy. In A.M. Wetherby & B.M. Prizant (Eds.), *Autism spectrum disorders: A transactional developmental perspective* (pp. 333–368). Baltimore: Paul H. Brookes Publishing Co.

Paul, R. (1995). *Language disorders from infancy through adolescence.* St Louis: Mosby.

Peterson, S., Bondy, A., Vincent, Y., & Finnegan, C. (1995). Effects of altering communicative input for students with autism and no speech: Two case studies. *Augmentative and Alternative Communication, 11,* 93–100.

Romski, M.A., & Sevcik, R.A. (1988). Augmentative communication system acquisition and use: A model for teaching and assessing progress. *NSSLHA Journal, 16,* 61–74.

Romski, M.A., & Sevcik, R.A. (1996). *Breaking the speech barrier: Language development through augmented means.* Baltimore: Paul H. Brookes Publishing Co.

Romski, M.A., Sevcik, R.A., Adamson, L.B., Browning, J., Williams, S., & Colbert, N. (1999, November). *Augmented communication input intervention for toddlers: A pilot study.* Poster session presented at the annual meeting of the American Speech-Language-Hearing Association, San Francisco.

Romski, M.A., Sevcik, R.A., & Forrest, S. (2001). Assistive technology and augmentative communication in inclusive early childhood programs. In M.J. Guralnick (Ed.), *Early childhood inclusion: Focus on change* (pp. 465–479). Baltimore: Paul H. Brookes Publishing Co.

Sevcik, R.A., & Romski, M.A. (1997). Comprehension and language acquisition: Evidence from youth with severe cognitive disabilities. In L.B. Adamson & M.A. Romski (Eds.), *Communication and language acquisition: Discoveries from atypical language development* (pp. 187–202). Baltimore: Paul H. Brookes Publishing Co.

Sevcik, R.A., & Romski, M.A. (2002). The role of language comprehension in establishing early augmented conversations. In D.R. Beukelman & J. Reichle (Series Eds.) & J. Reichle, D.R. Beukelman, & J.C. Light (Vol. Eds.), *Augmentative and alternative communication series: Exemplary practices for beginning communicators: Implications for AAC* (pp. 453–476) Baltimore: Paul H. Brookes Publishing Co.

Sevcik, R.A., Romski, M.A., & Adamson, L.B. (2001, March). *Toddlers with developmental disabilities who are not speaking: Receptive language skills and augmented language intervention outcomes.* Paper presented at the Gatlinburg Conference on Research and Theory in Mental Retardation and Developmental Disabilities, Charleston, SC.

Sevcik, R.A., Romski, M.A., Watkins, R., & Deffebach, K. (1995). Adult partner-augmented communication input to youth with mental retardation using the system for augmenting language (SAL). *Journal of Speech and Hearing Research, 38,* 902–912.

Warren, S., & Yoder, P. (1997). Emerging models of communication and language intervention. *Mental Retardation and Developmental Disabilities Research Reviews, 3,* 358–362.

Yoder, D., & Kraat, A. (1983). Intervention issues in nonspeech communication. In J. Miller, D. Yoder & R. Schiefelbsuch (Eds.), *Contemporary issues in language intervention* (pp. 27–51). Rockville, MD: American Speech-Language-Hearing Association.

Yoder, P., Warren, S., McCathren, R., & Leew, S. (1998). Does adult responsivity to child behavior facilitate communication development? In S.F. Warren & M.E. Fey (Series Eds.) & A.M. Wetherby, S.F. Warren, & J. Reichle (Vol. Eds.), *Communication and language intervention series: Vol. 7. Transitions in prelinguistic communication* (pp. 39–58). Baltimore: Paul H. Brookes Publishing Co.

6

Asymmetry in Input and Output for Individuals Who Use AAC

Martine M. Smith and Nicola Clare Grove

At least three factors can be presumed to influence the language acquisition process: the structural characteristics of the target language; the input provided to the language-learning child; and the uptake, or processing by the child of the input received. However, the relative importance of each of these influences is as yet unresolved (Harris, 1992; McDonald, 1997). A further matter of debate is the nature of the relationship between comprehension and production in language acquisition and the role children's production experiences play in their induction of the language rules of their community. This chapter considers the relationship between input and output for children who can hear and understand speech but who depend on alternative and augmentative communication (AAC), such as manual signs or graphic representations, for language production. For these children, there is an asymmetry between the modalities of input and output. We attempt to determine some of the clinical and educational implications of such asymmetry and consider how to address the gaps in our existing knowledge.

The population of individuals who use AAC systems is heterogeneous; generalizations, therefore, must always be tempered. Each individual presents a unique profile of abilities and challenges, of language learning opportunities and communication options, and of communication needs and learning supports. It is proposed here that the situation of individuals who benefit from nonspeech communication systems to augment their spoken communication may be fundamentally different from that of individuals for whom nonspeech modalities function as an alternative to spoken language. The particular focus of this chapter is on language development, as evidenced in the emergence of structural regularities in the use of manual or graphic signs. We are interested in how the atypical productive experiences of many individuals who use manual or graphic signs may influence the acquisition of language structure for at least some individuals with severe congenital speech impairments.

Communication is a transactional process—individuals mutually influence each other, as communication turns are negotiated between participants in a conversation. Communication context and partners can influence what is talked about, how much talk is produced, and how power relationships within a conversation are determined (e.g., Rondal, 1980; Snow, 1995). These influences may be even stronger in conversations where there is one participant with a severe speech impairment (Light, Collier, & Parnes, 1985a; Smith, 2003). However, there is no evidence to suggest that fundamental regularities of language structure are equally vulnerable to contextual influences. Thus, while acknowledging the importance of partner influences, it may be possible to explore aspects of the development of structure by considering the "talk" produced by individuals with the ability to hear and understand speech but who communicate expressively using manual or graphic signs and other modalities of communication.

Acquisition theories vary in their predictions of the extent of grammatical knowledge that children can acquire with atypical productive experience (Sutton, 1997). Theories that focus on input as a primary source for language acquisition (e.g., Crain & Fodor, 1993; Pinker, 1994) suggest that development should not be impeded if productive experiences differ from a presumed norm. By contrast, theories that emphasize a functional source of expressive language (e.g., Ninio & Snow, 1988) allow greater room for such experiences to influence the developmental process. Sutton (1997) pointed out that, even if receptive language is a sufficient basis for expressive language, people can make few assumptions about the grammatical knowledge of children who have significant speech production difficulties (Blockberger, 1997; see also Chapter 3). In fact, assumptions of any kind are difficult, given the heterogeneity of individuals who may require augmentation of their communication skills; however, there is growing evidence that many of these children have atypical patterns of expression when viewed in relation to typically developing speaking children. Furthermore, their patterns of expression share similarities across both graphic and manual modalities. Patterns reported include a tendency to rely on single-term utterances (Bruno, 1989; Spiegel, Benjamin, & Spiegel, 1993; von Tetzchner & Martinsen, 1996); relatively high frequency of word order errors (Grove, 1995; Grove & Dockrell, 2000; van Balkom & Donker-Gimbrère, 1996); and lack of internal morphological or clause structure (Grove, 1995; Grove et al., 1996; Smith, 1996). To fully explore the challenges facing individuals acquiring language using nonspeech modalities, we need to consider the differential effects of AAC system characteristics on a developing language system.

Typical Language Development

In typical language development, children must acquire mastery over both the conceptual aspects of language and the rule-governed computational domains of phonology, morphology, and syntax. The input they receive represents conceptual information in patterned structural forms. The child's task is to infer meanings and map those meanings onto the formal structures used for their expression, that is, to analyze the input not only for its conceptual content, but also its computational characteristics. Three aspects of experience are presumed to interact in this process: the structure of the ambient language, the input to the child, and the child's own processing mechanisms (Harris, 1992; McDonald, 1997), although the relative contribution of each aspect is the subject of some debate (e.g., Nelson, 1997; Piatelli-Palmarini, 1980, 1994).

Spoken language input is composed of organizational units far smaller than individual words—syllables and subsyllabic units such as individual phonemic segments. Evidence from both typical and atypical language development suggests that these sublexical properties, cued by prosodic and phonologic information in the input, can be used by the child to identify the basic units for analysis of morphology and syntax. They thus provide a critical launch pad into language structure (Bishop, 1997; Fee, 1997; Locke, 1996; McDonald, 1997; McGregor, 1997; Morgan, Meier, & Newport, 1987). In this context, Petitto argued that

> Humans are born with a nascent structure-seeking mechanism, blind to modality, which initially attends to and seeks to discover particular units with particular distributional patterns in the input. These units correspond in size and organization to syllabic units in language, as well as to other properties of natural language phonology. (1993, p. 97)

This potential for sublexical organization allows the child to induce structural properties and build a matching output system. As long as the data presented as input are perceivable, producible, and segmentable and uptake of the data is adequate, the process of acquisition should be unimpeded (Harris, 1992; Petitto, 1993). Even children developing in quite exceptional circumstances evidence patterns of acquisition very similar to those reported for typically developing children, suggesting that the structure-seeking mechanism is both robust and amodal in its operation. For example, children with hearing impairments who have signing parents acquire language in a typical way but in a visual-gestural modality (Bellugi, van Hoek, Lillo-Martin & O'Grady, 1988). Children with intellectual impairments may plateau at an early stage of language development but otherwise differ little from their typically developing peers (Fowler, 1998; Rondal, 1994), and children with Williams syndrome develop sophisticated syntax and morphology despite low levels of nonverbal cognition (Bellugi, Wang, & Jernigan, 1994). In all of the previous cases, however, there is symmetry in the modalities of input, uptake, and output. What is remarkable for most individuals using AAC is the complex relationship between the communication modalities available for their language input and for language production.

Language Development in AAC

Communication is a multi-modal process, both in typical and in exceptional circumstances; however, the burden of referential communication typically falls to one primary mode of communication, most commonly speech or manual sign. Meaning and communicative intent may well be modulated through the recruitment of additional modalities such as facial expression, prosody, or gesture, but such complementary and supplementary communicative systems are fundamentally different to formal linguistic systems in their organization and their function (McNeill, 1992; Petitto, 1993). Such complementary "division of labor" across modes of communication may be difficult both to distinguish and to maintain in children with significant speech impairments. Only since the late 1990s has attention been paid to the complex interrelationships between input–output modalities and comprehension–production systems in AAC use (Grove & Smith, 1997; Oxley & von Tetzchner, 1999; Smith, 1997, 1998). It seems clear that when adults with intact linguistic competence use signs or graphic representations to accompany their speech, they are coding selected words into a different modality. Whether the process is the same for the developing child using AAC is another question altogether.

One common hypothesis that informs much of the work in AAC draws on an underlying assumption that individuals with the ability to hear, use spoken language input to develop receptive language. Spoken receptive language in turn provides a basis for expressive language. The forms of representation that underlie both comprehension and production are therefore presumed to be derived from speech. From this perspective, the task for the nonspeech communicator is to recode a message from speech into an augmentative or alternative modality either at the point of transmission or between the stages of grammatical encoding and phonological encoding (Lloyd, Quist, & Windsor, 1990; Loncke, Vander Beken, & Lloyd, 1997). In the former speech-based model, a spoken message is mapped onto available lexical options in manual or graphic representations at the point of expression. In the latter case, internal abstract lexical representations may be bimodal, so that the formulation of the utterance may be bi- or multi-modal.

The process of recoding may influence communication patterns beyond the obvious formal characteristics of the message (i.e., signs rather than words). For example, in aided communication, rate of production may be dramatically slowed and gaze patterns may differ from spoken interaction; however, a speech-based model implies that these features are superficial and relatively trivial and that the underlying structure of the message remains unaffected by the modality of production. It follows from this assumption that the difference between a user who augments speech with manual or graphic signs and one who uses the latter modalities as a replacement or alternative for speech is merely a question of degree.

However, we suggest that the distinction is far from trivial and may, in fact, have profound implications for the language acquisition process. We consider first the input and output characteristics of communication systems available to individuals with severe speech impairments and explore the compatibility of system characteristics with the task of language construction.

Input Characteristics   Although it is widely accepted that, in principle, there should be some modeling of AAC modalities (Goossens' & Crain, 1988), in practice input to children using AAC is typically dominated by speech (Grove, 1995; Harris, 1982; Smith, 1998, for further discussion of the role of augmented input; see also Chapter 5). Communication partners may make no use of the AAC system at all or may represent occasional content words in graphic or manual form. Grove (1995) found that, when communicating with signers who had moderate intellectual impairments, teachers tended to use the full spoken form but produced one accompanying sign per clause. Wilkinson, Romski, and Sevcik (1994) reported that combinations of graphic representations in the input accounted for as little as 3% of all input for one individual who uses AAC, to a high of 14% for another youth. The input to most individuals who use AAC can therefore be characterized as full spoken language, with sporadic use of isolated lexical items in the alternative modality; however, when faced with the task of producing referential output, the relative dominance of modality must be revised by the individual who uses AAC (Smith & Grove, 1999; see Figure 6.1). In some instances, particularly with children with significant physical disabilities, no clear modality may be functionally dominant or children may attempt to recruit multiple modes in the service of linguistic communication (Heim & Baker-Mills, 1996; Light, Collier, & Parnes, 1985b; Smith, 1998; von Tetzchner, 1997).

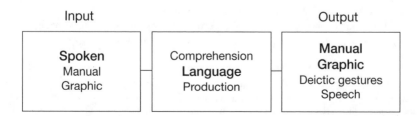

Figure 6.1.   Model of input–output relationships in AAC.

A further unknown is the uptake by an individual who uses AAC from the input provided. While it may well appear that speech is the dominant input modality, if the speech itself is not accessible to the individual who uses AAC, then the very reduced manual or graphic input may in fact be functionally dominant (Oxley & von Tetzchner, 1999; see also Chapter 5).

Output Characteristics   When faced with building an output system, individuals using AAC typically have either manual or graphic signs available to them, with occasional use of tactile signs.[1] There are certain key features that differ across manual signs and graphic representations and from the speech that they are designed to reproduce. In full sign language, signs have both morphological and syntactic structure. When used as lexical items, as in AAC, they may be rarely combined and may appear indistinguishable from holistic gestalts. However, they remain potentially contrastive at a phonological level because, like words, signs are composed of bundles of features. Also like words, signs are dynamic, taking on form as the articulators (hands) move and change shape and position. Thus, words and signs are subject to variations in production of certain dimensions of the message, within specified parameters, creating the potential for developmental change and creativity.

Unlike manual signs, graphic representations are static and may be highly pictorial, or more abstract, varying along the iconicity continuum (Stephenson & Linfoot, 1996). Although recent technological developments allow access to "dynamic" symbols, even in such cases, the movement applies to the symbol as a whole, rather than to specific parameters of symbols. The trend in intervention has been toward use of more pictorial and iconic systems, which appear easier to acquire in the initial stages of learning (Ecklund & Reichle, 1987; Mizuko, 1987; Mizuko & Reichle 1989; Yovetich & Young, 1989). The most sophisticated of these systems is Blissymbolics (Bliss, 1965). Blissymbolics is a semantically based system and has rules for combining symbols and for generating new lexical items. In addition, certain word-order constraints operate, with a general subject–verb–object ordering (Schlosser, 1997). Most other graphic systems have no such associated rules. In contrast to words and manual signs, graphic representations are not articulated, but rather are selected (via eye gaze, pointing, or other movement), from a predetermined array. They are inaccessible to direct manipulation or systematic change that originates from the user (as opposed to the designers of the system).

The characteristics of particular AAC systems should have an effect on the linguistic performance or productions of individuals who use AAC; how-

---

[1]Communication is multi-modal, and particularly for individuals with severe physical impairments, patterns of cross-modal organization and integration may be extremely complex. For the purposes of referential, rather than deictic communication, individuals are generally more constrained in the modes that they can use. The discussion here focuses on manual or graphic signs as potential candidates for linguistic organization, while recognizing that for some individuals these modes may only partly contribute to overall communication.

ever, if underlying representations are speech based and are re-coded into AAC modalities at the point of transmission, there should be a close match between the underlying spoken message and the output (manual or graphic), within the limits of the output system. Given appropriate contextual support and expectations for communication, those message elements that are available as lexical items in the alternative modality should be communicated in the order and degree of completeness in which they occur in the underlying message. Although it may not be possible to reproduce the morphology of the spoken language (because both manual signs and graphic representations may lack the equivalent inflections), word order should be preserved, unless there is specific linguistic motivation for altering word order.

DATA CONSIDERATIONS

Language Production in Alternative Modalities

Since the 1980s, increasing attention has been paid to detailed description of the output of individuals using AAC, as the focus has broadened from an initial emphasis on communicative efficiency (e.g., Light, 1988) to include a focus on language acquisition (Blockberger, 1997; Grove, 1995; Heim & Baker-Mills, 1996; Light, 1997; Smith, 1998; Soto & Toro-Zambrana, 1995; Sutton, 1997, 1999; van Balkom & Donker-Gimbrère, 1996). Although actual published data are still scarce, a number of examples of output in nonspeech modalities have been made available, and some of these examples are presented in Figures 6.2 and 6.3. The data presented have been gathered from a range of individuals, including hearing children with intellectual impairments using manual sign (Grove, 1995); hearing children with cerebral palsy whose intellectual abilities are unimpaired, using Picture Communication Symbols (PCS; Mayer-Johnson, 1981, 1985) (Smith, 1998) and traditional orthography (Smith, 2003); and hearing adolescents with cerebral palsy using a variety of graphic systems (van Balkom & Donker-Gimbrère, 1996). Input to all of the individuals is conventional spoken English. In the case of the signers, some key words are presented bimodally in speech and sign, but typically at the rate of only one sign per clause (see previous discussion).

Figure 6.2 presents data from Grove (1995), in which three hearing children with moderate to severe intellectual impairments used manual signs in conversation and story narration. All of the students had been learning signs for 3–11 years. Vocabulary knowledge was assessed through checklists compiled by teachers and speech pathologists. The students were reported to understand between 100 and 300 signs and to use between 35 and 250 signs productively. All but one had passed the 50-item stage, at which word combinations develop in children with the ability to speak. Data were elicited through natural conversations, narratives, and picture descriptions.

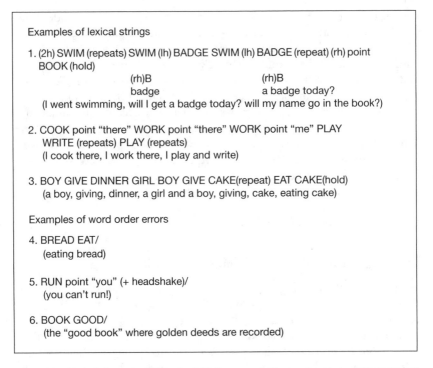

Examples of lexical strings

1. (2h) SWIM (repeats) SWIM (lh) BADGE SWIM (lh) BADGE (repeat) (rh) point
   BOOK (hold)

   | (rh)B | (rh)B |
   | badge | a badge today? |

   (I went swimming, will I get a badge today? will my name go in the book?)

2. COOK point "there" WORK point "there" WORK point "me" PLAY
   WRITE (repeats) PLAY (repeats)
   (I cook there, I work there, I play and write)

3. BOY GIVE DINNER GIRL BOY GIVE CAKE(repeat) EAT CAKE(hold)
   (a boy, giving, dinner, a girl and a boy, giving, cake, eating cake)

Examples of word order errors

4. BREAD EAT/
   (eating bread)

5. RUN point "you" (+ headshake)/
   (you can't run!)

6. BOOK GOOD/
   (the "good book" where golden deeds are recorded)

Figure 6.2. Manual sign output. *Note*: Capital letters are used to denote use of graphic or manual signs: Graphic signs are indicated using italic font (*PUT, CAR*); manual signs are not italicized (CUP, BOOK). Speech is written in lowercase. Hand use: (2h) = two hands; (lh) = left hand; (rh) = right hand. Point = index finger points: meaning of the point is in quotation marks. Manual gestures are not conventional signs. (*Source:* Grove, 1995.)

The first example in Figure 6.3 is taken from Smith (1998) in which an adolescent with cerebral palsy and relatively age-appropriate receptive language skills used PCS in a conversation describing an event during a recent outing. Examples 2 and 3, also from Smith (1998), feature Yvonne, age 6 years, 11 months, using PCS in a barrier game to describe pictures so her father can select a matching picture. Yvonne is assessed as functioning in the average cognitive ability range, and on the Test of Reception of Grammar (Bishop, 1982), she scored an age equivalent of 8.0. Her PCS board contains more than 250 symbols.

Examples 4 and 5 are from Smith (2003). Neill, an adolescent with cerebral palsy, uses traditional orthography. He used a DeltaTalker with Word-Strategy program and responded to specific spoken stimuli for each picture from the Renfrew Action Picture Test (Renfrew, 1988) presented.

The last three examples are from van Balkom & Donker-Gimbrère (1996) and describe the graphic output of four adolescents with cerebral palsy who

1. *SWEET HOUSE GREEN SHOP OUTSIDE BED*
   (I ate sweets outside lying down on the grass)

2. *BED UNDER BED BOOK SHOES*
   (shoes are under the bed)

3. *DRINK GIRL*
   (the girl is drinking)

   stimulus: what is the girl doing
4. the girl at on to the toys
   (the girl is holding a teddy)

   stimulus: tell me all about this picture
5. the boy hand to down fruit the woman a fruit bag
   (the boy is picking up fruit for the woman; the woman has a bag of fruit)

6. *CLEAN GIRL MUMMY DESK*
   (they—girl and mummy—clean the desk)

7. *GIRL BLUE BOX HELP BOY IN SHOPPING CAR*
   (the girl helps the boy putting the blue box in the shopping cart)

8. *TWO BED SLEEP BOY ONE GIRL WHITE BED BROWN BED*
   (the boy and the girl are sleeping in two beds: one in a white bed and the other in a brown bed)

Figure 6.3. Graphic output. *Note:* Capital letters are used to denote use of graphic or manual signs: Graphic signs are indicated using italic font (*PUT, CAR*); manual signs are not italicized (CUP, BOOK). Speech is written in lowercase. (*Sources:* Smith, 1998, 2003; van Balkom & Donker-Gimbrère, 1996.)

were selected because of their experience in graphic sign use. Their task was to describe pictures as if telling a story to a younger child. All necessary graphic signs were available to the students on their boards, and the therapist was asked to confirm each selection and then to paraphrase the completed utterance to allow confirmation by the student.

Despite the provision of spoken input, which conforms with strict morphological and syntactic regularities, the output in the AAC modalities does not reflect the structure of the spoken input. Three general patterns emerge in the data: limited use of multi-term constructions, word order differing from the input, and ambiguity of productive morphology.

Limited Use of Multi-term Constructions   For the students studied by Grove, the Mean Length of Sign Turn (MLST) was 1.84 (SD. 0.45, range 1.31–2.58) across a range of conversational opportunities—a finding echoed in many other studies of children using manual signs (e.g., Fenn & Rowe, 1984; Grove & McDougall, 1991; Udwin & Yule, 1990). Similarly,

Smith (1998) reported that Yvonne, a 6-year-old with age-appropriate receptive language abilities, typically produced only one PCS symbol per utterance,
with very occasional multi-term utterances despite having both the necessary
symbols available to her and at least some opportunities and encouragement
to use multi-term constructions. This finding mirrors reports from other research (Collins, 1996; Hjelmquist & Sandberg, 1996; Udwin & Yule, 1990; von
Tetzchner & Martinsen, 1996). Van Balkom and Donker-Gimbrère (1996) reported that for the 42 individuals who used AAC that they studied, "a large
majority never combined elements in order to create meanings they lacked in
their sign lexicons" and "more than half produced messages that on average
did not exceed two graphic signs in length" (p. 159).

Word Order Differs from the Input   Even in the limited transcripts provided in Figures 6.2 and 6.3, there is evidence of word order that
violates that of the spoken language of the environment. Word order appears
to be one of the earliest cues to meaning comprehended by young children
(Golinkoff, Pasek, Cauley, & Gordon, 1987), and word order violations are reported as occurring infrequently in typical language development, even in
children with cognitive impairments such as Down syndrome (Dooley, 1976;
Radford, 1990; Ramer, 1976). By contrast, in AAC output, reports of non-
English word order are not uncommon and examples of word order differences are evident in Figures 6.2 and 6.3 (Fenn & Rowe, 1984; Light, Remington, Clarke, & Watson, 1989; Wilkinson et al., 1994). Fifteen percent of the
output from the 10 children studied by Grove (1995) failed to respect English
word order, and for the children who had some intelligible speech, this was
true in both modalities. Errors mainly involved the placement of objects after
verbs, with no consistent ordering patterns discerned. These children were
clearly not inducing word order rules governing the placement of semantic patients from the input and translating these into sign: indeed, speech seemed
to follow sign, rather than the other way around.

A second feature of the multi-term utterances produced by these children is that many appear to be built from chained lexical items, rather than
embedded structures. This pattern is comparable to the performance of children at the earliest stage of word combinations (Brown, 1973; Lahey, 1988).

Thus, the data from at least some children using manual signs or communication boards suggest significant difficulty in making the transition to
multi-term utterances and more frequent rule violations than would be predicted based on patterns of typical development. Output in many cases is typ-
ified by lack of evidence of functional constituents and clause structure, which
is generally assigned through rich interpretation on the part of the communication partner.

Productive Morphology   Word order and clause structure are not
the only aspects of grammar which can function to modulate the meanings of

propositions. Traditional assessment measures such as mean length of utterance (MLU) also reflect the development of the internal complexity of words at the morphological level. It is difficult to establish evidence of morphological development for children using communication boards where lexical items must be selected from a predefined array. For example, although Yvonne is credited with production of SHOES in Figure 6.3, in fact, she has no access to a separate PCS representation for *shoe* versus *shoes*. Although for communication purposes, the utterance can be glossed as a plural, there is no independent evidence that she has acquired a rule.

The situation is not quite as clear for children using manual sign. In sign language, morphological marking most commonly takes place through changes to the forms of hand shape, location, movement or orientation, which result in changes to meaning (Brennan, 1992; Stokoe, Casterline, & Cronenberg, 1965). Grove (1995) analyzed the sign output of 10 children ages 10–16, with intellectual impairments. The findings suggest that it is possible for this group to modify the sublexical parameters of sign, even though they have not been exposed to any linguistic input in this modality. In this context, sign modifications were defined as changes to the citation form of lexical signs, which were consistent with meaning. Grove, Dockrell, and Woll (1996) cited three examples of this type of modification (see Figure 6.4).

Out of a total of 643 signs produced by the students, 24 signs were modified in ways that added meaning, suggesting some degree of creativity within the system. As Figure 6.4 illustrates, the aspects of the sign which were modified corresponded to the segmental properties of natural sign languages:

Robbie was presented with a picture of three men standing at a bus stop. He produced the manual sign MAN three times in succession. He seemed to be using repetition to pluralize meaning.

Brendan was describing how he had told his mother to stop talking to her friends and come home. He used the manual sign SHUT-UP, displaced from himself towards her, out of the normal signing space (a change in location). This seemed to carry the meaning, "I told you to shut up."

Michael was in the swimming pool and wanted people to notice a new achievement. He used the manual sign LOOK, which in the Makaton Vocabulary is an index finger moving outwards from the eye. Michael used two hands and reversed the movement towards himself, effectively conveying "All of you look at me!" by doubling the sign and changing its orientation.

Figure 6.4. Modifications to manual signs produced by hearing children with intellectual impairments. (From Grove, N., Dockrell, J., & Woll, B. [1996]. The two-word stage in manual signs: Language and development in signers with intellectual impairments. In S. von Tetzchner & M. Jensen [Eds.], *Augmentative and alternative communication: European perspectives* [pp. 108–109]. London: Whurr; reprinted by permission.)

hand shape, location, movement, orientation, and hand use and mainly conveyed differential information about the shapes and locations of objects and quality of actions (Brien, 1992; Stokoe et al., 1965). Thus, the types of meaning that were specified were those particularly suited to the visual-manual modality. It is not clear, however, whether this phenomenon is intrinsically linguistic. A number of criteria need to be met before modulations at the level of the word can be considered rule governed, including contrastivity, consistency, and productivity (Bates, Bretherton, & Snyder, 1988). In this case, the majority (18 of 24) of sign modulations met the criterion of contrastivity—a sign was produced in two different ways within the corpus, involving change to one parameter. The data were insufficient to determine either consistent or generative production; that is, we do not know if the children produced these variations consistently in association with the same linguistic context, nor whether modifications were generalized across classes of sign. For example, is that modulation for GIVE–small object also used in signs such as TAKE, CARRY, and HOLD? A conservative assessment of the data would suggest that the modifications are semantically driven and iconic in their origins. Nevertheless, they are clearly something more than holistic gestures, if we accept the criteria proposed by both Petitto (1993) and McNeill (1992), who maintained that gestures are holistic and nonsegmentable.

However modifications to signs are classified, it is apparent that these children were able to manipulate sublexical properties of signs in order to effect changes in meaning. In this respect, they appear to be producing modality-specific behavior more complex than the input provided to them, a phenomenon which has been observed in other cases of children using sign or gesture (Goldin-Meadow & Mylander, 1984, 1993; Newport, 1988).

Thus, overall many users of AAC demonstrate a pattern in which they produce strings of lexical terms, which in some instances can be glossed into a cohesive whole. There is little evidence of internal structural development, although there is evidence to suggest some morphological development in children using manual signs, certainly beyond that of the children using graphic representations. At the level of the clause, manual, graphic, and the accompanying spoken output look remarkably similar. Although these children can acquire a lexicon that is used productively, they appear to have real problems in generating grammatical structure or in mapping their grammatical structure into a nonspeech modality. It is apparent that predictions made on the basis of the speech re-coding model are not fulfilled for many of the individuals who have been studied.

Explanations of Patterns of Production

Several factors may contribute to the patterns of output reported for individuals who use AAC. Five possible explanations are considered here: 1) a drive for communicative efficiency; 2) the effects of a pragmatic style of communication; 3) the effects of a linguistic deficit; 4) the effects of re-coding from one modality to another; and 5) the effects of a modality asymmetry between input and output.

Communicative Efficiency   Under the communicative efficiency hypothesis, telegrammatic constructions produced by individuals who use AAC are seen as accommodating to the rate and vocabulary restrictions imposed particularly by graphic communication, with output biased towards "strings" of contentives, similar in many respects to pidgin languages (von Tetzchner, 1985). Although this argument is persuasive in relation to aided communication, it is difficult to see why similar patterns should occur with manual signs, where there is the potential to approximate spoken language rates and where limited sign output may even slow the rate of communication due to the consequent ambiguities that may arise (Klima & Bellugi, 1979). Ascribing patterns of output to a deliberate choice of discourse register suggests potential access to an unimpaired underlying speech-based message, although there may be no independent evidence that alternative registers are available. Alternatively, the pattern of output may reflect a particular stage of development, as suggested by Givón (1985).

Pragmatic Style of Communication   The pragmatic argument is similar to the Communicative Efficiency Hypothesis in that it proposes that the development of structure is constrained within the AAC modality because its function remains primarily communicative, rather than linguistic. Givón (1985) distinguished between an early pragmatic or paratactic mode of communication and a subsequent syntactic mode of communication. The former stage of development is characterized by a topic–comment structure, a slow rate of delivery, a low noun–verb ratio in discourse, and no use of grammatical morphology. A syntactic mode is built around a subject–predicate structure, with a fast rate of delivery, a higher noun–verb ratio in discourse, and extensive use of grammatical morphology. Children are presumed to actively construct their syntactic mode while retaining access to the pragmatic mode as a register of choice where communicatively appropriate. Children experiencing difficulty with the active construction of the syntactic mode may rely on pragmatic strategies combined with a lexicon primarily composed of content words. This pattern would place them in the second phase of language development in Locke's (1997) terms, characterized by semantic and pragmatic strategies for expressing themselves.

Certainly, some of the data from individuals who use AAC match the features of Givón's pragmatic mode, suggesting that either they are making a register choice to support communicative efficiency, or they have not as yet developed a syntactic mode. Some individuals such as Robbie, Brendan, and Michael (see Figure 6.4), who show evidence of a primitive inflectional morphology, may be moving from a paratactic towards a syntactic mode. More conservatively, their modifications may be viewed as iconic and deriving from the conceptual system. Either way, the emergence of modifications suggests a transitional phase of development between pragmatic and syntactic modes.

Givón's model is compatible in many ways with the observed patterns of linguistic output in manual and graphic signs; however, in itself it is an insufficient explanation because it still does not make clear why users apparently fail to avail themselves of the word order information provided in speech to construct utterances in manual signs or graphic representations. One explanation may be that some manual and graphic sign users have specific deficits in processing and abstracting relevant linguistic information from their environmental input.

Linguistic Deficit Hypothesis   The linguistic deficit hypothesis finds support from literature describing the features commonly found in children with impaired language skills, patterns which mirror those reported for individuals who use AAC: structural simplifications, omission of function words, and short utterances (e.g., Fletcher & Garman, 1995; Tyler & Sandoval, 1994). Descriptions of asymmetric language profiles are common in the literature on developmental language impairments (e.g., Adams, 1990; Camarata, Nelson & Camarata, 1994; Fey, Cleave, Long, & Hughes, 1993). Such findings may reflect the differential vulnerability of computational rather than conceptual dimensions of language (Bishop & Edmundson, 1987). The linguistic deficit hypothesis allows for the possibility that some aided communicators may develop appropriate expressive language (see Soto & Toro-Zambrana, 1995) but suggests that such progress will be constrained by the extent of the linguistic impairment, the related underlying neuropathology, and the vulnerability of particular aspects of morphological knowledge (Redmond & Johnson, 2001). There may be persuasive reasons for accepting a thesis of "within-person deficit." However, it is worth noting that in developmental language disorders, typically many different profiles of relative linguistic strengths and weaknesses are described, prompting suggestions of syndromes of disorder (e.g., Lees & Urwin, 1997; Rapin & Allen, 1987), such as lexical-syntactic deficit syndrome or semantic-pragmatic deficit syndrome. By contrast, the manual and graphic sign output of many individuals who use AAC can be characterized as a single deficit pattern, with primary limitations in syntactic organization and inflectional morphology. It is possible that linguistic limitations may influence the structure of graphic or manual sign output without necessarily representing significant difficulties with the generation of structure at all levels.

Recoding Argument   Unlike the linguistic deficit hypothesis, the recoding argument rests on the premise that that there is an intact linguistic system that provides an internal speech message to be re-coded into an alternative modality (Levelt, 1989); however, some individuals who use AAC may not have developed the metalinguistic skills required to re-code a speech-based message into a different modality. Alternatively, they may be constrained by the available lexicon in the target modality. Studies of typically developing preschool children and older school-age children have reported patterns of short utterances and non-English word order in graphic communication output, despite the children's intact spoken language skills (Smith, 1996; Sutton & Morford, 1998). In addition, a gradual approximation to spoken language word order as age of the children increased was noted in both studies, suggesting a possible role for metalinguistic skills in cross-modal translation. Sutton, Gallagher, Morford, and Shahnaz (2000) asked competent adult speakers to communicate messages containing either subject-relative or object-relative clauses using voice output communication aids (VOCAs) with limited PCS displays. Target sentence pairs included, for example: "The girl who pushes the clown wears a hat" and "The girl pushes the clown who wears a hat." Relative pronoun grammatical markers were not provided. Faced with the challenge of resolving ambiguity arising from the matching order of major constituents, many (36 of 43) of the participants chose to vary word order in order to retain a structural distinction across the sentence pairs, yielding apparent word order violations.

It is important to acknowledge however, that although there are superficial similarities between the output of the typically developing children and those using AAC, the integrity of the linguistic system can only be assumed for the former group. Several other questions remain unanswered. If the underlying process is one of recoding, what is the explanation for the differences between input structure and output structure beyond mere simplifications? Where in the recoding process does word order change and why? How can the apparent emergence of modality-specific inflections be accounted for? Elucidating the problem requires looking more closely at the asymmetry in modality between input and output.

Modality Asymmetry Argument   The modality asymmetry argument proposes that a fundamental problem for individuals who use AAC lies in the nature of the relationship between the modalities of input and output. Petitto (1993) suggested that the language acquisition process is driven in the first instance by an innate structure-seeking mechanism seeking particular types of units as input. For many individuals using AAC, the spoken input they receive provides all of the necessary organizational components for the induction of structure; however, when the task becomes one of generating output in an AAC modality, the match between the properties of the two systems may be incomplete. Figure 6.5 illustrates the potential properties that are available for the user to manipulate.

Graphic Representations   PCS constitute a set of lexical items. There are no formational constraints or standards of form governing creation of new symbols, and there are no sublexical parameters that can be manipu-

Properties	Lexical	Syntactic	Morphological inflectional	Phonological segmental	Phonological suprasemental
Natural languages spoken input	+	+	+	+	+
Graphic signs Picture Communication Symbols (PCS)	+	–	–	–	–
Blissymbols	+	?	?	?	–
Manual signs	+	–	+	+	+

Figure 6.5. Comparison of natural language and AAC systems. (*Source:* Smith & Grove, 1996.)
Key: + = has quality; – = doesn't have quality; ? = unclear.

lated for morphological inflection. PCS are intended to be used in the word order of the spoken language of the environment; there is not presumed to be any independent PCS syntax. PCS represent a "flat" modality, with no intrinsic suprasegmental features, although conceivably pause time or force of selection could be recruited for paralinguistic purposes. As a productive system, PCS offer a poor match with the features of a spoken or signed language base; in essence, PCS output can only be produced as chains of lexical items.

By comparison, Blissymbols present contrastivity at a sublexical level. Each symbol is constructed through the combination of individual meaningful elements. These elements are not analogous to a phonology because each carries meaning, and so they may best be described as a collection of morphological rather than phonological segments (Sutton, personal communication, 1996). Although parasitic to a large extent on spoken language and arguably largely iconic in form (Besio & Chinato, 1996), there are some explicit rules governing the ordering of symbols so that children have access to syntax-like constraints. Detailed evidence from users of Blissymbols is not available, but a study by Soto and Toro-Zambrana (1995) suggests that some users show some mastery of the morphosyntactic features available in the system. There is also anecdotal evidence of interference from the constituent order of Blissymbols in speech output. A young man with cerebral palsy whose first productive system was a Bliss chart subsequently used an electronic text-based communication aid in adulthood and was occasionally heard to use topic–comment structure and adjectives following nouns, mirroring his earlier Bliss output and possibly respecting the CLASSIFIER + MODIFIER order of Blissymbols (Cockerill, personal communication, 1996). This pattern suggests that his underlying linguistic representations may have been influenced at one point by the syntax of the graphic system, rather than the speech in the input. Of course, of relevance also in this context is the nature and focus of instruction in use of the graphic system. Individuals who use AAC systems may be atypically reliant on direct instruction, given the paucity of opportunities for incidental learning within their environment.

Manual Signs   In the context of AAC, manual signs are typically taught as isolated lexical items, and incidental sign input is sporadic. Therefore, there is almost no contrastivity presented to the child at a syntactic level; however, because the signs are derived from natural sign languages, latent sublexical properties may be perceived and taken up. The lexicon that the child sees and uses is contrastive in its combinations of hand shapes, movements, locations, and orientations. Signs appear to be stored separately from words in long-term memory by individuals with intellectual impairments (Reid & Kiernan, 1979), and it seems plausible to suggest that once the child's productive lexicon reaches a certain size, it will be represented as bundles of features (hand shapes, locations, movements, and orientations) rather than as distinct lexical items (McDonald, 1997). Locke (1997) suggested that this structure analysis system comes into play to locate recurring elements within and across utterances, so that each individual entry is "a unique recombination of a small set of phonemes." This shift in focus from whole gestalts to segments would explain how it is possible for signers to change meanings by introducing changes to form. Suprasegmental properties also seem to be available to signers, who may use both stress and holds of signs paralinguistically, although they may not be able to master the subtle pauses and changes of expression which signal distinctions in sentence types and propositional shifts (Grove, 1995).

To summarize, individuals who use AAC are in the unique position of being exposed to fully specified spoken language input, with a very much more restricted and lexically based input in another modality. In order to construct a productive as opposed to a receptive linguistic system, the individual who uses AAC must essentially extract principles from the complete input and realize those principles in the more restricted modality. This task requires that they induce the rules from one system and apply those rules in another, often very different system. The question then arises, if the formal properties of input and output modalities are different and the structure-seeking mechanism cannot find an appropriate match of sublexical units across modalities, how can development proceed? Perhaps an even greater puzzle is the question of how children actually produce AAC output, which is more complex either in terms of utterance length or in terms of morphological structure than the input they receive within that modality? One possible indicator may come from studies of children developing sign language.

Output as Input

Sign language research with deaf children of hearing parents (e.g., Goldin-Meadow & Mylander, 1993) seems to indicate that the "home-sign" systems produced by the children show hierarchical organization considerably more complex than the organization of the signed input they receive. Developments of this nature are taken as strong indicators of an innate language acquisition component at work, seeking structures of a particular kind and developing these structures into an organized hierarchy. But where does the structure-seeking mechanism focus its attention?

One suggestion comes from Elbers (1995), who reported on the developmental course of a self-created form, a word-blend produced by a Dutch child. The child created the word form and subsequently modified the form to match morphological constraints of Dutch. Elbers argued that the changes observed in the use of the word-blend can only be understood if the child's analysis of his own productions is viewed as central to the construction of a coherent system. She outlined four theoretical supports for the output as a source for input hypothesis:

> The Effort argument suggests that representations of sound/meaning pairs which derive from production will be better retained and so will be better available as input for analysis than those from comprehension. The No Guessing argument suggests that the sound/meaning pairs that originate in production will be less problematical than those from comprehension, and so will be more suitable as input for analysis. The Double Processing argument suggests that production offers more opportunity for on-line analysis than does comprehension. And finally, the Internal Speech argument suggests that production may offer a plausible mechanism for off-line analysis, i.e., internal speech. (Elbers, 1995, pp. 52–53)

Her suggestion is that a child's novel productions "need not only be a result of a process of analysis, but may also constitute an object for such processes" (p. 65). Platt and MacWhinney (1983) explored the same phenomenon with preschool children. They presented the children with sentences of varying types, some involving errors that the children themselves had been observed to produce and others with similar errors devised by the researchers or with no errors. The preschool children were significantly more likely to accept as correct those sentences containing self-generated rather than other-generated errors, suggesting, in Platt and MacWhinney's view that

> Children...seem frequently to learn their own solutions to language structure problems, to such an extent that these errors dominate for a while over the correct forms to which the child is more frequently exposed via reception. The primary source of the incorrect form must be the child himself. (1983, p. 412)

If children can use their own output as a source of input for further analysis, then this begins to account for some of the creative use of AAC systems. The morphological development reported by Grove et al. (1996) may be based on the child's analysis of his or her own attempts to express conceptual content. Elbers suggested that "if this idea is correct then the frequency of occurrence of forms in a child's output, rather than in adult input, should be an important determinant of what is analyzed and acquired" (1995, p. 66). This suggestion ties in well with the finding of Wilkinson and colleagues (1994) that although five of the seven "combiners" they studied were individually consistent in their ordering of constituents, the word order used varied across subjects and furthermore, within individuals, did not reflect the ordering presented in the input to any significant extent. The issue of frequency of occurrence also raises questions about the possible implications of the typically low rates of initiation of novel utterances by individuals using graphic signs (e.g., Kraat, 1987; Soto & Toro-Zambrana, 1995).

CLINICAL AND EDUCATIONAL IMPLICATIONS

We have argued here that the asymmetry across input and output modalities experienced by many individuals who use AAC may have significant effects on their development of language structure. If this position is correct, what are the clinical and educational implications that follow?

Symmetry Restored: Role of Voice Output Communication Aids

With advances in technology since the 1980s, many more individuals have had access to VOCAs. What impact might provision of voice output have for an individual using aided communication? Early provision of voice output may yield many benefits. It allows access to independent feedback regarding productions and opportunities for engaging in vocal play, nonsocial speech, and repetition. Independent voice output has been shown to be facilitative in supporting literacy skills (McGinnis & Beukelman, 1989) and in generating more positive attitudes to users (Gorenflo & Gorenflo, 1991), thus potentially increasing the range and number of social interaction contexts within which an aided communicator may gain experience using AAC. The provision of voice output may also help to make transparent the function of picture symbols as mediators. When the input is spoken and the output is spoken, the pictures on an overlay of a voice output device are simply a way of accessing speech. The pictures or icons on the overlay clearly are not intended as the communication message—the acoustic output is the message.

One aspect that may be crucial in determining the potential facilitative role of voice output devices is the extent to which these devices provide opportunities for users to manipulate constituents. The design of some systems has been heavily influenced by pragmatic considerations and script theory so that stored phrases are activated on the selection of a single graphic representation (Nelson, 1986). The gain in communicative efficiency might be at the cost of linguistic proficiency. Locke (1995) suggested that the production of scripts and formulaic utterances is characteristic of the second phase of language development, when social utterances are stored as whole items and processed by the right hemisphere. A child who only has access to scripts, even if these were spoken, might show a plateau in development at the paratactic stage of communication referred to by Givón (1985).

With individuals who are unable to access a device directly, it is not known whether the presumed advantage of such symmetry restoration outweighs the disadvantages of the complex motor and cognitive demands implicit in acquiring the requisite operational skills. Does provision of a voice output simply add another dimension to the communication process without necessarily enhancing that process?

Symmetry Restored: Matching Input and Output Characteristics

An alternative route to restoring symmetry may be to match as closely as possible the structural characteristics of communication systems provided for both input and output. The range of computational and conceptual characteristics available to children using nonspeech systems may vary quite considerably, depending on the properties of both the input and the output modalities and the nature of the input and output provided. An individual who uses AAC and can use some speech as output has the possibility of mirroring, in his or her output, the distribution of computational and conceptual aspects of language presented in input. By contrast, individuals who have no access to speech production, and for whom AAC modalities function as an alternative to speech, are faced with a much more challenging task: the cross-modal rule induction and application referred to previously. That is to say, the distinction between augmentative and alternative communication is a fundamental one.

In the case of alternative communication users, the match between the characteristics of their input and output communication systems, in their potential for hierarchical organization, and specifically for segmentation at a sublexical level (the syllabic units referenced by Petitto [1993]), may be decisive. AAC sets, which are presented lexically in the input and which do not offer sublexical units for analysis, are likely to be used lexically, as strings of contentives. Furthermore, the absence of sublexical elements may severely constrain innovation, the creativity that is a feature of typical language acquisition.

Creativity may still enter the system if a user's own productions serve as a source for further analysis. An increased focus on own productions may arise in situations where the output produced by an individual who uses AAC actually exceeds the input provided in the AAC modality by other communication partners, in terms of the overall frequency of occurrence of AAC forms; however, if the AAC signs are selected rather than produced, then the potential for the user to discover possible parameters of variation for the refinement of meanings expressed is significantly curtailed. It is likely that creativity will be limited to the domain of content. A child, for example, may develop considerable skill in flexibly using a restricted lexical set to communicate novel information through the use of analogy, antonyms, or other strategies to communicate vocabulary not specifically available on a board (see Chapter 12 for further discussion).

Decisions relating to system selection must therefore take into account not only the immediate communicative needs of an individual but also the longer-term development opportunities afforded by different systems. There may be many valid reasons for choosing a picture-based graphic system (including user preference, transparency for other communication partners, and attitudes of significant communication partners). What is important, however, is that within the decision-making process, consideration is given to language as well as communication issues.

IMPLICATIONS FOR
FUTURE RESEARCH AND PRACTICE

We have identified some of the ways in which the language output of children using manual signs and graphic symbols appears to diverge from what we might expect; however, it may be that the problems we identified are more apparent than real. Should the data presented in Figures 6.2 and 6.3 be taken as evidence of underlying language differences? Or are the differences simply artifacts of particular communication media and situational constraints? For example, Kraat (1991) wisely cautioned not to infer underlying language abilities on the basis of communication board output. Two questions then still remain: what should be inferred on the basis of the output, and how can abilities in any underlying spoken language system be explored? What other organizational structures should be explored?

In order to answer these questions, a research agenda that focuses on the gaps in the current knowledge base is necessary. Critically, in-depth information about the relative contributions of input, production, and modality to the processes of receptive and expressive language development is also needed.

Relationship Between Input and Output Systems

A major gap in knowledge concerns the underlying relationships between input and output systems for individuals using AAC. More in-depth information is needed regarding receptive and expressive language development. If the argument is that receptive language will provide the basis for expressive language development, then clearly far more meticulous attention needs to be paid to receptive language. In our research descriptions traditionally, the question of comprehension has been the Cinderella component in the story. This avoidance is understandable, given the difficulties in defining and assessing comprehension, even for individuals without additional impairments.

The challenge is to find a methodological approach that is appropriate to the individuals we serve.

Role of Production

Another major question relates to the role of production generally in language acquisition. This question typically has been explored primarily in relation to the role of overt articulation in language development. Evidence from a case study of a child with typical hearing but the inability to speak suggests that a receptive grammar can develop through comprehension without production (Stromswold, 1994). Similarly, the study of infants tracheotomised at birth, but with the ability to produce age-appropriate linguistic structures once the speech mechanism was restored, suggests that an expressive system can develop in the absence of overt articulation (Adamson & Dunbar, 1991). By contrast, Blockberger (1997) reported specific difficulties with comprehension and production of grammatical morphology in 20 children with severe speech impairments, compared with language-matched speaking peers. Redmond and Johnson (2001) suggested that there may be very specific interactions between severe speech impairments and particular grammatical structures. Access to a productive system may allow analysis of the self-generated units, which Elbers (1995) argued serve as a privileged source of information to a language acquisition system. While comparable analysis may well be possible in the absence of overt production, it may simply be more difficult and put further strain on the child's language resources. As previously mentioned, where graphic representations can only be selected and not produced through motor articulation, the implications are as yet unknown. A particular concern however must be the low rates of initiation of novel productions by children who use graphic signs.

Role of Translation

We have briefly discussed the view that AAC output largely represents an expression of a speech-based message, re-coded into another modality. If this hypothesis is correct, then the question arises as to whether cross-modal translation should itself be a focus of intervention for those who cannot produce speech. In other words, if the presumption of recoding is correct, should we attempt to build recoding skills to support both the development of an expressive speech-based system, as well as to support the user in the recoding process? It may well be that the gradual shift towards English word order in PCS output observed by Smith (1996) as the age of the preschool children increased reflected a difference in metalinguistic skills of translating. Perhaps what is needed is an explicit focus on the skill of translating from one modality to another, rather than a general focus on structure, with its implicit presumption of cross-modal translation.

Exploration of Modality Effects

Many researchers have raised the possibility that both the modality and the interaction context of most AAC communications are such that a simple application of a spoken language frame of reference may only serve to muddy the waters, rather than illuminate the process (Light, 1997; Smith, 1996; Soto, 1999; von Tetzchner & Martinsen, 1996). There is a pressing need for further investigation of the specific features of graphic and manual communication, exploring both the similarities and the differences of organizational structure across these contexts and speech. In sign languages, for example, the location of an object is usually specified before the object is located. This is visually coherent because otherwise the signed object would hang in space. We do not know if it is possible to develop a "grammar" of graphic representations. If it is, then graphic output across different spoken language contexts should show similar patterns. In other words, it should not matter if the ambient spoken-language word order is subject–verb–object as in English or verb–subject–object as is the case in Irish—the graphic output should respect the priorities of the graphic modality, rather than reflecting spoken language constraints. Logically, these contrasting organizational structures might be expected to differentially affect the language acquisition process. In order to explore such effects, we need to look for patterns that are suggestive of productive rule-governed behavior within the modality (see Grove, 1997).

One of the sources of information about computational skills that has been relatively under-explored is the area of literacy development. For individuals with no access to speech production, the mastery of an orthographic code allows a potential match between computational characteristics in the input and output systems. Careful exploration of patterns of written language output should allow us to see if the observed patterns of graphic representation use reflect the medium, rather than underlying language abilities. Literacy restores the match between computational characteristics of input and output. It is also the case that an alphabetic code offers the opportunity for restoring symmetry and for supporting the development of computational skills as an intervention approach.

Storage and Retrieval of Lexicon

Linked to modality effects are questions regarding the underlying representations in memory. Is there a single lexicon, with dual representation of both spoken and graphic or manual entries? In this scenario, message formulation within the AAC modality clearly occurs long before the articulation phase, so the process is one of AAC encoding, rather than re-coding. Alternatively, is the nonspeech lexicon separately stored and represented, analogous to a bilingual situation, so that creativity may develop across either lexicon? For graphic representations, a third option exists, in that the representations may arguably not be stored as representations at all, but simply exist as external phenomena that can be harnessed for communication purposes. Each of these conceptualizations raises different implications in terms of both language and communication development, yet we have little direction to guide our understandings.

Choice of Pictorial or Abstract Systems

To date, there is little scientific evidence on which to base a decision about system selection. Studies have suggested pictorial systems are easier to learn initially, but that pictorial cues may inhibit transfer to a more abstract, symbolic system of representation (Sheehy & Howe, 2001; Wu & Solman, 1993). There is therefore an initial learnability advantage for PCS over Blissymbols; however, no studies have provided any evidence to suggest that it is easier for children to use PCS than Blissymbols. In fact, Raghavendra and Fristoe (1995) reported that, although enhancing Blissymbols may support faster learning and improved symbol retention, these advantages did not transfer into more effective communicative use of symbols. Likewise, Smith (1996) found that preschool children did not automatically transfer their skills in pointing to the correct PCS to using those symbols for communication. Careful and rigorous study of the effects of the introduction of contrasting systems and their long-term impact is needed in addition to discovering the process that kick-starts the shift from mere identification of pictures or matching signs to referents to the communicative use of nonspeech representations (see Chapter 4). The question of learnability or retention may be less relevant than previously thought, if high learnability ratings do not translate any more easily to linguistic or communicative use. Other factors, such as the instructional approach and the opportunities for functional generalization of skills, may be more significant in promoting effective use.

Optimizing Input

We need guidance on the best way to optimize input information, in order to maximize uptake of language. There are questions regarding the relative benefits of modeling of AAC input, the benefits of including or omitting speech as input, and how to match input to presumed uptake demands. Some investigators (e.g., Remington & Clarke, 1993a, 1993b) have argued that dual input may increase task difficulty by requiring a dual focus. Paivio (1986) also suggested that different kinds of information may be better suited and prioritized in processing across modalities. Should input be provided only in the nonspeech modality? If we do so, does this approach make the cross-modal translation more opaque? It seems likely that the answers to at least some of these questions will differ, depending on whether the individual in question is using the nonspeech modality as an alternative or as an augmentative communication option—for example, those with no functional speech may need relatively more models of language in their chosen modality because they have fewer options for self-expression. There is a need for carefully controlled studies comparing the effects of multi-modal input and speech-only input on AAC output. Tentative steps along this road have already been taken (Iacono & Duncum, 1995; Iacono, Mirenda & Beukelman, 1993). Further research may allow clinical decisions to be made about the nature and extent of input that is maximally facilitative.

Methodological Issues

To date, most of our information derives from small numbers of individuals followed for a relatively brief period of time. Most studies represent a snapshot in time rather than a videotaped sequence. In this respect, our data are from relatively brief periods of observation when set in the context of language learning years; perhaps what we are reporting is a transitional stage. Some individuals using AAC develop a linguistic system based on spoken language with no apparent difficulties. For example, Bruno (1998, personal communication) describes F, a 6-year-old boy with cerebral palsy who produced the following utterances on his voice output device:

She had the least mistakes.
We had Annie's birthday party.
I am going to a basketball game with Anastasia.
We are going to see Anastasia's uncle's team.

Detailed descriptions of the experiences of such individuals, particularly with reference to the nature of the input provided to them and the output options offered to them, may shed some light on the degree of asymmetry that the process of language acquisition can tolerate and the features of AAC output systems that can be considered supportive of language acquisition. There is an urgent need for carefully controlled longitudinal studies that follow children through both their AAC language acquisition and also their literacy development. Such studies may allow us to see progression toward a linguistic system that mirrors more closely that of the community (see von Tetzchner & Grove, 2003).

FUTURE CHALLENGES

One of the consistent challenges in research in most areas of AAC relates to the relatively small number of individuals within this population and the heterogeneity among individuals who use AAC. The potential pool of data remains critically constrained, although it is also worth remembering that much of what is known about child language was derived from careful study of individual children. There is a clear need to enhance the emphasis on international collaboration and links to mainstream research. There is a growing impetus for sharing data across child language research, with the development of databases such as CHILDES (MacWhinney, 2000). A major barrier to sharing data is the development of agreed conventions for transcription that can capture the very different communication that can arise when there is one partner with a severe speech impairment and several modalities are harnessed for communication. How should units for analysis be defined (Smith & Grove, 2001)? Which units are the most appropriate for inclusion? How should data where information is carried simultaneously across multiple modalities be treated? What kind of analysis is appropriate, if the system of organization is not syntactically based? As Fletcher and Garman (1995) pointed out, questions such as these reflect more than "good housekeeping" but are of fundamental theoretical and practical significance.

Finally, at least three factors must be considered in exploring the process of language acquisition: the input to the child, the uptake by the child from that input, and the output produced by the child. Separating the effects of these three interactive dynamic elements is extraordinarily complex. It is possible, if not indeed likely, that all three elements are affected in the case of a child with a severe communication impairment. Researchers in child language are as yet unable to agree what constitutes input and therefore what role communication partners play in the process. For most individuals who use AAC, there is some element of neurological damage, often implicating both cognitive and sensory-perceptual processes, thus affecting possible uptake, while the child's own output itself may critically influence the nature of further input provided (Locke, 1995). Asymmetry in input and output modalities may potentially exert a relatively peripheral influence on the language acquisition process for individuals with access to spoken language input and the potential for some speech output; however, its impact may be profound for very many others. Although attention has focused to date on interaction patterns within the communication dyad of individuals who use AAC and speaking partners, there has been relatively little attention to the individual who uses AAC's own output as a potential source of further information not only for the communication partner, but also for the individual who uses AAC.

REFERENCES

Adams, C. (1990). Syntactic comprehension in children with expressive language impairment. *British Journal of Disorders of Communication, 25,* 149–171.

Adamson, L., & Dunbar, B. (1991). Communication development of young children with tracheostomies. *Augmentative and Alternative Communication, 7,* 275–283.

Bates, E., Bretherton, I., & Snyder, L. (1988). *From first words to grammar.* Cambridge, England: Cambridge University Press.

Bellugi, U., van Hoek, K., Lillo-Martin, L., & O'Grady, L. (1988). Dissociation between language and cognitive functions in Williams syndrome. In D. Bishop & K. Mogford (Eds.), *Language development in exceptional circumstances.* Edinburgh, Scotland: Churchill Livingstone.

Bellugi, U., Wang, P.P., & Jernigan, T.L. (1994). Williams syndrome: An unusual neuropsychological profile. In S. Broman & J. Grafman (Eds.), *Atypical cognitive deficits in developmental disorders: Implications for brain function.* Mahwah, NJ: Lawrence Erlbaum Associates.

Besio, S., & Chinato, M. (1996). A semiotic analysis of the possibilities and limitations of Blissymbols. In S. von Tetzchner & M. Jensen (Eds.), *Augmentative and alternative communication: European perspectives* (pp. 171–181). London: Whurr.

Bishop, D. (1982). *Test of Reception of Grammar.* Manchester: University of Manchester, Department of Psychology.

Bishop, D. (1997). *Uncommon understanding: Development and disorders of language comprehension in children.* Hove, England: Psychology Press.

Bishop, D., & Edmundson, A. (1987). Language-impaired 4-year-olds: Distinguishing transient from persistent impairment. *Journal of Speech and Hearing Disorders, 52,* 156–173.

Bliss, C. (1965). *Semantography (Blissymbolics).* Sydney: Semantography Publications.

Blockberger, S. (1997). *The acquisition of grammatical morphology by children who are unable to speak.* Unpublished doctoral dissertation, University of British Columbia, Canada.

Brennan. (1992). The visual world of BSL: An introduction. In D. Brien (Ed.), *A dictionary of British sign language.* London: Faber & Faber.

Brien, D. (1992). *A dictionary of British sign language.* London: Faber & Faber.

Brown, R. (1973). *A first language: The early stages.* Cambridge MA: Harvard University Press.

Bruno, J. (1989). Customizing a Minspeak system for a preliterate child: A case example. *Augmentative and Alternative Communication, 5,* 89–100.

Camarata, S., Nelson, K., & Camarata, M. (1994). Comparison of conversational recasting and imitative procedures for training grammatical structures in children with specific language impairment. *Journal of Speech and Hearing Research, 37,* 1414–1423.

Collins, S. (1996). Referring expressions in conversations between aided and natural speakers. In S. von Tetzchner & M. Jensen (Eds.), *Augmentative and alternative communication: European perspectives* (pp. 89–100). London: Whurr.

Crain, S., & Fodor, J. (1993). Competence and performance in child language. In E. Dromi (Ed.), *Language and cognition: A developmental perspective* (pp. 141–171). Norwood, NJ: Ablex.

Dooley, J. (1976). *Language acquisition and Down's syndrome: A study of early semantics and syntax.* Unpublished doctoral dissertation, Harvard University, Cambridge.

Ecklund, S., & Reichle, J. (1987). A comparison of normal children's ability to recall symbols from two logographic systems. *Language, Speech & Hearing Services in Schools, 18,* 34–40.

Elbers, L. (1995). Production as a source of input for analysis; evidence from the developmental course of a word-blend. *Journal of Child Language, 22,* 47–71.

Fee, E.J. (1997). The prosodic framework for language learning. *Topics in Language Disorders, 17*(4), 53–62.

Fenn, G., & Rowe, J. (1984). An experiment in manual communication. *British Journal of Disorders of Communication, 10,* 3–16.

Fey, M., Cleave, P., Long, S., & Hughes, D. (1993). Two approaches to the facilitation of grammar in children with language impairment: An experimental evaluation. *Journal of Speech and Hearing Research, 36,* 141–157.

Fletcher, P., & Garman, M. (1995). Transcription, segmentation and analysis: Corpora from the language impaired. In G. Leech, G. Myers, & J. Thomas (Eds.), *Spoken English on computer* (pp. 116–127). Essex: Longman Press.

Fowler, A.E. (1998) Language in mental retardation. In J. Burack, R. Hodapp, & E. Zigler (Eds.), *Handbook of mental retardation and development* (pp. 290–333). Cambridge, England: Cambridge University Press.

Givón, T. (1985). Function, structure and language acquisition. In D. Slobin (Ed.), *The crosslinguistic study of language acquisition* (Vol. II, pp. 1005–1027). London: Lawrence Erlbaum Associates.

Goldin-Meadow, S., & Mylander, C. (1984). Gestural communication in deaf children: The effects and noneffects of parental input on early language development. *Monograph in Social Research and Child Development, 17,* 527–563.

Goldin-Meadow, S., & Mylander, C. (1993). Beyond the input given: The child's role in the acquisition of language. In P. Bloom (Ed.), *Language acquisition: Core readings* (pp. 507–542). London: Harvester Wheatsheaf.

Golinkoff, R.M., Pasek, K.H., Cauley, K., & Gordon, L. (1987). The eyes have it: Lexical and syntactic comprehension in a new paradigm. *Journal of Child Language, 14,* 23–45.

Goossens', C., & Crain, S. (1988). *Augmentative communication: Intervention resource.* Wauconda, IL: Don Johnston Developmental Equipment.

Gorenflo, D.W., & Gorenflo, C.W. (1991). The effects of information and augmentative communication technique on attitudes towards nonspeaking individuals. *Journal of Speech and Hearing Research, 34,* 19–34.

Grove, N. (1995). *An analysis of the linguistic skills of signers with learning disabilities.* Unpublished doctoral dissertation, University College, London.

Grove, N. (1997) Gesture, language and multimodality: Implications for research and practice. In E. Björk-Åkesson & P. Lindsay (Eds.), *Communication . . . naturally: Theoretical and methodological issues in augmentative and alternative communication* (pp. 92–101). Västerås, Sweden: Mälardalen University Press.

Grove, N., & Dockrell, J. (2000) Multi-sign combinations by children with intellectual impairments: An analysis of language skills. *Journal of Speech, Language, and Hearing Research, 43,* 309–323

Grove, N., Dockrell, J., & Woll, B. (1996). The two-word stage in manual signs: Language development in signers with intellectual impairments. In S. von Tetzchner & M. Jensen (Eds.), *Augmentative and alternative communication: European perspectives* (pp. 101–118). London: Whurr.

Grove, N., & McDougall, S. (1991). Exploring sign use in two settings. *British Journal of Special Education, 18,* 149–156.

Grove, N., & Smith, M. (1997). Input output asymmetries in AAC. *ISAAC Bulletin, 50,* 1–3

Harris, D. (1982). Communicative interaction processes involving nonvocal physically handicapped children. *Topics in Language Disorders, 2,* 21–37.

Harris, M. (1992). *Language experience and early language development: From input to uptake.* Cambridge: MIT Press.

Heim, M., & Baker-Mills, A. (1996). Early development of symbolic communication and linguistic complexity through augmentative and alternative communication. In S. von Tetzchner & M. Jensen (Eds.), *Augmentative and alternative communication: European perspectives* (pp. 232–248). London: Whurr.

Hjelmquist, E., & Sandberg, A. (1996). Sounds and silence: Interaction in aided language use. In S. von Tetzchner & M. Jensen (Eds.), *Augmentative and alternative communication: European perspectives* (pp. 137–152). London: Whurr.

Iacono, T.A., & Duncum, J. (1995). Comparison of sign alone and in combination with an electronic communication device in early language intervention: Case study. *Augmentative and Alternative Communication, 11,* 249–259.

Iacono, T.A., Mirenda, P., & Beukelman, D. (1993). Comparison of unimodal and multimodal AAC techniques for children with intellectual disabilities. *Augmentative and Alternative Communication, 9,* 83–94.

Klima, E., & Bellugi, U. (1979). *The signs of language.* Cambridge, MA: Harvard University Press.

Kraat, A. (1987). *Communication interaction between aided and natural speakers: An IPCAS study report* (2nd ed.). Madison: University of Wisconsin, Trace Research & Development Center.

Kraat, A. (1991, August 16–17). Methodological issues in the study of language development among children using aided language: Reactant Paper 1. In J. Brodin & E. Björk-Åkesson (Eds.), *Methodological issues in research in augmentative and alternative communication* (pp. 118–123). Proceedings of the First ISAAC Research Symposium, Stockholm, Swedish Handicap Institute.

Lahey, M. (1988). *Language disorders and language development.* New York: Macmillan.

Lees, J., & Urwin, S. (1997). *Children with language disorders* (2nd ed.). London: Whurr.

Levelt, W.J. (1989). *Speaking: From intention to articulation.* London: MIT Press, A Bradford Book.

Light, J. (1988). Interaction involving individuals using augmentative and alternative communication: State of the art and future directions. *Augmentative and Alternative Communication, 4,* 66–82.

Light, J. (1997). "Let's go star fishing": Reflections on the contexts of language learning for children who use aided AAC. *Augmentative and Alternative Communication, 13,* 158–171.

Light, J., Collier, B., & Parnes, P. (1985a). Communicative interaction between young nonspeaking physically disabled children and their primary caregivers: Discourse patterns. *Augmentative and Alternative Communication, 1,* 74–83.

Light, J., Collier, B., & Parnes, P. (1985b). Communicative interaction between young nonspeaking physically disabled children and their primary caregivers: Modes of communication. *Augmentative and Alternative Communication, 1,* 125–133.

Light, P., Remington, B., Clarke, S., & Watson, J. (1989). Signs of language. In M. Beveridge, G. Conti-Ramsden & I. Leuchar (Eds.), *Language and communication in mentally handicapped people.* London: Chapman & Hall.

Lloyd, L.L., Quist, R., & Windsor, D. (1990). A proposed augmentative and alternative communication model. *Augmentative and Alternative Communication, 6,* 172–183.

Locke, J. (1995). Development of the capacity for spoken language. In P. Fletcher & B. MacWhinney (Eds.), *Handbook of child language* (pp. 278–302). London: Blackwell Press.

Locke, J. (1996). Why do infants begin to talk? Language as an unintended consequence. *Journal of Child Language, 23,* 251–268.

Locke, J. (1997). A theory of neurolinguistic development. *Brain and Language, 58,* 265–326.

Loncke, F., Vander Beken, K., & Lloyd, L. (1997). Toward a theoretical model of symbol processing and use. In E. Björck-Åkesson & P. Lindsay (Eds.), *Communication naturally: Theoretical and methodological issues in augmentative and alternative communication* (pp. 102–112). Västerås, Sweden: Mälardalen University Press.

MacWhinney, B. (2000). *The CHILDES project: Tools for analyzing talk* (3rd ed.) Mahwah, NJ: Lawrence Erlbaum Associates.

Mayer-Johnson, R. (1981). *The Picture Communication Symbols.* Solana Beach, CA: Mayer-Johnson Co.

Mayer-Johnson, R. (1985). *The Picture Communication Symbols* (Vol. II). Solana Beach, CA: Mayer-Johnson Co.

McDonald, J. (1997). Language acquisition: The acquisition of linguistic structure in normal and special populations. *Annual Review of Psychology, 48,* 215–241.

McGinnis, J.S., & Beukelman, D.R. (1989). Vocabulary requirements for writing activities for the academically mainstreamed student with disabilities. *Augmentative and Alternative Communication, 5,* 183–191.

McGregor, K. (1997). Prosodic influences on children's grammatical morphology. *Topics in Language Disorders, 17*(4), 63–75.

McNeill, D. (1992). *Hand and mind: What gestures reveal about thought.* Chicago: University of Chicago Press.

Mizuko, M. (1987). Transparency and ease of learning of symbols represented by Blissymbols, PCS and Picsyms. *Augmentative and Alternative Communication, 3,* 129–136.

Mizuko, M., & Reichle, J. (1989). Transparency and recall of symbols among intellectually handicapped individuals. *Journal of Speech and Hearing Disorders, 54,* 627–633.

Morgan, J.L., Meier, R.P., & Newport, E.L. (1987). Structural packaging in the input to language learning: Contributions of prosodic and morphological marking of phrases to the acquisition of language. *Cognitive Psychology, 19,* 498–550.

Nelson, K. (1986). Event knowledge and cognitive development. In K. Nelson (Ed.), *Event knowledge: Structure and function in development* (pp. 87–118). Mahwah, NJ: Lawrence Erlbaum Associates.

Nelson, K. (1997). Cognitive change as collaborative construction. In E. Amsel & K. Ann Renninger (Eds.), *Change and development: Issues of theory, method and application* (pp. 99–115). Mahwah, NJ: Lawrence Erlbaum Associates.

Newport, M. (1988). Constraints on learning and their role in language acquisition: Studies of the acquisition of American Sign Language. *Language Science, 10,* 147–142.

Ninio, A., & Snow, C. (1988). Language acquisition through language use: The functional sources of children's early utterances. In Y. Levy, I. Schlesinger, & M. Braine (Eds.), *Categories and processes in language acquisition* (pp. 12–30). Mahwah, NJ: Lawrence Erlbaum Associates.

Oxley, J., & von Tetzchner, S. (1999). Reflections on the development of alternative language forms. In F. Loncke, J. Clibben, H. Arvidson, & L. Lloyd (Eds.), *Augmentative and alternative communication: New directions in research and practice* (pp. 62–74). London: Whurr.

Paivio, A. (1986). *Mental representations: A dual coding approach.* Oxford: Oxford University Press.

Petitto, L. (1993). Modularity and constraints in early lexical acquisition: Evidence from children's early language and gesture. In P. Bloom (Ed.), *Language acquisition: Core readings* (pp. 95–126). London: Harvester Wheatsheaf.

Piatelli-Palmarini, M. (Ed.). (1980). *Language and learning: The debate between Jean Piaget and Noam Chomsky.* London: Routledge and Kegan Paul.

Piatelli-Palmarini, M. (1994). Ever since language and learning: Afterthoughts on the Piaget-Chomsky debate. *Cognition, 50,* 315–346.

Pinker, S. (1994). *The language instinct: The new science of language and mind.* London: Allan Lane, The Penguin Press.

Platt, C.B., & MacWhinney, B. (1983). Error assimilation as a mechanism in language learning. *Journal of Child Language, 10,* 401–414.

Radford, A. (1990). *Syntactic theory and the acquisition of English syntax.* Oxford: Basil Blackwell.

Raghavendra, P., & Fristoe, M. (1995). "No shoes; They walked away?": Effects of enhancements on learning and using Blissymbols by normal 3-year-old children. *Journal of Speech and Hearing Research, 38,* 174–188.

Ramer, A. (1976). Syntactic styles in emerging language. *Journal of Child Language, 3,* 49–62.

Rapin, I., & Allen, D. (1987). *Developmental dysphasia and autism in preschool children: Characteristics and subtypes.* Proceedings of the First International Symposium on Speech and Language Disorders in Children, London.

Redmond, S., & Johnson, S. (2001). Evaluating the morphological competence of children with severe speech and physical impairments. *Journal of Speech, Language, and Hearing Research, 44,* 1362–1375.

Reid, B., & Kiernan, C. (1979). Spoken words and manual signs as encoding strategies in short-term memory for mentally handicapped children. *American Journal of Mental Deficiency, 84,* 200–202.

Remington, B., & Clarke, S. (1993a). Simultaneous communication and speech comprehension. Part I: Comparison of two methods of teaching expressive signing and speech comprehension skills. *Augmentative and Alternative Communication, 9,* 36–48.

Remington, B., & Clarke, S. (1993b). Simultaneous communication and speech comprehension. Part II: Comparison of two methods of overcoming selective attention during expressive sign training. *Augmentative and Alternative Communication, 9,* 49–60.

Renfrew, C. (1988). *Action Picture Test.* Oxford, England: C.E. Renfrew.

Rondal, J. (1980). Father's and mother's speech in early language development. *Journal of Child Language, 7,* 353–369.

Rondal, J. (1994). Exceptional cases of language development in mental retardation: The relative autonomy of language as a cognitive system. In H. Tager-Flusberg (Ed.), *Constraints on language acquisition: Studies of atypical children* (pp. 155–174). Mahwah, NJ: Laurence Erlbaum Associates.

Schlosser, R.W. (1997). Nomenclature of category levels in graphic symbols. Part I: Is a flower a flower a flower? *Augmentative and Alternative Communication, 13,* 4–13.

Sheehy, K., & Howe, M. (2001). Teaching non-readers with severe learning difficulties to recognise words: The effective use of symbols in a new technique. *Westminster Studies in Education, 24*(1), 61–71

Smith, M. (1996) The medium or the message: A study of speaking children using communication boards. In S. von Tetzchner & M. Jensen (Eds.), *Augmentative and alternative communication: European perspectives* (pp. 119–136). London: Whurr.

Smith, M. (1997). The bimodal situation of children developing alternative modes of language. In E. Björck-Åkesson & P. Lindsay (Eds.), *Communication . . . naturally: Theoretical and methodological issues in augmentative and alternative communication* (pp. 12–18). Västerås, Sweden: Mälardalen University Press.

Smith, M. (1998). *Pictures of language: The role of Picture Communication Symbols in the language acquisition of children with severe speech and physical impairments.* Unpublished doctoral dissertation, Trinity College, Dublin.

Smith, M. (2003). Environmental influences on aided language development: The role of partner adaptation. In S. von Tetzchner & N. Grove (Eds.), *Augmentative and alternative communication: Developmental perspectives* (pp. 155–175). London: Whurr.

Smith, M., & Grove, N. (1996, August 7–10). *The bimodal situation of children learning language using AAC.* Paper presented at the Seventh Biennial Meeting of the International Society for Augmentative and Alternative Communication, Vancouver.

Smith, M., & Grove, N. (1999). The bimodal context of children acquiring language using manual and graphic signs. In F. Loncke, J. Clibbens, H. Arvidson, & L. Lloyd (Eds.), *Augmentative and alternative communication: New directions in research and practice* (pp. 8–30). London: Whurr.

Smith, M., & Grove, N. (2001). Determining utterance boundaries: Problems and strategies. In S. von Tetzchner & J. Clibbens (Eds.), *Understanding the theoretical and methodological bases of augmentative and alternative communication* (pp. 15–41). Proceedings from the Fifth ISAAC Research Symposium, Washington, DC, August 2000.

Snow, C.E. (1995). Issues in the study of input: Finetuning, universality, individual and developmental differences and necessary causes. In P. Fletcher & B. MacWhinney (Eds.), *The handbook of child language* (pp. 180–193). Oxford: Blackwell Press.

Soto, G. (1999). Understanding the impact of graphic sign use on the message structure. In F. Loncke, J. Clibbens, H. Arvidson, & L. Lloyd (Eds.), *Augmentative and alternative communication: New directions in research and practice* (pp. 40–48). London: Whurr.

Soto, G., & Toro-Zambrana, W. (1995). Investigation of Blissymbol use from a language research paradigm. *Augmentative and Alternative Communication, 11,* 118–130.

Spiegel, B., Benjamin, B.J., & Spiegel, S. (1993). One method to increase spontaneous use of an assistive communication device: A case study. *Augmentative and Alternative Communication, 9,* 111–117.

Stephenson, J., & Linfoot, K. (1996). Pictures as communication symbols for students with severe intellectual disability. *Augmentative and Alternative Communication, 12,* 244–256.

Stokoe, W., Casterline, D.C., & Cronenberg, C.G. (1965). *A dictionary of American Sign Language on linguistic principles.* Washington, DC: Gallaudet College Press.

Stromswold, K.J. (1994, November). *Language comprehension without language production.* Presented at the 19th Annual Boston University Child Language Conference.

Sutton, A. (1997). Language theory and intervention practice. In E. Björck-Åkesson & P. Lindsay (Eds.), *Communication naturally: Theoretical and methodological issues in augmentative and alternative communication* (pp. 33–47). Västerås, Sweden: Mälardalen University Press.

Sutton, A. (1999). Linking language learning experiences and grammatical acquisition. In F. Loncke, J. Clibbens, H. Arvidson, & L. Lloyd (Eds.), *Augmentative and alternative communication: New directions in research and practice* (pp. 49–61). London: Whurr.

Sutton, A., Gallagher, T., Morford, J., & Shahnaz, N. (2000). Relative clause sentence production using augmentative and alternative communication systems. *Applied Psycholinguistics, 21,* 473–486.

Sutton, A., & Morford, J. (1998). Constituent ordering in picture pointing sequences produced by speaking children using AAC. *Applied Psycholinguistics, 19,* 525–536.

Tyler, A., & Sandoval, K. (1994). Preschoolers with phonological and language disorders: Treating different linguistic domains. *Language Speech and Hearing Services in Schools, 25,* 215–234.

Udwin, O., & Yule, W. (1990). Augmentative communication systems taught to cerebral palsy children—a longitudinal study. 1: The acquisition of signs and symbols and syntactic aspects of their use over time. *British Journal of Disorders of Communication, 25,* 295–309.

van Balkom, H., & Donker-Gimbrère, M. (1996) A psycholinguistic approach to graphic language use. In S. von Tetzchner & M. Jensen (Eds.), *Augmentative and alternative communication: European perspectives* (pp. 153–170). London: Whurr.

von Tetzchner, S. (1985). Words and chips—pragmatics and pidginization of computer-aided communication. *Child Language Teaching and Therapy, 1,* 295–305.

von Tetzchner, S. (1997). Introduction to language development. In E. Björck-Åkesson & P. Lindsay (Eds.), *Communication naturally: Theoretical and methodological issues in augmentative and alternative communication* (pp. 8–11). Västerås, Sweden: Mälardalen University Press.

von Tetzchner, S., & Grove, N. (Eds.). (2003). *Augmentative and alternative communication: Developmental perspectives.* London: Whurr.

von Tetzchner, S., & Martinsen, H. (1996). Words and strategies: Conversations with young children who use aided language. In S. von Tetzchner & M. Jensen (Eds.), *Augmentative and alternative communication: European perspectives* (pp. 65–88). London: Whurr.

Wilkinson, K., Romski, M.A., & Sevcik, R.A. (1994). Emergence of visual graphic symbol combinations by youth with moderate or severe mental retardation. *Journal of Speech and Hearing Research, 37,* 883–895.

Wu, H.M., & Solman, R. (1993). Effective use of pictures as extra-stimulus prompts. *British Journal of Educational Psychology, 63,* 144–160.

Yovetich, W.S., & Young, T.A. (1989). The effects of representativeness and concreteness on the "guessability" of Blissymbols. *Augmentative and Alternative Communication, 4,* 35–39.

III

Operational Competence

7

Supporting Competent Motor Control of AAC Systems

Jutta Treviranus and Vera Roberts

Most children can use their voices to produce rudimentary music; however, when it comes to using an external musical instrument to create more than a cacophony of sounds, a great deal of instruction and practice is needed. Musicians also have very specific and individual preferences about the type of instrument they use and how it is designed. Like musicians, individuals who use augmentative and alternative communication (AAC) require specialized skills developed through intensive instruction and practice to effectively control their AAC systems. Due to the frequently limited number of voluntary actions available to them, individuals who use AAC must employ a more complex notation system. Furthermore, the process of controlling the instrument must leave them enough cognitive energy to compose the message. Given the enormous investment of time and energy needed to become a talented communicator and the critical function to be performed, it behooves us to carefully choose and personalize AAC systems.

A necessary foundation for competent communication is operational competence: the ability to effectively control the tool or tools used to communicate, whether these tools are a part of the body or an external device (Light, 1989). This chapter discusses research issues related to motor control of AAC tools. Cognitive and sensory/perceptual issues will be discussed in other chapters (see Chapters 8 and 9). Before we embark on a review of motor control, we must recognize that motor function is not a clearly circumscribed domain but is dependent on and influenced by a myriad of other factors, including emotional state, level of arousal, comfort, motivation or attitude toward a tool or a task, attention to a task, and/or understanding of a task. Research and intervention in this area must take these and other dynamically interacting factors into account.

In the following sections, we briefly summarize the clinical wisdom used to guide decisions regarding the motor control of AAC systems, identify ways in which this can be supported through objective assessments, and review research that is relevant to these decisions. Although this chapter discusses AAC system optimization for motor control, it should be recognized that in the process of designing the entire AAC system, other factors may take priority, and motor control may need to be compromised. These factors include cognitive demands, linguistic optimization, cosmesis, and other practical considerations.

RESEARCH IN THE MOTOR CONTROL OF AAC SYSTEMS

Research in the area of motor control of AAC systems is plagued by a number of challenges and problems. One challenge is that there is no homogeneous group of individuals with developmental disabilities who use AAC. Motor profiles, cognitive abilities, sensory-perceptual abilities, and socioemotional factors, which all affect motor performance, vary tremendously across individuals who use AAC. This makes it difficult to apply standard empirical research methodologies. Researchers are frequently unable to find enough research participants in a given geographic area who meet a common set of criteria. A second challenge is that the human resources and funding for research in the field are scarce. As a result, research in the field is disjointed geographically and temporally. It has neither the momentum nor the cumulative mass to move forward with any consistency. As a result, the knowledge base addressing issues related to motor control of AAC systems in 2002 is largely anecdotal or involves the results of studies related to the efficacy of a specific technology. Frequently, there is no control group or control condition in these studies and confounding factors are not adequately addressed. In some studies, conclusions about the efficacy of a tool are based on theoretical calculations and not on human trials. Consequently, for a large portion of the research, the results cannot be generalized and may not be predictive of motor performance for more than the specific individuals participating in the study. Results of the research must be applied very cautiously. Outcome measures showing high levels of device abandonment and underuse suggest that future research is urgently required to refine current practices and improve outcomes for individuals who use AAC (Collier, Norris, & Rothschild, 1990; Murphy, Markova, Collins, & Moodie, 1996).

Given the status of research that directly addresses motor control of AAC systems, AAC practitioners or support teams may need to draw on research in a number of related fields in which research is better supported or more mature. For example, human factors or the factors that affect human performance have been the subject of a well-established field of research. Human factors are defined as systematic approaches to improving the fit between the user and the tool or environment (Kantowitz & Sorkin, 1983). The field of human factors has examined human functioning in the performance of particular tasks in great depth. This knowledge has been applied to the design of products and environments that are used to perform specific goal-oriented tasks. While the field of human factors has primarily addressed the performance of individuals without disabilities, the knowledge gained can be cautiously applied or modified to gain insight into tool fit for individuals with disabilities. The related field of neuromotor therapy also has a modest body of research. Although much of this research is conducted by supporters or detractors of specific treatment regimes (e.g., Brooks-Scott, 1999; Sabbadini, Bonanni, Carlesimo, & Caltagirone, 2001), the insights into factors that improve neuromuscular control can be of benefit when determining an optimal AAC control system. Also of relevance is the largely applied research body addressing seating and positioning systems (Post, 1990).

Given the paucity of empirical research, the art and science of designing AAC control systems for individuals with developmental disabilities is based largely on clinical "wisdom." This wisdom is occasionally supported with single case studies or anecdotal descriptions, but rarely verified through repeatable research. Caution must be exercised as this unverified knowledge becomes the subject of numerous prescriptive clinical textbooks and more significantly the subject of exams for accreditation processes. Many textbooks have dropped the cautions and disclaimers of earlier publications and present the unsupported or poorly supported clinical assumptions as generalizable fact. The exams or accreditation processes enshrine these unsupported assumptions as indisputable principles of practice. The complexity of supporting the development of competent motor control of AAC systems may require the flexibility of unconstrained human judgment; however, we have a duty to recognize our assumptions and verify that they are accurate.

Since the 1970s, professionals in the field have collected the clinical wisdom of the time and synthesized it into assessment protocols, guidelines, or clinical manuals. For example, in 1983, Barker, Hastings, and Flanagan created the control evaluator and training kit. In the late 1980s, Lee and Thomas brought together a team of clinicians to develop a comprehensive assessment protocol, which they documented in a detailed manual on the assessment of control of computer based-technology for people with physical disabilities. Other comprehensive clinical manuals have included Cook and Hussey (1995) and Anson (1997).

For a field of research to grow and mature, it requires the ongoing discussion, debate, and knowledge building that occurs within a community of interest (McNaughton, Beukelman, & Dowden, 1999). To facilitate this process, the community requires a common, but evolving and flexible, frame of reference. This frame of reference serves to draw together the collective research findings. It serves not just as a communication tool but also as a tool to organize and structure collaboration.

A focus group of leaders in the field, conducted by Jennifer Angelo (2000), may be a good snapshot of the state of the science of interface design in AAC. The leaders were asked to generate a list of the most influential factors in switch selection. Rather than creating a systematic, logical list of factors, the experts composed a list representing a broad range of overlapping approaches and perspectives. The nature of the factors identified by these experts, the varying classification schemes and theories represented, and the lack of attention to objective measures suggest that switch assessment (and possibly other areas of practice) remains a "soft" individual art. The field appears not to have settled on common structures or theoretical viewpoints with which to frame dialogue.

MODELS OF MOTOR CONTROL

To frame or provide structure to our clinical wisdom about motor control of AAC systems, several authors have proposed frameworks or models that are adaptations of models from other relevant fields. The two models or frameworks of greatest relevance to motor control of a communication tool are Cook and Hussey's (1995) Human Activity Assistive Technology (HAAT) model and Gentile's (1987) Skill Acquisition Model.

The HAAT model was an adaptation of Bailey's Human Performance Model (1989) extended to encompass factors encountered by users of assistive technology. The HAAT served to frame the complex interrelationship between the human, the activity, the assistive technology, and the context. At the core of this model was the person's wish to perform an activity. The activity defines the goal of the assistive technology system, is accomplished by completing a set of tasks, and is carried out within a context. The activity and context determine the skills required to complete the activity. If there is a shortfall in the necessary skills, assistive technology may be used.

The Skill Acquisition Model, a system of movement classification, was an extension of Bernstein's (1967) systems model. The Skill Acquisition Model described skill as a goal-directed behavior that is guided by the consequences of the movement it produces. The goal of skill acquisition is to attain economy of effort by maintaining or changing movement attributes such as body orientation and object position. The Skill Acquisition Model emphasized the dimension of time and the maturation of the skill.

These models provide the bridge between the field of AAC and other relevant fields; they also provide a common framework to organize and relate the collective observations and insights gathered in the field. A creative combination of the two models may best represent the motor control challenges faced by individuals who use AAC.

MOTOR IMPAIRMENTS OF INDIVIDUALS WITH DEVELOPMENTAL DISABILITES WHO USE AAC

Before we embark on a discussion of research related to the design of AAC control systems, it would be useful to review the physical challenges faced by individuals with developmental disabilities who use AAC. Individuals with developmental disabilities who cannot use speech to communicate effectively are frequently also affected by neuromuscular or musculoskeletal problems that impede their motor control. Frequently, the cognitive impairments associated with developmental disability are one reason AAC is required; however, this section will only consider issues of AAC access relating to motor impairment (see Chapter 8 for further discussion of cognitive issues). The following is a discussion of common developmental disabilities with related motor issues and the considerations these motor issues bring to bear on AAC system access and selection.

Cerebral Palsy

Perhaps the most common developmental disability with associated motor impairment is cerebral palsy. Bobath (1991) and Cogher, Savage, and Smith (1992) noted the following characteristics. Cerebral palsy is characterized by hypertonia (increased muscle tension) or hypotonia (decreased muscle tension) or fluctuations between the two. All forms of cerebral palsy result from damage to regions of the brain involved in muscle control, coordination, and balance. Due to this brain damage, individuals with cerebral palsy are at increased risk for cognitive impairments and learning delays. Their ability to produce speech may be impaired, requiring the use of AAC. Generally, the impairment of the neuromuscular system that prevents speech production also impairs other regions of the body and makes the already complex task of selecting appropriate AAC systems all the more difficult.

The extent of motor system impairment caused by cerebral palsy is quite varied; one or more limbs may be affected or a specific region of the body may be affected (e.g., right side or lower body). In the case of the more common spastic cerebral palsy, the region affected is used to categorize the instance of cerebral palsy (e.g., hemiplegia, quadriplegia). Generally, the type of cerebral palsy is labeled by the manifestation of the disorder in the affected region, and the discussion unfolds following this classification of the disorder.

Hypertonic, or spastic, cerebral palsy is the most common form of the disorder and refers to the presence of constant tension in the muscles. This form is caused by damage to the cerebral cortex. Athetoid cerebral palsy involves uncontrolled, often erratic, movements. The most rare form of cerebral palsy is ataxic cerebral palsy, which features lack of balance and coordination and presence of tremors. Finally, mixed cerebral palsy involves a combination of two or three of the forms of cerebral palsy.

Spastic Cerebral Palsy   Not all individuals with cerebral palsy require AAC or require AAC all of the time. The remaining discussion will cover individuals for whom AAC systems are a requirement at least some of the time. When choosing the appropriate AAC systems for an individual who has cerebral palsy, the form of and regions affected by the cerebral palsy must be considered along with standard considerations of an AAC assessment such as age, communication needs/lifestyle, literacy level, and language skills.

When the individual has all or partial control of one upper limb, as is the case of hemiplegia or monoplegia, then AAC systems that require fine motor control or precise pointing may be appropriate. Gesture-based communication would be an appropriate complementary communication system for these individuals. Choices for aided AAC may include direct selection systems or standard keyboard entry; however, it should be noted that planning, control, and coordination of fine motor actions is often impaired in individuals who have cerebral palsy, and typical limb functioning and appearance may be misleading. Seating position is seldom an issue in this form of cerebral palsy nor is physical access (i.e., the ability to physically obtain the AAC system without assistance).

Individuals with diplegia will have more severe spasticity in the legs than arms. There is, however, some involvement of the upper limbs, and fine motor control is generally affected. Establishing the individual's range of movement and ability to coordinate movement will be key in any assessment to determine an appropriate aided AAC system. Individuals with diplegia may have concomitant tone problems in the trunk. For this reason, they may require special positioning or supports in order to sit with stability and may be able to stay in one position for only limited amounts of time. Furthermore, care must be taken to devise a system that will be physically accessible to the individual as often as possible with as little assistance as possible.

Athetoid Cerebral Palsy   Athetoid cerebral palsy is characterized by uncontrolled and erratic movements, especially of the hands and face; it is caused by damage to the basal ganglia in the midbrain. Individuals with this form of cerebral palsy have varied muscle tone and fluctuate between hypertonia and hypotonia. These fluctuations are largely responsible for the associated writhing and erratic movements and make control or coordination of movement for affected individuals extremely difficult. Individuals with athetoid cerebral palsy will also have difficulty holding an upright seating position with any degree of steadiness. The variability of muscle tone in individuals with this form of cerebral palsy makes assessment and selection of an AAC system particularly difficult.

Ataxic Cerebral Palsy   This form of cerebral palsy is characterized by lack of balance and coordination that results from damage to the brain's center for balance and coordination in the cerebellum. Also, tremors are often associated with this more rare form of cerebral palsy and fine motor skills are particularly affected.

Down Syndrome

Down syndrome is also a common developmental disability but with fewer motor issues than are associated with cerebral palsy. Winders (1997) and Smothers Bruni (1998) summarized the following characteristics. Typically, the individual with Down syndrome exhibits poor muscle tone (hypotonia) and loose-jointedness (hyperflexibility). Generally, individuals with Down syndrome require AAC for two reasons: 1) to scaffold language learning and production; and, 2) to augment unintelligible speech. Although physical characteristics of the formation of the tongue and palette are largely associated with speech difficulties in individuals with Down syndrome, studies indicate other contributing factors. Blackstone (1989), in summarizing this research, noted that the hypotonia associated with Down syndrome along with neurological impairment may hinder speech production as might brain morphology, processing difficulties, and memory deficits. Furthermore, these processing deficits may also interfere with writing and production of gestures or signs. Studies of gesturing ability showed that individuals with Down syndrome were slower and less consistent in the formation of gestures compared with their typically developing peers (Elliot, 1985; Frith & Frith, 1974).

Complex motor sequences may be more difficult for individuals with Down syndrome. For example, Elliot, Gray, and Weeks (1991) found that AAC systems involving pointing or keyboard entry may not be the most efficient choice for individuals with Down syndrome who use AAC and may require intense motor training. Furthermore, Anwar and Hermelin (1979) found that in a pointing task, children with Down syndrome had difficulty changing the angle of their pointing from straight ahead to slightly off-center. This finding is particularly important because this kind of motion may be required for typing or pointing to items in an array.

Autism, Pervasive Developmental Disorder – Not Otherwise Specified, and Asperger's Syndrome

Cohen and Volkmar (1997) and Anderson (1999) noted the following characteristics of individuals with autism and related disorders. These disorders are characterized by uneven gross and fine motor skills. Language skills are usually impaired in individuals with autism, and one in three will have no spoken communication at all. Similar impairments of language and communication may be evident in individuals with a diagnosis of pervasive developmental disorder–not otherwise specified (PDD–NOS). Individuals with Asperger's syndrome, however, generally have stronger language and communication skills. Issues of motor access to AAC are less frequently a problem for individuals who have a diagnosis of autism or PDD. However, an assessment of motor skills should still involve the expertise of an occupational or physical therapist to determine functional positioning and the ability to produce hand shapes, orientation, position and movement, and/or the appropriate access to aided AAC systems (Light, Roberts, DiMarco, & Greiner, 1998).

Rett Syndrome

Rett syndrome is a progressive disorder that is typically found only in females; it is believed to be fatal to male fetuses. Lindberg (1991), Hagberg (1994) and Cohen and Volkmar (1997) summarized the following characteristics of individuals with Rett syndrome. Girls with Rett syndrome have a loss of communication skills by 18 months, loss of purposeful use of the hands, and gait disturbances. Motor skill loss is followed by development of stereotypical hand movements such as tapping, flapping, or squeezing. Girls with Rett syndrome generally develop spinal curvature, rigid (inflexible) muscles, and contracted joints. Motor skills in these individuals are severely limited and are likely to deteriorate during adulthood. This deterioration may affect ability to maintain stability in an upright position as well as coordination of movement of limbs and head. The contracted joints and stereotypical movements associated with Rett syndrome may make reaching, pointing, and gesture formation extraordinarily difficult or impossible for the affected individual. Seating position will also likely be a concern due to associated muscle rigidity, poor circulation, and spinal curvature.

MOTOR SKILL ACQUISITION

In order to adequately support competent motor control of AAC systems, it is useful to understand research and theory related to skill acquisition. The ideal AAC system can be controlled without conscious awareness of the process or the motor steps involved (Light & Lindsay, 1991). As with speech, the communicator should be able to concentrate on the message and not the production. To reach this ideal, the individual must become highly skilled at controlling the AAC system, to the point where the required actions have become automatic or habituated (Treviranus, 1994).

Skill development requires a large investment of time and effort. Therefore, it behooves the AAC team to select the method of controlling the AAC system with great care. Unlike other aspects of the AAC system, such as output mode, the motor control acts should remain relatively stable. Changes to the method of controlling the tool may be likened to learning to touch-type with a completely new keyboard layout or learning to write with the opposite hand.

Two important precursors to motor skill acquisition are 1) understanding of the task and the motor steps needed to accomplish the task; and 2) trusting the tool or system (Newell, 1981; Treviranus, 1994). The individual's mental model of the motor task should be accurate and complete. Tasks inconsistent with an individual's mental model of a task are learned more slowly. For example, people who learned to type using a typewriter had difficulty learning the use of the "return" key on a word processor to only separate paragraphs rather than to separate each line of text. For these individuals, having text wrap to the next line without having to hit "return" was inconsistent with their previous model of the carriage return (Carroll & Olson, 1988). Trust is built on an accurate understanding of the system and on the trustworthiness or reliability of the system. Trust depends on how well the system meets the expectations the user has of it (Newell, 1981; Treviranus, 1994).

Stages of Skill Acquisition

Skilled behavior can only be achieved through many hours of practice. Most theorists agree that there are three distinct stages in learning a skill (Anderson, 1989; Fitts, 1964; Lane, 1987). In the first phase, the learner collects facts, background information, and general rules related to the skill. Performance of the task is slow and effortful, requiring the learner's full attention. The learner experiments with various strategies to approximate the desired behavior. In the second phase, the skill is refined. Task components become integrated and inefficient strategies are filtered out; however, task performance remains largely under conscious control. Noticeable gains in speed and accuracy are made during this stage. Performance gains begin to plateau at the end of this stage. The third stage is the longest stage. Through many repetitions of the task, with only gradual improvements, the learner achieves skilled, automatic performance. At this stage, the behavior no longer requires the user's full attention. The learner no longer relies on external feedback to guide behavior, but uses internalized patterns of expected events. The learner can generalize the behavior to similar tasks and fine-tune the behavior for efficiency in specific task situations.

For an individual who is learning to use automatic scanning, the first phase would be spent understanding the scanning pattern, learning the movement needed to activate the switch, becoming familiar with the timing needed to make a selection, determining strategies for error correction, and learning the layout of the keyboard. In the second phase, the individual who uses AAC would integrate the component skills into more fluid control of the interface. Rather than following the cursor visually, the user may learn to look at the desired item and hit the switch when it is highlighted. During this phase, missed selections and errors would decrease and higher scanning speeds would be tolerable. Task endurance would also increase. In the final phase, the user would begin to reduce visual vigilance of the scanning keyboard and make selections based on the familiar scanning pattern. Errors would be greatly reduced and error correction would cause less disruption. Conscious attention to the task of scanning would be decreased, allowing the user to concentrate on the message to be communicated. True skilled behavior is characterized by (Fisk, Oransky, Skedsvold, 1988; Lane, 1987; Logan, 1988; Salmoni, 1989; Treviranus, 1994)

1. Economy of effort (Far less energy and attention are required largely due to the automaticity of skill components. This also implies that the mechanisms for performing the task tend not to be readily available to conscious awareness.)
2. Consistency of performance
3. Adaptability (Performance mechanisms are automatically adjusted to compensate for a wide variety of task conditions.)
4. Speed
5. Dependence on internalized (or intrinsic) prompts and feedback rather than prompts and feedback from the environment or computer system (extrinsic prompts)
6. Ability to anticipate the actions of the system
7. Ability to multitask or carry on more than one activity at a time

Researchers agree that initial performance on a task is not a predictor of skilled performance (Lane, 1987). Therefore, it may be greatly misleading to decide which access system will ultimately lead to the best skilled performance based on initial performance. Certain access systems lend themselves better to skill development (e.g., access systems with consistent tasks as well as prompts and feedback that can be internalized). Similarly, certain actions are more conducive to skilled performance (e.g., actions that are not dependent on external prompting). For example, a comparison of initial performances using Morse code versus automatic scanning would be a misleading indicator of future skilled performances with these two systems. The AAC team must extrapolate the knowledge they have of the learner's abilities and needs to choose the optimum access system. If users have the prerequisite abilities to learn Morse code, they may be able to achieve far better performance using Morse code than using automatic scanning.

Similarly, training that promotes optimal initial performance may not necessarily be optimal for skill acquisition. Variations in the training task, interference or interruptions in the training schedule, and emphasis on discovery learning may result in poorer initial performance but in the development of more robust and transferable long-term performance (Gardlin & Sitterley, 1972; Lane, 1987; Lee & Magill, 1985; Logan, 1988).

The needs of the skilled user are very different from the needs of the novice user (Logan, 1988; Newell, 1981; Salmoni, 1989). Novice users are heavily reliant on external cues and feedback to guide their performance while skilled users rely on internalized or memorized cues. For example, a novice user of scanning would rely heavily on the visual highlighting of rows and items, whereas the skilled user of scanning would rely on familiarity with the scanning rhythm and the timing required to select each key. Skilled users can deal with complex choices, whereas novice users benefit from a staged introduction of choices. For example, the novice individual who uses AAC may need to use a series of logically branched keyboards with few items in each keyboard, whereas the skilled user may wish to have one large keyboard with all the choices represented.

UNAIDED AAC

Before any external communication tool is considered, the AAC team should determine the individual's ability to communicate without the use of an external device. Communication using only the body is referred to as unaided communication, whereas communication using an external (high-technology or low-technology) device is referred to as aided communication. Even individuals who rely heavily on external communication devices also use unaided communication. Methods of unaided AAC include gaze, pointing, physically leading a communication partner, gesture-based codes, and manual sign systems. In the mid-1970s, when the AAC field was in its infancy, the focus of studies was to show that individuals with severe developmental disabilities could indeed learn to communicate using some form of sign, symbol, or other AAC device (see Sevcik, Romski, & Adamson, 1999, for an overview). Since then, research on AAC use by individuals with developmental disabilities has assessed communication patterns (e.g., Romski, Sevcik, & Adamson, 1999; Schepis, Reid, & Behrman, 1996), communication efficacy (e.g., Sevcik et al., 1999), role of the communication partner (e.g., Hourcade & Parette, 2001), and methods of teaching communication acts (e.g., Mechling & Gast, 1997; Reichle & Johnston, 1999). As Sevcik and Romski (2002) noted, "The field's focus has moved away from an assessment of devices . . . and onto the development and refinement of effective interventions that promote functional communication use, along with broader issues of consumer advocacy and social policy" (p. 5).

Little research examines unaided AAC. In terms of functional communication, unaided AAC is often seen as limited because signs and gestures generally require a communication partner who is conversant in these symbols and their meanings. Indeed, research has found that individuals with communication devices were better able to convey their meaning with aided systems than with gestures alone (Romski et al., 1999). However, unaided systems are praised for their portability and physical accessibility/proximity. Regardless of advances in AAC technology, unaided AAC has a place in the communication toolbox of individuals with developmental disabilities.

The motoric dimension of sign formation has been divided into seven characteristics:

1. Production mode (degree of contact between the hands and/or body in formation of signs)
2. Symmetry (refers to two-handed signs with a symmetrical sign requiring both hands to form the same shape)
3. Handedness (left or right hand formation)
4. Visibility (ability to see the sign being made)
5. Reduplication (ability for others to reproduce the sign)
6. Complexity
7. Fluidity (transition from beginning to end hand shapes)

An overview of the research suggests that signs with hand/body contact are learned more easily, as are signs that are symmetrical (see Doherty, 1985, for an overview of research in these areas). Research into acquisition of signing skills should be expanded to investigate how these motoric characteristics affect cognitive load and muscle fatigue while communicating as well as efficacy of the communications.

AIDED COMMUNICATION

Despite the importance of unaided systems, many individuals with significant communication disabilities require aided AAC. Designing an aided AAC system that affords optimal motor control requires that the AAC team make a series of decisions or choices (Beukelman & Mirenda, 1998; Cook & Hussey, 1995; Lee & Thomas, 1989).

Although a number of cognitive, linguistic, and social factors will influence these decisions, we will restrict our discussion to optimization of motor control. Ideally, these decisions should be based on a motor ability profile, a series of objective criteria-based assessments followed by careful matching of resulting tool criteria with existing or customizable tools. In reality, the decision is frequently influenced by available technology and the AAC systems familiar to the team. The ideal tool configuration as determined by motor assessment often does not exist, or may exist in a tool that does not have other features that are needed for communicative competence.

The practice of basing assessment on readily available technology can create an unfortunate cycle. Assessing based on trial and error with available tools does not identify more optimal tool criteria, leading to a demand for only the tools already available and the perpetuation of an ever-shrinking feature set.

Once it has been decided that some form of aided communication is needed, the general choices related to motor control include

- What positioning system, if any, is needed in each communication context
- What control act will be used
- What input device is most effective
- What selection method is most effective
- What selection set layout is most efficient
- What mounting system is needed

Positioning

Proper positioning contributes to motor control by aligning the body, normalizing tone, and preventing discomfort, fatigue, and potential deformities (McEwen, 1997). Motor assessment for AAC system control cannot occur without first addressing proper positioning in each of the positions the individual will use throughout the day (Beukelman & Mirenda, 1998). Accurate control of distal joints is dependent on stabilization and support of proximal joints. Positioning must take into account conditions that trigger primitive reflexes. Control is optimized when muscle tone is normalized as much as possible (balancing hypertonicity versus hypotonicity, and extension versus flexion; McEwen, 1997). Occasionally, optimum postural control and positioning (according to neuromotor principles) is inconsistent with optimal positioning for AAC system control (Beukelman & Mirenda, 1998). At times, voluntary movement is so restricted that the AAC team has no choice but to choose a control action that may trigger primitive reflexes such as the asymmetrical tonic neck reflex (ATNR). The postural supports needed to control posture and muscle tone may also restrict movement needed to control an AAC device. In these situations, the team must make an informed choice, with full knowledge of the consequences of the choice. The topic of positioning for optimal AAC system control is covered very thoroughly in a number of clinical textbooks and will not be replicated in this chapter (Beukelman & Mirenda, 1998; Cook & Hussey, 1995; McEwen, 1997).

Control Act or Effector

Once the individual is well positioned, an inventory of voluntary, repeatable actions can be taken. The generally accepted hierarchy of access sites is:

hands and arms, then head, and last feet and legs (Lee & Thomas, 1989). Hands and arms are considered first because they are the most practical body part for pointing, they allow a great deal of fine motor control if unimpaired, and hand use tends to be more socially acceptable. An individual may be able to control several fingers or only a single digit; stabilizers such as splints or hand held pointers can be used. Head movement can be used to directly point to a target using mechanical or electronic pointers, or it can be used to activate several switches. Discrete, repeatable vocalizations can be used even if they cannot be understood (Treviranus, Shein, & Parnes, 1992). Puffing and sipping are also possible control acts, although these are rarely controllable by individuals who cannot speak due to neuromotor impairment. Controlled gaze can be an effective control mechanism for partner-assisted communication and can be used with electronic sensors to control computer-based AAC systems (Brandenburg & Vanderheiden, 1987).

Once an inventory of available voluntary movements is taken, these movements are usually ranked using a number of criteria. These criteria most commonly used include (Beukelman & Mirenda, 1998; Cook & Hussey, 1995; McEwen, 1997)

- Speed and accuracy of movement
- Ability to initiate the movement, control the movement throughout the range, and terminate the movement
- Strength and endurance
- Versatility

Versatility refers to a collection of practical factors, such as the likelihood that the action can be accurately detected by a switch or other interface, and the ability to use the action in different contexts and positions. The inventory and criterion ranking of available voluntary movements is used to help determine the selection method and the specific input device.

To gain insight into the qualities of human movement, several researchers in the assistive technology field have attempted to replicate research findings derived from human factors studies of users without disabilities in studies of individuals who use alternative access technologies. The most popular of these is the attempt to replicate or suggest adjustments to Fitts' law. Fitts (1964) found that speed of movement toward a target had a consistent relationship with the distance and size of the target. The smaller and further away the target is, the longer it takes to move to the target. This holds true whether movement is in a three-dimensional plane or a two-dimensional plane such as a computer screen (Jagacinski & Monk, 1985). It also holds true when using pointing devices such as helmet-mounted controls or hand-controlled joysticks. Radwin, Vanderheiden, and Lin (1990) found that, for individuals without disabilities, Fitts' law held when using a standard mouse or a head pointer, but average movement time was faster when using the mouse than when using the head pointer. They also found that Fitts' law held for two individuals with cerebral palsy using head pointers; however, movement time was greatly improved when these individuals were provided thoracic support throughout the continuum of target size and distance. These types of studies lead to further questions. Is there a consistent correlation between spacing of targets, and speed and accuracy? What influence does the number of joints to be controlled in the action have on Fitts' law (e.g., shoulder, elbow, and wrist versus elbow alone with wrist and shoulder stabilized)? Which is most predictive of speed and accuracy for individuals with neuromotor impairments: distance or size of targets? Future research is required to address these questions.

Input Device

The primary function of the input device is to accurately detect the control signal(s) made by the user. The simplest and most common input devices are mechanical microswitches or switch arrays. These can be used when the control act involves a movement that causes some body part to make contact with and move a switch surface. The following properties must be considered when determining the most suitable mechanical switch (Beukelman & Mirenda, 1998; Cook & Hussey, 1995; Lee & Thomas, 1989; McEwen, 1997):

- Size and shape
- Resistance or force required to activate the switch
- Travel of the switch or distance the switch must be moved to signal activation and whether there is a fixed or flexible end point
- Feedback provided
- Orientation
- Position

The body part making contact with the switch and the degree of control of the action determines the switch size, shape, and contact surface. Head contact would dictate a soft surface but does not require a large surface for targeting. The strength and range of the movement and the presence or absence of involuntary movements or tremors determines the resistance or force and travel required to activate the switch. Possible switch feedback includes the tactile and kinesthetic indicators provided by switch travel, resistance, and the switch end point; auditory feedback provided by the mechanical switch or added through the hardware or software the switch controls; and visual feedback provided by the AAC system. Membrane switches do not require any travel but also provide limited feedback. The switch or switch array should be oriented and positioned to accommodate the range and direction of the control act. The position of the switch must also balance the range of movement required by the switch position with the number of involuntary actions detected due to closer proximity of the switch to the resting position of the controlling limb.

The mounting of the input device must accommodate the position and orientation found best for accuracy, speed, and comfort. Mounting must also take into account practical considerations such as ease of set up, the various positions of the person, and the need for portability of the device (Beukelman & Mirenda, 1998; Cook & Hussey, 1995; Lee & Thomas, 1989; McEwen, 1997). The mounting system can also be used to provide stabilizers or guides to improve the accuracy of switch activation. The relative arrangement of multiple switches must take into account the actions required to release one switch and move to the next switch. For example, four switches can be arranged in many different ways, such as using a gated four-direction joystick in a square box surrounding the user's thumb or in a horizontal crescent array with vertical slots as stabilizers.

If the controlling act cannot be detected using a mechanical switch then other interfaces must be explored, including

- Pneumatic switches that are activated through puffing and sipping
- EMG switches that are activated through muscle contractions that do not cause movement of a body part
- Sound switches or voice switches that detect sounds or utterances of a specific quality
- Motion detectors or video processing systems that detect specific movement patterns (e.g., eye movement, head pointers) (Brandenburg & Vanderheiden, 1987)

Selection Method

The primary motor task to be accomplished in aided communication is to indicate a selection or a series of selections that comprise a message. The most direct and simple method of indicating a selection is to point to the desired item (direct selection; Vanderheiden, 1984). Pointing can be achieved with various body parts and with the aid of sticks or pointers that extend reach. If an individual cannot reliably point to an adequate number of selections, then coding or scanning is used. Coding entails sequencing the items that can be directly selected as a code for a larger set of selectable items. Scanning entails giving a timed response to choices offered sequentially.

Direct Selection   Clinical knowledge holds that direct selection is the simplest and most generally familiar method of indicating a choice. Most studies indicate that direct selection is also less cognitively demanding than scanning. Ann Ratcliff (1994) compared the performance of 100 typically developing children from first through fifth grade using direct selection and scanning. The children made significantly more errors using scanning than direct selection. The difference between direct selection and scanning became more pronounced as the difficulty level of the comprehension task increased. This finding was supported by Mizuko, Reichle, Ratcliffe, and Esser (1994) who studied the short-term visual memory differences when using direct selection and row–column scanning in typically developing 4-year-olds. Short-term visual memory was significantly reduced when using scanning. This bias toward direct selection holds even when assessment protocols would predict otherwise. Horn and Jones (1996) compared the response accuracy, acquisition rate, and response time of a child with severe physical limitations when using scanning and direct selection. Results indicated that direct selection was more effectively used even though pre-assessment information predicted that scanning should be a more appropriate technique.

Direct selection, if within the user's capabilities, is also faster. Users of direct selection can reach from 30 to 60 selections per minute, whereas users of scanning systems are usually restricted to fewer than 10 selections per minute (Goodenough-Trepagnier, 1980; Trefler & Crislip, 1985).

To determine whether direct selection is an option and to optimize the direct selection interface, the individual's pointing range and resolution must be assessed (Beukelman & Mirenda, 1998; Cook & Hussey, 1995; Lee & Thomas, 1989; McEwen, 1997). Range refers to the area that can be reached with a pointing action whether with a limb, one or more digits, a pointer of some sort (e.g., head, mouth, or chin pointers), or eye gaze. Resolution refers to the number of discrete targets that can be accurately selected within that range. Resolution may vary across the available range. Range and resolution can be improved by manipulating the position and orientation of the target surface, and by providing stabilizers (e.g., grasping the edge of the target surface and sliding to targets along the edge). The range dictates the overall size and shape of the keyboard; the resolution determines the size and spacing of the targets.

When computer-based or electronic AAC systems are used, once a target is reached, the user must also signal the selection. Depending on the keyboard used, this is done by pressing a key, pausing or sustaining a pointer over the target for a given interval, performing a gesture, or activating a switch. To improve accuracy, a number of selection characteristics can be manipulated; these include the key pressure, the key delay or duration the key must be depressed before a selection is signaled, the key travel, and the key feedback. When indicating a selection by dwelling over a target, the duration of the dwell, the parameter of the dwell area, and the feedback to indicate that the dwell timing has been initiated and completed can be manipulated. When indicating a selection using a gesture (specific movement of the pointer) or switch activation (e.g., mechanical switch, vocalization, blink, puff or sip), the choice of the switch or gestures and various parameters of the switch or gesture used can be manipulated (see the section called Input Device for further discussion). Systems are available that make it easier to select the likely key by using the relative probability that one key will be selected over another. These systems may reduce the dwell time of the probable target, draw the cursor toward the target (causing the target to be "magnetic"), or increase the active area of the target (see the section called Disambiguation).

Ideally the assessment should not be constrained in the range of keyboard sizes, shapes, target properties, or input techniques tested, but should be guided solely by the individual's abilities. In reality, AAC teams do not have the assessment tools or the actual technologies available for prescription to fully explore the user's capabilities. Given what is known about body mechanics, the rectangular, flat, targeting surface of most keyboards is not the ideal direct selection interface. A curved keyboard surface that follows the radius of the arm or a kidney-shaped keyboard would seem more appropriate if using single-digit pointing. Parallel rows of uniform keys are also not ideal. Most individuals have varying levels of resolution across the range they are able to reach reliably. Clinical experience also holds that keys with kinetic, tactile, and auditory feedback are preferred by users with neuromotor impairments. Ironically, membrane keyboards or touch screens are becoming more popular.

Scanning   At the other end of the selection technique continuum is scanning. Direct selection is operationally simple but requires the greatest physical control. Scanning is operationally complex and extremely slow but requires minimal physical control (Ratcliff, 1994). Scanning is an option when a communicator can only point to, or reliably make contact with, one or two discrete targets. Scanning refers to the process whereby a person or device sequentially presents choices or groups of choices to the communicator, who signals when the desired item is reached. In computer-based scanning, the options are usually highlighted by a cursor moving in an established pattern over an array of items on the computer screen. The user controls the cursor by activating or releasing one or more switches. Large sets of items are often arranged into subgroups; the user first chooses the group to which the desired item belongs, and then the item itself.

The cursor movement can be ongoing (automatic scanning), activated by a single switch hit[1] (automatic stop scanning), stepped forward by repeated switch hits (step scanning), or occur only when the switch is depressed (inverse scanning). A selection can be signaled by hitting the same switch, hitting

---

[1]Although the term *switch hit* is used, this can be replaced with *switch activation* to refer to nonmechanical switches such as sound switches, EMG switches, and eye blink switches.

a second switch, releasing the switch, releasing the switch and waiting a predetermined interval, or releasing the switch and hitting a second switch (Lee & Thomas, 1989).

To determine which scanning type is best, a number of skills can be objectively measured. These skills include reaction time as it relates to timed activation of a switch and timed release, the ability to sustain hold on a switch, the ability to move rapidly and accurately between switches, and the ability to hit the switch repeatedly (Beukelman & Mirenda, 1998; Cook & Hussey, 1995; Lee & Thomas, 1989; McEwen, 1997). Automatic scanning requires accurate timing in activating the switch. Many individuals with neuromotor impairments experience increased muscle tone and spasticity when anticipating the need to act, making it difficult to activate a switch. If this is the case, inverse scanning may be easier as it requires timed release of a switch. If timed release is not reliable, two-switch inverse scanning may be considered as scanning toward a target can be resumed if the switch is released too soon, given that the second switch is used to indicate a selection. If timing of any kind is very difficult, step scanning is a slow and tedious alternative; however, as the user develops greater skill, the transition from step scanning to inverse scanning is a natural progression that requires minimal adjustment in either the conceptual model or the motor pattern.

The pattern or order in which selectable items are presented can also be varied. These scanning patterns include linear scanning (one item at a time), row–item scanning (first rows and then items within rows), group–row–item scanning (groups of rows, then rows, and then items within rows) and quadrant scanning (quarters of the keyboard and then the quarters of the quarter; Lesher, Moulton, & Higginbotham, 1998). The balance of wait time versus switch hits required to make a selection can be varied by adjusting the scanning pattern. Group–row–item scanning, compared with linear or row–item scanning, reduces the average number of items scanned in waiting to select any one item but increases the number of switch hits and the complexity of the process. Through mathematical analysis, it is evident that a square arrangement of the keyboard is most efficient for row–column scanning.

Users who have three to five voluntary movements that they can sustain and accurately release may be able to use directed scanning, where a cursor is driven across the matrix of selectable items to the intended item and a selection is indicated. This method may provide greater speed and directness than traditional scanning (Treviranus & Drynan, 1990; Vanderheiden, 1984).

With all scanning techniques, the scanning speed can be adjusted. The speed–accuracy tradeoff associated with adjusting the scanning speed must take into account the individual's tolerance for inaccuracy. The speed can be continuous or variable. A scanning delay or a slower rate when restarting at the beginning of the array allows the user to adjust following a selection and find the next desired item. Some keyboards allow the user to accelerate toward the desired item and then invoke a slower scanning speed when the desired item is in proximity (Treviranus & Drynan, 1990).

Depending on the scanning pattern, certain keys in the array are reached quicker than others. In standard row–column scanning, the upper left-hand corner is scanned first and the lower right-hand corner last (See Figure 7.1). Selectable items can be arranged to take advantage of this order by placing the most important or most frequently chosen items in the upper left-hand corner. For a directed-scanning system the most efficient array varies depending on several factors: whether the cursor returns to the center following a selection or remains in the same position, whether the cursor can "wrap" around the edges or stops at the edge of the keyboard, and whether or not diagonal movements are possible by holding two switches at the same time (see Figure 7.2).

1	2	3	4	5	6	7	8
2	3	4	5	6	7	8	9
3	4	5	6	7	8	9	10
4	5	6	7	8	9	10	11
5	6	7	8	9	10	11	12
6	7	8	9	10	11	12	13
7	8	9	10	11	12	13	14
8	9	10	11	12	13	14	15

Figure 7.1. Row–column scanning. Cells are ranked according to the number of scanning steps that must be taken to arrive at the cell. To improve efficiency, items of higher priority can be arranged in more quickly scanned cells.

x + 5	x + 5	x + 5	x + 5	5	x + 5	x + 5	x + 5	x + 5
x + 5	x + 4	x + 4	x + 4	4	x + 4	x + 4	x + 4	x + 5
x + 5	x + 4	x + 3	x + 3	3	x + 3	x + 3	x + 4	x + 5
x + 5	x + 4	x + 3	x + 2	2	x + 2	x + 3	x + 4	x + 5
5	4	3	2	1	2	3	4	5
x + 5	x + 4	x + 3	x + 2	2	x + 2	x + 3	x + 4	x + 5
x + 5	x + 4	x + 3	x + 3	3	x + 3	x + 3	x + 4	x + 5
x + 5	x + 4	x + 4	x + 4	4	x + 4	x + 4	x + 4	x + 5
x + 5	x + 5	x + 5	x + 5	5	x + 5	x + 5	x + 5	x + 5

Figure 7.2.   Directed scanning. Cells are ranked for a directed scanning keyboard in which the cursor returns to the center following a section. Cells that can be reached using only one movement are ranked higher. *X* refers to the individual difficulty rating associated with moving from one controlling act to another.

Lesher and colleagues (1998) found that frequency-based arrangements resulted in significant switch savings; however, the motor efficiency gains must be weighed against the cognitive costs of arranging vocabulary items according to frequency, rather than in logical familiar sequences (Light & Lindsay, 1991).

Additional Approaches

If a communicator is not able to effectively point to more than a few items, is scanning the only choice? Three approaches can be used to bridge the gap between direct selection and scanning (Treviranus, 1994; Vanderheiden, 1984).

One approach is to use a form of coding in which two or more direct selections are used to choose each item. The sequence of actions required to choose an item can be either cued or memorized. In the second approach, the user chooses a group of items and relies on the computer to guess (or "disambiguate") which item within the group is intended. Thus, the user makes fewer selections to choose each item, unless the computer guesses incorrectly. The last approach is to combine direct selection and scanning in one device. Thus, users directly select to the extent of their abilities and then scan to choose items that they are unable to select; or select from a larger group and then scan items within that group (hybrid selection; Treviranus et al., 1992). Although these approaches have been sporadically implemented in AAC devices since the 1980s, they are far less popular and common than scanning or direct selection systems. This is unfortunate as a large proportion of individuals who are unable to use direct selection may have more controllable actions than the one or two acts required in scanning; these individuals may benefit from coded access, disambiguation, or hybrid access.

Coded Access   For the purposes of this chapter, we wish to distinguish between coding, such as Morse code, in which a series of relatively meaning-free actions are combined to select an item, and coding, such as abbreviation expansion, numeric encoding, or iconic encoding (also referred to as retrieval techniques), in which symbolic items are combined to form a code for the desired message. For the purposes of our discussion, the former will be termed *primary coding* and the latter *secondary coding.* Only primary coding will be discussed in this chapter; secondary coding or retrieval techniques will be covered in other chapters.

The most commonly available primary code is Morse code. In traditional Morse code, the alphanumeric characters and commands are selected by entering a variable length code of two elements frequently referred to as *dits* and *dahs.* Users must reliably control the timing of one or two actions in order to distinguish dits from dahs. As the code is of variable length, all elements of the code must be entered within a set time interval. In single-switch Morse code, dits and dahs are distinguished by holding the switch for a short and a long duration respectively.

A number of Morse code variations have been developed to adapt Morse code to the motor characteristics of individuals with neuromotor impairments. Vanderheiden (1984) proposed a selection technique that uses three reliable actions to control Morse code and eliminates the timing requirements usually associated with Morse code. The user does not use the duration of switch activation to distinguish between dits and dahs but instead activates one of two switches (i.e., a dit switch and a dah switch). In addition, the elements of the code do not need to be entered during a set time interval. The third switch is used to signal the completion of the code. A successful variant of this approach to Morse code is the use of a three-state switch (i.e., left, off, and right) such as a lever to replace the first two switches, allowing the user to activate the second switch with the same action used to deactivate the first switch. If only two actions are available, the second action can be used to either signal the end of the code sequence or to enter the second duration.

To reduce the need to memorize the code, a number of devices have provided the Morse code user with a traversable visual map of the code. The choices are displayed in a binary tree structure. The user guides the cursor to the selection by activating the appropriate switch at each branching (Beukelman & Mirenda, 1998). Although the code is visually mapped out, the visual scanning and tracking demands of the technique may make it difficult to accurately control for individuals who have perceptual and visual-motor deficits.

Morse code, when mastered, is a potentially fast and efficient means of computer input; however, several factors restrict its use (Brandenburg & Vanderheiden, 1987). Some users have difficulty meeting the motor demands of Morse code, even when modified to reduce timing requirements. Effective use of Morse code is dependent on the user's ability to memorize the codes; the training requirements to learn Morse code are frequently unrealistic in today's assessment and training environments (Beukelman, Yorkston, & Dowden, 1985). Morse code is also dependent on literacy skills. Even when the codes are reassigned to symbols, children often have difficulty in understanding the operational demands. Morse code in its traditional form is designed for skilled, literate users. The initial learning load is very high and must be mastered before the access technique can be used effectively (Treviranus, 1994).

There are approaches to coded access in addition to Morse code. For example, the eight positions of a joystick or an eight-switch array have been used as an alternative to Morse code. As the number of possible code elements is increased, the length of each code can be reduced (Cantor, 1998).

A form of coding prevalent prior to 1990 was the use of a manual eye-gaze frame referred to as an Etran (Trefler & Crislip, 1985). Users pointed with their eyes to a group of items on the eye-gaze frame, subsequently indicating which item was intended within the group by gazing to another group which indicated the location, color, or number of the item (Beukelman et al., 1985). Anecdotal reports argue that this is an efficient selection method; the primary limitation is the listener. Because listeners must decode the message, even trained listeners may be unable to keep up with skilled users (Trefler & Crislip, 1985). Electronic systems have been modeled on the Etran. These systems overcome the reduced reliable resolution of eye gaze by grouping selectable items into eight groups of eight items. The user first gazes at the appropriate group and then at the group that corresponds to the position of the desired item within the group. In most implementations the display remains static. The gaze is detected remotely by a built-in camera system (Brandenburg & Vanderheiden, 1987).

Coded access has been the subject of several studies in the larger commercial realm. For example, research has explored a coding system for users who can accurately target to a telephone keypad (Witten, 1982). In most keypads, three letters of the alphabet are assigned to each of nine keys. The simplest application of the keypad requires two keystrokes to select each letter (Witten, 1982). The user selects the key to which the desired letter is assigned and then one of the remaining three keys to indicate which of the three letters is intended. This technique has been developed further to eliminate the need to make a second selection through disambiguation (see the section on Disambiguation for further discussion).

Researchers have argued that coded selection techniques are potentially far more efficient than scanning (Goodenough-Trepagnier, 1980; Vanderheiden, 1984). Coded access is also far more conducive to motor skill development and automaticity as the cues and prompts needed to control the system can be internalized; however, use of traditional coding systems is restricted due to one or more of the following reasons (Treviranus, 1994):

- The initial training demands are high because the user must memorize a code.
- The system is based on traditional orthography and therefore requires well-developed literacy skills.
- The user must be able to time his or her response.
- The possible controlling actions monitored by the device are limited (e.g., eye gaze, pressing keys on a telephone keypad).

Disambiguation   The second approach to access using less precise pointing actions involves prediction of the intended choice by the computer. This method is referred to as *disambiguation*. The most successful model of disambiguation is the communication that occurs between individuals using graphic communication displays and their familiar listeners. Frequently, these individuals get their message across with very ambiguous, imprecise pointing (augmented with facial expression, body gestures, and vocalizations). The familiar listener disambiguates the imprecise pointing actions by using what they know about the individual (what they usually speak about) and the context and by observing the individual's pointing actions (where they seem to be pointing to or heading toward).

There are also electronic systems that incorporate disambiguation. Foulds, Soede, and van Balkom (1987) further developed the telephone keypad interface, described previously, using disambiguation. In this system, a computer predicts which of the three letters is intended given information about the occurrence of letter combinations and sequences in the English language. Arnott and Javed (1992) used a similar approach on a standard computer keyboard by disabling all but twelve keys. In trials with four clients with cerebral palsy over a 5-week period, they found that the clients made up to 50% fewer typing errors when using the "reduced keyboard."

Linguistic prediction programs typically make use of knowledge of previous messages and the immediate context of the message, but commercially available computer access systems do not record the pointing action, only the final key press or completed dwell time (i.e., keeping the pointer on the desired target for a predetermined time). Researchers at the Hugh MacMillan Centre and Lyndhurst Spinal Cord Centre, however, have investigated the use of a computer monitoring and access technique called *dynamic competition selection,* which mimics a familiar listener by also monitoring the pointing action (Nantais, Shein, Milner, & O'Beirne, 1991). The system sets the sensitivity for selection of each element based on both lexical probability distributions based on previously entered selections and pattern analysis of the pointing motion itself. Specifically, pointing motions using a head pointer are monitored. This information is used by a "neural-net" program that learns about the user's pattern of movement. Once trained to recognize motions, the neural-net can suggest the likelihood of an element being targeted or simply passed over. The system then allows likely elements to be more easily selected, and makes selection of unlikely elements more difficult by manipulating the dwell time for selection. This technique is therefore more tolerant of imprecise pointing than standard keyboards. Although attempts have been made to mimic the familiar listener in disambiguating imprecise pointing, there is as yet no computer-based system that is as effective as a familiar listener.

Hybrid Access   If direct selection is potentially faster than scanning but direct selection is beyond the pointing abilities of many individuals who use AAC, a combination of direct selection and scanning may more closely match a user's motor skills. Treviranus and colleagues (1992) investigated a hybrid access system that allowed a child with repeatable discrete utterances to directly select high-frequency words or groups of vocabulary using voice recognition and then scan to vocabulary that could not be directly selected. A variation of this system would be to combine direct pointing to a group of items with scanning within the group. This system could be further enhanced by allowing direct selection of predicted or high frequency items as well as groupings of remaining items, combined with scanning within the selected group.

Dynamic Visually Cued Coding   Given that many AAC devices now include dynamic displays, there is a class of selection techniques that has not been explored. These selection techniques bridge the gap between scanning and direct selection and address the restricting factors presently associated with coded access systems. These are coded access systems that are dynamically, visually cued.

The simplest form of this coding is a quartering keyboard (Treviranus, 1992, 1994). In a quartering keyboard, all of the selectable items are divided into four quarters. The user points to the quarter containing the target item. That quarter then expands to fill the whole keyboard and is again divided into four quarters. The user then chooses the quarter containing the desired

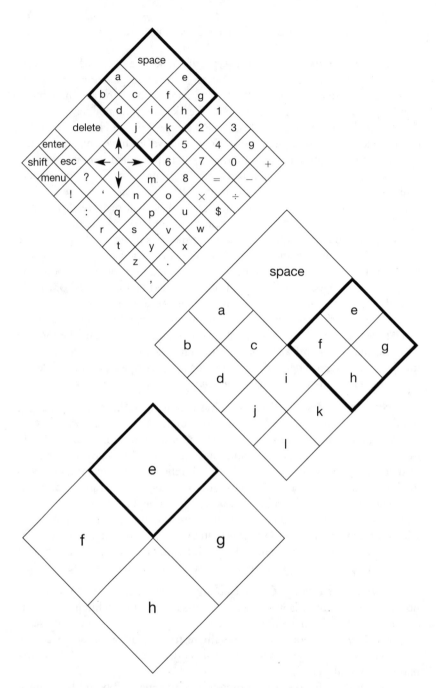

Figure 7.3. Diagonally oriented quartering keyboard to accommodate head movement in four directions. The selected squares can 1) be expanded to fill the screen if imprecise pointing is used (see above) or 2) they can remain in the same location if switches are used (see opposite). (From Treviranus, J. [1992]. *Quartering, halving, gesturing: Computer access using imprecise pointing*. Proceedings of the 15th Annual Conference of RESNA, Toronto, Canada; adapted by permission.)

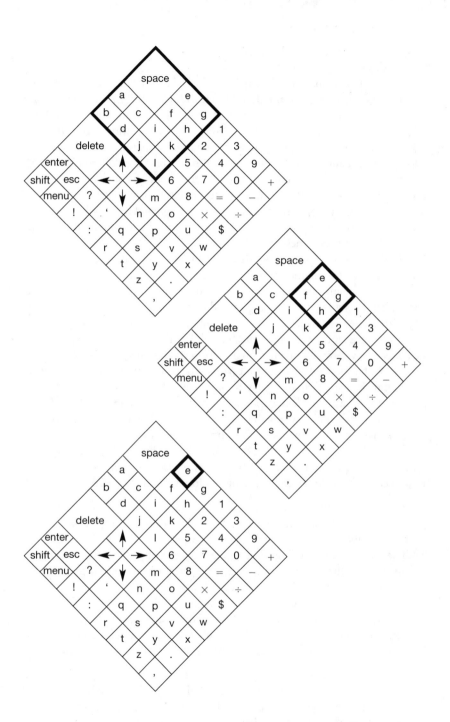

225

item as before and that quarter expands to display one item per quarter. The user then points directly to the desired item. Thus, a user who can only point to four targets can accurately pick one of 64 items with three selections. Each selection act involves locating the desired choice and pointing to it. If the keyboard is accessed using a head pointer, it can be displayed as a diamond to allow control using vertical and horizontal head movements (see Figure 7.3), rather than diagonal movements. If the user is not accessing a touch screen but is using a head pointer or other mouse emulator, once the user has pointed to the desired group or item, a selection can be signaled by pressing a switch, vocalizing (to activate a sound switch), or pausing over a square for a predetermined time (dwell time).

This selection technique lends itself well to simple gestural input. Using the example of the diamond keyboard accessed using a head pointer, each quarter of the diamond can be bisected with a vertical or horizontal line. A selection can be signaled by passing over the line and back to the center of the keyboard. The desired item is therefore selected by a series of three horizontal and/or vertical head movements. The size of the movements required can be adjusted by moving the lines further from the middle of the keyboard.

As with other coding techniques, this type of selection technique lends itself well to motor habituation. Treviranus (1994) found that, over 1–2 years, users became less and less dependant on visual cues and visual feedback. Users reached the point where the selectable items no longer needed to be visible; the users chose items using fluid habitual gestures.

The various permutations of this selection technique have not been explored. A wide array of user-optimized coding schema and selection techniques could be developed by varying the following three factors:

- The discrete signals: the number of discrete signals or targets that make up the elements of the code (e.g., X keys on a keyboard, X number of switches, or X number of switches each with two durations)
- The code length: the length of the sequence of signals that will comprise the codes in the coding system (e.g., an item can be chosen by pressing targets 4 times or by hitting a switch twice).
- Variable/uniform length of code: whether the length of the sequence is uniform or variable (e.g., in the same coding scheme a frequently chosen item could be entered by activating only one or two targets whereas a less frequently chosen item could be entered by activating four targets).

The coding scheme allows the quicker selection of more frequently chosen items when a variable code length is used. This method is visually represented by varying the number of items in each group such that frequently selected items would be in a group with few items.

The coding scheme can be matched to the user's skills and needs by varying these factors. The number of items that can be selected is determined

Table 1

○○							

○ e				− t			
○○ i		○− a		−○ n		−− m	
○○○ s	○○− u	○−○ r	○−− w	○−− d	−○− k	−−○ g	−−− o

○○○ h	○○○○− v	○○−○ f	−−○○ z	○−○○ l	−○−○− ( )	○−−○ p	○−−− j	−○○○ b	−○○− x	−○−○ c	−○−− y	−−○○ z	−−○− q	○○−−○○ ?	−−−− Ch

Table 2

− t							
−○ n				−− m			
−−○ d		−○− k		−−○ g		−−− o	
−○○○ b	−○○− x	−○−○ c	−○−− y	−−○○ z	−−○− q	○○−−○○ ?	−−−− Ch

Table 3

−○ n			
−−○ d		−○− k	
−○○○ b	−○− x	−○−○ c	−○−− y

Table 4

−○− k	
−○−○ c	−○−− y

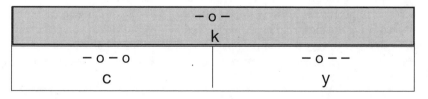

Figure 7.4. Visually cued two-switch Morse code. Motor control of the keyboard does not differ from traditional three-switch Morse code.

227

by the number of possible discrete signals and the code length. (In a scheme of uniform code length, the number of items is equal to the number of signals to the power of the number of elements in the code. For example, if the user can point to 4 targets and she points three times to complete a code, she can select 64 items or 4^3).

Thus, a visually cued equivalent to two-switch Morse code could be devised (see Figure 7.4). The discrete signals would be two, plus a signal to indicate the completion of a code. The code length would be variable, with one to six signals. Unlike traditional Morse code, the user could begin using the system without memorizing the code. Unlike the tree representation of Morse code referred to earlier, the user can maintain the desired final selection in view at all times.

A coding scheme can be represented to the user in deceptively simple ways using dynamic visual cuing. The visual cuing allows the user to regard the code as simply selecting the group or key containing the desired item more than once. Each time a group is selected that group expands to become the entire keyboard until there is only one item on each key (see Figures 7.5 and 7.6). Because a dynamic keyboard is used, the range and resolution of the user's limited pointing abilities can be accommodated. The size, spacing, location, and layout of the target areas can be manipulated.

Unlike Morse code, these dynamic visually cued coding keyboards can be populated with pictures, symbols, words, or phrases. If the user is literate the code length can be reduced using disambiguation (see Figure 7.6). Thus, the communicator does not specify the letter *e* but the group containing the letter *e* (e.g., the group *e, d, g*). The computer tries to "guess" which letter is intended, either directly after the letter is entered or once the end of the word is indicated by a space or punctuation. Thus, the length of the code can be reduced by one or two elements. In order to aid the computer in guessing the most likely letter, letters can be grouped to decrease the likelihood that any two letters in the group will occur in the same place (Silverman & Treviranus, 1994). As with other selection techniques, a key can be used to retrieve another keyboard with other sets of vocabulary items.

These selection techniques (e.g., coded access, disambiguation, hybrid access) can potentially address some of the shortfalls of scanning access without requiring the motor skills of direct selection. To date, this area is relatively unexplored with very few commercial or research technologies implementing these techniques. Clearly, future research is required to investigate applications of these techniques.

Errors

An often ignored but important aspect of control system design is the handling of errors. It has been observed that recovery from errors can cause sig-

yes	no	Do you have?			
go fish		bird	cat	dog	donkey
		fish	giraffe	horse	monkey
		mouse	pig	panther	rat
		sheep	snake	whale	zebra

bird	cat	dog	donkey
fish	giraffe	horse	monkey
mouse	pig	panther	rat
sheep	snake	whale	zebra

panther	rat
whale	zebra

Figure 7.5. Keyboards can be populated with words, phrases, pictures, or symbols. In this case, the user can target four large targets and makes a selection by choosing the desired square three times.

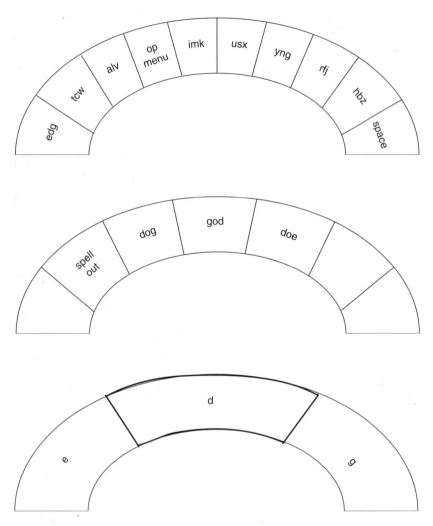

Figure 7.6. The keyboard shape is designed to match the user's optimal range. Disambiguation is used to determine which word is being constructed using ambiguous selections of keys with more that one letter. In this case, the system offers three possible words (dog, god, doe) or the option to manually choose the correct letter (spell out).

nificant reductions in the fluency of access. A selection error not only causes communication to slow down but also causes distraction from the intended message and the communication task. Error management is therefore an important component of system design. These management techniques include: striking the correct balance between speed and accuracy when adjusting features such as scanning speed; designing the system such that the consequence of an error at any one step in the process is minimized; and, most important, creating easy techniques to correct errors. The correct balance of speed and

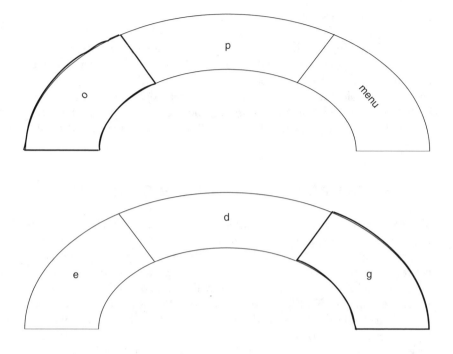

accuracy depends on the individual, the context, and the task. We are much more forgiving of errors in an e-mail than in a cover letter, and certain communicators are more tolerant of errors than others. Each step in making a selection provides another opportunity for an error; however, more steps may reduce the consequence of any one error. Take the example of automatic scanning. If the scanning pattern is group–row–item, there is the opportunity to choose the wrong group, the wrong row, and the wrong item. If the scanning pattern is row–item, there is only the opportunity to choose the wrong row and item; however, if the two arrays have the same number of items each error in row–column scanning has much greater consequence than in group–row–item scanning as the individual must wait for the cursor to scan a much larger group of items with each error. Ideally, the communicator should have an easy, one-step method of reversing or undoing the consequences of an erroneous action (e.g., an undo switch, an escape cell in the scanning array, or a signal such as an extended switch hold to reverse the preceding selection). It is important that error correction is designed so that more errors are not made in the process of correcting errors.

Integrating Motor Considerations with Other Considerations

Determining the best positioning system, control act, input device, selection method, selection set layout, and mounting system from a motor control perspective allows the AAC team to draft the functional requirements for a low-technology or high-technology AAC device. These functional requirements need to be adjusted to take into account cognitive, linguistic, and socio-emotional considerations as well. Even if the individual is supplied with an ideal AAC control system, the assessment and prescription process has been wasted if the system is rejected due to complexity, cosmesis, or unrealistic demands on the listener.

ASSESSMENT, RESEARCH AND PRODUCT DESIGN

The disparity between design principles, derived from research and clinical practice, and evolving product design conventions is a distressing trend in the area of motor access to AAC that highlights the need for greater collaboration between researchers, clinicians, and product designers. Feature sets and options on AAC systems are shrinking rather than expanding. The situation is reminiscent of the QWERTY keyboard. The QWERTY keyboard layout was originally designed to slow down typists using mechanical typewriters. Keys frequently occurring together were separated so that the typewriter strikers would not jam. The QWERTY arrangement of keys is therefore a poor design and far less efficient than other layouts for today's keyboards; however, it has become a convention. A great deal of manufacturing and training has been invested in the QWERTY keyboard layout, making it virtually impossible to replace. Similarly, conventions are becoming established in alternative access that are not based on sound design principles and may become difficult to change. For example, clinical wisdom and human performance research shows that control is more accurate if switches have kinetic feedback and travel; however, membrane switches without travel or feedback are becoming more popular in AAC systems because of their relativly low cost and ease of manufacturing.

For the general population, in which the range of needs is fairly constrained and the controlling acts available are many, a reduced set of device control options is only inconvenient. There is usually another way to complete the same task. For individuals who require AAC systems, a large range of interface choices is critical because the needs of this group are very diverse. The controlling acts available to any one individual may be very limited and the tasks achieved using alternative access techniques are typically critical tasks. Furthermore, because of the critical functions addressed by the AAC system, the risk of repetitive strain injury may also be greater. The need for a variety of options is therefore much greater for individuals using AAC systems.

In addition to a broad range of interface choices to meet the broad range of motor skills, a new way of transferring the user interface from AAC system to AAC system must be devised so that the user does not need to master a new control system to take advantage of technical advances. This would require de-coupling the interface from the device functionality or allowing sufficient interface flexibility to replicate the user's familiar interface. The same service should be available to individuals who use AAC that keyboard manufacturers have delivered to QWERTY keyboard users, albeit for more optimized interfaces.

To ensure that the field does not stagnate with a limited set of conventions within AAC systems, there must be strong links between 1) assessment and prescription, 2) research and outcome measures, and 3) product design and development. Research, assessment findings, and outcome measures should drive product design, not the other way around. Assessment and prescription should not be constrained by available products or product conventions. Research that guides product development should go beyond testing of specific devices to testing new overall device strategies. Long-term performance with an AAC system should be considered in evaluating its efficacy, not just initial performance. To influence and steer technical development, the field needs to conduct outcome measures, comparative evaluations, and clinical feedback. This requires greater collaboration among researchers, clinicians, and product manufacturers to develop a more solid empirical base on which to build future technological developments.

Among the priorities for future research in the area of motor control of AAC systems are

1. The investigation and development of systems that support skilled motor control and support the transfer of mastered skills from one AAC system to another, as well as the investigation of predictors of skilled performance

2. Research to support the development of intelligent assistance that emulates the familiar partner but does not undermine the interface predictability required for motor habituation

3. The evaluation and development of access methods that allow the individual to make better use of all available voluntary actions, including profiling of the range of voluntary actions and their characteristics to realistically guide product design in the field

4. The investigation of training strategies that encourage long-term skill integration

5. The investigation of the effects of repetitive movement on individuals who use AAC and methods of preventing associated injuries

AAC REPLICATING RESEARCH NETWORKS

The research agenda required to fill the gaps in knowledge and to support the assumptions made in clinical practice are vast and overwhelming. Given the extremely heterogeneous group served and the scarcity of funding and human resources in the AAC field, researchers may need to develop and adopt alternative research paradigms in order to accomplish their research agendas.

The ubiquitous use of the web and e-mail in the field offers the opportunity to network with peers on a more consistent and far-reaching basis than ever before. This networking capability has been used by a number of communities of interest to achieve tasks that were previously impossible or difficult to do by any one member in isolation (McNaughton et al., 1999). The characteristics of the AAC field make it a prime candidate for networked collaboration. Expertise is very specialized and distributed; there are very few people practicing in the field, and research in the field has been chronically underfunded and understaffed. Research in the field also requires a high level of expertise and cannot be easily assigned to novices. Research participants are widely distributed geographically and differ greatly in the needs and skills that influence their performance. All of these factors pose significant challenges to advances in research. Rather than making do with the resources and strategies used in the past, the AAC field needs to consider new strategies and research paradigms. One alternative is to leverage the networks available to collectively amass the data needed to arrive at research conclusions that can be generalized. By systematically integrating single-subject or within-subject research methodologies into assessment and prescription processes and documenting the outcomes, the field and communicators who use AAC would be well served.

Many clinicians and clinics have adopted objective measurement tools and instruments for deriving outcome measures in their clinical practice (Petty, 1999). These tools are used to guide individual prescriptions, to inform AAC system design, and to justify funding. Thus, there is a large amount of valuable data generated on a daily basis. If harmonized, synthesized, and analyzed, these data could be used to establish well-supported guidelines for the field. Unfortunately, there is no consistency across clinics in the instruments used or how they are applied, and data collected are rarely shared outside the individual service body.

O'Keefe, Jutai, Marshall, Lindsay, Schuller, and Schlosser (1998) addressed the issue of insufficient research participants by developing a database of individuals who use AAC who would be willing to participate in research. Although making it easier to recruit subjects, this database does not address the lack of funding or human resources that plagues most AAC research units.

What is needed is a distributed clinical research replication network with a common clinical database, adoption of a common set of assessment instruments, and consistent application of those instruments. Fuhrer (1999) alluded to this approach for outcome measures research and suggested that Clinical Improvement Methodology would act as an ideal tool. The primary focus of Clinical Improvement Methodology is in cost control and service evaluation and as such does not afford the flexibility needed to answer pertinent clinical questions that may be counter to cost reduction goals; however, this type of network can be used as a model and adapted to answer specific research questions that cannot be adequately addressed by a single researcher due to lack of access to sufficient participants. Funding and administrative structures would need to be adjusted to make this type of collaboration possible. Health administrators would need to be convinced that the potential gains in service efficacy and client satisfaction would offset the cost of clinical personnel time. A networking tool would need to be adapted to meet the needs of such collaboration.

Once such a network is established, the collaborative would need to agree on research goals and specific research questions. Participant criteria and a carefully delineated, easily replicated research methodology could be designed. The design would need to be a fast and simple methodology that could be integrated into an AAC control assessment or follow-up. As part of the clinical reporting process, the research data could be submitted to a shared database. Once adequate data were collected, the results could be synthesized and analyzed by a designated team. Candidate research questions for this type of network might include the following:

- What is the average optimal range and resolution for individuals who use AAC who can directly select using a single digit?
- What effect does variable scanning speed have on speed and accuracy in single-switch row–column scanning?
- Is it better to widely space targets or provide shoulder and elbow stabilization with closely grouped targets for participants with spastic cerebral palsy who use direct selection?
- What scanning and direct selection speed can individuals who use AAC reach following 1 year of AAC use?

Although this type of network would be beneficial to all aspects of AAC, it is particularly useful in the area of motor control by participants with developmental disabilities. Motor characteristics are extremely heterogeneous. The likelihood that two individuals with similar motor characteristics are available to participate in research in a single research facility may be very slim. A network that includes numerous facilities in widely distributed geographic regions is more likely to succeed in collecting the data needed to draw meaningful research conclusions. Given the research impediments faced in the AAC field, this collaboration may be the only way to adequately support or dispute assumptions and principles of practice.

CONCLUSION

In 1997, Janice Light suggested that what was needed in the AAC field was an equivalent to Velcro. For well over a century, children had been laboriously learning to tie their shoes. Proficient management of shoelaces was seen as a developmental milestone and a subject of early education—until Velcro was invented and Velcro closings for shoes became widely available. We have not yet discovered a Velcro for AAC device control. The operational requirements of AAC control remain laborious, the training demands remain very high, and the rewards of mastery remain very disappointing. Worse yet, researchers have not even developed a shoelace equivalent. Although tying a shoelace is a consistent task that, when mastered, can be transferred to a multitude of shoes encountered in a lifetime, AAC tool control is inconsistent and the skills acquired are often not transferable to the next AAC device prescribed. Rather than conducting the type of exploration that would be required to discover Velcro, the field appears to be settling into a set of device conventions that are counter to even the very limited research conclusions available.

To advance the field, researchers need to explore the boundaries of what individuals who use AAC are capable of, not just immediately, but also with training. They must understand the goal or destination of intervention better and explore new ways of arriving at that goal without being constrained by existing technologies. Researchers should explore what makes achieving the task easier and what makes it harder, and for whom. They must recognize the assumptions that guide their practice and systematically test those assumptions. Researchers also need to explore other fields of research and development to see if they can re-purpose approaches in the field. With the existing resources available, researchers cannot achieve this agenda. Given the dilemma of assigning limited human resources either to AAC assessment, prescription and training, or to research, researchers may need to find ways to do both. By designing assessment, training, and follow-up in such a way that they can also act as research replication, they leverage the human resources available.

Making the choices necessary to design an individual's AAC control system is a high-stakes process with long-term and far-reaching repercussions. To ensure that our choices do not squander the individual's limited time and energy and put their chances of becoming competent communicators at risk, we must equip ourselves with a body of well-supported knowledge and well-designed access tools. Only by creating a network of collaborators, including researchers, clinicians, users, product developers, and experts in other fields, can we build the knowledge needed to make these critical decisions intelligently.

REFERENCES

Anderson, J.R. (1989). Acquisition of cognitive skill. *Psychological Review, 89,* 369–406.

Anderson, J. (1999). *Sensory motor issues in autism.* San Antonio, TX: Psychological Corp.

Angelo, J. (2000). Factors affecting the use of a single switch with assistive technology devices. *Journal of Rehabilitation Research and Development, 31,* 5.

Anson, D.K. (1997). *Alternative computer access*. Philadelphia: F.A. Davis.

Anwar, F., & Hermelin, B. (1979). Kinaesthetic movement after-effects in children with Down's syndrome. *Journal of Mental Deficiency Research, 23*, 287–297.

Arnott, J.L., & Javed, M.Y. (1992). Probabilistic character disambiguation for reduced keyboards using small text samples. *Augmentative and Alternative Communication, 8*, 215–223.

Bailey, R.W. (1989). *Human performance engineering* (2nd ed.). Upper Saddle River, NJ: Prentice Hall.

Barker, M.R., Hastings, W.R., & Flanagan K. (1983). The control evaluator and training kit: An assessment tool for comparative testing of controls to operate assistive devices. In *Proceedings of the Sixth Annual Conference on Rehabilitation Engineering* (pp. 159–161). Washington, DC: Rehabilitation Engineering Society of North America.

Bernstein, N. (1967). *The co-ordination and regulation of movements*. New York: Pergamon.

Beukelman, D.R., & Mirenda, P. (1998). *Augmentative and alternative communication: Management of severe communication disorders in children and adults* (2nd ed.). Baltimore: Paul H. Brookes Publishing Co.

Beukelman, D., Yorkston, K., & Dowden, P. (1985). *Communication augmentation: A casebook of clinical management*. San Diego: College-Hill Press.

Blackstone, S.W. (1989). Visual scanning: Training approaches. *Augmentative Communication News, 2*(4), 3.

Bobath, K. (1991). Neurophysiological basis for the treatment of cerebral palsy. In *Clinics in developmental medicine* (No. 75, 2nd ed.). Philadelphia: Lippincott Williams & Wilkins.

Brandenburg, S., & Vanderheiden, G. (1987). Communication, control, and computer access for disabled and elderly individuals. *Resource Book 1: Communication aids*. Boston: College-Hill Press.

Brooks-Scott, S. (1999). *Handbook of mobilization in the management of children with neurologic disorders*. Boston: Butterworth-Heinemann.

Cantor, A. (1998, March). *Avoiding the mouse-trap: An evaluation of keyboard-only access to Windows*. Presentation at the California State University–Northridge conference, Los Angeles.

Carroll, J.M., & Olson, J. R. (1988). Mental models in human-computer interaction. In M. Helander (Ed.), *Handbook of human-computer interaction* (pp. 45–65). Amsterdam: Elsevier Science Publishers.

Cogher, L., Savage, E., & Smith, M.F. (1992). *Cerebral palsy: The child and young person*. London: Chapman & Hall Medical.

Cohen, D.J., & Volkmar, F.R. (1997). *Handbook of autism and pervasive developmental disorders*. New York: John Wiley & Sons.

Collier, B., Norris, L., & Rothschild, N. (1990). Technology—what's working, what's not and why? *Augmentative and Alternative Communication, 6*, 119.

Cook, A.M., & Hussey, S.M. (1995). *Assistive technologies: Principles and practice*. St. Louis, MO: Mosby.

Doherty, J. (1985). The effects of sign characteristics on sign acquisition and retention: An integrative review of the literature. *Augmentative and Alternative Communication, 1*, 108–121.

Elliott, D. (1985). Manual asymmetries in the performance of sequential movement by adolescents and adults with Down syndrome. *American Journal of Mental Deficiency, 90*, 90–97.

Elliot, D., Gray, S., & Weeks, D.J. (1991). Verbal cuing and motor skills acquisition for adults with Down syndrome. *Adapted Physical Activity Quarterly, 8*, 210–220.

Fisk, A.D., Oransky, N.A., & Skedsvold, P.R. (1998). Examination of the role of "higher-order" consistency in skill development. *Human Factors, 30,* 567–581.

Fitts, P.M. (1964). Perceptual-motor skill learning. In A.W. Melton (Ed.), *Categories of human learning.* San Diego: Academic Press.

Foulds, R.A., Soede, M., & Van Balkom, H. (1987). Statistical disambiguation of multicharacter keys applied to reduce motor requirements for augmentative and alternative communication. *Augmentative and Alternative Communication, 3,* 192–195.

Frith, U., & Frith, C.D. (1974). Specific motor disabilities in Down's syndrome. *Journal of Child Psychology & Psychiatry & Allied Disciplines, 15,* 293–301.

Fuhrer, M.J. (1999, November 24–26). *Assistive technology outcomes research: Impressions of an interested newcomer.* Proceedings of the International Conference on Outcome Assessment in Assistive Technology, Oslo, Norway.

Gardlin, G.R., & Sitterley, T.E. (1972). *Degradation of learned skills—A review and annotated bibliography.* Seattle: Boeing.

Gentile, A.M. (1987). Skill acquisition: Action, movement and neuromotor processes. In J. Carr & R. Shepherd (Eds.), *Movement science: Foundations for physical therapy in rehabilitation.* Rockville, MD: Aspen.

Goodenough-Trepagnier, C. (1980). *Rate of language production with a SPEEC nonvocal communication system* (pp. 92–93). Proceedings of the First International Conference on Rehabilitation Engineering, Toronto, ON.

Hagberg, B. (1994). *Rett syndrome: Clinical and biological aspects.* (Clinics in Developmental Medicine, No. 127). Cambridge, England: Cambridge University Press.

Horn, E.M., & Jones, H.A. (1996). Comparison of two selection techniques used in augmentative and alternative communication. *Augmentative and Alternative Communication, 12,* 23–31.

Hourcade, J.J., & Parette, P. (2001). Providing assistive technology information to professionals and families of children with MRD: Interactive CD-ROM. *Education and Training in Mental Retardation and Developmental Disabilities, 36,* 272–279.

Jagacinski, R.J., & Monk, D.L. (1985). Fitts' law in two dimensions with hand and head movements. *Journal of Motor Behavior, 17,* 77–95.

Kantowitz, B.H., & Sorkin, R.D. (1983). *Human factors: Understanding people–system relationships.* New York: John Wiley & Sons.

Lane, N.E. (1987). *Skill acquisition rates and patterns: Issues and training implications.* New York: Springer-Verlag.

Lee, K.S., & Thomas, D.J. (1989). *Control of computer-based technology for people with physical disabilities: An assessment manual.* Toronto: University of Toronto Press.

Lee, T.D., & Magill, R.A. (1985). Can forgetting facilitate skill acquisition? In D. Goodman, R.B. Wilberg, & I.M. Franks (Eds.), *Differing perspectives in motor learning, memory, and control* (pp. 3–21). Amsterdam: Elsevier Science Publishers.

Lesher, G.W., Moulton, B.J., & Higginbotham, D.J. (1998). Techniques for augmenting scanning communication. *Augmentative and Alternative Communication, 14,* 81–101.

Light, J. (1989). Toward a definition of communicative competence for individuals using augmentative and alternative communication systems. *Augmentative and Alternative Communication, 5,* 137–144.

Light, J. (1997). Communication is the essence of human life: Reflections on communicative competence. *Augmentative and Alternative Communication, 13,* 61–70.

Light, J., & Lindsay, P. (1991). Cognitive science and augmentative and alternative communication. *Augmentative and Alternative Communication, 7,* 186–203.

Light, J.C., Roberts, B., DiMarco, R., & Greiner, N. (1998). AAC to support receptive and expressive communication for people with autism. *Journal of Communication Disorders, 31,* 153–180.

Lindberg, B. (1991). *Understanding Rett syndrome: A practical guide for parents, teachers, and therapists.* Toronto: Hogrefe & Huber.

Logan, G.D. (1988). Automaticity, resources, and memory: Theoretical controversies and practical implications. *Human Factors, 30,* 583–598.

McEwen, I.R. (1997). Seating, other positioning and motor control. In L. Lloyd, D. Fuller, & H. Arvidson (Eds.), *Augmentative and alternative communication: A handbook of principles and practices* (pp. 280–298). Needham Heights, MA: Allyn & Bacon.

McNaughton, D., Beukelman, D., & Dowden, P. (1999). Tools to support international and intercommunity collaboration in AAC research. *Augmentative and Alternative Communication, 15,* 280–288.

Mechling, L.C., & Gast, D.L. (1997). Combination audio/visual self-prompting system for teaching chained tasks to students with intellectual disabilities. *Education and Training in Mental Retardation & Developmental Disabilities, 32*(2), 138–153.

Mizuko, M., Reichle, J., Ratcliff, A., & Esser, J. (1994). Effects of selection techniques and array sizes on short-term visual memory. *Augmentative and Alternative Communication, 10,* 237–244.

Murphy, J., Markova, I., Collins, S., & Moodie, E. (1996). AAC systems: Obstacles to effective use. *European Journal of Disorders of Communication, 31,* 31–44.

Nantais, T., Shein, F., Milner, M., & O'Beirne, H. (1991). *Dynamic competition selection technique for computer access.* Proceedings of the 14th Annual Conference of Rehabilitation Engineering and Assistive Technology Society of North America (RESNA), Kansas City, MO.

Newell, K.M. (1981). Skill learning. In D. Holding (Ed.), *Human skills* (pp. 203–226). New York: John Wiley & Sons.

O'Keefe, B., Jutai, J., Marshall, P., Lindsay, P., Schuller, R., & Schlosser, R. (1998). Database for the identification of AAC users for participation in research, product development, and service delivery. *Augmentative and Alternative Communication, 14,* 115–116.

Petty, L. (1999). Computer access evaluations and quantitative measurement. *American Journal of Occupational Therapy, 9,* 4.

Post, K.M. (1990). *Evaluation and intervention techniques in seating and mobility: Technology review '90: Perspectives on occupational therapy practice.* Rockville, MD: American Occupational Therapy Association.

Radwin, R.G., Vanderheiden, G.C., & Lin, M.I. (1990), A method for evaluating head-controlled computer input devices using Fitts' Law. *Human Factors, 32*(4).

Ratcliff, A. (1994). Comparison of relative demands implicated in direct selection and scanning: Considerations from normal children. *Augmentative and Alternative Communication, 10,* 67–74.

Reichle, J., & Johnston, S. (1999). Teaching the conditional use of communicative requests to two school-age children with severe developmental disabilities. *Language, Speech and Hearing Services in Schools, 30,* 324–334.

Romski, M.A., Sevcik, R.A., & Adamson, L.B. (1999). Communication patterns of youth with mental retardation with and without their speech-output. *American Journal on Mental Retardation, 104,* 249–259.

Sabbadini, M., Bonanni, R., Carlesimo, G.A., & Caltagirone, C. (2001). Neuropsychological assessment of patients with severe neuromotor and verbal disabilities. *Journal of Intellectual Disability Research, 45,* 169–179.

Salmoni, A.W. (1989). Motor skill learning. In D.H. Holding (Ed.), *Human skills* (2nd ed., pp. 197–226). New York: John Wiley & Sons.

Schepis, M., Reid, D.H., & Behrman, M. (1996). Acquisition and functional use of voice output communication by persons with profound multiple disabilities. *Behavior Modification, 20,* 451–460.

Sevcik, R., & Romski, M. (2002). AAC: More than three decades of growth and development. *The ASHA Leader, 5*(19), 5.

Sevcik, R.A., Romski, M.A., & Adamson, L. (1999). Measuring AAC interventions for individuals with severe developmental disabilities. *Augmentative and Alternative Communication, 15,* 38–54.

Silverman, C., & Treviranus, J. (1994). *Harnessing the potential of scripting languages for clients with disabilities.* Proceedings of the Ninth Annual Conference on Technology and Persons with Disabilities, Los Angeles.

Smothers Bruni, M.A. (1998). *Fine motor skills in children with Down syndrome: A guide for parents and professionals.* Bethesda, MD: Woodbine House.

Trefler, E., & Crislip, D. (1985). No aid, an Etran, a Minspeak: A comparison of efficiency and effectiveness during structured use. *Augmentative and Alternative Communication, 1,* 151–155.

Treviranus, J. (1992). *Quartering, halving, gesturing: Computer access using imprecise pointing.* Proceedings of the 15th Annual Conference of Rehabilitation Engineering and Assistive Technology Society of North America (RESNA), Toronto, Canada.

Treviranus, J. (1994). Mastering alternative computer access: The role of understanding, trust and automaticity. *Assistive Technology, 6,* 26–41.

Treviranus, J., & Drynan, D. (1990). *Indirect selection techniques: A comparison.* Proceedings of the Fourth International Society on Augmentative and Alternative Communication Conference, Stockholm, Sweden.

Treviranus, J., Shein, F. & Parnes, P. (1992). *Using speech recognition to augment alternative access.* Proceedings of the Seventh Annual Conference, Technology and Persons with Disabilities, Los Angeles.

Vanderheiden, G. (1984). *A unified quantitative modeling approach for selection based augmentative communication systems.* Unpublished dissertation, Department of Technology in Communication Rehabilitation and Child Development, University of Wisconsin, Madison.

Winders, P.C. (1997). *Gross motor skills in children with Down syndrome: A guide for parents and professionals.* Bethesda: MD: Woodbine House.

Witten, I.H. (1982). *Principles of computer speech.* London: Academic Press.

8

Cognitive Skills and AAC

Charity Rowland and Philip D. Schweigert

The relationship between communication skills and cognitive skills has been the topic of a large body of research. In this chapter, we briefly review this research as it pertains to augmentative and alternative communication (AAC) systems, individuals who use AAC, and clinicians. We discuss ways to accommodate cognitive considerations within the context of AAC intervention and suggest directions for future research.

RELATIONSHIP BETWEEN LANGUAGE AND COGNITION

The possible relationships between language and cognition have fueled extensive research in the realm of child development. The major controversy in this area (succinctly reviewed by Notari, Cole, & Mills, 1992) involves the degree to which cognition influences language development or language influences cognitive development. In other words, are skills in one domain precursors or prerequisites to skills in the other domain?

Research Involving Children without Disabilities

Most of the relevant research involves young children without disabilities who are just learning to express themselves using language. One body of research has examined relationships between language development and the attainment of Piagetian sensorimotor stages as demonstrated through performance on object permanence, "means–ends," tool use, symbolic play, and imitation tasks (e.g., Bates, 1979; Lifter & Bloom, 1989; McCune, 1995; McCune-Nicolich, 1981; Shore, 1986; Steckol & Leonard, 1981; Terrell, Schwartz, Prelock, & Messick, 1984; Ungerer & Sigman, 1984). Although a number of correlational relationships have been demonstrated in the child without disabilities, causal relationships have not been proven. Taken as a whole, this research has supported no strong conclusions.

Another body of research has examined the relationship between the child's understanding of nonlinguistic concepts and the ability to express those concepts using language (e.g., Corrigan, 1978; Gopnik & Meltzoff, 1986; Reznick & Goldfield, 1990). Rice (1983, 1989) insisted that there is not an isomorphic mapping of nonlinguistic concepts onto linguistic structure or semantics. Her review of this research and the possible models of interaction that might characterize the relationship between linguistic and cognitive domains led her to conclude that no single model adequately represents the complexity of the relationship.

Research Involving Children with Disabilities

A few researchers have conducted studies on the relationship between language and cognition in individuals with mental retardation (e.g., Abbeduto, Davies, & Furman, 1988; Abbeduto, Furman, & Davies, 1989; Kahn, 1984; Lobato, Barrera, & Feldman, 1981; Rast & Meltzoff, 1995) and in children with pervasive developmental disorders (e.g., Atlas & Lapidus, 1988). Such research from the field of special education generally echoes the evidence collected from children without disabilities: Correlational relationships have been demonstrated between cognitive and linguistic attainments, but no causal relationships have been established.

Effect of This Research on AAC Services

Despite cautions from Corrigan (1979), who questioned the validity of generalizing from such studies to clinical interventions, findings of correlational relationships were widely assumed to be causal and were in fact widely applied and incorporated into decision-making approaches to AAC (e.g. Owens & House, 1984; Shane, 1981), resulting in the adoption of cognitive prerequisites for speech-language services (as described in Notari et al., 1992). It is not surprising that apparent relationships between spoken language and cognitive development in typically developing children might have been assumed to apply directly to the development of alternatives to speech. The roots of AAC lie in the development of alternative language systems for individuals who have difficulties with the physical aspects of speech, the assumption being that the user's cognitive and sensory systems are intact. It would be natural to assume that prerequisites to speech might also be prerequisites to other forms of language in an individual whose only barrier to speech is a physical limitation.

The AAC Community Rebels

The field of AAC has changed rapidly, becoming ever more inclusive in terms of its constituency. AAC services now encompass users who demonstrate the full range of cognitive, sensory, and social/emotional causes for their communication disorders, with or without physical reasons for not using speech. The scope of AAC intervention has broadened to include all forms and levels of communication, including presymbolic means of communication (Mirenda, 1993). AAC researchers and clinicians have coalesced into a community with a strong identity that produces its own research based on experience in serving individuals who use AAC (Beukelman, 1993; Zangari, Lloyd, & Vicker, 1994). The community has recognized the dangers of extrapolating results from basic research on typically developing (and speaking) children to clinical interventions for the many populations of individuals who use AAC. It is not surprising, therefore, that in the late 1980s the AAC community became disenchanted with the presumed connection between cognition and language.

A number of researchers from the AAC community aired their skepticism regarding the relevance of cognitive skills to AAC services. Snyder-McLean, McLean, and Etter (1988) cited a number of reasons why it is inappropriate to use assessments of Piagetian sensorimotor stages (and specifically the Uzgiris-Hunt scales) to describe the functioning of individuals with disabilities. Social/expressive skills are seriously confounded with cognitive skills; speech is required to pass many items; and many scales include only a small number of items. Snyder-McLean and colleagues concluded that "we cannot predict any one client's communication level on the basis of his or her sensorimotor stage level(s)" (1988, p. 12).

Kangas and Lloyd (1988) thoroughly reviewed the question of cognitive prerequisites to language intervention for individuals who may potentially use AAC. They found that despite very weak evidence to support a cognitive basis for language even in children without disabilities, the assumption had exerted a strong and deleterious effect on individuals who may potentially use AAC. Some clinicians were waiting passively for cognitive skills to develop or attempting to teach "prerequisite" cognitive skills, needlessly denying or delaying communication services. Romski and Sevcik suggested that there were no clear prerequisites for AAC intervention, especially because AAC includes gestural/vocal communication, stating that "Some of these cognitive milestones are simply not necessary to begin an initial communication repertoire, while others are important, but can be incorporated into the intervention protocol" (1988, p. 41). Notari, Cole, and Mills reviewed the evolution of the "cognitive referencing" model of eligibility for speech-language services and labeled the approach "an oversimplified application of current theory" (1992, p. 28). It seems that the notion of cognitive prerequisites to AAC intervention has by now been laid to rest, at least among the research community.

Data on Children Who Are AAC Candidates

Something that has been missing in this debate is data on the cognitive skills of children who are AAC candidates and who may not develop language skills that take the form of speech. We have reviewed assessment data collected on a large number of children who participated in our research and demonstration projects between 1987 and 2001 to shed light on the relationship between five Piagetian cognitive skills and the presence of symbolic communication skills. These data are unique in that the participants are all nonverbal children who are candidates for AAC. First, we eliminated any children with total blindness (who could not be expected to imitate a visual model) and children with severe orthopedic involvement (that would compromise their ability either to produce imitative behaviors or to demonstrate cognitive attainments that require object manipulation). Then, we narrowed our investigation to children for whom assessments of both cognitive and communicative skills that had been administered within the same month were available. This resulted in a sample of 45 children ages 3–12 years. These children experienced a wide range of disabilities including autism, sensory impairments, cognitive limitations, and orthopedic impairments that were related to a variety of causes including cytomegalovirus, traumatic brain injury, and many rare congenital syndromes such as Rett, Refsum, Williams, and Pierre-Robin syndromes.

Each participant was characterized as having symbolic communication skills (involving any sort of symbol) or not, as revealed by data from the Communication Matrix (Rowland, 1990, 1996), the Generic Skills Inventory (Snyder-McLean, Sack, & Solomonson, 1995) or the Generic Skills Assessment Inventory (McLean, Snyder-McLean, Rowland, Jacobs, & Stremel-Campbell, 1981). Sources of information for cognitive skills were the Generic Skills Inventory (Snyder-McLean et al., 1995), the Generic Skills Assessment Inventory (McLean et al., 1981), the Battelle Developmental Inventory (Newborg, Stock, & Wnek, 1984, 1988), the Callier-Azusa Scale–G (Stillman, 1978), or the School Inventory of Problem Solving Skills (Rowland & Schweigert, 1997). These instruments were examined for specific items that required imitation skills, object permanence, means–ends, tool use, or symbolic play. Participants were given credit for having a cognitive skill or symbolic communication if that skill was assessed as either emerging or mastered (if such a distinction was made). If several different items related to one of the Piagetian skills (e.g., object permanence is implied in making detours, circumventing barriers, and searching for and locating hidden objects), participants were given credit if they demonstrated at least 50% of those items at either emerging or mastered levels. Because the various assessment instruments did not necessarily contain items related to all five of the Piagetian cognitive skills of interest, n for the six comparisons made varies from 45 to 23.

Data that would support a strong precursor or prerequisite relationship between symbolic communication skills and specific Piagetian skills would include instances where the participant either demonstrated both skills or demonstrated neither skill. Data that would challenge the notion of a strong relationship between skills would include "mismatches" between any two skill domains (i.e., instances where the participant demonstrated one skill but not the other). These are the data that are presented in Table 8.1. Table 8.1 shows the percent of participants who demonstrated symbolic communication skills but did not demonstrate each of the five Piagetian cognitive skills and the percent of participants who demonstrated each of the cognitive skills but did not demonstrate symbolic communication skills.

The cognitive skills associated with the largest percentage of mismatches with symbolic communication skills were imitation and symbolic play. A total of 46% of the participants showed a mismatch between imitation and symbolic communication skills, and the mismatches were virtually evenly divided between the two types of mismatches. The concept of imitation as necessary to language learning derives from the fact that speech is most easily learned through the imitation of auditory/visual models and is not easily imparted except through demonstration. Infant research has shown that typically developing neonates imitate facial expressions and that infants imitate vocal sounds (Kuhl & Meltzoff, 1996; Meltzoff & Moore, 1997). The ability to imitate is clearly a useful learning strategy that teachers may target. When speech is not the targeted mode, however, other forms of teaching do work and may work better. Presymbolic means of communication (gestures and vocalizations) are likely to occur naturally and through a process of operant conditioning may become intentionally communicative; physical prompting of ges-

Table 8.1.   Mismatches between five Piagetian cognitive skills and symbolic skills

Cognitive skill	n	Symbolic communication present but cognitive skill absent	Cognitive skill present but symbolic communication absent	Total mismatches
Imitation	45	24%	22%	46%
Object permanence	31	16%	10%	26%
Means–ends	31	32%	6%	38%
Tool use	31	35%	3%	38%
Symbolic play	23	48%	9%	57%

Source: Rowland and Schweigert (2001).

tural communication is also possible. Reichle stated, "Although imitation is probably the most straightforward method of acquiring new forms of vocal mode communication, it is not necessarily the quickest route to acquiring vocabulary in the gestural and graphic modes, where a number of other response prompts, including physical prompting, can be used" (1991, p. 42).

Fully 57% of participants showed a mismatch involving symbolic play and symbolic communication. Most of the discrepancies involved participants who demonstrated symbolic communication but did not demonstrate symbolic play. Symbolic play is highly dependent on motivation and experience, and its absence may say more about preference and social/emotional development than about any underlying symbolic ability. Thus, conclusions based on assessments of symbolic play skills are questionable for populations who may have little inclination toward such play schemes, regardless of their cognitive abilities. Ungerer and Sigman (1984) hinted at this confound in their study of play and language, commenting on the fact that children who are likely to relate to other children through play are also those who are likely to use language to relate to them.

The remaining three Piagetian cognitive skills all showed considerable percentages of mismatches related to symbolic communication. For both means–ends and tool use, the total percentage of mismatches was 38%, and for object permanence, it was 26%. For all three of these skills, the mismatches primarily involved participants who demonstrated symbolic communication but did not demonstrate the cognitive skill (as is also the case for symbolic play).

This meta-analysis is tentative and is weakened by the disparate measures of cognitive skill; the lack of reliability measures related to their administration; and the fact that we have, in some instances, inferred the relationship between assessment items and the five Piagetian cognitive skills. The data, however, confirm our suspicions that there is no simple relationship between symbolic communication skills and these cognitive skills.

WHAT DOES THE AAC COMMUNITY REALLY NEED TO KNOW ABOUT COGNITIVE DEVELOPMENT?

Although arguments about the relationship between cognition and language may be moot for now, the previous discussion leaves us to wonder what relevance cognitive skills do have to our endeavors. Language development is essentially a cognitive achievement, and because language is assumed to describe experience, then it is ridiculous to believe that there is not a connection of some sort. In this section, we shift our perspective to consider aspects of cognitive development that are related to communication in general. The discussion is based on the presumption that communication is a generic skill that includes presymbolic communication as well as speech and the various alternative symbolic systems. To set the stage for this discussion, the basic elements of a generic communication act are reviewed.

Elements of a Generic Communication Act

A communication act involves four observable elements, as illustrated in Figure 8.1: a sender, a receiver, a topic (or referent), and a means of expression (which may be presymbolic or symbolic). These are physical elements requiring attentional and motor skills to coordinate. Communication development involves the progressive distancing between these four elements (Werner & Kaplan, 1963). The physical distance between sender and receiver increases as the individual progresses from gestural means of communication that require close contact with the receiver to more distal gestures (e.g., pointing) and eventually to speech or other abstract symbolic means, which may be conveyed at even greater distances. Topic development involves progressive distancing between the sender and the topic or referent. Initial topics are strictly internal and related intimately to the self (hunger, pain), but they soon expand to include external topics that are related to one's own needs (food, blanket). Environmental topics soon appear, at first restricted to referents that are present (the cat sleeping on the rug), but eventually expanding to include referents

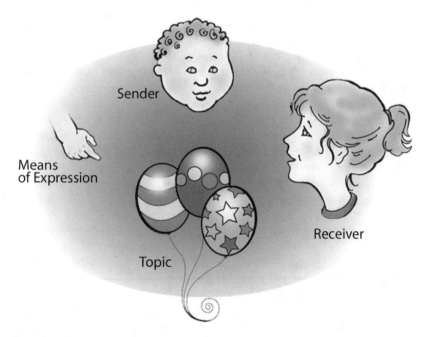

Figure 8.1. Four elements of a generic communication act.

that are absent (Mom at the office) or completely abstract (emotions). The distance between the topic and the means of expression increases conceptually (as opposed to physically) over time. Initially, the topic of communication is indicated through physically contacting it, later through concrete representations of its physical properties (iconic gestures or sounds, pictures) and finally through abstract representations that bear no physical similarity to their referents (spoken words, manual signs).

Individuals who have significant orthopedic impairments may have difficulty with the progressive distancing of these four elements. The means of expression may be limited and may preclude means that involve physical distance between the elements of the exchange. Individuals who have significant intellectual limitations may not be able to understand means of expression (such as symbols) that allow greater conceptual distance between the four elements. Individuals who have sensory impairments may not realize that potential topics or receivers are present or may have difficulty attending jointly to both. AAC should ameliorate the barriers to progressive distancing between sender, receiver, topic, and means of expression imposed by physical, intellectual, or sensory limitations.

Beyond the observable elements that make up a communicative exchange is the specific meaning intended by the sender, such as making a request or protesting or directing the receiver's attention to something. As communication skills develop, the number of intended meanings that may be relayed increases. The sender's intended meaning does not necessarily accord with the meaning ascribed to the message by the receiver. For instance, a child might push a toy across the table, attempting to convey the message "Turn it on for me," but the receiver might interpret the message as "I don't want this." Misinterpretations of intended meaning are especially common for individuals who may potentially use AAC because communicative behavior may be unclear or a communication device may not incorporate any markers of intended meaning. For instance, an utterance emanating from a voice-output device is produced with the same intonation, regardless of whether it is intended as a request or a comment, and an individual who points to a picture of the playground may be asking to go there or directing the receiver to look at something happening there.

Six Cognitive Factors Related to AAC

The aspects of cognitive development that appear to have high relevance to AAC systems may be roughly divided into factors related to awareness, communicative intent, world knowledge, memory, symbolic representation, and metacognitive learning strategies. These six aspects are discussed next in relationship to the four elements of a generic communication act. Table 8.2 provides a definition and major components for each of the six factors addressed in this section.

Table 8.2. Six cognitive factors related to AAC

Factor	Definition	Major components
Awareness	Perception of internal and external stimuli leading to understanding of causal relationships between them	Self versus all else People versus objects Nonsocial contingency awareness Social contingency awareness Theory of mind
Communicative intent	Understanding that specific behaviors directed toward another person may convey meaning and may result in a specific response	Preintentional communication Intentional communication
World knowledge	Understanding of relationships between the self and environmental entities based upon perceived value of previous experiences and leading to expectations regarding future behavior	Relationships between self and objects Relationships between self and people Relationships between objects Relationships between people Motivation
Memory	Ability to store information and impressions and to retrieve them at a later time	Information storage • Five sensory stores • Short-term or working memory • Long-term memory Information retrieval • Recognition • Recall
Symbolic representation	Nature of the relationship between symbols and referents	Concrete symbols Abstract symbols
Metacognitive skills	Understanding of own learning strategies that may be used to manipulate learning combined with processes (conscious and unconscious) that regulate behavior	Metalinguistics Metamemory Executive functions

Awareness Even before an individual can coordinate the four elements of a communication act, awareness of some very basic environmental distinctions must be obtained. First, there must be an awareness of "self" versus the rest of the world—in other words, "I am one thing, and everything else in the environment is somehow external, separate, and different from myself." A certain amount of experience with the environment generally leads to the development of contingency awareness—the realization that a specific behavior has a specific consequence. The baby who figures out that a certain arm movement causes a mobile suspended over the crib to move has acquired *nonsocial* contingency awareness. Similarly, the baby may learn that certain behaviors make Dad (and other people) do certain things, demonstrating an awareness of *social* contingencies. Intentional communication involves an awareness that people are different from objects and that people respond to certain behaviors in ways that objects do not. In other words, it is worthwhile to vocalize in the presence of a person, but not in the presence of objects (although the development of technology and the advent of "smart" interfaces may rapidly obviate this difference). Social contingency awareness implies that the individual purposefully directs behavior toward another person (although a specific topic may not yet be evident). Once basic environmental discriminations and contingency awareness have been achieved, then environmental awareness also affects the extent to which the sender is aware of topics for communication and of the presence of potential communication partners (receivers).

These very basic levels of awareness cannot be taken for granted in individuals who have sensory limitations, especially if these are combined with cognitive limitations. Clearly, sensory impairments may have a significant impact on the ability to notice environmental events and comprehend causal relationships between them. Orthopedic limitations may also restrict personal experience of contingent relationships or may make it difficult for individuals to physically demonstrate their understanding of a contingent relationship, resulting in the faulty assumption that the individual does not understand.

A much higher level of awareness than contingency awareness involves understanding the perceptions and thoughts of other people. Meltzoff (1999) endorsed the construct of "theory of mind," basing his discussion on the explosion of recent research that suggests the cognitive precocity of the human infant. Theory of mind refers to an understanding that other people have thoughts, desires, goals and intentions of their own. He considers this awareness a building block for communication. It will be interesting to see how this construct influences future discussions of the development of communication.

Communicative Intent Awareness of social contingencies is the foundation for communicative intent. The intent to communicate on the part of the sender distinguishes a purposeful communicative act from one that merely serves to communicate because the receiver (mis)interprets the expressive behavior as conveying intended meaning. Behaviors that are produced without communicative intent—or indeed without any intent—are often interpreted as communicative (as when the baby, pricked by the diaper pin, cries and the mother interprets the cry as a deliberate request for help).

An important component of presymbolic communication intervention involves responding to preintentional behaviors as if they were communicative in order to shape them into intentional communicative behavior; in other words, presymbolic behavior may legitimately be treated as if communicative intent is present, when it is not. Expanding the scope of AAC to embrace presymbolic interventions that involve reinforcing preintentional communication may have had the unanticipated effect of obscuring the importance of communicative intent. Intentional communication implies not only intentional behavior, but also behavior that is produced with communicative intent. This is not a trivial distinction. Behavior that has communicative intent is intentional behavior that is purposefully directed toward another person with intended meaning. It requires dual orientation—orientation to both the communication partner and the topic or referent.

Grove, Bunning, Porter, and Olsson (1999) provided a thought-provoking analysis of the development of communicative intent as it relates to individuals with the most profound disabilities. They pointed out that when communicative intent is not yet developed (or when the severity of orthopedic limitations makes intent unclear), the caregiver's response to potentially communicative behaviors affects the evolution of communicative intent in the individual. Even once communicative intent is assumed, a communicative exchange may rely on the social negotiation of meaning between sender and receiver because the expressive behaviors and their intended meaning may never be clear. Caregivers must depend on their own inferences and intuition to ascribe meaning, creating an unusual degree of interdependency between sender and receiver.

A spate of research has illuminated the relationship between communicative intent and communication development in children with disabilities. Stephenson and Linfoot (1996a) examined the relationship of communicative intent to the acquisition of graphic symbols in studies by other researchers and determined that when communicative intent was absent, the acquisition of a large number of graphic symbols was unlikely to occur. They compared the acquisition of just a few graphic symbols to the nonspeech vocalizations and gestures of an infant that seem to have specific meaning but are not truly referential. They also pointed out that using an aided AAC system requires in essence triple orientation—orientation toward the receiver, the topic, and the AAC system. Iacono, Carter, and Hook (1998) discussed the issue of intentionality in depth, suggesting the importance of accurately assessing communicative intent in the course of planning intervention. Yoder and Warren (1999) found a strong relationship between intentional communication and later language acquisition in children with developmental disabilities and determined that maternal responsivity mediated this relationship. In addition, Calandrella and Wilcox (2000) found correlations between intentional nonverbal communication and language development 6 and 12 months later in children with developmental delay. Interestingly, they also found a relationship between some signals involving only single orientation (attention to objects, but not to adults) and later language scores.

In a study of 41 children with a wide range of severe disabilities who shared a lack of symbolic communication, we found that those who were less adept in terms of intentional presymbolic communication made slower progress toward the goal of symbolic communication (Rowland & Schweigert, 2000b). Of those who had intentional communication prior to intervention, 100% acquired some form of symbolic communication. Of those without intentional communication prior to intervention, 38% did not acquire any symbolic communication skills at all. The remaining 62% did acquire some symbolic communication skills but required extensive instruction in the use of presymbolic communication prior to acquiring those skills.

World Knowledge

Once communicative intent has been achieved, then intentional communication involves the relaying of our own experience and knowledge to other people, as well as the gaining of knowledge from others. General experience in and of the world provides an understanding of the relationships between things, between the self and others, and between other people. Meltzoff (1999) unveiled a "theory–theory" of developmental psychology—a theory that children develop their own theories about how the world works and correct and refine these theories as their experience deepens. Such theories serve as the basis for regulating communicative interactions with people. General world experience provides a common platform of behavioral expectations that individuals count on to govern interactions, as well as a common knowledge base that facilitates meaningful conversations even between strangers. In individuals with physical, sensory, and cognitive limitations, this common knowledge base cannot be taken for granted.

World knowledge involves one overriding factor that affects all types of AAC intervention. That factor is motivation, which evolves from the learner's world experience and his or her desire to repeat valued or pleasurable experiences and to avoid unpleasant ones. Without high levels of motivation, individuals are unlikely to learn to use any AAC system. Contexts for learning should be compelling and the topics and vocabulary embedded in an AAC system should be valuable and useful to the learner in order to capitalize on the motivation developed through world experience. AAC systems also address a different aspect of motivation—the motivation bred by success. Often, individuals who may potentially use AAC have had extensive experience in failing to communicate effectively using conventional means. The motivation to attempt to communicate may be compromised by this history of failure, leading in some cases to impaired mastery motivation and learned helplessness (Seligman, 1975). Appropriate AAC systems should increase the motivation to communicate because they make it easier for the user to do so.

Memory   All learning requires memory. Contingency awareness is not established, nor is world knowledge gained without the capacity to store information and to build on remembered experiences. Once communicative intent is acquired, increasingly sophisticated memory skills are required to establish a repertoire of effective communication skills. Light and Lindsay (1991) provided a thorough discussion of the perspective on memory promoted by the cognitive science movement and its implications for AAC (Gardner, 1985). Memory is commonly divided into three components: sensory stores, short-term memory, and long-term memory.

Sensory Stores   A sensory information store for each sense initially filters information, storing input temporarily for up to several seconds. The individual with sensory impairments who uses AAC may experience limitations in one or more of these sensory stores, preventing information from reaching deeper memory systems. Attentional deficits may also prevent information from entering sensory stores.

Short-Term Memory   Working or short-term memory gradually increases in capacity to 7 plus or minus 2 items during the course of childhood. Its capacity may be extended through rehearsal, external memory aids, and the overlearning of information that results in automaticity. Clearly, short-term memory is in operation as communicative exchanges are executed, whether presymbolically or symbolically, and with or without communication devices. Short-term memory would be necessary to coordinate the orientations and behaviors inherent in a communicative exchange, particularly where more than one symbol must be sequenced. Limitations in attention span, a tendency to perseverate on thoughts or actions, and physical impairments may impose delays in sequencing behaviors that may outstrip the limits of short-term memory. The addition of an aided AAC system to the elements requiring coordination in a communicative act may also strain the bounds of an individual's short-term memory.

Long-Term Memory   Long-term memory is used to store knowledge about procedures, facts, biographic information, language, and the world in general relatively permanently. Various categories of memory stores have been postulated (e.g., declarative versus procedural, episodic versus semantic). Individuals who have experienced traumatic brain injury, stroke, or dementia may experience specific decrements in these stores. Individuals who are candidates for AAC may have better memory for certain types of information than for others, and this fact should be a consideration in the choice of AAC systems and vocabulary. Various types of encoding may be used to store knowledge in memory and various strategies may be used to retrieve knowledge from long-term memory. Recognition memory—the capacity to determine whether a perceived stimulus is familiar or unfamiliar—is functional from birth. Recognition memory allows people to profit from experience by identifying similarities between current stimuli and previous experiences (McShane, 1991). Recall memory is a more difficult two-stage process. Recall memory may be improved by the conscious application of memory-enhancing strategies. Clearly, the individual's long-term memory capacity is a factor in the memorization and retrieval of symbolic and presymbolic means of expression.

Memory is also differentially implicated in the various methods of accessing symbols in high- and low-technology symbol systems. The influence of different ways of displaying graphic symbols and moving from one set to another in electronic devices has been investigated by Mizuko, Reichle, Ratcliff, and Esser (1994); Oxley and Norris (2000); and Reichle, Dettling, Drager, and Leiter (2000). The cognitive demands of many high-technology devices are quite high (independent of the symbol system embedded into the device), including the need to memorize what messages are available and the need to learn how the messages are associated with cues (e.g., pictures).

Symbolic Representation   Symbols, as the term is used here, are publicly used representations of meaning (as opposed to unobservable mental representations involved in encoding or manipulating information). In order to move beyond communication that depends on very direct actions and connections between the four elements of a communication act, the memories of world knowledge must be translated into some sort of code. That code will involve symbols that stand for referents and that imply a certain level of representation—a specific degree or type of relatedness between symbol and referent.

As communication develops, the conceptual distance between symbol and referent increases as the means of expression becomes more abstract. The meaning of spoken words, because they are abstract symbols, must be committed to long-term memory. Alternative symbol systems have been described in the AAC literature as varying according to their iconicity. A number of studies have been conducted of the transparency/translucency of manual signs, Blissymbols, and other graphic symbol systems (Carmeli & Shen, 1998; DePaul & Yoder, 1986; Fuller & Lloyd, 1991; Fuller & Stratton, 1991; Mizuko, 1987; Yovetich & Young, 1988). Clearly, the assumption is that symbols bearing a more iconic relationship with a referent will be easier to learn initially and their meaning will be easier to deduce, even where memory does not serve well. Many individuals who use AAC will learn to use more concrete levels of representation—very commonly, pictures and even three-dimensional objects that have an intrinsic perceptual relationship to their referents independent of memorized associations. The level of representation inherent in the symbol may be a valuable facilitator of learning. One can teach someone to use pictures or objects as symbols through repeated association and practice (Romski & Sevcik, 1988; Stephenson & Linfoot, 1996b), but the task is far easier if the individual understands the representation inherent in the symbol. Warren and Yoder (1998) and Wilcox and Shannon (1998) discussed the importance of timing intervention that targets linguistic (or symbol-based) communication in synchrony with an individual's maturational capability and specifically the ability to understand a given level of symbolic representation.

A small body of research has been conducted on the development of picture representation skills and their influence on learning, which is reviewed by Sevcik, Romski, and Wilkinson (1991; see also Chapter 4). Picture recognition precedes the use of pictures as symbols in children without disabilities. A number of studies have described participants with disabilities who had picture-matching skills but could not use the information in pictures, as well as participants who could use pictorial information but couldn't match pictures (Stephenson & Linfoot, 1996b). DeLoache and Burns (1993) suggested that children first recognize pictures (pointing to and labeling them); then interpret them (deriving information about the real world from them); and finally learn that they can be used to represent specific reality (using them for symbolic communication). Sevcik and colleagues (1991) concluded that individuals who use AAC may learn specific object–picture relationships without having generalized object–picture matching skills and that the generalized skill may develop as a result of learning some specific relationships.

Metacognitive Skills The acquisition of a symbol system allows people to publicly describe and consider their experiences, including internal experiences such as how they learn and remember things. Metacognitive skills allow people to reflect on their own cognitive processes. These skills include metalinguistics (the ability to contemplate personal use and learning of language), metamemory (the ability to contemplate personal memory strategies), and executive functions (processes that are involved in the self-regulation of motor and mental behavior). These abilities are always useful but become critical when the means of expression is complex and the array of topics is large.

The more structurally complex the language system that is being learned, the more helpful it is to have metalinguistic and metamemory skills. Users of high- or low-technology AAC systems that require the organization and navigation of large vocabularies of abstract symbols clearly benefit from good metalinguistic skills. Metalinguistic skills would presuppose the presence of abstract language skills, at least on a receptive level. Oxley and Norris (2000) listed a whole host of specific metacognitive skills that may be used to support the memorization of message location in a high-technology system, including using nonspecific markers and picture cues; using spatial information; clustering, sorting, and categorizing information; and using verbal and imaginal mnemonics. Search strategies that may help with message retrieval include trial-and-error searching and systematic and logical searching. As suggested by Light and Lindsay (1991), explicitly teaching the specific organizing, memorization, or scanning skills required by a system may better prepare learners to use very complex systems.

Executive functions regulate the deployment of attention and the planning and inhibition of behavior. These processes allow people to monitor their performance and adjust their learning strategies as needed. Executive processes may operate with or without the person's awareness (McShane, 1991). Conscious executive processes may be harnessed to improve learning.

MATCHING COGNITIVE REQUIREMENTS OF AAC SYSTEMS TO THE COGNITIVE SKILLS OF THE LEARNER

The previous discussion has suggested ways in which certain aspects of cognitive development may be related to generic communication acts. The following discussion addresses how the six cognitive factors described previously may relate to four broad classes of AAC systems. Table 8.3 summarizes the major points of this discussion. An additional set of issues relate to the manner in which symbol systems are displayed and accessed in high- and low-technology systems: these issues, which primarily involve memory and its organization, are treated separately in this section. Finally, we discuss the influence of the user's prior experiences with communication systems.

Presymbolic Communication

Presymbolic communication refers to intentional communication that does not involve symbol-to-referent correspondence. It includes postural change, limb movements, gestures, nonspeech vocalizations, and facial expressions. It also includes the use of single-purpose switches (as when an individual with severe orthopedic impairments uses a single switch to gain attention). Presymbolic communication is most clearly affected by contingency awareness, communicative intent, and memory.

Awareness   To communicate intentionally, even without symbols, an awareness of one's ability to affect the behavior of another person must be achieved. If this social contingency awareness is not already present, then it

Table 8.3. Relevance of six cognitive factors to four major classes of AAC systems

Cognitive factor	Presymbolic communication	Two- and three-dimensional symbols (low- or high-tech methods)	Aided abstract symbols (print, Blissymbols, other abstract graphic codes)	Unaided abstract symbols (speech or manual sign)
Awareness	Continency awareness may be taught if not present.	Assumed	Assumed	Assumed
Communicative intent	May be taught if not present	Assumed	Assumed	Assumed
World knowledge	Contexts should be highly motivating to the learner.	Topic/vocabulary should be valued and useful to learner. Individual symbols should be based on user's own experience.	Topic/vocabulary should be valued and useful to learner.	Topic/vocabulary should be valued and useful to learner.
Memory	Very low requirements	Recognition memory In some cases symbol meaning may be deduced without prior memorization.	Recognition memory	Recall memory
Symbolic representation	None	Concrete Symbol-to-referent correspondence may be taught if not present, but best to start with existing representational skill level. Symbols should be discriminable.	Abstract Blissymbols have some iconicity, but overall quite abstract.	Abstract
Metacognitive skills	Not needed	Not needed	Very useful, in some cases necessary	Very useful, in some cases necessary

257

may be taught. If nonsocial contingency awareness exists, then it may be used as an avenue to the attainment of social contingency awareness (Schweigert, 1989; Schweigert & Rowland, 1992). Even in cases where there is little tolerance for interaction with other people, there is generally something in the environment to which access may be controlled by another person, thus rendering that person a valued communication partner.

Communicative Intent   Communicative intent evolves at the point that interaction with other people takes on dual orientation (to both receiver and topic or referent). The individual who initially lacks dual orientation may be taught to use specific presymbolic behaviors to coordinate attention to other people and specific topics or referents. Communicative intent may then provide a framework for the subsequent acquisition of symbolic communication skills (Rowland & Schweigert, 2000b).

Memory   While all communication requires both short- and long-term memory, the memory load is not high for presymbolic communication. Short-term memory is necessary to coordinate attention to communication partners and topics and to produce behaviors that connect the two. Gestures are generic communication behaviors without specific referents, so a few gestures go a long way. A small repertoire of gestures stored in long-term memory may be used over and over again so that overlearning is likely to occur.

Communication Using Two- and Three-Dimensional Symbols

Two- and three-dimensional symbols, also called tangible symbols, have a concrete relationship to their referents based on common perceptual features (Rowland & Schweigert, 2000a, 2000b). A number of authors have addressed the use of three-dimensional *objects of reference* (Bloom, 1990; Ockelford, 1992), most frequently within the context of activity boxes, anticipation shelves, or calendar systems (Joffee & Rikhye, 1991; Stillman & Battle, 1984; Ulmholtz & Rudin, 1981) and often targeting individuals with deafblindness (Engleman, Griffin, & Wheeler, 1998). The use of three-dimensional object symbols has in the past been most commonly associated with receptive communication, although they are at least equally useful for expressive communication. Picture symbols (line drawings and photographs) are more commonly used as symbols for both expressive and receptive communication (Bondy & Frost, 1994; Heller, Allgood, Ware, & Castelle, 1996; Johnson, 1994; Schwartz, Garfinkle, & Bauer, 1998), often in conjunction with a voice-output device (Heller, Alberto, & Bowdin, 1995; Stephenson & Linfoot, 1996a, 1996b). Two- and three-dimensional symbols make relatively low demands on the user's cognitive abilities as compared with abstract symbols. They require levels of communicative intent, memory, and representational ability that build on the awareness, world knowledge, and memory required for presymbolic communication.

World Knowledge   For the user of two- and three-dimensional symbols, world knowledge may be an especially salient factor. Although many individuals are able to understand the representational aspects of generic photographs or line drawings that may be purchased commercially, many others will not. For those individuals, symbols may be constructed to conform to their own world knowledge, emphasizing the properties (whether visual or tactile) that are meaningful to their specific experience (Rowland & Schweigert, 2000a, 2000b). The features of a symbol that are meaningful to one person may be less than meaningful to someone else, depending on the individual's sensory abilities and experience with both referent and symbol. For instance, one teacher described a little girl who could understand and use photographs that depicted herself interacting with specific referents but didn't seem to understand photographs of the referents alone or of other people interacting with them.

Communicative Intent   A child who does not understand that holding out an empty cup (a presymbolic gesture) may cause Mom to fill the cup with more milk is not likely to learn to hold out a symbol for milk to request a refill. Our research has shown that individuals who already have intentional presymbolic communication (either acquired spontaneously or through deliberate instruction) are generally successful at learning to use two- and three-dimensional symbols, as contrasted with individuals without communicative intent, as described previously (Rowland & Schweigert, 2000b). Where intentional presymbolic communication skills are not present, they may be taught.

Memory   Two- and three-dimensional symbols are permanent. Thus, recognition memory is used to determine which of the presented symbols are needed to communicate a specific meaning. As explained previously, recognition is an easier task than is recall. It is also possible that an individual may derive so much information from the iconic properties of these symbols that the meaning will be obvious even without prior memorization; examples might include using a shoelace to represent a shoe, or using a photograph of the user's own dog to represent the dog. Even where a variety of interpretations for a symbol might be possible (as in a generic drawing of a dog to represent the user's dog), the iconic qualities provide clues to its meaning, narrowing down the possible referents and lessening the demand on long-term memory.

Symbolic Representation   Some individuals may learn to use some symbols strictly through paired association and without understanding the inherent relationship between symbol and referent; however, it is likely that learning will occur more quickly if there exists a generic understanding of the level of symbolic representation. The level of representation inherent in two- and three-dimensional symbols varies along a continuum from an identical object used as a symbol to a black-and-white line drawing of a generic example of the referent, with other levels of representation (e.g., partial objects, colored photographs) ranging along the continuum between these points. Thus, varying levels of symbolic representation may be accommodated by different types of two- and three-dimensional symbols.

It is important to note that comprehension of a specific level of representation cannot be assumed in any particular individual based solely on etiology or the presence or absence of specific impairments. For instance, miniature objects are sometimes assumed to be an appropriate level of representation for individuals who don't understand two-dimensional representations, either because of cognitive limitations or visual impairments. Mirenda and Locke (1989) and Stephenson and Linfoot (1996b) have noted the difficulty that individuals who have severe intellectual impairments may have in using miniature objects as symbols. We have also noted the fallacies inherent in assuming that individuals without sight can understand the representational value of miniature objects (Rowland & Schweigert, 2000a).

Aided Abstract Symbol Systems

Some AAC systems involve abstract symbols such as written words or Blissymbols that are permanent and displayed in static arrays. These symbol systems place greater demands on memory and involve a higher (more abstract) level of representation than do two- and three- dimensional symbols.

Memory   Abstract symbols do not have a clear iconic relationship to referents. Therefore, their meaning must be memorized without benefit of inherent cues. Repeated practice may result in overlearning, and automaticity may help in retrieval. Retrieval, however, is typically accomplished through the recognition of the correct symbols out of an array—an easier task than recall memory.

Symbolic Representation   The comprehension of abstract symbols is obviously more difficult than that of concrete symbols. Written symbols bear no physical similarities to referents. Blissymbols (McNaughton & Kates, 1980) and some other graphic codes do have iconic qualities that the user may utilize to learn and memorize their meaning; however, these meanings are not immediately obvious to the new user (they are translucent at best), and the relationship must be learned. We include them here under our discussion of abstract symbols for this reason.

Metacognitive Skills   Aided systems that involve large vocabularies present real challenges to metacognitive skills. The user must understand the method of partitioning vocabulary into useful chunks and the system for navigating through the vocabulary. For very complex systems, metacognitive skills are probably necessary; in any case, metacognitive skills will speed the learning process as a new system is acquired.

Unaided Abstract Symbol Systems

Unaided systems that involve abstract symbols include speech and, for the AAC candidate, the various forms of manual sign language.

Memory   Memory requirements for speech and sign language are high because the symbols must be recalled, rather than recognized out of a display of permanent symbols. Nevertheless, children often acquire large spoken and signed vocabularies very rapidly. Overlearning and automaticity are extremely valuable in acquiring enough manual signs to generate fluent messages, but even a small vocabulary of signs may be useful. Some manual signs are iconic (either transparent or translucent), and these may be more easily recalled. In addition, it is possible to create iconic gestures on the spur of the moment when the official sign is not known or remembered (e.g., patting the chair to indicate "sit down").

Symbolic Representation   The level of symbolic representation varies among individual signs. Although some signs are very concrete (transparent or translucent), most are abstract. Different signing systems also vary in terms of the degree to which they stress semantic and syntactic features of language (see Beukelman & Mirenda, 1998, for a review of the various manual sign systems).

Metacognitive Skills   Although metacognitive skills are always useful, it is likely that modest vocabularies of abstract symbols may be learned without any ability to reflect on their use. The larger the vocabulary and the more complex the language use, the more important metacognitive skills become.

Cognitive Skills Related to the Display and Access of Symbols

When symbol systems are embedded into some sort of aided system, there are a number of variables related to the display and access to it that should be considered in terms of underlying cognitive requirements. These factors relate primarily to memory and metalinguistic skills and are different for low- and high-technology systems. These considerations should be overlaid on top of the considerations outlined in Table 8.3 that relate to the type of symbols embedded in the system.

Low-Technology Systems   In low-technology systems, permanent symbols may be presented in large arrays or small arrays or even one symbol at a time. It is possible that an individual could understand the meaning of a number of symbols presented separately, but when they are placed together in the same array, they may be so similar that it is difficult to discriminate between them. Thus, symbols must be chosen or constructed that are easily discernable from one another. Discriminability will depend on the sensory and perceptual skills of the individual learner. Larger displays are clearly more efficient, but the larger the display, the greater the discrimination skills required and the greater the memory demands in terms of understanding what one symbol means as opposed to another. The size of an array may be gradually increased until it is clear that maximum efficiency of selection has been reached. In many cases, books of symbols are developed with a number of related symbols on each page. Vocabulary is then increased by adding pages to the book, each containing the same optimum number of symbols. Tabs with symbolic or color cues to show where to find specific sets of vocabulary may aid in navigating through the book.

One issue that frequently arises in the use of low-technology displays of permanent symbols is the user's ability or willingness to scan the options: It is impossible to make an informed choice without knowing what the options are. The user with visual impairments may have to learn to scan the display tactually. Even individuals who have good sight may need a great deal of encouragement before they will thoroughly scan an array of symbols visually. Finally, some individuals who have perfectly functional vision may, for one reason or another, perform better with the benefit of the added information provided by a tactual scan.

The fact that symbols in an aided system are able to be manipulated may be an important factor in learning to use them. Symbols may be placed next to (or onto) the referent, accenting the association between symbol and referent. A literal association is thus possible between symbol and referent, which may make learning and memorizing the correspondence more rapid. Manipulable symbols also make the exchange of information obvious and literal, as when the user hands a picture or object symbol to the communication partner to make a request. For some individuals, this feature may be key in reinforcing the need to involve another person in a communicative exchange.

High-Technology Devices   The use of high-technology devices involves some of the same display and scanning issues of low-technology systems but also raises a number of new issues related to cognitive requirements. Different physical access techniques, chosen to accommodate the user's physical abilities, are associated with different cognitive demands (see Chapter 7 for further discussion of access issues). Some systems allow direct selection of symbols. The user with extremely limited motor control may rely on visual or auditory scanning of symbols, requiring only a minimal motor response to indicate when the correct symbol has been reached. The assumption has been that scanning places greater demands on memory because it is slow (requiring more sustained short-term memory) and is also cognitively complex.

A small body of research has involved the comparison of scanning techniques with direct selection techniques in children without disabilities. Ratcliff (1994) compared visual row–column scanning to direct selection and determined that row–column scanning was more difficult, presumably partly because it is more cognitively complex than direct selection. Mizuko, Reichle, Ratcliff, and Esser (1994) compared linear scanning (direct selection) with row–column scanning and found that when the array size was 40 symbols, direct selection was related to better performance on a short-term visual memory task (although the performance difference disappeared with a smaller 30-symbol array). AAC systems that utilize word or character prediction capitalize on the relative probabilities of word/character combinations and reduce the number of "switches" (user actions) required to complete words or phrases. Lesher, Moulton, and Higginbotham (1998) conducted studies of scanning configurations involving different combinations of access method, matrix layout, and prediction methods, comparing the switch savings implied in simulated applications of each.

When vocabulary becomes large enough to exceed the limitations of a manageable single array, then it must be organized into categories of some sort. This categorization should reflect the user's own world knowledge and experience. Light and Lindsay (1991) pointed out that the models of the world constructed by individuals who use AAC may not be the same as those of the person who organizes vocabulary for them. Clearly, it is important to involve the user in the organization of vocabulary if at all possible. Where multiple sets or layers of symbols are involved, there must be some way to move from one to another. Ideally, this is accomplished at the will of the user (as when the user presses a key that allows access to a different set of words), but sometimes this is the task of the communication partner (as when the partner must change the overlay on a voice output communication aid to make a new set of symbols accessible). Frequently, the organization of symbols requires the learning of some sort of code that is used to access the different chunks of vocabulary. The code may involve picture or color cues, numbers, words, or alphabetic codes. The more abstract the codes for the different sets of symbols, the greater are the memory demands. For complex systems, the user who has the metacognitive skills necessary to understand the organization of vocabulary and to deliberately practice the retrieval skills needed to access it will be far ahead.

All of these issues should be considered when high-technology AAC devices are prescribed. Too often, high-technology AAC devices are prescribed based solely on the physical limitations of the user and without regard to the cognitive requirements implicit in the system.

Effect of Learning History

The degree to which a learner already possesses a receptive or expressive symbolic communication system affects the learning of a second symbolic system. The individual who uses AAC who is learning to use a new symbolic communication system in the absence of any existing receptive or expressive symbolic system may be characterized as a first-language learner. If he or she already has receptive language and/or has already learned to use some other symbolic system expressively, he or she may be characterized as a second-language learner. The difference between first-language learning and second-language learning is profound. For the second-language learner, the whole notion of using symbols to communicate is well established. The learning of new symbols is accelerated because there are old symbols to which the new ones may be associated; furthermore, generic strategies for learning symbols may already be in place. Individuals with good language comprehension skills may be told what symbols mean, how they relate to the existing receptive language code, and how to use the new system. Thus, a child with total blindness who understands and uses speech may use Braille as a code for the familiar spoken sounds, just as the child with sight uses written letters as a code for familiar spoken sounds. For the first-language learner, however, the whole concept of communicating through symbols is new. The child with blindness without a receptive or expressive language system has nothing to which he or she can relate symbols in Braille and is unlikely to connect the raised dot patterns to referents. Learning each new symbol may be a daunting conceptual and memory task, potentially made easier if the symbol is inherently similar to the referent in some way.

Many individuals who use AAC understand speech and are in essence second-language learners, already immersed in a first language. Speech comprehension is helpful both as a language on which to map a new code and as a receptive strategy. Romski and Sevcik (1992, 1993) studied beginning versus advanced symbol achievement patterns for individuals with and without speech comprehension and determined that although receptive speech was helpful, it was not necessary for symbol acquisition. DeLoache and Burns (1993) concurred. One strategic error that we have witnessed regularly is the provision of an initial AAC system that consists entirely of some way of indicating "yes" and "no." On the surface, this seems like an economical, flexible, and powerful way to give the learner communicative control; however, an individual without receptive language skills who is unable to comprehend the questions to which "yes" and "no" are appropriate answers cannot use a yes/no response meaningfully (although using a "yes" or "no" response merely to indicate acceptance or rejection of a proffered item can be accomplished without understanding language).

Another area where learning history may come into play is in the demonstration of *fast mapping*. Fast mapping is the ability to learn new symbols with very little exposure to them (Crais, 1992) and is a feature of good teaching strategies recommended by Beukelman and Mirenda (1998). Romski, Sevcik, Robinson, Mervis, and Bertrand (1995) demonstrated fast mapping in students with mental retardation who learned to use graphic symbols in a short-term follow-up study. Wilkinson and Green (1998) studied fast mapping as it relates to the short-term retention of receptive vocabulary in children with mental retardation, noting the possible effect of memory limitations on this skill. We found that 80% of participants in a recent study who learned to use two- and three-dimensional symbols became fast mappers (Rowland & Schweigert, 2000b). Explicit associations between symbols and referents may facilitate fast mapping, as may extensive exposure and practice.

CLINICAL IMPLICATIONS: UNDERSTANDING IS THE KEY

In this section, we discuss three major aspects of clinical practice that are suggested by an approach that is informed by the cognitive implications of AAC use. Clinical practice that is cognitively grounded would ask a number of questions about understanding.

- Is the selection of the AAC system based on a full understanding of the cognitive requirements of the system, the user's own cognitive skills, and how congruent these are?
- How does the clinician know that the user understands the symbolic representation inherent in the system?
- Is the learner given the degree of experience needed to understand how to use the new system in all available contexts?

These three questions speak to an approach that is based on an adequate assessment of relevant communicative and cognitive skills, documentation of the user's comprehension of any symbolic representation involved in his or her system, and the provision of adequate practice to facilitate the learning and memory needed to master the system.

Understanding the User's Skills: Meaningful Assessment

Although we do not believe that there are any prerequisites for communication intervention, we do believe in a logical sequence of intervention. A logical intervention sequence would build on existing skills, allowing communication at the current level of competence while working systematically toward higher levels of competence. Such an approach would recognize the importance of contingency awareness, communicative intent, and symbolic representation and would be based on a thorough assessment of these aspects of the user's current communicative and cognitive skills. Iacono and colleagues (1998) suggested techniques for assessing communicative intent in children with severe and multiple disabilities and discussed the dangers of basing intervention on an inaccurate assessment of its presence or absence. They argue that "If interventionists were to consider the level of intentional functioning of their students, then the level of symbol use expected could be more clearly defined and more realistic functional goals could be set" (1998, p. 160).

Parents and professionals are understandably anxious to aim for the most conventional communication system possible. If speech does not appear to be an option currently, then systems involving the use of abstract symbols are attractive, and voice output devices can be especially seductive. Unfortunately, the selection of an AAC system is not always based on what the user's current abilities are. The consequence of overestimating a user's current abilities is that we will target an AAC system for which the user does not have the skills needed for mastery. The danger of aiming too high is failure, leading to frustration on the part of teachers and students and potentially dampening motivation or even contributing to learned helplessness (Seligman, 1975). The consequence of underestimating a user's current abilities is that we will target an AAC system that is easily used but doesn't provide the full communicative power of which the user is capable. The danger of aiming too low is that unnecessary time is spent while the user shows how easily he or she can use the system and demonstrates the need for a more complex system. This seems to us the lesser danger. Clearly, however, the best scenario is one that involves neither over- nor underestimation, but embraces the user's current skills as a basis for learning more complex skills.

AAC systems are sometimes prescribed solely on the basis of the physical limitations of the individual (and without regard for cognitive considerations) or on the basis of a diagnosis (as when children with autism are automatically given picture communication systems). Beukelman and Mirenda (1998) noted that there exist no formal tests that predict the ability to use any specific AAC device or system and stressed the need to evaluate the skills of the learner and then to compare these to the learning requirements of systems to ensure an appropriate fit. Thorough assessment may provide insight into the major cognitive factors from Table 8.2 that may influence the choice of AAC systems. These considerations, based on current functional communicative and cognitive skills, will be far more illuminating than the individual's disabilities or etiology (Rowland & Schweigert, 2000b).

At the minimum, assessment should reveal whether the individual has contingency awareness, presymbolic intentional communication, and understanding of any levels of symbolic representation. Some communication assessments that would provide such information include the Communication Matrix (Rowland, 1990, 1996), Dimensions of Communication (Mar & Sall, 2000), and the Communication and Symbolic Behavior Scales (Wetherby & Prizant, 2003). Fairly extensive probes of an individual's ability to understand the relationships between various levels of representation may be in order if symbolic systems are being contemplated. Franklin, Mirenda, and Phillips (1996) studied different symbol matching assessment protocols and learned that different protocols produce different results in participants with disabilities versus participants without disabilities and in participants with verbal label comprehension versus those without. Beukelman and Mirenda (1998) noted that an individual may be able to match on a visual level without truly understanding symbol-to-referent relationships, but that a lack of matching skills should not necessarily preclude the use of symbols. One approach developed to assess an individual's symbolic representation skills through symbol-to-referent matching tasks is the Levels of Representation Pre-Test described in Rowland and Schweigert (2000a).

Monitoring the User's Understanding of the System

An intervention approach that pays full accord to cognitive implications would incorporate procedures to monitor the user's comprehension of symbols. Although it would seem to be of fundamental importance, this is a factor that is often ignored in clinical protocols, as when learners are allowed to use symbols without ever demonstrating their comprehension of them. In other cases, the user's comprehension is checked only well into the intervention, by which time the learner may have already fallen into the habit of using symbols without understanding their meaning. Assuming that comprehension exists when it does not is not in the user's best interests. The user learns that it really does not make much difference which symbol he or she chooses, especially if all the symbols represent desirable options. As a result, the instructor does not know whether the learner understands the meaning of the individual symbols or not. This situation will be difficult to remedy if it is allowed to persist for any length of time.

For beginning users of alternative symbol systems, comprehension checks may be systematically embedded into the teaching of each new symbol. Rowland and Schweigert (2000a, 2000b) provided suggestions for conducting comprehension checks. Even after users have demonstrated their understanding of an array of symbols, a change in instructional variables, such as size or organization of the array or a change in the level of representation, may cause confusion. A comprehension check may be reinserted into the instructional procedure whenever such variables are adjusted to gauge whether or not the learner can handle the change in the protocol.

Providing Adequate Practice to Ensure Learning

Light and Lindsay (1991) cautioned that achieving correct performance does not necessarily lead to the automaticity that makes symbolic communication efficient. They warned that users may need to invest in hundreds of practice trials to get there. Unfortunately, many instructional protocols stop when some criterion of error-free performance is achieved, never offering the degree of practice necessary to achieve overlearning and automaticity. Light and Lindsay also noted a tendency to change AAC systems frequently, which reduces the likelihood of overlearning. We, too, have often witnessed new AAC systems introduced every year as a student progresses from one classroom to the next. When students have to learn to use a new system every year, it is unlikely that they will be able to take advantage of fast mapping. Sticking with the same AAC system once initial success is achieved (rather than pushing immediately on to a more abstract system) may encourage more rapid vocabulary growth by virtue of fast mapping.

The typically developing child spontaneously rehearses newly acquired words, practicing them over and over many times a day. One way to increase the frequency of spontaneous practice is to provide topics and vocabulary of maximal interest to the individual who uses AAC. Regardless of the AAC system in question, learning will occur more rapidly when valuable reasons to communicate are built into the system through topics and vocabulary that are highly motivating (partly because the learner is more likely to want to use the system spontaneously). It is through knowledge of the individual's level of awareness and world experiences that one may determine optimum contexts for communication learning, motivating topics for communication, and the vocabulary appropriate to those topics. It may be difficult to determine highly motivating topics for individuals who have profound limitations. If interviewing family members and teachers does not reveal compelling contexts and topics for communication, then structured preference probes may be necessary (Gast et al., 2000; Piazza, Fischer, Hagopian, Bowman, & Toole, 1996; Rowland & Schweigert, 1993c). For the individual who has strong interest in the physical world but little interest in communicating with other people, those strong interests may be used to scaffold and facilitate communicative interactions.

Unfortunately, simply providing highly motivating contexts and vocabulary will not necessarily result in adequate practice of new communication systems. In most instances, clinicians must ensure the provision of many deliberate opportunities to use new systems and vocabulary. Ideally those opportunities will be embedded into the regular activities of school, home, and community environments. A number of authors have described methods of targeting AAC use in typical activities (e.g., Calculator & Jorgensen, 1991; Hamilton & Snell, 1993; Rowland & Schweigert, 1993a, 1993b).

CONCLUSION

The area of cognitive development as it relates to AAC is an important though relatively unexplored one. Although we are still far from establishing firm connections between specific cognitive abilities and language development in individuals who use AAC, we are closer to a systematic approach to intervention. Studies confirming relationships between intentional presymbolic communication and symbolic communication in children with disabilities have contributed to a clearer understanding of a logical intervention sequence (Calandrella & Wilcox, 2000; Rowland & Schweigert, 2000b; Yoder & Warren, 1999, 2001). We have a better idea of where intervention should begin to be successful and of the route that may be taken to attain higher levels of communication using augmentative and alternative communication systems.

A number of avenues for future research are suggested by the research reviewed here. An assessment protocol that would reveal the cognitive abilities (such as the six factors delineated in previous sections) that are explicitly related to the use of specific AAC systems would be a useful adjunct to existing assessments of communication-related skills. Choosing an AAC system with full knowledge of the cognitive skills required to use it would increase the likelihood of understanding and success on the part of the user. Challenges to this endeavor include our lack of knowledge regarding exactly how cognitive skills develop in nonverbal children, how to measure such skills, and the influence of motivation on the assessment and performance of cognitive skills.

Although there has been a spurt of recent interest in communicative intent, further research in this area that addresses the development of intent in children with severe disabilities in particular is indicated. Expansion of the research to address the topic of persistence and mastery motivation and their relationship to the development of communicative intent would be especially helpful.

In terms of symbolic representation, a great deal of research has been conducted on the development of picture understanding and the use of pictures to convey meaning in children with and without disabilities. Much less has been conducted on the use of three-dimensional representations. Research on the development of understanding of the representative value of objects in children with and without disabilities would be useful.

Understanding of memory and its application to AAC also deserves further study. Further research might help us to identify more precisely the memory requirements necessary to access different AAC systems and to coordinate the production of messages using those systems. It would be useful to understand the difference in memory limitations involved in populations who have congenital impairments as compared with those who have acquired impairments that have affected memory and resulted in impaired communication skills. It is likely that the implications of impaired memory skills on the prescription of AAC systems would be different for a child who has never experienced language than for an adult who has sustained a head injury or for an elderly individual with dementia.

Finally, there are endless population-specific questions that could be asked. How does the prolonged motor planning time needed by children with

Rett syndrome influence their ability to coordinate the four elements of a communication act? Does the motor planning time needed outstrip their memory capacity? Can the superior skills that children with autism might possess in the realm of negotiating the physical environment be used to scaffold the acquisition of skills for negotiating the social environment? Could individuals with Alzheimer's disease who have impaired communication skills benefit from using the AAC systems developed for younger people who have never used speech?

All of these areas are fraught with methodological complications. The conduct of experimentally rigorous and substantive studies involving the behavior and education of individuals who have severe disabilities is logistically difficult and presents ethical dilemmas. Much of the research that has been conducted addressing cognitive abilities and specific AAC systems has been conducted on children without disabilities, which has caused its share of controversy in the AAC research community (Bedrosian, 1995; Higginbotham, 1995; Higginbotham & Bedrosian, 1995; Krogh & Lindsay, 1999). All of the research suggested previously would, in our view, require validation based on individuals who use or may potentially use AAC.

REFERENCES

Abbeduto, L., Davies, B., & Furman, L. (1988). The development of speech act comprehension in mentally retarded individuals and nonretarded children. *Child Development, 59,* 1460–1472.

Abbeduto, L., Furman, L., & Davies, B. (1989). Relation between the receptive language and mental age of persons with mental retardation. *American Journal on Mental Retardation, 93,* 535–543.

Atlas, J.A., & Lapidus, L.B. (1988). Symbolization levels in communicative behaviors of children showing pervasive developmental disorders. *Journal of Communication Disorders, 21,* 75–84.

Bates, E. (1979). *The emergence of symbols: Cognition and communication in infancy.* San Diego: Academic Press.

Bedrosian, J.L. (1995). Limitations in the use of nondisabled participants in AAC research. *Augmentative and Alternative Communication, 11,* 6–10.

Beukelman, D.R. (1993). AAC research: A multidimensional learning community. *Augmentative and Alternative Communication, 9,* 63–68.

Beukelman, D.R., & Mirenda, P. (1998). *Augmentative and alternative communication: Management of severe communication disorders in children and adults* (2nd ed.). Baltimore: Paul H. Brookes Publishing Co.

Bloom, Y. (1990). *Object symbols: A communication option.* Sydney, Australia: North Rocks Press.

Bondy, A., & Frost, L. (1994). The picture exchange communication system. *Focus on Autistic Behavior, 9*(3), 1–19.

Calandrella, A.M., & Wilcox, M.J. (2000). Predicting language outcomes for young prelinguistic children with developmental delay. *Journal of Speech, Language and Hearing Research, 43,* 1061–1071.

Calculator, S.N., & Jorgensen, C.M. (1991). Integrating AAC instruction into regular education settings: Expounding on best practices. *Augmentative and Alternative Communication, 7,* 204–214.

Carmeli, S., & Shen, Y. (1998). Semantic transparency and translucency in compound Blissymbols. *Augmentative and Alternative Communication, 14,* 171–183.

Corrigan, R. (1978). Language development as related to stage 6 object permanence development. *Child Language, 5,* 173–189.

Corrigan, R. (1979). Cognitive correlates of language: Differential criteria yield differential results. *Child Development, 50,* 617–631.

Crais, E. (1992). Fast mapping: A new look at word learning. In R. Chapman (Ed.), *Processes in language acquisition and disorders* (pp. 159–185). St. Louis: Mosby.

DeLoache, J., & Burns, N.M. (1993). Symbolic development in young children: Understanding models and pictures. In C. Pratt & A.F. Garton (Eds.), *Systems of representation in children: Development and use* (pp. 91–112). New York: John Wiley & Sons.

DePaul, R., & Yoder, D.E. (1986). Iconicity in manual sign systems for the augmentative communication user: Is that all there is? *Augmentative and Alternative Communication, 2,* 1–10.

Engleman, M.D., Griffin, H.C., & Wheeler, L. (1998). Deaf-blindness and communication: Practical knowledge and strategies. *Journal of Visual Impairment and Blindness* 783–798.

Franklin, K., Mirenda, P. & Phillips, G. (1996). Comparisons of five symbol assessment protocols with nondisabled preschoolers and learners with severe intellectual disabilities. *Augmentative and Alternative Communication, 12,* 63–77.

Fuller, D.R., & Lloyd, L.L. (1991). Toward a common usage of iconicity terminology. *Augmentative and Alternative Communication, 7,* 215–220.

Fuller, D.R., & Stratton, M.M. (1991). Representativeness versus translucency: Differential theoretical background, but are they really different concepts? A position paper. *Augmentative and Alternative Communication, 7,* 51–58.

Gardner, H. (1985). *The mind's new science: A history of the cognitive revolution.* New York: Basic Books.

Gast, D., Logan, K., Jacobs, H., Murray, A., Holloway, A., & Long, L. (2000). Pre-session assessment of preferences for students with profound multiple disabilities. *Education and Training in Mental Retardation and Developmental Disabilities, 35,* 393–405.

Gopnik, A., & Meltzoff, A.N. (1986). Relations between semantic and cognitive development in the one-word stage: The specificity hypothesis. *Child Development, 57,* 1040–1053.

Grove, N., Bunning, K., Porter, J. & Olsson, C. (1999). See what I mean?: Interpreting the meaning of communication by people with severe and profound intellectual disabilities. *Journal of Applied Research in Intellectual Disabilities, 12*(3), 190–203.

Hamilton, B.L., & Snell, M.E. (1993). Using the milieu approach to increase spontaneous communication book use across environments by an adolescent with autism. *Augmentative and Alternative Communication, 9,* 259–272.

Heller, K.W., Alberto, P.A., & Bowdin, J. (1995). Interactions of communication partners and students who are deaf-blind: A model. *Journal of Visual Impairment and Blindness,* 391–401.

Heller, K.W., Allgood, M.H., Ware, S.P., & Castelle, M.D. (1996). Use of dual communication boards at vocational sites by students who are deaf-blind. *RE:view, 27*(4), 180–190.

Higginbotham, D.J. (1995). Use of nondisabled participants in AAC research: Confessions of a research infidel. *Augmentative and Alternative Communication, 11,* 2–5.

Higginbotham, D.J., & Bedrosian, J.L. (1995). Participant selection in AAC research: Decision points. *Augmentative and Alternative Communication, 11,* 11–13.

Iacono, T., Carter, M., & Hook, J. (1998). Identification of intentional communication in students with severe and multiple disabilities. *Augmentative and Alternative Communication, 14,* 102–114.

Joffee, E., & Rikhye, C.H. (1991). Orientation and mobility for students with severe visual and multiple impairments: A new perspective. *Journal of Visual Impairment and Blindness, 85*(5), 211–216.

Johnson, R. (1994). *The picture communication symbols combination.* Solana Beach, CA: Meyer-Johnson Co.

Kahn, J. (1984). Cognitive training and initial use of referential speech. *Topics in Language Disorders, 6,* 14–28.

Kangas, K.A., & Lloyd, L.L. (1988). Early cognitive skills as prerequisites to augmentative and alternative communication use: What are we waiting for? *Augmentative and Alternative Communication, 4,* 211–221.

Krogh, K.S., & Lindsay, P.H. (1999). Including people with disabilities in research: Implications for the field of augmentative and alternative communication. *Augmentative and Alternative Communication, 15,* 222–233.

Kuhl, P.K., & Meltzoff, A.N. (1996). Infant vocalizations in response to speech: Vocal imitation and developmental change. *Journal of the Acoustic Society of America, 100,* 2425–2438.

Lesher, G.W., Moulton, B.J., & Higginbotham, D.J. (1998). Techniques for augmenting scanning communication. *Augmentative and Alternative Communication, 14,* 81–101.

Lifter, K., & Bloom, L. (1989). Object knowledge and the emergence of language. *Infant Behavior and Development, 12,* 395–423.

Light, J., & Lindsay, P. (1991). Cognitive science and augmentative and alternative communication. *Augmentative and Alternative Communication, 7,* 186–203.

Lobato, D., Barrera, R.D., & Feldman, R.S. (1981). Sensorimotor functioning and prelinguistic communication of severely and profoundly retarded individuals. *American Journal of Mental Deficiency, 85,* 489–496.

Mar, H., & Sall, N. (2000). *Dimensions of communication.* Paterson, NJ: St. Joseph's Children's Hospital.

McCune, L. (1995). A normatic study of representational play at the transition to language. *Developmental Psychology, 31,* 198–206.

McCune-Nicolich, L. (1981). Toward symbolic functioning: Structure of early pretend games and potential parallels with language. *Child Development, 52,* 785–797.

McLean, J.E., Snyder-McLean, L., Rowland, C., Jacobs, P., & Stremel-Campbell, K. (1981). *Generic skills assessment inventory.* Parsons: Bureau of Child Research, University of Kansas.

McNaughton, S., & Kates, B. (1980). The application of Blissymbolics. In R.L. Schiefelbusch (Ed.), *Nonspeech language and communication* (pp. 303–322). Baltimore: University Park Press.

McShane, J. (1991). *Cognitive development: An information processing approach.* Oxford: Basil Blackwell.

Meltzoff, A.N. (1999). Origins of theory of mind, cognition and communication. *Journal of Communication Disorders, 32,* 251–269.

Meltzoff, A.N., & Moore, M.K. (1997). Explaining facial imitation: A theoretical model. *Early Development and Parenting, 6,* 3–9.

Mirenda, P. (1993). AAC: Bonding the uncertain mosaic. *Augmentative and Alternative Communication, 9,* 102–114.

Mirenda, P., & Locke, P. (1989). A comparison of symbol transparency in nonspeaking persons with intellectual disabilities. *Journal of Speech and Hearing Disorders, 54,* 131–140.

Mizuko, M. (1987). Transparency and ease of learning of symbols represented by Blissymbols, PCS, and Picsyms. *Augmentative and Alternative Communication, 3,* 129–136.

Mizuko, M., Reichle, J., Ratcliff, A., & Esser, J. (1994). Effects of selection techniques and array sizes on short-term visual memory. *Augmentative and Alternative Communication, 10,* 237–244.

Newborg, J., Stock, J.R., & Wnek, L. (1984, 1988). *Battelle Developmental Inventory.* Itasca, IL: Riverside Publishing.

Notari, A.R., Cole, K.N., & Mills, P.E. (1992). Cognitive referencing: The (non) relationship between theory and application. *Topics in Early Childhood Special Education, 11*(4), 22–38.

Ockelford, A. (1992). *Objects of reference.* London: RNIB.

Owens, R.E., Jr., & House, L.I. (1984). Decision-making processes in augmentative communication. *Journal of Speech and Hearing Disorders, 49,* 18–25.

Oxley, J.D., & Norris, J.A. (2000). Children's use of memory strategies: Relevance to voice output communication aid use. *Augmentative and Alternative Communication, 16,* 79–94.

Piazza, C., Fischer, W., Hagopian, L., Bowman, L., & Toole, L. (1996). Using a choice assessment to predict reinforcer effectiveness. *Journal of Applied Behavior Analysis, 29,* 1–9.

Rast, M., & Meltzoff, A.N. (1995). Memory and representation in young children with Down syndrome: Exploring deferred imitation and object permanence. *Development and Psychopathology, 7,* 393–407.

Ratcliff, A. (1994). Comparison of relative demands implicated in direct selection and scanning: Considerations from normal children. *Augmentative and Alternative Communication, 10,* 67–74.

Reichle, J. (1991). Defining the decisions involved in designing and implementing augmentative and alternative communication systems. In J. Reichle, J. York, & J. Sigafoos (Eds.), *Implementing augmentative and alternative communication: Strategies for learners with severe disabilities.* Baltimore: Paul H. Brookes Publishing Co.

Reichle, J., Dettling, E.E., Drager, K.D.R., & Leiter, A. (2000). Comparison of correct responses latency for fixed and dynamic displays: Performance of a learner with severe developmental disabilities. *Augmentative and Alternative Communication, 16,* 154–162.

Reznick, J.S., & Goldfield, B.A. (1990). *Rapid change in language acquisition during the second year: Naming explosion or knowing explosion?* Unpublished manuscript.

Rice, M.L. (1983). Contemporary accounts of the cognition/language relationship: Implications for speech-language clinicians. *Journal of Speech and Hearing Disorders, 48,* 347–359.

Rice, M.L. (1989). Children's language acquisition. *American Psychologist, 44,* 149–156.

Romski, M.A., & Sevcik, R.A. (1988). Augmentative and alternative communication systems: Considerations for individuals with severe intellectual disabilities. *Augmentative and Alternative Communication, 4,* 83–93.

Romski, M.A., & Sevcik, R.A. (1992). Developing augmented language in children with severe mental retardation. In S.F. Warren & J. Reichle (Series and Vol. Eds.), *Communication and language intervention series: Vol. 1. Causes and effects in communication and language intervention* (pp. 113–130). Baltimore: Paul H. Brookes Publishing Co.

Romski, M.A., & Sevcik, R.A. (1993). Language comprehension: Considerations for augmentative and alternative communication. *Augmentative and Alternative Communication, 9,* 281–285.

Romski, M.A., Sevcik, R., Robinson, B., Mervis, C., & Bertrand, J. (1995). Mapping the meanings of novel visual symbols by youth with moderate or severe mental retardation. *American Journal on Mental Retardation, 100,* 391–402.

Rowland, C. (1990, 1996). *Communication matrix*. Portland: Oregon Health Sciences University.

Rowland, C., & Schweigert, P. (1993a). *Analyzing the communication environment: An inventory of ways to encourage communication in functional activities* [Manual and videotape]. Tucson, AZ: Communication Skill Builders.

Rowland, C., & Schweigert, P. (1993b). Analyzing the communication environment to increase functional communication. *Journal of The Association for Persons with Severe Handicaps (Special Issue on Communication), 18,* 161–176.

Rowland, C., & Schweigert, P. (1993c). *The early communication process using microswitch technology* (Manual and videotape). Tucson, AZ: Communication Skill Builders.

Rowland, C., & Schweigert, P. (1997). *School inventory of problem solving skills*. Portland: Oregon Health Sciences University.

Rowland, C., & Schweigert, P. (2000a). *Tangible symbol systems* (2nd ed.). Portland: Oregon Health Sciences University.

Rowland, C., & Schweigert, P. (2000b). Tangible symbols, tangible outcomes. *Augmentative and Alternative Communication, 16,* 61–78.

Rowland, C., & Schweigert, P. (2001). [Comparisons of communication and cognitive skills in children with severe disabilities]. Unpublished raw data.

Schwartz, I.S., Garfinkle, A.N., & Bauer, J. (1998). The Picture Exchange Communication System: Communicative outcomes for young children with disabilities. *Topics in Early Childhood Special Education, 18*(3), 144–159.

Schweigert, P. (1989). Use of microswitch technology to facilitate social contingency awareness as a basis for early communication skills: A case study. *Augmentative and Alternative Communication, 5,* 192–198.

Schweigert, P., & Rowland, C. (1992). Early communication and microtechnology: An instructional sequence and case studies of children with severe/multiple disabilities. *Augmentative and Alternative Communication, 8,* 273–286.

Sevcik, R.A., Romski, M.A., & Wilkinson, K.M. (1991). Roles of graphic symbols in the language acquisition process for persons with severe cognitive disabilities. *Augmentative and Alternative Communication, 7,* 161–170.

Seligman, M. (1975). *Helplessness: On depression, development and death*. San Francisco: W.H. Freeman.

Shane, H. (1981). Decision making in early augmentative communication system use. In R. Schiefelbusch & D. Bricker (Eds.), *Early language: Acquisition and intervention* (pp. 389–425). Baltimore: University Park Press.

Shore, C. (1986). Combinational play, conceptual development, and early multiword speech. *Developmental Psychology, 22,* 184–190.

Snyder-McLean, L., McLean, J.E., & Etter, R. (1988). Clinical assessment of sensorimotor knowledge in nonverbal, severely retarded clients. *Topics in Language Disorders, 8,* 1–22.

Snyder-McLean, L., Sack, S.H., & Solomonson, B. (1995). *Generic Skills Inventory*. Tucson, AZ: Communication Skill Builders.

Steckol, K.F., & Leonard, L.B. (1981). Sensorimotor development and the use of prelinguistic performatives. *Journal of Speech and Hearing Research, 24,* 262–268.

Stephenson, J., & Linfoot, K. (1996a). Intentional communication and graphic symbol use by students with severe intellectual disability. *International Journal of Disability, Development and Education, 43,* 147–165.

Stephenson, J., & Linfoot, K. (1996b). Pictures as communication symbols for students with severe intellectual disability. *Augmentative and Alternative Communication, 12,* 244–255.

Stillman, R.D. (Ed.). (1978). *Callier-Azusa Scale–G*. Dallas: Callier Center for Communication Disorders, University of Texas at Dallas.

Stillman, R.D., & Battle, C.W. (1984). Developing prelanguage communication in the severely handicapped: An interpretation of the Van Dijk method. *Seminars in Speech and Language, 5,* 159–170.

Terrell, B.Y., Schwartz, R.G., Prelock, P.A., & Messick, C.K. (1984). Symbolic play in normal and language-impaired children. *Journal of Speech and Hearing Research, 27,* 424–429.

Umholtz, R., & Rudin, D. (1981). *Teaching time concepts through the use of concrete calendars*. Austin: Texas School for the Blind.

Ungerer, J.A., & Sigman, M. (1984). The relation of play and sensorimotor behavior to language in the second year. *Child Development, 5,* 1448–1455.

Warren, S.F., & Yoder, P.J. (1998). Facilitating the transition from preintentional to intentional communication. In A.M. Wetherby, S.F. Warren, & J. Reichle (Eds.), *Communication and language intervention series: Vol. 7. Transitions in prelinguistic communication* (pp. 365–384). Baltimore: Paul H. Brookes Publishing Co.

Werner, H., & Kaplan, B. (1963). *Symbol formation*. New York: John Wiley & Sons.

Wetherby, A.M., & Prizant, B. (2003). *Communication and Symbolic Behavior Scales manual: Normed edition*. Baltimore: Paul H. Brookes Publishing Co.

Wilcox, M.J., & Shannon, M.S. (1998). Facilitating the transition from prelinguistic to linguistic communication. In A.M. Wetherby, S.F. Warren, & J. Reichle (Eds.), *Communication and language intervention series: Vol. 7. Transitions in prelinguistic communication* (pp. 385–416). Baltimore: Paul H. Brookes Publishing Co.

Wilkinson, K.M., & Green, G. (1998). Implications of fast mapping for vocabulary expansion in individuals with mental retardation. *Augmentative and Alternative Communication, 14,* 162–170.

Yoder, P.J., & Warren, S.F. (1999). Maternal responsivity mediates the relationship between prelinguistic intentional communication and later language. *Journal of Early Intervention, 22,* 126–136.

Yoder, P.J., & Warren, S.F. (2001). Relative treatment effects of two prelinguistic communication interventions on language development in toddlers with developmental delays vary by maternal characteristics. *Journal of Speech, Language and Hearing Research, 44,* 224–237.

Yovetich, W.S., & Young, T.A. (1988). The effects of representativeness and concreteness on the "guessability" of Blissymbols. *Augmentative and Alternative Communication, 4,* 35–39.

Zangari, C., Lloyd, L.L., & Vicker, B. (1994). Augmentative and alternative communication: An historic perspective. *Augmentative and Alternative Communication, 10,* 27–59.

9

Visual Issues and Access to AAC

Tracy M. Kovach and Patricia Bothwell Kenyon

The importance of functional vision in selection and use of augmentative and alternative communication (AAC) systems often has been overlooked (Bailey & Downing, 1994; Blackstone, 1994). Most AAC systems use visual symbols, whether unaided (e.g., gestural codes or manual sign systems) or aided (e.g., representational or abstract symbols) to represent spoken language. For individuals who require AAC, having a visual impairment can have a significant impact on the successful development of operational competence. For these individuals, the need for system modifications and/or adapted implementation strategies must be acknowledged and put into practice for the development of effective and functional communication outcomes. This chapter discusses the relationship between functional vision and AAC and the strategies to accommodate visual impairments alone and in conjunction with severe physical impairments.

INCIDENCE AND DEMOGRAPHICS

According to the Centers for Disease Control and Prevention (2001), nearly 1 in every 1,000 American children has low vision or is legally blind. Medical developments since the 1970s in developed nations have reduced the incidences of visual impairment and blindness from infections and poor nutrition. Two thirds of the children with visual impairments in developed nations have one or more other disabilities.

According to a comprehensive study of children 3–10 years of age by the Metropolitan Atlanta Developmental Disabilities Surveillance Program (MADDSP), visual impairment occurs in 0.8 children per 1,000 and cerebral palsy occurs in 2.4 per 1,000 children (Centers for Disease Control and Prevention, 2001). Data from this study also indicated that 48% of children with visual impairments have cerebral palsy. Conversely, 70% of the children with

277

cerebral palsy were identified as having visual impairments. This finding is consistent with other reported studies indicating that the incidence of visual impairments in children with developmental delay and cerebral palsy ranges from 48% to 75% (Black, 1980; Miller, Menacker, & Batshaw, 2002; Schenk-Rootlieb, van Nieuwenhuizen, van der Geual, Wittebol-Post, & Willemse, 1992).

Several other trends were identified by the MADDSP study as well. Only 17% of the children with visual impairments were diagnosed prior to 2 years of age, which raises concerns about the effect that undiagnosed, uncorrected poor vision may have on language development. By 5 years of age, 70% of children with visual impairments had been identified. It is likely, however, that a disproportionate percentage of the unidentified children are children with cerebral palsy. Traditional acuity testing for very young children with significant physical impairments and/or with mental retardation can be very difficult because these children cannot give the feedback necessary for accurate testing (Brodsky, Baker, & Hamed, 1996). Advances in visual assessment for these children will hopefully improve early identification of visual impairments. For example, studies using a combination of visual evoked potentials (VEP) and preferential looking techniques can obtain more complete assessment of children who otherwise cannot give subjective responses (e.g., Orel-Bixler, Haegerstrom-Portnoy, & Hall, 1989).

TYPES OF VISUAL IMPAIRMENTS

Vision is defined as "the special source by which objects, their form, color, position, etc., in the external environment are perceived, . . . the act function, process, or power of seeing, sight" (Cline, Hofstetter, & Griffin, 1980, p. 696). A person's sense of vision provides him or her with experiences and knowledge that are difficult to gain through other sensory channels. Sonksen, Levitt, and Kitsinger summarized the unique impact that vision has on development:

> Vision has long been considered the most important input modality for normal development. Although sound, like light, spans space, only sight presents the world in a perspective which remains to be examined again: sounds come and are gone and touch does not span space. Both therefore are inferior to sight as learning modalities. (1984, p. 273)

It is important to understand that the range and severity of vision loss and visual impairments can vary greatly (Sacks, 1998). A summary of various types of visual impairments and their definitions can be found in Table 9.1.

Visual Acuity

Visual acuity is the "acuteness or clearness of vision (especially of form vision), which is dependent on the sharpness of the retinal focus, the sensitivity

Table 9.1.   Categories of visual impairments

Categories of visual impairment	Definition	Subtypes
Refraction	Caused when cones and lens do not bring images into sharp focus on the retina	*Myopia (nearsightedness)* Cornea excessively curved, lens is too strong, or eye is elongated Images of distant objects are not focused directly on retina and appear blurry
		Hyperopia (farsightedness) Cornea relatively flat, eye not as long as normal, or focusing power of eye is weak Objects focused at point behind retina, resulting in straining to focus on nearby objects
		Astigmatism Shape of cornea not quite right; rays passing through it not properly focused Both near and far objects may appear blurry Often appears in combination with near- or farsightedness
		Anisometropia Significant difference between the refractive power of each eye (e.g., one eye nearsighted, other eye farsighted)
Structural impairments	Caused when one or more parts of the eye's optical, movement, or nerve systems are poorly developed, damaged, or not functioning properly	*Optic nerve or visual pathway* Atrophy or underdevelopment of optic nerve, resulting in various degrees of vision loss
		Amblyopia Eye turns out or wanders, suppressing vision in that eye Variety of causes due to one eye having better acuity Can be caused by strabismus
		Cataracts Cloudiness of crystalline lens of the eye Found in some types of syndromes
		Oculomotor difficulties Affects ability of eyes to focus on one object and fuse the images into one Strabismus: one or both eyes turned inward or outward Nystagmus: rhythmic jiggling of eyes; eyes move but child sees stationary picture

(continued)

Table 9.1.   *(continued)*

Categories of visual impairment	Definition	Subtypes
Cortical visual impairment (CVI)	Temporary or permanent visual impairment caused by damage to the posterior visual pathways and/or occipital lobes of the brain	Leading cause of visual loss for children with neurological issues Degree of neurological damage and visual impairment depends on time of onset, and location and intensity of insult Visual systems of brain do not consistently understand or interpret what the eyes see

From King, J. (2000). *The Bridge School classroom strategies: Vision and AAC, 2.* Hillsborough, CA: The Bridge School; adapted by permission.

of the nervous elements, and time interpretation faculty of the brain" (Cline et al., 1980, p. 9). There are three commonly used categories for visual acuity impairments (Bishop, 1991; Corn, 1985; Individuals with Disabilities Education Act [IDEA] of 1990, PL 101-476; Miller et al., 2002):

- *Legal blindness:* Sight that is equal to or less than 20/200 (a person can see at 20 feet what an unaffected person can see at 200 feet) in the best eye with correction or a visual field that is no greater than 20°
- *Partial sight:* Sight that is 20/200 to 20/70 with best correction
- *Low vision:* Severe visual impairment even after correction with a need to be assisted by aids or modifications to permit function

Most often, acuity measures are related to refractive or ocular/lens issues, and eyeglasses are worn for correction.

Impairments Resulting from Central Nervous System Damage

Cortical Visual Impairment   Children using AAC systems often have multiple disabilities as the result of central nervous system damage, which puts them at high risk for cortical visual impairment (CVI), the most common visual impairment in developed countries (Brodsky et al., 1996; Good, Jan, DeSa, Barkovich, Groenveld, & Hoyt, 1994). CVI essentially results from damage to areas of the central nervous system that are responsible for interpreting or registering visual sensory information; that is, visual perception is impaired or lost secondary to damage to the geniculate and/or extra geniculate pathways (lateral geniculate body, optic radiations, and primary visual cortex). This damage prevents the proper reception and/or interpretation of visual stimuli. Individuals with CVI may experience bilateral loss of vision, yet have a normal pupillary response. Furthermore, an eye examination may display no other abnormalities (Good et al., 1994; Lambert, 1995).

Vision in children with CVI may vary from moment to moment, depending on a variety of factors (Brodsky et al., 1996; Good et al., 1994; Jan, Groenveld, Sykanda, & Hoyt, 1987):

- Changes in the environment
- Familiarity of task, objects, and/or people
- Lighting
- Stresses the child is experiencing
- The child's attention
- Seizure activity
- Fatigue

These factors will all affect visual performance significantly more in children with CVI than in typically developing children (Anthony, 1990; Good et al., 1994; Jan et al., 1987; King, 2000). This variability is often confusing to caregivers and professionals, as children may perform tasks without difficulty one day, or even one hour, and not the next. Children with CVI will often be able to find and/or grasp familiar objects without "looking" or navigate through a room without bumping into furniture or objects. Because these children sometimes appear to have such functional vision, others may think that they are, at other times, being uncooperative or not trying hard enough. It is important to remember that what may appear to be a lack of motivation may, in reality, stem from the inherent visual variability of CVI.

One characteristic of CVI resulting from central nervous system damage that may have a significant impact on use of AAC systems is that of visual field deficits. The visual field is the area of physical space visible to an eye (Good et al., 1994). Visual field deficits result in "blank" areas within the visual field. The person with field deficits is usually unaware that they are not seeing objects or space in the affected area.

Another characteristic particularly important to AAC systems is color vision. For children with CVI, color vision is an ability that is frequently preserved, and in particular, certain colors such as yellow, red, and orange are often relatively well perceived and can be used to capture visual attention (Geilhaus & Olson, 1993; Good et al., 1994).

The ability to identify shapes may also be preserved in CVI. Objects that are familiar will have increased recognition. Thus, children will benefit significantly from repeated exposure to objects they use for learning. Repetition is very important for children with cortical visual impairment and helps explain their acknowledgment of and preference for familiar objects over new or unfamiliar ones.

Using central vision may be difficult for children with CVI (King, 2000). Behaviorally, this means that children may not look directly at an object or person but instead will use their peripheral vision to locate, see, and guide object grasping (Sacks, 1998). They also may not make direct eye contact with people, a very important nonverbal communication skill. Observation of responses to caregivers' comments such as "look at me" or "look here" may be a clue that the child is having difficulty using central vision.

Children with CVI may also demonstrate a preference for a nontraditional head position or posture because they are experiencing field cuts, are experiencing difficulties with ocular motor control, or are using their peripheral vision. Demanding a proper head position and eye-to-eye or eye-to-object central vision focus may decrease functional visual abilities (Sacks, 1998).

In additionally, CVI can result in a reduced ability to visually perceive an entire "picture." Visual figure ground, or the ability to screen important versus extraneous visual information, is often impaired (Good et al., 1994; Sacks, 1998). An environment that is visually rich, or full of information, may interfere with visual function in children with CVI. Behaviorally, these children may come very close to an object to screen out the background information, thereby increasing their ability to visually attend.

Light in the environment may also be problematic for children with CVI. Both photophobia and light gazing are commonly noted, either of which may interfere with visual performance (Good et al., 1994; Jan & Groenveld, 1995). Photophobia is a hypersensitivity to light; however, children with CVI may also overly attend to bright sources of light such as skylights, windows, or even the sun, which can interfere with attention to other visual stimuli (Sacks, 1998). Light sources, visual stimulation, and reduction of visual clutter are important considerations when setting up learning environments to maximize functional visual abilities for children with CVI.

Other Visual Impairments   In addition to being at high risk for CVI, children with neurological damage may also demonstrate other visual impairments that significantly affect vision. Children born prematurely can develop retinopathy of prematurity (ROP), which is caused by vascular damage to the retina of preterm infants. Associated complications with ROP include nearsightedness (myopia), strabismus, glaucoma, and blindness (Miller et al., 2002). Strabismus is a condition where binocular vision, the ability to use both eyes together, is not present. Imbalances in eye musculature or significant farsightedness are two common causes of strabismus. If unidentified and untreated, these can lead to amblyopia (low or reduced visual acuity not correctable by refractive means and not attributable to other apparent structural or pathological anomalies). In the case of strabismus, the reduced visual acuity in one eye is secondary to nonuse or prolonged suppression; such a period of nonuse causes the brain to essentially "turn off" one eye. The rate of occurrence for strabismus for children with cerebral palsy is 30%–50% (Duckman, 1979; Jones, 1983; Nelson, Calhoun, & Harley, 1991).

Visual accommodation is the ability of the lens to change its curvature to change the focal point of the eye and can be severely impaired with central nervous system damage (Duckman, 1979). When visual accommodation is impaired, the individual will have difficulty holding an object in focus as it moves farther from or closer to the eyes. Visual accommodation also allows a person to focus on a relatively close object and then quickly focus on a more distant object without difficulty. Examples of using visual accommodation skills include looking back and forth between a person and a communication device, a computer screen to a keyboard, and a desktop to a blackboard. Children with cerebral palsy have been found to have significant accommodative insufficiency, as high as 100% (Duckman, 1979); as a result, they are often unable to make shifts in their visual focusing. Using an aided AAC system frequently requires shifts in focus or redirected eye gaze. This may be extremely difficult or impossible for some children who have cerebral palsy (Cook & Hussey, 1995).

Table 9.2 summarizes the characteristic differences between ocular and cortical visual impairments. It is important to note that a child may experience multiple types of visual impairments. For example, a child with cerebral

Table 9.2. Characteristic differences between pure ocular and cortical visual disorders

Characteristics	Ocular disorder	Cortical visual disorder
Eye examination	Usually abnormal	Normal
Visual function	Consistent	Highly variable
Visual attention span	Usually normal	Markedly short
Sensory nystagmus	Present when congenital and early onset	Not present
Poorly coordinated eye movements	Present when congenital and early onset	Usually normal
Rapid head shaking (horizontal)	Occasionally	Never
Compulsive light gazing	Rarely	Common
Light sensitivity	Dependent on the eye disorder	Occurs in ⅓ of cases
Eye pressing	Common; used for magnification	Common; used for magnification, reduction of crowding, or both
Color preservation	Dependent on the eye disorder	Preserved
Appearance	Appears visually impaired	Usually normal
Peripheral field loss	Occasionally	Nearly always
Presence of additional neurological disabilities	Fairly common	Nearly always

palsy may have CVI but also may require corrective lenses due to a refractive impairment.

IMPORTANCE OF VISION FOR LANGUAGE AND COMMUNICATION DEVELOPMENT

The impact of low or no vision on the development of language is profound (Jan, Sykanda, & Groenveld, 1990; Kekelis & Prinz, 1996; Preisler, 1995; Reynell, 1978; Sonksen et al., 1984; Troster & Bramberg, 1993). Preisler's work has revealed that language development in children with severe visual impairments is more delayed than in children with hearing impairments (Preisler, 1995). Infants with visual impairments miss interpersonal cues that typically take place between an infant and caregiver, in part because the baby who is visually impaired cannot observe and learn the traditional nonverbal cues from the caregiver (Priesler, 1995; Sonksen et al., 1984). In turn, caregivers miss the communication efforts of the young infants because of the nontraditional nature of the cues from the baby. For example, blind infants may become very still when interested in an external stimuli compared to sighted infants who will look to the stimuli, turn their heads, and have increased arm and leg motions (Priesler, 1995; Sonksen et al., 1984).

Communication related to objects such as person–person–object communication does not occur, as young children with visual impairments are unaware of the objects in the environment. Furthermore, parents of children with visual impairments are less likely than parents of typically developing children to label objects in the environment (Priesler, 1995). Even the simple nonverbal action of pointing to an object does not develop in blind children or children with severe visual impairment (Preisler, 1995).

Early Object Learning

For children with sight, the majority of initial learning about their environment and objects in it is visually and tactilely driven (Bigelow, 1991; Ruff, 1980). Research indicates that refined manipulation of objects develops with the ability of infants to look at objects (Fraiberg, 1977; Hatwell, 1990; Rochat, 1989). The manual manipulation of objects in conjunction with vision allows the tactile and kinesthetic information to be paired with the visual information to integrate and to form more complete object concepts. The infants can learn about the object's consistency when seen from different orientations because they can rotate the object, move around, or tilt their heads.

Ruff (1980) found that infants' active manipulation of objects is a critical component for learning about objects. Other research has suggested that for young children, visual learning is more rapid than haptic (tactile) learning, with haptic and visual learning not becoming equally efficient until adolescence (Juurmaa & Lehtinen-Railo, 1988). These results have important implications for children with central nervous system damage and significant visual impairments and motor deficits that prevent active manipulation of objects and sensory feedback; however, the full implications of these findings are not completely understood. It is known that children with severe visual and motor impairments have impaired stereognostic skills (e.g., impaired haptic object identification; Bolanos, Bleck, Firestone, & Young, 1989; Reitan, 1971; Solomons, 1957; Tachdjian & Minear, 1958). Thus, for children with central nervous system damage and impaired vision and motor-sensory skills, there is reason for significant concern when considering the development of object concepts and their importance in language development.

By 12 months of age, typically developing children develop three-dimensional spatial knowledge through self-initiated movement and visual fixation (Bigelow, 1991). Furthermore, vision is used to confirm the position of nearby sound sources very early in infancy. Thus, auditory object orientation is tutored by vision. For a child with visual impairments, learning about the environment and object concepts has to be developed through auditory and tactile perception (Sonksen et al., 1984). For example, for the concepts of "in" and "out," size and shape are visually coordinated in the sensorimotor stage. The child with severe visual impairments does not have an opportunity to observe these qualities over and over again, as does the child with sight, resulting in a diminished experience with the object world.

Vision also reinforces auditory object identification and localization in the child with sight. A child hears a sound and looks to see what has made it. The child looks and subsequently sees an object that is constant over space and in time. In contrast, sound exists only temporarily. Children with significant visual impairments who must develop auditory object permanence, without the benefit of vision, may experience significant delays in the development of object concepts (Sonksen et al., 1984).

Early Motor Learning

Early motor learning in children with visual impairments is different from that of typically developing children (Bigelow, 1991; Reynell, 1978; Sonksen et al., 1984; Troster & Bramberg, 1993). Young children with visual impairments have a delayed knowledge about the body, resulting in decreased hand play and use as early as 10–12 weeks of age (Sonksen et al., 1984). While children with sight begin to show refined and directed hand motions at 10–12 weeks, children with visual impairments show a general decrease in hand use. Through observation, infants who can see begin to realize the potential of different body parts for functional activities (e.g., arms for prehension and manipulation, legs for mobility). Children with visual impairments do not have this opportunity for learning.

Visual cues support early knowledge of vertical orientation. Vision fine-tunes the vestibular/proprioceptive input and links the body's sensory awareness with the outside world. Initially, it is the visual system that initiates postural control; the vestibular/proprioceptive system takes over at a later developmental stage. Thus, the visual system is very important in postural righting and control necessary for many learning tasks (Troster & Bramberg, 1993).

Children with severe visual impairments may also experience significant delays in their ability to transition from one posture to another. Blind children develop the ability to hold a static posture equally as well as children with sight, but their visual system does not provide the same drive to explore the environment; thus, they have a delay in movements that are self-initiated (Adelson & Fraiberg, 1974).

Because these major areas of development are affected in children with visual impairments, the development of concepts such as spatial awareness, spatial relations, interpersonal interaction skills, object permanence, object concepts, symbolic representation, and language are all negatively impacted. These limitations add to the challenges of developing AAC systems, which typically consist of visual representations of language and communication, such as natural gestures, sign language, or picture, letter, or word boards (Kovach & Kenyon, 1998).

INTERVENTIONS TO ENHANCE VISUAL FUNCTIONING

Fortunately, most individuals with visual impairments have some functional vision. The literature suggests that even low vision will make a significant difference on the impact of the delays discussed in the previous section (Reynell, 1978). Thus, it is important to use strategies that will enhance the use of residual vision whenever possible (Bailey & Downing, 1994). When considering how to enhance residual vision, it is important to understand the visual problem and determine if it is an ocular vision loss, cortical visual impairment, or both (Jan et al., 1990; Tierney & King, 1998). (See Table 9.1.)

There are no set interventions for any given impairment; each child will be different and will present different needs and skills. Table 9.3 provides guidelines for interventions that might enhance visual function. For example, enlarging an image, a traditional adaptation, may be helpful for some children; however, it may increase the visual confusion for a person with a field cut. Children with CVI will show a better visual response to brightly colored objects than to the classical contrast approach of black and white or pastel colors (Good et al., 1994). Given the varied effects of different types of visual im-

Table 9.3. Suggested interventions to enhance visual function

Visual element	Considerations to improve visual attending
Color	Use bright primary colors to attract visual attention. Red, orange, and yellow are colors that may be particularly effective.
Size	Match size to visual abilities (e.g., enhance size for poor acuity; do not enhance for significant field cuts or tunnel vision)
Contrast	Use high contrast such as white on black or black on yellow; use contrasting colors Use focused illumination to increase contrast between objects
Lighting, glare	Decrease all sources of glare
Light gazing	Use environments that do not have sources of bright, intense light
Photophobia	Use environments that do not have sources of bright, intense light
Distance	Position objects and AAC systems at the user's preferred distance to accommodate visual abilities
Positioning	Use positions/positioning systems that provide a good base of support to facilitate visual function
Tracking difficulties	Extend the time and practice provided to learn scanning skills and locations
Complexity	Introduce parts of objects/symbols that make up a whole Begin with simplified designs, symbols, and choices Progress to more complex ones Emphasize particular lines to emphasize specific aspects of symbols
Familiarity	Attention is enhanced with familiarity. Use increased repetition with novel objects/symbols
Multisensory approach	Introduce sensory stimuli one modality at a time Slowly combine input modalities

pairment, it is critical that enhancing strategies and visual abilities are individually matched. Some of the basic visual elements that can be considered when trying to enhance visual responsiveness are color, size, contrast, lighting, distance and positioning, motion, complexity, and familiarity. (Readers are also referred to Tierney and King's *Guidelines for Custom Visual Displays* and *Visual Profile* in King, 2000.)

Color

Color encompasses several elements: *aspects of hue,* or the attribute of the color sensation (i.e., red, green, blue); *saturation,* or the amount of black, white, or gray within a color; and *brightness,* or the luminance intensity of the color. According to the theory of visual functioning, pastels are less stimulating than the brightness of primary colors (Geilhaus & Olson, 1993). This is something toy manufacturers have known for a long time and have utilized in their product development. When using color with communication symbols, rich colors may pull visual attention more effectively. As previously mentioned, color perception may remain intact for children with CVI. For some children, color perception may be important to AAC symbolic comprehension and memory.

Size

Size becomes a complex issue when working with individuals with visual impairments who require AAC systems. It is critical that visual abilities are fully understood and that this knowledge is used to guide appropriate system development. If children have poor acuity, larger AAC symbols may be better; however, if children have a significant field cut or tunnel vision, larger AAC symbols mean that more information may be lost into the "unseen" space. Children with CVI, unless they also have acuity issues, generally do not need enlargement to enhance functional vision.

Contrast

There are several aspects to be considered in the area of visual contrast. First, there is a contrast that comes from the difference in brightness of two objects. Examples are black letters on a white background and other reversed image symbols. Another type of contrast is related to the amount of light reflected off one area versus another. For example, increasing illumination by using a high-intensity reading lamp shining on an object to which a child needs to attend will increase the light reflecting off that object. Thus, "spotlighting" objects about which the child is learning may be helpful. Backlighting available on various AAC systems also increases contrast and illumination (Bailey & Downing, 1994; Geilhaus & Olson, 1993; Sacks, 1998).

Lighting

As mentioned previously, different lighting techniques can be used to increase contrast. It is also important to observe other effects of light, such as glare from windows or other sources that may obscure objects on computer and/or AAC device screens. Similarly, the presence of windows in the room that give an intense area of light may prevent visual attention to other objects. Having a child face a window may reduce glare on a device's screen but may make it difficult for a child to screen the window light out of his or her visual field (Jan, Groenveld, & Anderson, 1993; Sacks, 1998;). Children with CVI may be photophobic and may require environments that do not have bright lights. They may also be drawn to stare at bright light sources such as windows or fluorescent lights. Ideally, intervention would eliminate or reduce these light sources to enhance visual function.

Distance and Positioning

Typically developing infants at birth have visual acuity of 20/400 or see at 1 foot what an adult with normal sight sees at 20 feet; an infant of 3 months sees at 4 feet what the adult sees at 20 feet. By 2 years of age, a typically developing child has 20/20 vision (Greenwald, 1983.) The optimal distance to position an object from a visually impaired child, however, will vary with the size of the object and with the child's visual deficit. Children with ocular disorders may come physically close to objects to "magnify" them. Children with CVI may come close to fill their visual field with the object or picture and thus reduce the competing visual input in the background (Anthony, 1990; Jan et al., 1995). Observing the child's preferences may give important clues to the child's needs. Consideration must be given to the optimal distance for objects, AAC symbols, or aided communication device being used. The system may need to be visually close to the child until familiarity is established and then moved to a distance to enable more appropriate social interaction.

Another consideration is for the physical positioning needs of the child. The difficulties children with cerebral palsy may have with ocular motor control may mean that they need to use an upper gaze or a lower gaze to see an object. Perhaps they see objects best when placed in the upper right quadrant versus anyplace else. It is important to explore what the visual field preference is for the child.

Tracking and Visual Attending

Children with visual problems resulting from neurological deficits may have difficulty fixing and/or tracking moving objects secondary to decreased ocular motor control. This may have implications for the expectation that a child track the scanning lights on a device; however, movement of an object in their peripheral vision may stimulate a visual response from a child with CVI. Visual attending requires complex hemispheric control and requires the conscious or purposeful fixation of the eyes to an object (Good et al., 1994). This may be very difficult for children with central nervous system damage. As a result, they may require extended time and practice to learn AAC system use.

Complexity

The complexity of the visual stimulus may also have an impact on the child's ability to understand and use AAC systems. Complexity of graphic symbols involves the amount of information, the number of semantic elements, or, as some have defined it, the relationship of figure information to the background of the symbol (Lloyd, Fuller, & Arvidson, 1997). For the purposes of this chapter, complexity refers to the actual visual field or object being viewed. In this context, the following issues must be considered when developing visual images on AAC systems:

- Amount of detail of the AAC symbols
- Number of symbols in the visual field
- Balance between visual complexity and an optimal number of choices for communication purposes

In some cases, emphasis on certain lines (e.g., making particular lines bolder than others) may enhance the visual quality and emphasize pertinent qualities, thus simplifying the visual input (Bailey & Downing, 1994; Levack, Stone, & Bishop, 1994)

Familiarity

Children with visual impairments often show a marked preference for familiar objects and can interact with them more easily. Repetitive practice with objects and symbols is extremely important for children with visual impairments. A thorough familiarity with the parts of objects facilitates understanding of the gestalt of these objects. Thus, children with visual impairments need repeated exposure to all objects as part of their general learning environment as well as objects directly related to their communication needs in order to maximize performance (Bailey et al., 1994; Levack et al., 1994).

Other Adaptations

The benefit of using a multisensory approach to learning should always be considered for children with multiple disabilities; however, children with physical and sensory deficits may have a varying tolerance for the ability to integrate more than one sense and motor act at a time. When learning to be operationally competent in AAC system use, these children may not be able to look and listen (or look, listen, and press a switch) at the same time. In other words, a multisensory approach may actually be overstimulating. These children may need to perform tasks separately and sequentially, as opposed to simultaneously. They may look briefly, then listen, then organize a motion. Their response and activation time, therefore, may be very delayed, and their learning curve for a motor response may be dramatically delayed. In addition, their response to sensory input may be qualitatively different from children without visual impairments. For example, they may become very still and quiet when they are listening, which should not be misinterpreted as disinterest or an inability to perform.

IMPACT OF SEVERE VISUAL AND PHYSICAL IMPAIRMENTS ON AAC SYSTEM DEVELOPMENT

For individuals who use AAC, visual impairments may co-occur with a number of other disabilities. Some children who require AAC have both visual and auditory impairments, known as dual sensory impairment (DSI). It is not within the scope of this chapter to address the needs of this population; however, a number of researchers have developed excellent resources that provide insights into the visual component of DSI (e.g., Mar & Sall, 1994; Mathy-Laikko et al., 1989; Rowland, 1990; Rowland & Schweigert, 1989, 2000; Thorley, Ward, Binepal & Dolan, 1991).

Another category of multiple impairments that presents significant challenges to AAC development is that of severe visual impairment associated with severe physical impairment. One of the most common congenital causes of severe physical impairments is cerebral palsy (Mirenda & Mathy-Laikko, 1989). The prevalence of visual impairments with cerebral palsy should come as no surprise, as central nervous system damage is the cause of both cerebral palsy and certain visual impairments such as CVI. Individuals with severe speech, physical, and visual impairments require access to AAC to facilitate communicative competence. Included in this group are many who require alternative access to AAC systems (LaFontaine & DeRuyter, 1987). One method of alternative access that may be appropriate for these individuals, given their visual impairments, is auditory scanning.

Auditory Scanning

When speech, physical, and visual abilities are impaired, AAC system development is complex. For some children who have severe motor impairments, direct selection is not a viable means of accessing an AAC device; these children typically rely on some type of scanning. (See Chapter 7 for further discussion of specific access methods.)

Scanning is a complex task involving motor, cognitive, linguistic, and visual perceptual skills (Blackstone, 1989; Piche & Reichle, 1991; Ratcliff, 1994). Although visual scanning access accommodates the user's motor limitations, it requires significant visual skills. Visual scanning requires an individual to see and understand the symbol representations, follow a series of indicators that sequentially and systematically present choices, and anticipate and time a motor response to activate a switch for choice selection. When an individual must use scanning to access AAC but does not possess the visual skills required for visual scanning, auditory scanning may be a viable alternative (Blackstone, 1989). Auditory scanning is a method for accessing AAC system content when choices for content selection are presented using a verbal auditory cue, which typically consists of a word, phrase, or sentence. Clinical management of auditory scanning can be complicated when trying to define and develop levels of auditory representation and organization of system content.

There is very little information in the research literature about the development and use of auditory scanning as an access method for AAC systems. In the mid- to late 1990s, four national symposia on auditory scanning were held at The Children's Hospital in Denver, Colorado, to provide a forum for individuals with an interest in auditory scanning to share information and discuss successes and concerns. A web site and listserv[1] that focused on auditory scanning were developed for the primary purpose of promoting ongoing interest and information exchange about issues relating to auditory scanning.

Auditory scanning involves more than just the interface between a person and an AAC system; it is even more complex than visual scanning (Kovach & Kenyon, 1998). The lack of published research that considers auditory scanning may, in part, be due to

- Limited recognition of the benefits of auditory scanning access and limited understanding of populations who would benefit from auditory scanning
- Limited understanding of applications of auditory scanning
- The complexities involved in working with individuals with multiple disabilities who might benefit from auditory scanning
- Limited understanding of how to represent and organize AAC system content with auditory cues or "symbols"
- The significant variability across individuals who have multiple disabilities in terms of their cognitive, linguistic, motor, and visual abilities and needs

Individuals Who May Benefit from Auditory Scanning

The interest in auditory scanning and its potential benefits has increased significantly in the past decade. The increased availability of an auditory scanning feature on many electronic AAC systems in the 1990s has heightened awareness of its application beyond that for individuals with significantly compromised visual skills. Although auditory scanning is most applicable for individuals who have significant motor impairments with accompanying visual impairments, auditory scanning also may be used with individuals who have intact vision. For these individuals, auditory scanning may enhance visual scanning by

- Emphasizing or teaching the scanning pattern
- Helping the individual learn the names of the symbols
- Helping the individual maintain attention to the visual scanning pattern by pairing auditory and visual signals

---

[1]Readers are referred to the Auditory Scanning and Augmentative and Alternative Communication web site, http://espse.ed.psu.edu/spled/mcn/auditoryscanning/home.html.

- Enhancing visual interaction with communication partners and the environment by allowing users to listen to the scanning pattern rather than having to focus visual attention on a visual scanning pattern

Skills Needed for Auditory Scanning

Certain skills and abilities are needed to successfully use and benefit from auditory scanning. Although the range of these skills varies greatly, success in functional use of auditory scanning is generally dependent on four factors:

1. Physical ability to operate a mechanism (usually a single switch) to make a selection from a series of choices presented
2. Comprehension of spoken words as selection choices for intentional communication
3. Memory for selections previously and subsequently made to compose a message
4. Comprehension of content categorization cues that represent the message

As in all areas of AAC, proficiency in these areas is not a prerequisite to the application of auditory scanning, and these skills may develop as auditory scanning access is developed.

One of the few and earliest accounts of AAC system development using auditory scanning was described by Beukelman, Yorkston, and Dowden (1985). This case study exemplified the unique needs of an individual with severe speech, physical, and visual impairments, the challenges in addressing those needs, and the degree of success towards achieving operational competence. Blischak (1995) also described the unique and multiple dimensions of AAC implementation for a child using auditory scanning access. One challenge frequently noted in these types of anecdotal reports is the user's need to focus attention on the auditory cues rather than on his or her environment and communication partners. Blischak (1995) argued that for people with visual impairments who rely on their auditory channel to monitor their environment, this requirement might be difficult as well as uncomfortable because it creates conflict between listening to the scanning cues and listening to the communication partner and other auditory signals important for interaction and communication.

Careful consideration must be given to visual, auditory, cognitive, language, and motor skills necessary in auditory scanning implementation. Unfortunately, it is often difficult to assess these skills in individuals who have severe speech impairments and even more challenging for those with additional physical and visual impairments. Buzolich, King, and Baroody (1991) used an auditory scanning assessment tool to evaluate many of these skills using auditorily scanned stimuli. Unfortunately, this tool is unpublished (M.J. Buzolich, personal communication, 2000), and as of 2003, there are no other known assessment instruments for auditory scanning.

Surprisingly little is known about those who are already using auditory scanning. Blackstone, Kovach, and Light (reported by Blackstone, 1998b) surveyed 16 professionals who had experience using auditory scanning systems. These professionals reported on 28 individuals who used auditory scanning strategies primarily due to visual impairments (mean age = 12 years of age). Only 18% of the individuals who required AAC were reported to have completed any formal visual testing to determine their residual visual skills or the characteristics of their visual impairments. Additionally, little information was available about their cognitive or language skills. Motor skills were more thoroughly assessed, for the primary purpose of determining appropriate methods for scanning access; motor skills were not assessed with regard to knowledge about the subjects' visual, cognitive, or language skills, all of which can have a significant impact on motor control (Buzolich et al., 1991). No hearing impairments were reported. Information about speech reception, speech discrimination, and auditory memory skills was not gathered. The survey yielded no reports of attempts to modify formal assessment measures. For the most part, information in all of these areas was reportedly obtained through informal observation.

These data illustrate the disturbing lack of systematic assessment of skills in areas that significantly affect decisions about use of visual enhancements and/or auditory scanning. Modifying formal assessment measures raises questions about the validity of results, particularly in light of the language learning differences of children with severe visual impairments. Furthermore, limited information is available to establish the reliability and validity of the types of informal observations typically used to assess visual, cognitive, language, and motor skills.

During the 1999 Auditory Scanning Symposium, a protocol for documenting observations of these skills in a systematic manner was developed. Readers are referred to the Auditory Scanning and Augmentative and Alternative Communication web site for the protocol (http://espse.ed.psu.edu/spled/mcn/auditoryscanning/home.html). This protocol provides a method to structure observations of the performance of individuals who may benefit from auditory scanning. The data collected will assist clinicians in identifying skills necessary for more effective AAC system development. Future research is required to clearly delineate valid and reliable decision-making processes to help in determining the appropriate selection and customization of auditory scanning systems.

Components of Auditory Scanning in AAC Systems

As with any AAC system, auditory scanning systems should be customized to meet the individual's needs and skills. Designing and customizing auditory scanning systems is a complex multidimensional process. Decisions must be made with respect to numerous system components based on the user's needs and skills, including the auditory cue provided, the organization of the messages or content, and the rate of scanning access. Each of these issues is considered in the sections that follow.

Auditory Cues   An important component of any scanning method is the presentation or announcement of the selection option. In nonelectronic scanning systems, choice options are presented using objects or picture representations of messages by a communication partner or facilitator. This technique is often referred to as "partner-assisted scanning" (Quist & Lloyd, 1997). When choice options are presented orally (as in auditory scanning), this technique is referred to as "partner-assisted auditory scanning" (Blackstone, 1998a; Porter, 1989). It is also sometimes referred to as dependent auditory scanning. In electronic AAC systems using visual scanning, choices are presented automatically using system features such as light indicators that correspond to visual representations. In some systems, visual representations are highlighted as they are scanned. Sometimes, an audible tone or beep accompanies each designated choice option as it is visually presented, but these sounds have no specific meaning and serve primarily as auditory feedback indicating scanning movement or a choice being selected. Electronic AAC systems with auditory scanning typically use the system's speech output feature to announce the selection option in single word or phrase format but are otherwise identical to visual scanning. Although dependent on the user's residual vision and the system's features, a visual representation is usually indicated along with the verbal announcement.

The announcement of the selection option in all scanning systems is considered a *prompt*. This visual and/or auditory prompt alerts the user that selection options are forthcoming; however, in auditory scanning, the prompt has more accurately become know as an auditory *cue* because it not only announces to the user the location of the choice option but also provides information about the content of the message and guides system navigation for further choice selection. For example, the auditory cue "beverage" alerts the user to a choice option and to the fact that if selected, the subsequent content and selections will be types of beverages (e.g., milk, soda, juice). Conversely, the user must know and remember that to retrieve the message "milk," selection of the auditory cue "beverage" is necessary. If the user wants to find the target message "milk," hearing the auditory cue "beverage" will direct subsequent selections to the desired target message.

The auditory cue, in most systems, is customized for the individual user. Often, the type of auditory cue is dependent on the user's knowledge of the system content and the level at which the auditory cue is meaningful as an indicator of the system content. It can be a letter, word, phrase, or sentence. The type of cue is determined by the user's needs, the vocabulary organization and layout, and the system's parameters.

For individuals with intact vision, symbols on communication systems are meaningful representations of the system content, whether using direct selection or scanning access. The degree to which the auditory cue is "symbolic" has created much discussion. For example, if the auditory cue is identical to the message, (i.e., auditory cue is "milk" and, when selected, the speech output message is the word "milk") is the auditory cue symbolic, or is it simply an announcement of the selection option?

There are several types of auditory cues used for auditory scanning access. Table 9.4 summarizes these cues and their clinical applications.

Orthographic Auditory Cues Orthographic auditory cues include the oral presentation of the names of letters, numbers, and punctuation markers.

Table 9.4. Types of auditory cues and clinical applications

Type of cue	Definition	Example	Clinical applications
Orthographic cues	A letter represents a word, phrase, or sentence; also includes oral spelling	Cue: "W" Message spoken: "I want it"	Appropriate for word prediction, abbreviation expansion Used for oral spelling of individual words
Content cues	The most meaningful or salient part of a message	Cue: "drink" Message spoken: "I'm thirsty. Get me a drink."	Appropriate when direct relationship between cue and referent is needed or desired
Name/label cues	The name or label of the visual representation	Visual representation: rainbow Cue: "rainbow" Message spoken: "Colors"	Assists with visual perception of symbols Can represent multiple meanings for iconic encoding Use caution in assigning names to visual images that are seen differently, if at all, by individuals with visual impairments
Category cues	A word or phrase that represents related content	Cue: "beverages" Messages offered for selection: "juice," "milk," and "hot chocolate"	Eliminates need to scan through all choice options Must understand relationship between category cue and items within category

These types of cues are provided when an individual is writing using traditional orthography, using abbreviation expansion, or using word prediction.

Content Auditory Cues   A content auditory cue is a cue that is part of the message content; it is often the most salient part of the message. For example, if the message were a sentence such as "I'm thirsty. Get me a drink," the content cue would be the part of the message that is most meaningful for that user (i.e., drink). If the message is a single word versus a phrase or sentence, then the content cue is simply that word. For example, if the system content has single words such as "juice," "happy," and "hello" and the intended message is "hello," the content auditory cue for that message might simply be "hello." Content cues may be appropriate for individuals who need a direct relationship between the cue and the referent. Content cues might also be considered a "name/label" type of auditory cue, if the message is the same as the visual symbol referent. For example, the single-word message "cat" might be visually represented by the picture of a cat, so the auditory cue "cat" would be both a content and name/label cue.

Name/Label Auditory Cues   Name/label cues are auditory cues that are the labels or names of the visual symbols or representations of AAC system content. For example, the messages "juice," "happy," and "hello," might be represented by pictures of a glass filled with orange liquid, a happy face, and a hand waving, respectively. In these cases, the name or label auditory cues would then be the names of the pictures (i.e., glass, happy face, hand waving). For individuals with some vision, this type of cue may help focus attention and clarify their visual perception of the representation or visual symbol. As long as there is a one-to-one ratio of name/label cue to content and content is limited, these cues are likely to be scanned linearly. As system content increases and the time to scan through cues increases, it is important to organize both the cues and system content in a way that decreases the time it takes to scan to the desired message.

One way to decrease the time to scan to a message is to make available a limited set of cues that are then selected in a designated sequence to produce system content. This is the same concept that is used in iconic encoding, in which a system has a limited set of representations, with the location of these representations remaining constant (Baker, 1982). Each representation, identified by its name, has multiple associations, and selection of representations in different sequences produces different content. The length of the sequences is dependent on the number of selections available and the depth of their meanings. Using this encoding method and system organization structure, cognitive and memory demands are increased for recall of the meanings for the representations and the sequences for message selection; however, because there is a limited set of options to be sequenced and their presentation order is consistent, the user may be able to learn and remember the location of the options more easily and may therefore be able to anticipate the scanning and selection sequences (Reichle, Dettling, Drager, & Leiter, 2000). For auditory scanners, having fewer cues to scan through is an advantage but having fewer cues may require increased length of sequences in order to produce more system content. Participants at the 1997 Auditory Scanning Symposium have referred to this organizational architecture as being *wide*.

The extent to which an auditory cue can adequately represent multiple meanings, which are largely based on visual associations and experiential learning, has not been explored in the research. Auditory cues are almost always selected by sighted individuals. Individuals with visual impairments, even those with some residual vision, may have very different comprehension of objects and pictures than individuals with intact visual functioning. Caution should therefore be taken in assigning a name cue to a visual representation that the user may "see" differently, if at all. It should not be assumed that the name of the visual representation will be a meaningful auditory cue for an individual with a significant visual impairment, just because it is auditory and the user can hear it. For example, if the visual symbol for the message "color" is a picture of a rainbow and the auditory cue is the name of that picture (i.e., rainbow), is this name meaningful for the individual who has never clearly seen a rainbow? Given that visual knowledge is not only dependent on an intact visual system but also on development and experiential knowledge, meaning of auditory cues that are based upon names of visual representations must be carefully considered (Hellerstein, 1998). As previously indicated, it is critical to take into account a full understanding of the complexity of the user's visual impairments and the impact of these impairments on object knowledge and conceptual development.

Representing concepts meaningfully via verbal auditory cues remains one of the most significant challenges in auditory scanning system development (Blackstone, 1998a). It may also be the key factor that has hampered development of AAC systems that are more than just visual scanning systems with verbal cueing capabilities. Kovach (1989) reported a case study in which the auditory cue was the name of the symbol used on the visual display (e.g., the auditory cue "rainbow" was used for the picture of a rainbow). The user's understanding of the multiple and associated meanings for each corresponding auditory cue was developed in two ways. First, visual enhancements were used (in this case, enlarged) and then described in detail prior to using them on the AAC device. Second, the user participated in extended sessions of experiential learning which included physical assistance in manipulating three-dimensional replicas of the symbols, when possible, and engaging in meaningful and contextually based activities in which their meanings were explored and expanded. Several years later, this user reported at the 1998 Audi-

tory Scanning Symposium that these exercises were often recalled when trying to remember the content represented by specific symbols.

Categorical or Thematic Auditory Cues   An alternative to the development of multiple meaning auditory cues is organization of auditory cues using
a group–item method, similar to that used in visual scanning (Vanderheiden
& Lloyd, 1986). A group–item scanning method requires that the system content be organized in a specific manner. For example, each group might represent related content, such as "beverages" or "food" (if using a taxonomic organization). Each item in a group would then represent specific beverages (e.g.,
juice, milk, pop) or foods (e.g., sandwich, soup, salad). This scanning method
works well when using a system with a dynamic display. Initially, a linear scanning method for a limited number of choice options representing content in
related groups is displayed on the first page or main page. When one choice
is selected, a new display of items related to that selected choice is displayed
or a subgroup of related content options is scanned. This method of grouping
and subgrouping continues until the target content item is reached, which is
faster than if all items were scanned individually.

In auditory scanning, the auditory cue that represents the group or category of selection options is referred to as a *categorical cue*. Here, the auditory cue
reflects the hierarchical structure of the system content, and the individual
must understand that structure to access the vocabulary within each group.

It is important to understand that for an individual relying only on the
auditory cue, categorical cues may have no inherent meaning. Auditory cues
are heard one after the other, regardless of how the cues are presented (i.e.,
cues for groups are presented followed by items within the groups, which
sounds the same as if cues are presented in a simple linear fashion). Various
scanning patterns and dynamic display pages are visual concepts. For the individual relying on auditory scanning, it is the auditory cues that provide information about the way in which system content is categorically organized.
The auditory cue becomes extremely important because it is the only means
by which content information can be located. In visual scanning, even though
access to a specific choice is determined by the scanning pattern, the user can
see the choices available within a specific content theme, thus creating a spatial orientation of cue to content. In auditory scanning, the auditory cue to
content orientation is strictly temporal. In visual scanning, the user can see his
or her selections and how certain selections may alter available system content
for subsequent selections. In auditory scanning, the user has only a single cue
that disappears, except in memory, to guide him or her in system navigation.
The transitory nature of the auditory cue makes the organization of the system's content and how it is announced critical to the auditory scanner's ability to locate and retrieve content efficiently.

Research has shown that if more than four symbols are scanned sequentially, it is faster to use a row–column (group–item) scanning method (Venkatagiri, 1999). This means that many more categories and subcategories are needed to accommodate increased content. The result, described by participants at the 1997 Auditory Scanning Symposium, is a system with an architectural structure that is *deep*. Venkatagiri (1999) and others pointed out that row–column (group–item) scanning requires at least twice as many motor responses. In other words, the deeper the system is, the greater the number of switch activations to reach the final message. In addition, Ratcliff (1994) suggested that although row–column (group–item) scanning may reach the target representation faster, it is also less direct; therefore, the link from the user to the output is less logical because each switch hit does not actually make the final output selection. The deeper the hierarchical structure (i.e., more categories or levels), the more cognitively complex, and the greater the motor and memory demands (Beukelman & Mirenda, 1998; Mizuko et al., 1994).

Category auditory cues typically consist of single word cues but can also consist of a phrase or sentence. There are numerous ways of categorizing cues (Blackstone, 1998a). Content and corresponding auditory cues can be categorized in terms of activities (music, gym, recess); environments (home, school, community); grammatical structure (nouns, verbs, adjectives); or any other way that may group system content (e.g., people, places, things; things to say; things to play with; things I like). It is essential that the category cue for the system content is meaningful and that the user understands that these categories represent and refer to groups of upcoming predetermined system content. Otherwise, the auditory cue is only a prompt and does not serve as a meaningful indicator of the forthcoming selection options and system content.

Categorical cues provide more than a prompt for the location of system content; for some individuals, these types of cues also suggest possible messages to communicate. For example, auditory cues such as, "I want to play with something," "Let's go somewhere," and "I need something," may provide the individual with suggestions of messages they could communicate. When a selection is made for "I want to play with something," the system may then scan, "Let's play house" and "Let's play with the trucks." If "Let's play house" is selected, the system may then scan "doll," "bed," "chair," and so forth. This is not dissimilar from low-technology systems when choices are offered to the individual, as in "Do you want the red one, the white one, or the black one?" or when using 20 questions such as "Is it something to wear; is it something for your feet, hands, head?"

For some individuals, categorical cues that are phrases or sentences eventually may be reduced in length and replaced with their most salient key word. In the previous example, the first level of cues (i.e., "I want to play with something," "Let's go somewhere," "I need something") might be reduced to single word category cues such as "play," "go," and "needs," respectively. As vocabulary needs increase, system content can then be added in each of these categories. Because categorical cues are now words, not sentences, the time required in scanning is also reduced.

Auditory Cues Silenced   The need for the user to hear the auditory cue is obvious. For the communication partner, however, audible auditory cues may not necessarily be helpful. Although auditory cues may facilitate system use and message delivery rate, they may also create chaotic interactive communication, particularly if the communication partner is unfamiliar with this method of access. For example, if an unfamiliar communication partner hears a content auditory cue, he or she may mistake the cue for the intended message and respond accordingly. If the individual proceeds and selects the originally intended message, the partner may think the individual is ignoring the partner's response, or worse, think that the individual is unable to manage his or her communication system competently. Alternatively, communication partners who are familiar with the individual and his or her method of communication may use the auditory cue to predict what the user wishes to say by hearing only the auditory cue, thereby speeding up the rate of communication. Also, when communication partners hear an auditory cue, it provides for them an opportunity to prompt or encourage a message selection by the user. This can be helpful for users who are just learning their system content or may need to be reminded of the possible things to say in a given situation.

Options for silencing the auditory cue when using nonelectronic partner-assisted auditory scanning are limited to reducing the volume or providing the cue directly in the user's ear in an effort to prevent others from hearing it. Many electronic AAC systems provide an option for the auditory cue to be transmitted through one speaker and the message through another speaker. Systems using synthesized speech also often provide the option of a different voice, volume level, and speech rate for the auditory cue. Different volumes, voices, and speech rates for the auditory cue can provide a way for the user, as well as the communication partner, to discriminate cueing versus communication output. Having an earpiece plugged into the speaker announcing the auditory cue (e.g., standard and inexpensive headphones or ear buds that plug into any tape recorder) enables the user to hear the auditory cue yet differentiate and focus on the voice output for their intended expressive communication. Customized ear molds into which ear buds are inserted have been made for some users (Dreith, personal communication, February 2001), and can be made easily by an audiologist. This provides the delivery of the auditory cue without external headphones or ear buds that easily fall off or become displaced.

Content Organization and Auditory Design Layout   In both visual and auditory scanning access, message location and retrieval is often a slow and tedious process (Beukelman & Mirenda, 1998; Quist & Lloyd, 1997).

This is primarily because the user must wait for the prompt associated with the desired selection to be presented before a selection to produce the desired message can be made. If the number of symbols on a system is fairly limited, cues are presented one after the other until the desired choice is available for selection (linear scanning). Although having the most frequently used choices scanned first enhances message retrieval rate, other techniques must be employed when the individual requires access to more extensive vocabulary (Vanderheiden & Lloyd, 1986). Methods that group choices together, such as row–column or group–item scanning, must be used to organize the content in ways to increase the speed of choice presentation and selection (Beukelman, Yorkston, & Dowden, 1985; Mizuko, Reichle, Ratcliff, & Esser, 1994; Ratcliff, 1994).

As of 2003, little is known about optimal organizations of content for individuals who use auditory scanning. Light (1992) proposed that there are five possible approaches to content organization of AAC systems: taxonomic, schematic, semantic-syntactic, alphabetic, and idiosyncratic. Fallon and Light (2000) reported on the methods of content organization that children typically use. In this study, typically developing 4- and 5-year-old children organized line drawings representing a variety of language concepts. Results of this study suggested that typically developing children at this age organize concepts using a schematic approach the vast majority of the time. The application of this information to those with severe speech, physical, and visual impairments using auditory scanning is not yet clear; it is important that more research be done in this area to help guide the development of effective and efficient AAC systems.

In most AAC systems, the design layout is an important consideration. In auditory scanning systems, the organization of the content representations is more temporal than spatial. In this type of temporal organization, representations are presented sequentially. Thus, the design layout reflects the content organization and is critically linked to the way in which it is meaningfully presented to the user for message location and retrieval. This organizational structure is related to the types of auditory cues provided. It impacts the rate at which messages can be retrieved as well as the knowledge and memory of where specific messages are located and the encoding strategies used for message retrieval.

The cognitive and memory requirements for individuals using scanning access to AAC systems is significant. After a message is conceived, it must then be held in memory while being constructed using a laboriously slow process of content presentation and selection that requires focused attention and concentration. Information processing theory suggests a limited capacity for cognitive functions, especially those involving working memory (Oxley & Norris, 2000). With auditory scanning, there is no visual record available that documents for the user what has been selected during a message formulation task. Message formulation places high demand on cognitive attention and working memory for anyone using AAC; these demands are further increased because the individual is required to remember what was scanned and selected as well as the cue that directs him or her to what needs to be selected next. Auditory cues play a critical role in assisting users in the retrieval of information from the auditory scanning system by providing cues to the organizational structure of the content.

Issues related to information processing and cognitive science, such as working memory capacity, world knowledge, and internal models of the way our world works, are important considerations when working with individuals who require auditory scanning. A full discussion of these issues is unfortunately beyond the scope of this chapter. Readers are referred to Light and Lindsay (1991) and Chapter 8 for an overview of cognitive issues and their importance and relevance to AAC. Oxley and Norris' (2000) discussion of memory strategies that are relevant to children's use of AAC provided further insights. Of particular interest is the role that auditory cues (particularly content cues) have with recognition memory and the impact that category cues have on the development of internal linguistic organizational structures and schema (see Table 9.4). These relationships, as well as other interrelationships between cognitive science and AAC learning, memory, and message retrieval for auditory scanning, are as yet unexplored.

Rate of Auditory Scanning and Message Retrieval   The rate of auditory scanning and message retrieval is dependent on four factors: scan rate, length of auditory cue, rate of speech output for auditory cue, and user selection rate. In most electronic AAC systems, the actual scan rate has a wide range, from fractions of seconds to multiple seconds. The length of the auditory cue will influence scanning rate. Producing an entire sentence will take longer than a single word. Although in some electronic systems, the rates for the speech output of the auditory cue and the spoken message are the same, these rates can be set independently of one another in many systems. Therefore, an auditory cue can be spoken at a very fast rate, whereas the message can be spoken at a more natural speech rate. Finally, consistent with all AAC systems, message retrieval rate is dependent on the rate at which the user actually makes an intended selection. This rate is significantly decreased for any scanning access method, including auditory scanning.

In many systems, if the auditory cue is interrupted with a switch activation while it is being spoken, the announcement of the cue will be halted and the system will interpret it as a selection for that location and proceed accordingly. If the individual only needs to hear the first part of the auditory cue to obtain the necessary information about location and content, interrupting the auditory cue presentation with switch activation thus eliminates the need for the entire auditory cue announcement, which may increase message retrieval rate.

The way content is organized may help or hinder the rate of message retrieval. If content is categorized in ways that enable presentation of selection options efficiently and without lengthy sequences of options to scan, then content can more quickly be retrieved. Although critical to effective use of AAC systems, enhancement of message retrieval rate using auditory scanning has not been investigated.

The rate and method of synthesized speech output influences comprehension (Higginbotham & Baird, 1995). Adults with typical speech, hearing, and cognitive function comprehend synthesized speech output better in higher quality synthesizers. Due to the processing skills required, comprehension is improved with a slower than normal speech presentation rate, and single word comprehension is improved when there are up to 10 seconds between the words. The effect of these findings on the synthesized speech presentation of the auditory cue has not been addressed in the literature.

Device Selection Considerations

Development of appropriate electronic communication systems is based on an individual's needs and abilities and the device parameters and features that best address those. Some special considerations in the selection of auditory scanning systems include the following:

- The availability of different voices for scanning and for message delivery
- Flexibility in the type and length of auditory cues
- The scanning pattern (e.g., group–item)
- Scanning selection control techniques (e.g., step, automatic)
- Single- or multiple-switch access
- Customization of the scanning speed
- Number of rescans (i.e., how many times the scanning pattern will be repeated if no selection is made)
- Automatic or switch-activated scan restarts (i.e., how to get the system to start scanning)
- Associated auditory signals (e.g., "beeps" coinciding with visual scanning and switch activation)
- Visual display features and available visual enhancements (e.g., screen size, back lighting, symbol size, color, shape, borders)
- Static versus dynamic display

These must *all* be considered when developing auditory scanning AAC systems. Because users' needs and abilities change, AAC systems with the most flexibility in the areas identified are often most desirable and can be justified even at a very early stage in AAC system development because they can be modified as needed.

Decisions and recommendations for specific AAC devices for individuals using auditory scanning are often made based on the organizational structure of the system content and which system best supports it. In truth, when vision is so impaired that only the auditory cue is used for system access and no residual visual enhancements are beneficial, the display type of the system (i.e., fixed versus dynamic display) may make very little difference to the auditory scanner. Frequently, a combination of categorical, content, and name cues are used on both fixed and dynamic display systems. For example, with dynamic display systems, category cues are used until the target selection is made, and then a name or content cue is used; for example,

"animals" (category cue) → "pets" (category cue) → "cat" (name or content cue)

Similarly, in fixed display systems, even those in which iconic encoding strategies are used, the initial selections are basically category cues, and final selections are often content or name cues. For example, the message "apple" is retrieved by selecting the picture of apple three times; first, as a category cue for "food," second as a subcategory cue for "fruit," and finally the third selection is for the name cue of "apple."

It is critical to consider the way in which meaningful auditory cues guide users in the organization and retrieval of system content. For auditory scanners, operational competence may be intertwined with linguistic competence and comprehension of the auditory cue itself. The motor, memory, and cognitive advantages and disadvantages of auditory scanning with a fixed display that utilizes iconic encoding versus a dynamic display that employs a complex categorical structure must be explored. Although some have studied issues of fixed versus dynamic display types (e.g., Reichle et al., 2000), investigation has not extended to visual or auditory scanning. Determining the most efficient organization of the content using categorical, content, or name cues for message retrieval rate enhancement is critical.

Challenges to further development of auditory scanning systems include how to most effectively code vocabulary with an auditory cue while at the same time maximizing any residual visual abilities and how to organize and encode vocabulary (Blackstone, 1998a). Clearly, research in several areas of auditory scanning is needed to guide system development and implementation.

FUTURE RESEARCH DIRECTIONS

With so little research in the area of auditory scanning, questions abound. Although research priorities in the field of AAC as a whole have been identified, the needs of individuals with visual and motor impairments have, to date, been largely overlooked (Beukelman & Ansel, 1995). More information is needed to improve the application of auditory scanning access as well as to guide AAC system development that more specifically addresses the unique needs of individuals with severe speech, physical, and visual impairments. Areas identified for investigation through the Auditory Scanning Symposia, auditory scanning listserv discussions, and ongoing communication with clinicians who have been interested and involved in the application of auditory scanning access for these individuals include 1) vision and language learning; 2) auditory "symbolization"; 3) auditory processing and enhancements; 4) auditory imagery in message retrieval; and, 5) the impact of auditory versus visual "symbols" on language comprehension and message retrieval rate. Some thoughts about the importance of research in these areas follow.

Vision and Language Learning

Language characteristics of children who are blind include 1) an absence of gestures and other expressions that facilitate a caregiver's interpretation of preferences; 2) lack of coordinated eye, finger, and hand pointing that provide opportunities for caregivers to refer to external events and objects; and 3) "diminished opportunities to learn and to understand interpersonal rules in communication, the relation between objects and symbols as well as knowledge about the environment" (Preisler, 1995, p. 107). Preisler suggested that for young children with blindness, there is a need for their caregivers to become their "visual interpreters of the world" (p. 107).

Wills (1979) suggested that it is logical that children who are blind have difficulties in language development because so much of language deals with visual aspects of objects (e.g., color, shape). She pointed out that children who are blind have trouble organizing their experiences and "seem to use speech, almost as the sighted use vision, as a tool with which to recognize and build up an image of their world" (p. 115). Speech and language, then, may be a way of compensating for visual deficits. For children with severe speech impairments in addition to visual deficits, however, the use of language to build conceptual knowledge is challenging. When a child has severe physical disabilities, tactile exploration of the world is severely limited as well. How do children with severe speech, physical, and visual impairments develop conceptual knowledge, and what are the best ways to support this development?

In addition to using speech and language to help organize experiences, children who are blind "use sound for the purposes of categorization" (Wills, 1979, p. 94). What are the best ways to support the development of categorical knowledge for children with visual impairments, and what categorical cues are the most effective for accessing AAC? For example, for a child who requires auditory scanning, should categorical information be stressed to teach the use of categorical auditory cues? Such "categorical talk" about a toy car might sound like this: " A *car* is a *vehicle,* just like a truck, train, and boat. Would you like to play with a *vehicle?* Which *vehicle* would you like to play with?" How might this categorical learning affect the use of auditory scanning systems? Would it be easier to forego the use of a visual symbol for a more abstract referent if an auditory symbol could be more directly meaningful, regardless of visual skills or deficits?

For some, learning visual representations for spoken language may be similar to learning a second language. Once this visual language is learned, using it to encode spoken language might be considered a form of code switching, or alternating between the use of two languages, which requires a high degree of competence in both (Reyes, 1995). It may be easier for some children, then, to simply learn the auditory cue "help" than an abstract visual representation that requires code switching. Some individuals may benefit from a combined visual and auditory representational system. If so, what types of message content or referents are best represented visually, and which ones auditorily?

Auditory Symbolization

Auditory scanning systems involve auditory cues to guide the user in message retrieval and system operation. However, are auditory cues *symbols?* Is there an *auditory symbol set?* Because of the importance of visual representation in AAC systems, much attention has been given to visual symbols and symbol sets. For example, visual symbol characteristics have been described and taxonomies have been developed (Fuller, Lloyd, & Schlosser, 1992; Fuller, Lloyd, & Stratton, 1997; Lloyd & Fuller, 1986). Research has focused on the degree of iconicity, or the "visual relationship of a symbol to its referent," (Lloyd & Blischak, 1992, p. 106), as well as the degree to which iconicity aids in the learning and memory of symbols, or the *iconicity hypothesis* (Fristoe & Lloyd, 1979). Iconicity, by definition, involves a *visual* relationship to a referent. Is there an equivalent relationship for auditory symbols? The concept of iconicity has implications for individuals dependent on auditory cues. What is the nature of the relationship between various types of auditory cues and their real-world referents as understood by individuals with visual impairments? What is the relative "iconicity" of different types of auditory cues? Which auditory cues are most appropriate for whom and under what circumstances? If auditory cues are symbolic, how should auditory symbol sets change based on changes in users' linguistic and operational competence? What effects do these changes have on learning of auditory symbols (i.e., auditory cues) and system content? What are the most appropriate approaches to content organization within auditory scanning systems? Future research is required to answer all of these questions.

Auditory Processing

Vision plays a critical role in learning, language, and AAC system use. It is always important to explore techniques to enhance visual stimuli for individuals with visual impairments so that visual information may be more meaningful in AAC systems. Consideration should also be given to ways in which auditory stimuli, specifically the auditory cues for individuals using auditory scanning, can be enhanced to make them more meaningful. As Wills (1979) suggested, sound can be very important for children with severe visual impairments. Future research is required to determine whether auditory features such as pitch and volume can be used as meaningful enhancements to verbal auditory cues for individuals who use auditory scanning.

Research indicates that children process linguistic and auditory characteristics together, not separately, when they process speech. Jerger and colleagues (1993, 1994) studied the influence of the semantic and auditory dimensions of speech in children with typical hearing (60 children from 3;3 to 7;1 years of age) and children with hearing impairments (20 children from 3;3 to 10;9 years of age) using a pediatric auditory Stroop task. In this task, children were asked to attend only to the voice-gender of speech targets while ignoring the semantic content. The relationship between the semantic and auditory dimensions of the speech targets was manipulated. For example, a male voice said "mommy," representing a conflicting relationship; "ice cream," representing a neutral relationship; and "daddy," representing a congruent relationship. Based on reaction time in identifying the voice-gender, Jerger and colleagues found that: children with typical hearing responded slower when the semantic and auditory dimensions were conflicting; they could not ignore the semantic content in these speech targets (i.e., male voice saying "mommy"); they responded faster to congruent speech target relationships (i.e., male voice saying "daddy"). Children with hearing impairments also responded faster with congruent relationships but were less affected by the conflicting relationships than their hearing counterparts. These results suggest that it may be possible to capitalize on congruent semantic/auditory links to optimize auditory cues in scanning systems for individuals with significant visual and physical impairments. Future research is required to delineate how auditory dimensions (e.g., pitch) might be used to facilitate learning and memory of verbal auditory cues or system content. Perhaps meaning could be assigned to speech volume or pitch to help the individual who uses AAC organize and remember system content. For example, if the content for positive "feelings" (e.g., happy, laugh, excited) were spoken in a high-pitched voice and the content for negative "feelings" (e.g., sad, cry, worried) were spoken in a low-pitched voice, could the user more quickly access this content? What effect might this auditory enhancement have on learning and memory?

If the verbal auditory cue is not in itself symbolic, would the addition of an auditory feature (e.g., tone) make it symbolic? The use of tones to meaningfully represent language is certainly not a new concept. Tones have been used for Morse code since the early 1800s in the form of electrical or auditory signals. In Morse code, only two auditory signals, "dots" and "dashes," are used in sequences to represent letters, numbers, and punctuation. There is limited documentation demonstrating the successful use of Morse code for individuals with severe speech, physical, and visual impairments (Beukelman, Yorkston, & Dowden, 1985; Blischak, 1995). Clearly, there are significant literacy and memory components involved in learning the codes for letters to spell using Morse code; these components may overwhelm many young children with visual and physical impairments needing AAC access; however, Beukelman, Yorkston, and Dowden (1985) demonstrated that children with cerebral palsy were able to learn Morse code if they had a third-grade spelling level.

Irrespective of the literacy requirements, the notion that a series of tones could be used for system access is something to be considered. Tones directly entered into a communication system to access specific content would provide a potentially powerful rate enhancement alternative to auditory or visual scanning. For example, Weiss (1998) proposed a strategy using an adaptation of Morse code in which keys on a device were accessed by two switches. One switch on the left (equivalent to a "dot") and one switch on the right (equivalent to a "dash") were activated in a specific sequence to access key locations where content was then accessed. For example, a "dot, dash," or left, then right switch activation, directed the system to a location that generated a specific message. Further expansion of this idea suggested the possibility of using a system in which selection of a series of tones would access a specific category of information. For example, a "dot, dot, dot " (i.e., Morse code for the letter "s"), or series of three left switch activations, might direct the user to system content that had to do with school. Once in that content area, a "dash, dash," (i.e., Morse code for the letter "m"), or a series of two right switch activations, might direct the user to content related to math. Even if the final selection required scanning auditory cues, the time saved to get to that level could be significant and worth exploring for some auditory scanners.

The transient nature of auditory scanning requires users to focus their attention on the auditory cues, remember the cues that were previously selected, and anticipate those yet to come, rather than focus their attention on their communication partner and environment. In auditory scanning systems, there is no auditory equivalent to a visual display that maps users' previous and future paths of encoding. Therefore, it is important to consider ways to enhance auditory cues so that they are more memorable for determining the users' encoding paths. The addition of sound cues to the verbal auditory cue might help users determine if they were at the first, second, or third level of selection. For example, the pitch of the first level of verbal auditory cues might be low, the second high, and the third even higher. The pitch differences would provide feedback to users indicating their location within a hierarchical organization structure. This type of auditory enhancement can be compared to that provided by the auditory tones when dialing a touch-tone telephone; the feedback from these tones allows the user to recognize the "misdialing" of a familiar phone number immediately when the number doesn't "sound" right. In fact, it is reported that veteran Morse code users learn Morse code through "code training" that involves more of a total gestalt learning than a translation of character to code (Finley, 1995). More research is needed to investigate how components of sound, alone or combined with verbal cues, might be beneficial not only in the area of learning and memory but also in possibilities for providing direct selection access options to learners with physical and visual impairments.

Another area to be explored in attempting to enhance auditory cues, make them more permanent, and decrease the learning and memory demands for users is to have other sensory information associated with the cues. Unfortunately, use of tangible symbols and touch, demonstrated as an effective implementation strategy in AAC systems for individuals with dual sensory impairments, is not an option for most auditory scanners due to their associated severe physical impairments (Rowland & Schweigert, 1989, 2000); however, it may be possible to provide other types of sensory input that would help make auditory cues more meaningful. For example, the user might feel a vibration on the stomach when the "food" cue is presented auditorily or selected. The addition of this sensory stimulation to the auditory cues might provide a more lasting memory of the location within the system's architecture for the auditory scanner.

Finally, it is worth noting that successful use of auditory scanning systems depends on the users' ability to perceive, comprehend, and respond to the auditory cues presented. It is well documented that children with cerebral palsy have a high incidence of hearing impairment (Pellegrino, 2002). Despite this fact, professionals rarely mention hearing ability, particularly speech reception and discrimination, in formal or observational assessment reports of children who rely on auditory scanning (Blackstone, 1998b). Auditory skills must be assessed and considered in the development of AAC systems for those with severe speech, physical, and visual impairments.

The auditory skills required of individuals who use electronic auditory scanning systems are even more complex. Typically, the auditory cues in electronic systems are produced with the same speech synthesizer that produces the message output. Research suggests there are differences in the quality, voice selection, rate, and method of speech presentation using speech synthesizers and that these factors affect intelligibility and comprehension (e.g., Higginbotham & Baird, 1995; Higginbotham, Drazed, Kowarsky, Scally, & Segal, 1994; Higginbotham, Scally, Lundy, & Kowarsky, 1995; Mirenda & Beukelman, 1987). Given that children who require auditory scanning may be at increased risk for hearing impairments and given the demands of comprehension of synthesized speech, it is important that future research consider techniques to adapt auditory cues in terms of the synthetic speech voice, volume, and rate of presentation to maximize perception and comprehension by auditory scanners.

Auditory Imagery

Auditory imagery is another possible method for enhancing memory for auditory cues and content. "Mental imagery can be a powerful aid for human memory" (Tinti, Galati, & Vecchio, 1999, p. 579). Visual imagery, which has been studied more extensively than auditory imagery, has been shown to aid in learning and recall; however, Tinti and colleagues also recognized the importance of auditory imagery in memory. They demonstrated that individuals who are blind appeared to use auditory imagery for memory equally as well as sighted individuals used visual imagery. Not surprisingly, they also found that individuals who are blind did better on memory tasks when asked to use auditory imagery than they did when asked to use visual imagery to assist their memory (Tinti et al., 1999). Sharps and Price (1992) defined auditory images as the characteristic sounds produced by stimulus items. They found that "pictures and characteristic sounds were associated with significantly better recall than were verbal labels alone, indicating that auditory imagery has mnemonic value similar to that of visual imagery" (Sharps & Price, 1992, p. 81).

Tracy and Barker (1993) demonstrated that words that easily produced mental images were recalled more easily that those that did not; they concluded that word imagery was the best predictor of word recall. They emphasized that "Imagery is dependent upon perceptual experiences that one can attach to the stimuli" (Tracy & Barker, 1993, p. 157). For example, for typically developing individuals, a word such as *beach* might produce more visual images than auditory images, whereas *wind* might produce equal if not more auditory images. A person who has never experienced a trip to the beach might not generate the same visual or auditory images as a person who has spent several days there. Center, Freeman, Robertson, and Orthred (1999) found that individuals can be taught to use visual imagery and that visual imagery training improved their listening, comprehension, and reading. These results suggest that memory for auditory cues may be enhanced through the development of auditory imagery, and that using verbal auditory cues that promote auditory imagery, developed through experiential learning, might increase the auditory scanner's ability to learn and remember auditory cues as representative of communicative content. Further study in this area is needed. Research is also required to evaluate the effectiveness of different techniques to teach auditory cues, particularly with young children or with those who have cognitive impairments. For example, would the verbal auditory cue for *go* be more easily learned and remembered if it had an associated car sound with it? Once the auditory imagery had been established to aid in content retrieval, these associated sounds might be eliminated.

Auditory Cues and Language Comprehension

Although most attention has focused on techniques to maximize the design and use of auditory scanning systems, it is critical to remember that the end goal of providing these systems is to facilitate language development and functional communication. Future research is required to consider the impact of auditory scanning on language and communication. Romski and Sevcik (1996) described the ways in which the use of AAC systems contributes to functional communication and language development for individuals with cognitive impairments. They reported that visual-graphic symbols could be used for expressive communication and that as a result of their use, symbol comprehension also increased (Romski, Sevcik, & Pate, 1988; Romski & Sevcik, 1989). Romski and Sevcik (1993) further suggested that speech comprehension might be a critical factor in the development of AAC system use, primarily because the relationship between a referent and its symbol (the spoken word) is already established, thus facilitating the acquisition of a meaningful visual symbol. It is interesting to consider whether it is necessary for users to learn a new visual representation (a graphic symbol) if the spoken one is already understood. Could the spoken symbol be used to retrieve AAC system content through auditory scanning instead?

The presentation of an auditory cue may have the potential to do more than represent communication system content, or locate communicative content. It may become a language development strategy by verbally suggesting potential messages to communicate. This possibility is not unlike the situation where an adult asks a child a question and, receiving no response, presents choices to the child. For example, a young child might indicate to his mother that he is "hungry," either verbally or through nonverbal means such as gesturing or looking at the refrigerator. The mother asks the child what he would like to eat, but the child does not respond, perhaps because he doesn't know, can't remember the options, or doesn't have the vocabulary to indicate the preference. The mother then provides him with choices such as, "Do you want a hot dog, soup, or a peanut butter and jelly sandwich?" Once the child recognizes and comprehends these choices, particularly within the context of being hungry, he is then able to respond, "Hot dog." What is the role of a similar form of auditory prompting in AAC systems, and how might such a form of prompting translate into increased language learning? For example, an individual who uses AAC might have a number of general categories represented visually (using the visual enhancements described previously); when selected, each of these would provide options for further communication using auditory prompts. In this example, multiple modes (visual, auditory) are used to represent the referents. This approach may have merit; however, much more investigation of this strategy is warranted to determine the actual skills required for its use. Iacono, Mirenda, and Beukelman (1993) explored the use of multimodal techniques for communication on a limited basis and cautioned that use of multiple modes may actually be more complex than unimodal techniques for AAC development and use, at least in some situations.

Future Research Challenges

Future research in the area of auditory scanning is urgently required to determine effective practice. This research poses many challenges due to the significant variability in skills and abilities, particularly in the degree of physical and visual impairments, and the low incidence of those with severe speech, physical, and visual impairments for whom the application of auditory scanning is appropriate. Some ways to overcome these barriers may be to design research protocols that can be replicated across centers in order to pool subjects and aggregate findings (see Chapter 7 for further discussion). Networking of clinicians and potential researchers with interest in this field has begun through the auditory scanning web site and listserv. There are also many aspects of auditory scanning and the use of auditory cues that can be explored with individuals having a variety of disabilities or no disabilities at all (e.g., typically developing children, blind children with no speech or physical impairments).

In addition to studies focused on the needs of individuals with severe physical and visual impairments, future research should also consider the potential benefits of auditory scanning with other populations. For example, future research should consider applications of auditory cues (verbal or nonverbal) as a means of access and message retrieval for individuals with a broader range of needs, including those for whom auditory scanning may be an access enhancement, rather than a necessity. Many disciplines and areas of study outside the field of AAC (e.g., cognitive science, auditory imagery, auditory processing) may contribute important information relevant to auditory scanning and AAC. Finally, there is a need for greater collaboration between clinicians and AAC manufacturers in order to develop the means (beyond those available in systems at this time) to study the use of verbal and nonverbal auditory cues. AAC manufacturers must be willing to develop system prototypes to be evaluated with a variety of individuals needing an auditory presentation of system content. They must be willing to make system modifications to address the unique and variable needs of individuals who require auditory scanning.

Summary

Progress has been slow in addressing the needs of individuals with severe speech and visual impairments. Accommodations for visual deficits, including modifications of visual representations, have and continue to be important options for consideration in use of nonelectronic as well as electronic systems. Although current electronic AAC systems provide increased and improved visual enhancements, there appears to be a lack of understanding of the significance of vision in AAC system development and use. When individuals have severe physical impairments accompanied by severe speech and visual impairments, efforts to address these unique needs have focused on using existing adaptations for physical access (i.e., visual scanning), with the addition of a verbal auditory prompt that assists the user in locating a specific message and/or subsequent communicative content. Auditory scanning has been virtually unexplored in terms of its potential benefits and its applications to individuals with severe speech, visual and physical impairments who use AAC.

This chapter attempts to highlight some strategies and techniques in the area of access to AAC systems and development of operational competence for individuals with visual impairments. This area is complex but there may be an interface between operational and linguistic competence that is rich in opportunities for exploration to improve outcomes for individuals with speech, visual, and physical impairments.

REFERENCES

Adelson, E., & Fraiberg, S. (1974). Gross motor development in infants blind from birth. *Child Development, 45,* 114–126.

Anthony, T. (1990). *Cortical impairment: An overview.* Unpublished manuscript.

Bailey, B.R., & Downing, J. (1994). Using visual accents to enhance attending to communication symbols for students with severe multiple disabilities. *RE:view, 26*(3), 101–118.

Baker, B. (1982). Minspeak: A semantic compaction system that makes self-expression easier for communicatively disabled individuals. *Byte, 7,* 186–202.

Beukelman, D.R., & Ansel, B.M. (1995). Research priorities in augmentative and alternative communication. *Augmentative and Alternative Communication, 11,* 131–134.

Beukelman, D.R., & Mirenda, P. (1998). *Augmentative and alternative communication: Management of severe communication disorders in children and adults* (2nd ed.). Baltimore: Paul H. Brookes Publishing Co.

Beukelman, D., Yorkston, K., & Dowden, P. (1985). *Communication augmentation: A casebook of clinical management.* Austin, TX: PRO-ED.

Bigelow, A. (1991). Locomotion and search behavior in blind infants. *Infant Behavior and Development, 15,* 179–189.

Bishop, V.E. (1991). Preschool visually impaired children: A demographic study. *Journal of Visual Impairment and Blindness, 85,* 69–74.

Black, P.D. (1980). Ocular defects in children with cerebral palsy. *British Medical Journal, 281*(6238), 487–488.

Blackstone, S. (1989). Clinical news: Considerations for training visual scanning techniques. *Augmentative Communication News, 2*(4), 3–5.

Blackstone, S. (1994). Upfront. *Augmentative Communication News, 7*(5), 1–2.

Blackstone, S. (1998a). Clinical news: Auditory scanning. *Augmentative Communication News, 11*(4 & 5), 1–4.

Blackstone, S. (1998b). For consumers. *Augmentative Communication News, 11*(4 & 5), 7–10.

Blischak, D. (1995). Thomas the writer: Case study of a child with severe physical, speech, and visual impairments. *Language, Speech and Hearing in Schools, 26*(1), 11–20.

Bolanos, A.A., Bleck, E.E., Firestone, P., & Young, L. (1989). Comparison of stereognosis and two-paired discrimination testing of the hands of children with cerebral palsy. *Developmental Medicine and Child Neurology, 31,* 371–376.

Brodsky, M.C., Baker, R.S., & Hamed, L.M. (1996). The apparently blind infant. In M.C. Brodsky, R.S. Baker, & L.M. Hamed (Eds.). *Pediatric neuro-opthalmology* (pp. 1–41). New York: Springer Verlag.

Buzolich, M.J., King, J.S., & Baroody, S.M. (1991). Acquisition of the commenting function among AAC users. *Augmentative and Alternative Communication, 7,* 88–99.

Center, Y., Freeman, L., Robertson, G., & Orthred, L. (1999). The effect of visual imagery training on the reading and listening comprehension of our listening comprehenders in year 2. *Journal of Research in Reading, 22,* 241–256.

Centers for Disease Control and Prevention. (2001). *Vision impairment among children: Metropolitan Atlanta Developmental Disabilities Surveillance Program (MADDSP).* Retrieved January 15, 2001, from http://www.cdc.gov/nceh/cddh/dd/ddvi.html.

Cline, D., Hofstetter, H.W., & Griffin, J.R. (1980). *Dictionary of visual science.* Radner, PA: Chilton Book Co.

Cook, A.M., & Hussey, S.M. (1995). *Assistive technologies: Principles and practice.* St Louis: Mosby.

Corn, A.L. (1985). Strategies for the enhancement of visual function in individuals with fixed visual deficits: An interdisciplinary model. *Rehabilitation Literature, 46,* 8–11.

Duckman, R. (1979). Incidence of visual anomalies in a population of cerebral palsied children. *Journal of American Optometric Association, 50,* 607–614.

Fallon, K., & Light, J. (2000, August). The semantic organization patterns of young children: Implications for AAC. In *Proceedings of ISAAC 2000, The Ninth Biennial Conference of the International Society for Augmentative and Alternative Communication.* Washington, DC.

Finley, D. (1995). *So you want to learn Morse code: How to avoid frustration, minimize the pain and gain full HF privileges.* Retrieved February 1, 2001, from http://www.ees.nmt.edu/sara/sara/finley.morse.html.

Fraiberg, S. (1977). *Insights from the blind.* New York: Basic Books.

Fristoe, M., & Lloyd, L.L. (1979). Nonspeech communication. In N.R. Ellis (Ed.), *Handbook of mental deficiency: Physiological theory and research* (2nd ed., pp. 401–430). Mahwah, NJ: Lawrence Erlbaum Associates.

Fuller, D., Lloyd, L., & Schlosser, R. (1992). Further development of an augmentative and alternative communication symbol taxonomy. *Augmentative and Alternative Communication, 8,* 67–74.

Fuller, D., Lloyd. L., & Stratton, M. (1997). Aided AAC symbols. In L. Lloyd, D. Fuller, & H. Arvidson (Eds.), *Augmentative and alternative communication: Principles and practice* (pp. 48–79). Needham Heights, MA: Allyn & Bacon.

Geilhaus, M.M., & Olson, M.R. (1993). Using color and contrast to modify the educational environment of visually impaired students with multiple disabilities. *Journal of Visual Impairment and Blindness,* 19–20.

Good, W.V., Jan, J.E., DeSa, L., Barkovich, A.J., Groenveld, J.M., & Hoyt, C.S. (1994). Cortical visual impairment in children. *Survey of Ophthalmology, 38*(4), 351–364.

Greenwald, M.J. (1983). Visual development in infancy and childhood. *Pediatric Clinics of North America, 30,* 977–993.

Hatwell, Y. (1990). Spatial perception by eyes and hand: Comparison and cross-modal integration. In C. Bard, M. Fleury, & L. Hay (Eds.), *The development of eye–hand coordination across the life span.* Columbia: University of South Carolina Press.

Hellerstein, L. (1998). *Identification and treatment of visual perceptual problems.* Paper presented at the 1998 Auditory Scanning Symposium, Denver, CO.

Higginbotham, D.J., & Baird, E. (1995). Analysis of listeners' summaries of synthesized speech passages. *Augmentative and Alternative Communication, 11,* 101–112.

Higginbotham, D.J., Drazed, A.L., Kowarsky, K., Scally C., & Segal, E. (1994). Discourse comprehension of synthetic speech delivered at normal and slow presentation rates. *Augmentative and Alternative Communication, 10,* 191–202.

Higginbotham, D.J., Scally, C., Lundy, D., & Kowarsky, K. (1995). Discourse comprehension of synthetic speech across three augmentative and alternative communication (AAC) output methods. *Journal of Speech and Hearing Research, 38,* 889–901.

Iacono, T., Mirenda, P., & Beukelman, D. (1993). Comparison of unimodal and multimodal AAC techniques for children with intellectual disabilities. *Augmentative and Alternative Communication, 9,* 83–94.

Individuals with Disabilities Education Act (IDEA) of 1990, PL 101-476, 20 U.S.C. §§ 1400 *et seq.*

Jan, J.E., & Groenveld, M. (1993). Visual behaviors and adaptations associated with cortical and ocular impairment in children. *Journal of Visual Impairment and Blindness, 87,* 101.

Jan, J.E., & Groenveld, M. (1995). Visual behaviors and adaptations associated with cortical and ocular impairments in children. *The National Newspatch* (available from the Oregon School for the Blind).

Jan, J.E., Groenveld, M., & Anderson, D.P. (1993). Photophobia and cortical visual impairment. *Developmental Medicine and Child Neurology, 35,* 473–477.

Jan, J.E., Groenveld, M., Sykanda, A.M., & Hoyt, C.S. (1987). Behavioral characteristics of children with permanent cortical visual impairments. *Developmental Medicine and Child Neurology, 29,* 571–576.

Jan, J.E., Sykanda, A., & Groenveld, M. (1990). Habilitation and rehabilitation of visually impaired and blind children. *Pediatrician, 17,* 202–207.

Jerger, S., Elizondo, R., Dinh, T., Sanchez, P., & Chavira, E. (1994). Linguistic influences on the auditory processing of speech by children with normal hearing or hearing impairment. *Ear and Hearing, 15,* 138–160.

Jerger, S., Stout, G., Kent, M., Albritton, E., Loiselle, L., Blondeau, R., & Jorgenson, S. (1993). Auditory Stroop effects in children with hearing impairment. *Journal of Speech and Hearing Research, 36,* 1083–1096.

Jones, M. (1983). Cerebral palsy. In J. Unibreit (Ed.), *Physical disabilities and health impairments: An introduction* (pp. 41–58). New York: Macmillan.

Juurmaa, J., & Lehtinen-Railo, S. (1988). Cross-modal transfer of forms between vision and touch. *Scandinavian Journal of Psychology, 29,* 95–110.

Kekelis, L.S., & Prinz, P.M. (1996). Blind and sighted children with their mothers: The development of discourse skills. *Journal of Visual Impairment and Blindness, 90,* 423–436.

King, J. (2000). *The Bridge School classroom strategies: Vision and AAC, 2.* Hillsborough, CA: The Bridge School.

Kovach, T.M. (1989). Development and use of the Light Talker with the physically and visually challenged nonverbal child. In *Minspeak conference proceedings*. Wooster, OH.

Kovach, T., & Kenyon, P. (1998). Auditory scanning: Development and implementation of AAC systems for individuals with physical and visual impairments. *ISAAC Bulletin, 53*, 1–3, 7.

LaFontaine, L.M., & DeRuyter, F. (1987). The nonspeaking cerebral palsied: A clinical and demographic database report. *Augmentative and Alternative Communication, 3*, 153–162.

Lambert, S.R. (1995). Cerebral visual impairment. In K.W. Wright (Ed.), *Pediatric ophthalmology and strabismus* (pp. 801–805). St. Louis: Mosby.

Levack, N., Stone, G., & Bishop, V. (1994). *Low vision: A resource guide with adaptations for students with visual impairments* (2nd ed.). Austin: Texas School for the Blind and Visually Impaired.

Light, J. (1992, November). *Cognitive science: Implications for clinical practice in augmentative and alternative communication*. Paper presented at the annual convention of the American Speech-Language-Hearing Association, San Antonio, TX.

Light, J., & Lindsay, P. (1991). Cognitive science and augmentative and alternative communication. *Augmentative and Alternative Communication, 7*, 186–203.

Lloyd, L., & Blischak, D. (1992). AAC terminology policy and issues update. *Augmentative and Alternative Communication, 8*, 104–109.

Lloyd, L., & Fuller, D. (1986). Toward an augmentative and alternative communication symbol taxonomy: A proposed superordinate classification. *Augmentative and Alternative Communication, 2*, 165–171.

Lloyd, L., Fuller, D., & Arvidson, H. (Eds.). (1997). *Augmentative and alternative communication: A handbook of principles and practices*. Needham Heights, MA: Allyn & Bacon.

Mar, H., & Sall, N. (1994). Programmatic approach to use of technology in communication instruction for children with dual sensory impairments. *Augmentative and Alternative Communication, 10*, 138–150.

Mathy-Laikko, P., Iacono, T., Ratcliff, A., Villarruel, F., Yoder, D., & Vanderheiden, G. (1989). Teaching a child with multiple disabilities to use a tactile augmentative communication device. *Augmentative and Alternative Communication, 5*, 249–256.

Miller, M.J., Menacker, S.J., & Batshaw, M.L. (2002). Vision: Our window to the world. In M.L. Batshaw (Ed.), *Children with disabilities* (5th ed., pp. 165–192). Baltimore: Paul H. Brookes Publishing Co.

Mirenda, P., & Beukelman, D. (1987). A comparison of speech synthesis intelligibility with listeners from three age groups. *Augmentative and Alternative Communication, 3*, 120–128.

Mirenda, P., & Mathy-Laikko, P. (1989). Augmentative and alternative communication applications for persons with severe congenital communication disorders: An introduction. *Augmentative and Alternative Communication, 5*, 3–13.

Mizuko, M., Reichle, J., Ratcliff, A., & Esser, J. (1994). Effects of selection techniques and array sizes on short-term memory. *Augmentative and Alternative Communication, 10*, 237–244.

Nelson, L.B., Calhoun, J.H., & Harley, R.D. (1991). *Pediatric ophthalmology* (3rd ed.). Philadelphia: W.B. Saunders.

Orel-Bixler, D., Haegerstrom-Portnoy, G., & Hall, A. (1989). Visual assessment of the multiply handicapped patient. *Optometry and Visual Science, 66*, 530.

Oxley, J.D., & Norris, J.A. (2000). Children's use of memory strategies: Relevance to voice output communication aid use. *Augmentative and Alternative Communication, 16*, 79–94.

Pellegrino, L. (2002). Cerebral palsy. In M.L. Batshaw (Ed.), *Children with disabilities* (5th ed., pp. 443–466). Baltimore: Paul H. Brookes Publishing Co.

Piche, L., & Reichle, J. (1991). Teaching scanning selection techniques. In J. Reichle, J. York, & J. Sigafoos (Eds.), *Implementing augmentative and alternative communication: Strategies for learners with severe disabilities* (pp. 257–274). Baltimore: Paul H. Brookes Publishing Co.

Preisler, G.M. (1995). The development of communication in blind and in deaf infants—similarities and differences. *Child: Care Health and Development, 21*(2), 79–110.

Porter, P.B. (1989). Intervention in end stage of multiple sclerosis: A case study. *Augmentative and Alternative Communication, 5,* 125–127.

Quist, R., & Lloyd, L.L. (1997). Principles and uses of technology. In L.L. Lloyd, D.R. Fuller, & H.H. Arvidson (Eds.), *Augmentative and alternative communication: A handbook of principles and practices* (pp. 107–127). Needham Heights, MA: Allyn & Bacon.

Ratcliff, A. (1994). Comparison of relative demands implicated in direct selection and scanning: Considerations from normal children. *Augmentative and Alternative Communication, 10,* 67–74.

Reichle, J., Dettling, E.E., Drager, K.D.R., & Leiter, A. (2000). Comparison of correct responses and response latency for fixed and dynamic displays: Performance of a learner with severe developmental disabilities. *Augmentative and Alternative Communication, 16,* 154–163.

Reitan, R.M. (1971). Sensorimotor functions in brain-damaged and normal children of early school age. *Perceptual and Motor Skills, 33,* 655–664.

Reyes, B.A. (1995). Considerations in the assessment and treatment of neurogenic communication disorders in bilingual adults. In H. Kayser (Ed.), *Bilingual speech-language pathology: An Hispanic focus* (pp. 153–182). San Diego: Singular Publishing Group.

Reynell, J. (1978). Developmental patterns of visually handicapped children. *Child: Care, Health and Development, 4,* 291–303.

Rochat, P. (1989). Object manipulation and exploration in 2 to 5 month old infants. *Developmental Psychology, 25,* 871–874.

Romski, M.A., & Sevcik, R.A. (1989). An analysis of visual-graphic symbol meanings for two nonspeaking adults with severe mental retardation. *Augmentative and Alternative Communication, 5,* 109–114.

Romski, M.A., & Sevcik, R.A., (1993). Language comprehension: Considerations for augmentative and alternative communication. *Augmentative and Alternative Communication, 9,* 281–285.

Romski, M.A., & Sevcik, R.A. (Eds.). (1996). *Breaking the speech barrier: Language development through augmented means.* Baltimore: Paul H. Brookes Publishing Co.

Romski, M.A., Sevcik, R.A., & Pate, J.L. (1988). Establishment of symbolic communication in persons with severe retardation. *Journal of Speech and Hearing Disorders, 53,* 94–107.

Rowland, C. (1990). Communication in the classroom for children with dual sensory impairments: Studies of teacher and child behavior. *Augmentative and Alternative Communication, 6,* 262–274.

Rowland, C., & Schweigert, P. (1989). Tangible symbols: Symbolic communication for individuals with multisensory impairments. *Augmentative and Alternative Communication, 5,* 226–234.

Rowland, C., & Schweigert, P.H. (2000). Tangible symbols, tangible outcomes. *Augmentative and Alternative Communication, 16,* 61–78.

Ruff, H.A. (1980). The development of perception and recognition of objects. *Child Development, 51,* 981–992.

Sacks, S.Z. (1998). Educating students who have visual impairments with other disabilities: An overview. In S.Z. Sacks & R.K. Silberman (Eds.), *Educating students who have visual impairments with other disabilities* (pp. 3–38). Baltimore: Paul H. Brookes Publishing Co.

Schenk-Rootlieb, A.J.F., van Nieuwenhuizen, O., van der Geual, Y., Wittebol-Post, D., & Willemse, J. (1992). The prevalence of cerebral visual disturbance in children with cerebral palsy. *Developmental Medicine and Child Neurology, 34,* 473–480.

Sharps, M.J., & Price, J.L. (1992). Auditory imagery and free recall. *Journal of General Psychology, 119,* 81–87.

Solomons, H.C. (1957). *A developmental study of tactual perception in normal and brain injured children.* Unpublished doctoral dissertation, Boston University.

Sonksen, P.M., Levitt, S., & Kitsinger, M. (1984). Identification of constraints acting on motor development in young visually disabled children and principles of remediation. *Child: Care, Health and Development, 14,* 273–286.

Tachdjian, B.G., & Minear, W.L. (1958). Sensory disturbances in the hands of children with cerebral palsy. *Journal of Bone and Joint Surgery, 40A,* 85–90.

Thorley, B., Ward, J., Binepal, T., & Dolan, K. (1991). Communicating with printed words to augment signing: Case study of a severely disabled deaf-blind child. *Augmentative and Alternative Communication, 7,* 80–87.

Tierney, D., & King, J. (1998). Augmentative alternative communication for children with visual impairment. In *Biennial International Society for Augmentative and Alternative Communication Conference Proceedings* (pp. 426–427). Dublin, Ireland: Ashfield Publications.

Tinti, C., Galati, D., & Vecchio, M.G. (1999). Interactive auditory and visual images in persons who are totally blind. *Journal of Visual Impairment and Blindness, 93*(9), 579–583.

Tracy, R.J., & Barker, C.H. (1993). A comparison of visual versus auditory imagery in predicting word recall. *Imagination, Cognition and Personality, 13*(2), 147–161.

Troster, H., & Bramberg, M. (1993). Early motor development in blind infants. *Journal of Applied Developmental Psychology, 14,* 83–106.

Vanderheiden, G.C., & Lloyd, L.L. (1986). Communication systems and their components. In S. Blackstone (Ed.), *Augmentative communication: An introduction* (pp. 49–161). Rockville, MD: American Speech-Language-Hearing Association.

Venkatagiri, H.S. (1999). Efficient keyboard layouts for sequential access in augmentative and alternative communication. *Augmentative and Alternative Communication, 15,* 126–134.

Weiss, L. (1998). The Zygo Macaw and Morse code. *Morsels, 4*(1), 1–3.

Wills, D.M. (1979). Early speech development in blind children. *Psychoanalytic Study of the Child, 34,* 85–117.

IV

Social Competence

10

Pragmatic Development in Individuals with Developmental Disabilities Who Use AAC

Teresa A. Iacono

In its simplest form, pragmatics refers to the communicative functions of language (Gallagher, 1991). Such a definition belies the complexity of the area of communication known as pragmatics, comprising prelinguistic behaviors that drive the emergence of language, as well as the use of language to serve communicative goals (Dore, 1974; McTear & Conti-Ramsden, 1992). Any attempt to document pragmatic development will follow a chronology of

1. Emergence of *primitive* (Dore, 1974) or *prelinguistic* speech acts (Bates, Camaioni, & Volterra, 1975)
2. Appearance of early requests and comments (Wetherby, Cain, Yonclas, & Walker, 1988)
3. Expansion of pragmatic functions as language skills develop (Wetherby et al., 1988)
4. Use of language for discourse or conversation (Damico, 1985; McTear & Conti-Ramsden, 1992)

Movement through this chronology presents individuals with developmental disabilities who rely on augmentative and alternative communication (AAC) with a series of challenges. The methods with which individuals who use AAC and their communication partners meet these challenges will shape their patterns of communication at each stage of pragmatic development.

This chapter explores how the communication characteristics of individuals who use AAC are affected by processes occurring at each stage, according to the research base in typical and atypical communication development. Topics include information on 1) strategies that will enhance pragmatic development in light of known risk factors, 2) gaps in the research literature on understanding of pragmatic development in individuals who use AAC,

323

and 3) directions for strategies to address these research gaps for both theoretical and clinical benefit.

COMMUNICATION CHARACTERISTICS

Of concern in the AAC literature has been the passive role during dyadic interactions of individuals who use AAC (Basil, 1992; Buzolich & Lunger, 1995; Calculator & Dolloghan, 1982; Dattilo & Camarata, 1991; Harris, 1982; Light, 1988; Light, Collier, & Parnes, 1985a). Children using communication boards within a classroom setting studied by Harris (1982), for example, presented a profile of nonparticipation in which teachers dominated all communicative interactions by taking more and longer turns, thereby initiating most interactions; in contrast, the children adopted a role of respondent, producing little more than one-word responses to teacher initiations. According to Harris, this passivity was in sharp contrast to the participatory pattern of similar-aged children in the published literature. Studies since the work of Harris (1982) have documented similar profiles of passivity in children using AAC (e.g., Basil, 1992; Light et al., 1985a; von Tetzchner & Martinsen, 1996). Of further concern to Harris was the failure of her children to interact with peers; this concern has also been echoed in more recent research (e.g., Hunt, Alwell, & Goetz, 1991).

Conversational asymmetry between individuals with developmental disabilities who use AAC and speaking partners appears to continue to adulthood (Buzolich & Wiemann, 1988; Dattilo & Camarata, 1991). Explanations for the problems faced by individuals who use AAC in engaging equally with nondisabled partners in conversations have included inherent problems in conversations involving the use of AAC systems (Farrier, Yorkston, Marriner, & Beukelman, 1985). Technological advances have failed to provide the speed, ease of message access, and message appropriateness required to engage efficiently in conversations (Todman, Rankin, & File, 1999). In addition, researchers and clinicians have identified the need to teach both the individuals who use AAC and their partners strategies that facilitate interactions (Light, Binger, Agate, & Ramsay, 1999; Light, Dattilo, English, Gutierrez, & Hartz, 1992; von Tetzchner & Martinsen, 1996). Such strategies have been implemented in an attempt to reduce the dominance of the speaking partner and increase the conversational control exerted by the individual who uses AAC.

PRAGMATIC DEVELOPMENT

Despite the concern over their interactional skills, there has been little focus on the pragmatic development of individuals who use AAC in the published literature. As a result of this paucity of research, information must be gleaned from a literature base that extends beyond AAC. Knowledge of typical pragmatic development provides a basis for understanding areas of difficulty for individuals with various disabilities. Research into pragmatic development of individuals with developmental disorders, such as intellectual disabilities, autism, cerebral palsy, and multiple disabilities, including dual sensory impairment, provides a basis from which to begin the process of exploring pragmatic development in individuals who use AAC.

Early Social Interactions and the Emergence of Intentional Communication

Studies of parent–infant interactions have documented a synchrony of activity, whereby parents carefully study their infant's facial expressions and movements and respond to vocalizations as though they were social signals (Locke, 1993). The infant appears to take an active role in these interactions, as a result of an innate drive to engage in social interaction (Bruner, 1981; Locke, 1993; Siegel-Causey & Guess, 1989). According to Locke these early "conversational exchanges," occurring within a nurturant relationship, result in an attachment between the infant and parent. Locke argued that the linguistic significance of these early interactions, particularly those between mothers and infants (the major focus of research) is that "When infants become *attached* to their mothers many language-critical processes are encouraged: the desire to engage in playful vocalization, including vocal exploration, the emergence of turn taking and dialogue structure, and the desire to imitate vocal patterns" (1993, p. 107). The impact on the mother is to provide learning opportunities, encouraging communicative signals through the use of eye contact, gestures, and vocalization to signal a focus of attention (Bruner, 1981; Locke, 1993).

As infants become more intentional in their acts, displaying means–end behavior and coordinating their use of gestures, vocalizations, and eye-gaze, their signals become clearer, making it easier for adults to assign an intention to their communicative attempts (Bates, Begnini, Bretherton, Camaioni, & Volterra, 1977, 1979; Warren & Yoder, 1998; Yoder & Feagans, 1988). Adult responsiveness to these behaviors is thought to facilitate the infant's development of *illocutionary* behaviors (typically from 10 to 11 months of age, distinguished from the previous precommunicative *perlocutionary* stage by the directing of behaviors toward the adult with the intention of having an effect on the receiver (Bates et al., 1975; Bruner, 1974; Sugarman, 1984). In particular, gestures and vocalizations are used to elicit an adult's assistance in achieving a goal (*protoimperatives*) or to direct an adult's attention as a way of sharing information (*protodeclaratives*; Bates et al., 1979). The final stage is that of *locutionary* behaviors (from about 12 months of age); these behaviors are linguistic forms used to convey intentions.

According to Bruner (1981), important to the movement through these stages is the establishment of joint attention between parent and infant, whereby parents obtain cues as to their infant's focus of attention, providing responses and linguistic models within formats that constrain the context to a familiar routine, thereby increasing the saliency of the linguistic input. In this way, the parent scaffolds the learning situation (Bruner, 1974). Bruner (1981) noted the responsivity of parents to their infants in these communication exchanges. He argued that a parent's communication is linked closely to that of the child's; in particular, child initiations result in greater responsivity by the parent. A parent's ability to respond to an infant's early initiations is enhanced by an increase in the infant's rate of communicative signals, which co-occurs with the ability to coordinate attention between a referent and adult and to combine gestures and vocalizations from around 9 months of age (Sugarman, 1984; Warren & Yoder, 1998; Wetherby et al., 1988; Wetherby, Yonclas, & Bryan, 1989). These behaviors add clarity to the child's communicative attempts, assisting parents to recognize them as intentional communication.

Patterns in Developmental Disability

In the social interactions between infants and caregivers, caregiver responses to precommunicative signals, such as vocal turn-taking and imitating a facial expression, are thought to enhance cause–effect learning, thereby teaching an infant to exert control over the environment (Yoder, Warren, McCathren, & Leew, 1998). Infants with severe disabilities may fail to exert such control because of caregivers' problems in reading their early signals or the infants' inability to act on objects (Kraat, 1985; Watson, 1966). According to Watson (1966), the result is a failure to develop *contingency awareness,* or the understanding of the relationship between the infant's behaviors and effects on the environment. This failure to develop contingency awareness has been thought to affect later learning: The infant fails to develop motivation to act on the environment, thereby initiating a cycle of learned helplessness (Schweigert, 1989; Seligman, 1975). A potential long-term effect of learned helplessness is passivity in communication or even a failure of intentional communication to develop (Basil, 1992).

The ability to respond to prelinguistic signals and determine their intentions is dependent on the communication partner's ability to read them. Iacono, Carter, and Hook (1998) demonstrated the difficulty of the process of reading potentially communicative behaviors of children with severe physical impairments and secondary disabilities (intellectual and sensory). They attempted to elicit communicative behaviors from four young girls using sampling procedures that relied on establishing and then disrupting routine activities with each child. Although the girls responded to communicative events (e.g., being offered a nonpreferred item), the identification of intentional communication proved difficult because very few of their responses conformed to published criteria for demonstration of intentionality (e.g., Wetherby et al., 1988). Instead, the girls produced high rates of nonintentional communicative acts. These communicative acts were not technically intentional in that they failed to meet criteria of coordinated attention between an adult and referent accompanied by an unconventional gesture or vocalization, or the direction of conventional gestures or symbols to an adult (Wetherby et al., 1988). Nonetheless, they could be assigned communicative functions (i.e., they were perlocutionary acts), as determined by the researchers through a process of consensus coding. Iacono and colleagues argued that demonstration of behaviors critical to meeting criteria of intentionality, in particular coordinated attention, could be beyond the physical and sensory abilities of some children with severe and multiple disabilities. Instead, indicators such as the persistence of behaviors (even those that are idiosyncratic), rate, and modality-specific functions may provide caregivers with more accurate means of assigning meaning to prelinguistic signals.

There have been few studies directed at investigating the difficulties communication partners might experience in interpreting the prelinguistic behaviors of children with severe physical impairments and the potential disruption of parent–child interactions. From a review of early studies, Kraat (1985) suggested that, from an early age, severe physical impairments limit the infant's ability to take an active role in interactions. There are indications in the literature that, although young children with severe physical impairments rely on vocalizations, eye-gaze, and gestures in their interactions with communication partners (e.g., Bode, 1997; Harris, 1982; Heim & Baker-Mills, 1996; Light, Collier, & Parnes, 1985c; Miller & Kraat, 1984), these signals may be ignored or incorrectly interpreted because of their unintelligibility.

It is also possible that signals without a clear communicative intent may be "overinterpreted," as was indicated in a study by Yoder and Feagans (1988). These researchers asked mothers of 11-month-old infants with varying levels and types of disability (intellectual and physical) to observe videotaped interactions between themselves and their infants, and between other mother–child dyads. Some mothers were found to overattribute meaning to the behaviors of their own and other children with disabilities, often interpreting subtle signals that did not meet criteria for intentionality as communicative. What is not clear from this study is whether overinterpretation of prelinguistic behaviors is beneficial by reinforcing communicative attempts or if it may result in a failure of the infant to improve the clarity and conventionality of his or her signals (Yoder & Feagans, 1988). The relevance of Yoder and Feagans' findings to parent–child interactions is unknown, however, because such overattribution may occur only when the adult is an observer (as when viewing a videotape) rather than an active participant.

For infants with developmental disabilities other than physical impairments who may eventually require AAC systems, the information on pragmatic development is similarly sketchy to that of children with physical impairment. In addition, at times, conflicting evidence is presented. Nevertheless, children with various disabilities appear to have characteristics that impede the readability of their signals (Dunst, 1985). McCollum and Hemmeter (1997) summarized research indicating that children with Down syndrome, for example, demonstrate differences in eye contact and vocalizations and problems with social initiation in comparison with children without disabilities.

According to a transactional model of communication development (e.g., McLean & Snyder-McLean, 1978), child behaviors and characteristics have an impact on adult behaviors and style of interaction. This model would account for what appears to be a very controlling style by mothers of children with Down syndrome as compared with mothers of children without disabilities in dyadic interactions with their children. In particular, these mothers have been found to issue a high proportion of directives (Landry, Garner, Pirie, & Swank, 1994; Mahoney, Fors, & Wood, 1990; Roach, Barratt, Miller, & Leavitt, 1998). Mahoney and colleagues (1990) noted that this directive style was evident in the tendency of mothers of children with Down syndrome to request actions that were not related to the child's current focus of attention and were at developmental levels at the upper limits of their ability or potential. They argued that this style was indicative of the parents' intention to instruct the child, rather than engage in social interaction. In contrast, findings by Landry and colleagues (1994) and Roach and colleagues (1998) indicated that directives in the form of requests functioned to encourage play with objects to which children attended or to provide structure. According to McCollum and Hemmeter (1997), maternal directiveness is an outcome of child passivity during interactions (in line with the transactional model), which is not necessarily detrimental to communication development. A study by Crawley and Spiker (1983) revealed a pattern of directiveness but high sensitivity amongst some mothers in their interactions with their children with Down syndrome, for example. These mothers issued directives for actions relating to their child's focus of attention and responded to initiations with communication expansions.

From their review of research, McCollum and Hemmeter (1997) argued that attempts to engage children who are noncommunicative or whose signals are difficult to interpret tend to result in a directive style. It would seem that a style that is both directive and responsive has the potential to enhance communication development, rather than hinder it (Akhtar, Dunham, & Dunham, 1991; McCathren, Yoder, & Warren, 1995). This premise appears to underlie interventions focused on increasing prelinguistic, but intentional, communication acts (e.g., Warren, Yoder, Gazdag, Kim, & Jones, 1993), vocabulary (e.g., Warren, 1992), and early language (e.g., Hemmeter & Kaiser, 1994; Warren & Bambara, 1989).

Development of Functional Communication

Protodeclaratives and protoimperatives function to regulate the behavior of others and to establish joint attention, respectively (Bruner, 1981). These early request and comment functions continue to dominate as children move from prelinguistic, to linguistic, and then to multiword stages of development, which are distinguished by an expansion of functions and the development of increasingly advanced language forms (Wetherby & Prizant, 1989; Wetherby et al., 1988). According to Bruner (1981), early functions fall into three broad categories: 1) behavioral regulation, including requests for objects and actions and protests; 2) social interaction, including requests for social routines, showing off, greeting, calling, acknowledging, and requesting permission; and 3) joint attention, including comments, requests for information, and clarifications. As communication and language skills develop, more detailed taxonomies, which include discourse functions beyond initiation and response (see Chapman, 1981) become applicable in describing the range of potential communicative functions across developmental stages (McTear & Conti-Ramsden, 1992; Prutting & Kirchner, 1983).

Patterns in Developmental Disability   Patterns in developmental disability include prelinguistic functions and expansion of functions.

Prelinguistic Functions   Restrictions in communicative functions may become apparent even at the prelinguistic stage for children and even adults with developmental disabilities. Smith and von Tetzchner (1986) compared the pragmatic skills of 17 Norwegian children with Down syndrome with 18 children without disabilities, matched on mean age (13 months). The children with Down syndrome were found to produce few behaviors to signal joint attention but were similar to the children without disabilities in their use of imperatives (requests). In contrast, Mundy, Kasari, Sigman, and Ruskin (1995), in examining nonverbal communication in children with and without Down syndrome at two assessment periods (13 months apart), found deficits in the production of nonverbal requests but not joint attention in the group of children with Down syndrome. They explained the differences between these results and the patterns seen by Smith and von Tetzchner (1986) in terms of methodological differences. Smith and von Tetzchner measured pragmatic skills on the basis of qualitative ordinal scales; in contrast, Mundy and colleagues quantified use of nonverbal communication in response to structured communication opportunities. In addition, Smith and von Tetzchner provided only three opportunities for each pragmatic function examined, in comparison to the numerous opportunities provided children by Mundy and colleagues. Such methodological differences might also explain the difference between Mundy and colleagues' results and earlier studies, such as those indicating a paucity of joint attention in children with Down syndrome (see McCollum & Hemmeter, 1997). The specific difficulty with requests found by Mundy and colleagues (1995) replicated findings in previous studies by Mundy, Sigman, Kasari, and Yirmiya (1988) and Wetherby and colleagues (1989) and appears to be predictive of later language delays (Mundy et al., 1995).

Children with autism present a contrasting profile to those with Down syndrome in their prelinguistic communicative functions. Studies by Camaioni (1992), Tomasello and Camaioni (1997), and Wetherby and colleagues

(1989) have indicated a particular problem in the development of joint attention. Mundy, Sigman, and Kasari (1990) investigated the early communication of 15 children with autism and concomitant intellectual disabilities, who displayed little or no expressive language skills. The children were compared with groups of mental age– and language-matched children with intellectual disabilities only. The children with autism displayed a marked impairment in gestural joint attention when compared with both intellectual disability groups. Although fewer requests were also noted, the difference between the autism and language-matched intellectual disability group was not significant. Wetherby and colleagues (1989) reported similar findings from their study of the pragmatic skills of small groups of children with autism, children with Down syndrome, children with specific language impairments, and children without disabilities.

Little is known of the prelinguistic communication functions of children with physical impairments as a result of a lack of research in this area. An ongoing 5-year longitudinal study of nonspeaking children with physical impairments by Cress and colleagues is redressing this gap in the literature (Cress, 1999; Cress et al., 1999). Cress (1999) reported on the results of three monthly home visits over an 18-month period with 18 children (ages 12–24 months) and their parents. During these visits, the children were administered a series of assessments, including the Communicative and Symbolic Behavior Scales (CSBS; Wetherby & Prizant, 2003). Results from administering the communicative temptations of the CSBS indicated significantly poorer scores on joint attention than on behavioral regulation. According to Cress (personal communication, July 19, 2001), the children all received speech-language pathology services, which tended to focus on teaching requests to satisfy wants and needs. It is possible, therefore, that the children's early intervention influenced their stronger performance on behavioral regulation in comparison to joint attention. Alternatively, the differences seen might reflect developmental differences. Camaioni (1992) argued that the referencing of joint attention to share information with another person, as in declarative pointing (protodeclarative), requires an understanding and concern for a person's internal state. Such an understanding would appear to be more advanced developmentally than is communication for behavioral regulation, such as the instrumental use of pointing (protoimperative) in which the person is regarded simply as a means of obtaining an end. Particular difficulty with joint attention has been thought to arise from an underlying deficit in social cognition (e.g., Mundy et al., 1990), which interferes with the development of "theory of mind": that is, the ability to represent the mental states of other people (Camaioni, 1992; Sarria, Gomez, & Tamarit, 1996).

A similar hypothesis of a deficit in social understanding may also hold for the delay in joint attention seen in children with physical disabilities (Cress, 1999; Cress et al., 1999). Preliminary work by Dahlgren, Falkman, Dahlgren

Sandberg, and Hjelmquist (1998) suggested that deficits in theory of mind are not restricted to autism but extend to other groups with communication impairments, including children with cerebral palsy. Support for this hypothesis is not evident in the work of Cress and colleagues (Cress, 1999; Cress et al., 1999); however, Cress and colleagues (1999), in a further report on the children with physical impairments, found that the children were sociable, presumably demonstrating high rates of social/affective behaviors (gaze shifts and negative and positive affect) on the CSBS (Wetherby & Prizant, 2003).

An alternative hypothesis to that of a deficit in theory of mind was offered by Cress (1999). She argued that the children in her study produced few joint attention acts because the physical cost was too high in relation to the outcome. According to Cress and colleagues (1999), the children were willing to make a physical effort, through the combined use of gestures and vocalizations, to obtain the partner's attention and communicate a request for a tangible outcome; they were less willing to make this effort to engage in communication with only a social outcome.

Problems in early pragmatic skills may manifest as a plateau or cessation in development, in addition to a comparative deficiency in particular functions or speech acts. For individuals with severe to profound intellectual disabilities, for example, communicative functions may not extend beyond illocutionary forms of requests and comments. Ogletree, Wetherby, and Westling (1992) investigated the prelinguistic communication of 10 noninstitutionalized children, ages 6–12 years, with profound intellectual disabilities. The children demonstrated mostly regulatory behaviors and a paucity of joint attention. This pattern appears to continue into adulthood, according to the results of studies of adults with severe and profound intellectual disabilities by Cirrin and Rowland (1985); McLean, McLean, Brady, and Etter (1991); McLean and Snyder-McLean (1987); and McLean, Brady, McLean, and Behrens (1999).

Despite their limited communication repertoires, the children studied by Ogletree and colleagues did demonstrate a hierarchy of ability. Children who produced communicative acts at rates of greater than one per minute used distal gestures to reference objects away from themselves and combined vocalizations with gestures. These children demonstrated a trend of more communicative functions than did those who produced communicative acts at a lower rate, used contact gestures only, and produced few vocalizations. This difference in repertoire of functions between users of contact versus distal gestures was more pronounced in findings of McLean and colleagues for adults with severe to profound intellectual disabilities (McLean et al., 1991; McLean et al., 1999).

Gestures provide individuals without speech skills a means of expressing a range of communicative functions. Wetherby and colleagues (1989) noted that children with Down syndrome demonstrated the same communicative functions as children without disabilities at similar prelinguistic levels; the difference was in the reliance of children with Down syndrome on gestures, sometimes, in combination with vocalizations, whereas the children without disabilities used more isolated vocalizations. Similarly, the children with autism relied on gestures in their communication acts, but with few accompanying vocal acts, with those produced characterized by a lack of consonants. Miller and Kraat (1984) described the attention-getting behaviors of a 5-year-old boy with cerebral palsy, which frequently comprised vocalizations combined with arm-pointing. Other reports of children with physical impairments have also indicated a reliance on gestures, either alone or accompanied by vocalizations in communication acts (Bode, 1997; Harris, 1982; Heim & Baker-Mills, 1996; Light et al., 1985c).

In light of the role that gestures play in early communication across groups of children with and without disabilities, analysis of gesture types in relation to communicative functions may provide greater specificity in identifying levels of communication or readiness for symbolic intervention, particularly in children with limited or no speech. McLean and colleagues (1991, 1999) identified the two types of gestures described by Ogletree and colleagues (1992) in prelinguistic adults and children with severe intellectual disabilities. Contact gestures were produced while touching a referent or communication partner or within 6 inches of the referent; distal gestures were produced at least 6 inches from the referent or communication partner. Individuals who produced contact gestures only were less communicative, producing fewer intentional communicative acts, protodeclaratives and protoimperatives, and word-like vocalizations than those who produced distal gestures. McLean and colleagues (1999) also found that both children and adults producing distal gestures demonstrated the same rate of communication and range of functions as did symbolic communicators in their study. The researchers argued that distal gesturing demonstrates distancing from the object, a process that is thought to occur in the transition from presymbolic to symbolic communication and results from a shift in viewing objects as things to be acted on to objects as things of contemplation (Werner & Kaplan, 1984).

Pointing, one type of distal gesture, was examined in children with Down syndrome by Franco and Wishart (1995). Pointing is produced by typically developing infants primarily in referential/declarative contexts, in which the intent is to share information with a communication partner, whereas reaching is produced only in imperative/instrumental contexts, in which the aim is to engage the assistance of a communication partner to attain a goal. Franco and Wishart found that the children with Down syndrome (ages 21–47 months) demonstrated a similar pattern to that of typically developing children but at a higher rate and over a longer developmental period. Also, the children engaged in more frequent looking in association with their pointing as a visual check of their communication partner. They explained this pattern in terms of the children with Down syndrome's 1) experiences in failed communication attempts, resulting in an awareness of the need to monitor the partner in order to achieve efficient communication; and 2) lack of access to speech (e.g., "look") as a more efficient means of ensuring a partner's attention.

The pattern of frequent visual checks with pointing seen by Franco and Wishart (1995) suggests a fairly sophisticated understanding of communication. It is also a pattern that was observed by Cress and colleagues (1999) in their children with physical disabilities, particularly those who stayed at prelinguistic or transitional stages. These gaze shifts apparently were not the types of coordinated gaze that move from the communication partner, to the referent, and back to the partner to signal an intentional communicative act (Sugarman, 1984). Therefore, they may have served the same function of checking the partner's reactions to their gestural plus vocal behaviors as they did for the children with Down syndrome studied by Franco and Wishart.

Chan and Iacono (2001) conducted a detailed analysis of the gestural development in children with Down syndrome. Over a 5-month period, three preschool girls at a prelingistic stage of development were assessed in structured and unstructured communication sampling conditions. During this time, the girls demonstrated a range of gesture types, including 1) conventional gestures, which were highly conventional manual behaviors, unrelated to objects (e.g., waving "bye-bye," social games); 2) deictic gestures, which were nonsymbolic demonstrative or referential gestures (i.e., pointing, showing, giving, reaching, and taking); 3) enactive naming, which were manual behaviors related to objects (e.g., drinking from a cup) and indicated the child's recognition or classification of an object; and 4) symbolic gestures, which related to objects, but occurred with a substitute object or with a placeholder (e.g., making a "sawing" motion with a ruler). These gestures were used to convey different pragmatic functions, with the most common being comments, requests, and acknowledgements. During the 5 months, there was a decrease in the use of conventional and deictic gestures, and, for two of the girls, an increase in enactive naming. These two girls also demonstrated an overall increase in their rate of intentional communicative acts, with rates of at least one per minute associated with the appearance of signed, and to a lesser extent, spoken word production.

Chan and Iacono's (2001) findings suggest that changes in types of gestures accompanied by increased rates of communication may signal a readiness for symbolic communication. For children with typical development, the appearance of naming gestures seems to co-occur with the emergence of word production, whereas average rates of one intentional communication act per minute appear necessary for the transition from prelinguistic to symbolic communication (Bates et al., 1979; Wetherby et al., 1989; Wetherby & Prizant, 2003). McLean and colleagues (1999), however, found that the development of gestures that were independent of objects in the context of high rates of communication did not guarantee this transition in their groups of children and adults with severe intellectual disabilities. The researchers were puzzled by the failure of these participants to develop symbolic communication. Information on participants' intervention histories, in particular, whether augmentative forms of communication had been implemented, might have provided some insight into their lack of symbolic development. For these individuals, AAC may have provided an accessible modality needed for the transition to symbolic communication.

Expansion of Functions   Pragmatic development beyond the prelinguistic stage is supported by the development of language skills. Wetherby and colleagues (1988), for example, found that, as children without disabilities moved from the use of single words to multi-word language, their functional communication repertoire expanded. In particular, joint attention acts of requesting information and providing clarification, and social interaction acts of calling, requesting information, and acknowledging were produced by children with multi-word language, but not by children with prelinguistic or single word communication.

The potential for children with developmental disabilities and no or limited speech to expand their functional communication repertoire is dependent on the ability of their AAC system to support such expansion. Little is known about the range of speech acts produced by children who learn aided or unaided systems. Many interventions for children with severe disabilities have focused on teaching initial request functions to children with autism (Carr & Kologinsky, 1983; Layton, 1988; Salvin, Routh, Foster, & Lovejoy, 1977), intellectual disabilities (Mirenda & Santogrossi, 1985; Reichle & Johnston, 1999; Stephenson & Linfoot, 1995), and multiple disabilities, including physical impairments (Glennen & Calculator, 1985; Locke & Mirenda, 1988; Mathy-Laikko et al., 1989; Wacker, Wiggins, Fowler, & Berg, 1988). In contrast, there are few reports of AAC supporting other functions. An exception is a study by Rowland and Schweigert (2000) into the growth in symbolic communication of 41 children with various handicapping conditions following AAC intervention over a 3-year period. Tangible symbols were taught to the children by direct care staff, using naturalistic and spontaneous strategies in activities embedded in everyday routines. Rowland and Schweigert reported that although only request functions were initially targeted, other functions such as comments/labels, confirmation/negation, and refusal/rejection emerged in children who acquired symbols rapidly.

In an unpublished early report, Blackstone and Cassatt (1983) indicated that 15 young children with cerebral palsy using aided AAC systems demonstrated all communicative functions assessed using routine and nonroutine activities. These functions occurred using either aided AAC or other modalities. Unfortunately, published reports since then have suggested a more restricted repertoire (Basil, 1992; Harris, 1982; Light Collier, & Parnes, 1985b; Udwin & Yule, 1991). Light and colleagues (1985b) conducted an early detailed study of the functional communication skills of children who use AAC. Eight children with cerebral palsy, ages 4–6 years, who used aided AAC systems, participated in free play with caregivers and structured eliciting activities with a clinician. During the free play activities, many (39%) of the children's communication acts served to confirm or deny their caregivers' interpretations of their messages. Other functions also occurred as a response to caregiver demands: for example, 18% of child communications provided specific requested information and 5% provided clarification. In contrast, only 15% of their communicative acts served to request objects, activities, or attention. In the eliciting activities, the children produced a greater range of communicative functions, including greetings, closing, and social routines. The differences across the two conditions suggested that opportunities for specific functions play a role in a child's demonstration of their functional communication repertoire.

Udwin and Yule (1991) attempted to document, during an 18-month period, the pragmatic development of two groups of 20 children with cerebral palsy, ages 3;6–9;8 years: One group was learning Bliss, and the other was learning signs according to the Makaton Vocabulary (Grove & Walker, 1990). The children were assessed at 6-month intervals using a semi-structured conversation with an adult (Udwin & Yule, 1991). Although the children used signs or symbols to convey a variety of functions (15 in all) from the first assessment session, four communicative acts accounted for most Blissymbols (86%) and sign (89%) use. These acts were in response to *wh*- questions, labeling, requests for action, and descriptions of events. In addition, no noticeable growth in pragmatic development was evident during the 18-month period. Udwin and Yule argued that the deficits in functional use of AAC were a result of a combination of factors, including 1) the children's limited cognitive and social experiences, 2) their lack of motivation to communicate, 3) the nature of communication acts directed towards them by parents and teachers, and 4) limitations in the AAC systems causing slow rates of communication and access to limited vocabulary.

The focus of Udwin and Yule's (1991) study was the use of AAC modes. As a result of this focus, information was not provided on functions produced using other modes. Results from previous studies would indicate that analysis of gestures, vocalizations, eye-gaze, and facial expressions would have provided a more comprehensive picture of the children's functional communication (e.g., Harris, 1982; Heim & Baker-Mills, 1996; Light et al., 1985c). In addition, it is possible that the "semi-structured" interactions provided opportunities for some, but not other communicative functions. Other studies of children with cerebral palsy (Blackstone & Cassatt, 1983; Light et al., 1985b; McConachie & Ciccognani, 1995), intellectual disability (Iacono, Waring, &

Chan, 1996; McLean et al., 1999; Wetherby et al., 1989), and children with typical development (Ogletree et al., 1992; Wetherby et al., 1989) have shown differences in the communicative functions sampled in structured versus unstructured contexts.

The failure of the children studied by Udwin and Yule (1991) to develop their pragmatic skills was consistent with an overall lack of progress in their language skills (Udwin & Yule, 1990). Information from typical development indicates that growth in linguistic skills co-occurs with expansion of pragmatic skills as children are able to more effectively and efficiently meet their communication needs (McTear & Conti-Ramsden, 1992; Wetherby et al., 1988; Wetherby & Prizant, 1989). Little research involving individuals who use AAC has provided information on the codevelopment of pragmatic and language skills, although some reports suggest a relationship between the two (e.g., Heim & Baker-Mills, 1996; Kaul, 1999), and the interaction between different types of competencies was detailed by Light (1989).

Kaul (1999) conducted a direct investigation into the relationship between linguistic and pragmatic skills development. Participants in this study were five speaking and five nonspeaking children (ages 7–10 years) with cerebral palsy from families whose first language was Hindi. The nonspeaking children used picture (line drawings) and/or written word boards. Language and pragmatic assessments were conducted four times over a 9-month period. Two interventions were implemented. The first intervention immediately followed the first assessment (videotaped interactions with facilitators). The children's communication boards were modified by 1) increasing vocabulary in line with their tested receptive vocabulary; 2) adding grammatical markers of auxiliaries, person–number–gender, and case, organized according to Hindi morphology and syntax; and 3) changing the formats of displays to multipage theme boards for easier direct access by the children. Eight months later, a second assessment was conducted (again videotaped interactions), followed by the second intervention. In this intervention, facilitators were trained to use strategies to encourage the children to participate in interactions. Six months later, a third assessment was conducted, followed 3 months later by a final assessment.

Kaul's (1999) baseline measures (the first assessment) indicated differences between the two groups of children in communicative functions. For the children who used AAC, communication functioned most commonly to respond to partners' requests for information and confirmation: that is, giving information, acknowledging, confirming, and denying. In contrast, the speaking children demonstrated a larger range of communicative functions. These results are congruent with those of previous studies (e.g., Light et al., 1985b). In addition, the longitudinal nature of Kaul's investigation provides information on the developmental pattern of the children's communication skills. Following the modifications to their communication boards, the children increased their use of vocabulary and grammatical markers, a pattern that continued until the final assessment (i.e., after facilitator training and a period of 9 months). Concomitant increases were seen in the amount of communication produced and an expansion of pragmatic functions. According to Kaul's data, the growth in linguistic skills was associated with the expansion of communicative functions, and also with changes in the children's discourse skills.

Development of Discourse Skills

The development of pragmatic skills beyond basic functions facilitates the child's ability to engage in discourse, in particular to use communication in conversational interactions. As children move beyond the two-word stage, basic taxonomies that identify only initiations and responses (e.g., that used by Wetherby et al., 1988; Wetherby et al., 1989) fail to capture the range of conversational devices required for efficient and effective conversations. Protocols, such as that by Dewart and Summers (1988), address skills in initiating and responding to conversational repairs and terminating and joining conversations, as well as initiation and maintenance (see McTear & Conti-Ramsden, 1992, for an overview of pragmatic assessment protocols).

These skills appear to emerge as early as 2 years of age, although qualitative differences may distinguish younger from older children. McTear and Conti-Ramsden (1992), for example, reviewed studies indicating that although 2-year-olds may be able to take their turns in conversations, they lack the ability to anticipate the previous speaker's utterance completion and engage in turn-overlaps that characterize the conversations of more linguistically proficient speakers. Similarly, children as young as 18 months of age are able to initiate dialogue, using simple devices such as "What's that?" learned from routine interactions with adults (Halliday, 1975); however, the ability to presuppose the listener's perspective and knowledge and thereby choose appropriate topics and methods of introducing them relies on a combination of social and linguistic skills (McTear & Conti-Ramsden, 1992).

These social and linguistic skills are also implicated in the ability of children to recognize and resolve breakdowns in communication. According to McTear and Conti-Ramsden (1992), this ability involves knowing what aspects of a message were inadequate and the steps needed to repair the message. In a study by Garvey (1977), children as young as 3 years of age both responded to different types of requests for clarification and requested clarification of their communication partners. Older children demonstrated an increase in the number of strategies available to them for clarification and in the linguistic sophistication of the strategies used. Similarly, results of a study by Gallagher (1981) indicated that as language skills develop, children are able to increase the specificity of their revisions (i.e., providing only the information required by the listener). In reviewing research into the development of clarification skills in children, McTear and Conti-Ramsden (1992) found that the efficiency with which breakdowns are repaired increases with linguistic skills, probably as a result of developing understanding of what part of the message needs repairing and access to more sophisticated strategies.

Patterns in Developmental Disability   An implication of the close relationship between linguistic and social skills is that children with language delays will be at risk of problems in social interactions. Research involving children with specific language impairment (SLI; see Fujiki & Brinton, 1994) indicates the difficulty they face in joining peer interactions and responding to peer bids. The nature and reasons for these difficulties appear complex, not least because of individual differences in linguistics skills and social environments both within and across disability groups. According to a review by Miller (1987), for example, individuals with Down syndrome have demonstrated the ability to respond appropriately to partners' requests for clarification, use a variety of strategies for initiation of conversations, and use other features of appropriate conversational interaction. These studies have shown a tendency to use gestures over linguistic means, as an apparent method of compensating for spoken language deficiencies.

Beyond basic interaction skills, information on discourse skills of individuals with intellectual disabilities who use AAC is lacking. An exception is a study by Calculator and Dollaghan (1982) in which adults with severe intellectual disabilities who used AAC and lived in a residential setting were found to engage rarely in conversations. Their role in conversations was to respond to staff initiations, with the few initiations of the adults who used AAC often going unnoticed by staff. There is a similar lack of information on the discourse skills of individuals with autism who use AAC. Exceptions include a study by Loveland, Landry, Hughes, Hall, and McEvoy (1988). Children and adolescents with autism, in comparison with groups of younger children with language delays and typical development, showed a pattern of being less likely to respond to interactions, take fewer turns using vocalizations and gestures, and initiate less frequently. Other studies involving children with speech have focused on the uses of echolalia, demonstrating that it serves both interactive and noninteractive functions in autism (Prizant & Wetherby, 1985).

In contrast to research involving people with intellectual disabilities or autism, conversational interaction skills of individuals with physical disabilities who use aided AAC, both children (e.g., Basil, 1992; Harris, 1982; Light et al., 1985a) and adults (e.g., Buzolich & Wiemann, 1988; Calculator & Luchko, 1983; Dattilo & Camarata, 1991), have received a great deal of attention in the AAC literature. This focus appears to have originated in the early concern about the problems that individuals who use aided AAC have in maintaining an active role in conversational interactions (Kraat, 1985). In their study of young children with cerebral palsy using communication boards, Light and colleagues (1985a), for example, identified the following discourse pattern between the children and their caregivers: 1) caregivers took approximately twice as many turns as did the children; 2) the children fulfilled only half of their turn opportunities, responding only when obliged to do so by the caregiver's previous utterance; and 3) in the few situations in which the children initiated a topic, they relied on the caregiver to expand their utterances, which comprised single words. Light and colleagues also noted the caregivers' inability to tolerate silences, resulting in their frequent talking and continual attempts to maintain the conversational flow.

The asymmetry of interactions between individuals who use AAC and conversational partners is reminiscent of the dominant style of parents documented in studies of interactions between children with developmental disabilities and their mothers (McCollum & Hemmeter, 1997), and suggestions of a detrimental outcome for the child's communication development (Marfo, 1992). Close examination of the patterns described by Light and colleagues (1985a) and others (e.g., Basil, 1992; Harris, 1982), however, reveal adults' attempts to obtain the child's active involvement in a continuing conversation. Light and colleagues, for example, noted the highly transactional nature of the caregiver–child interactions, with caregivers responding to and accommodating children's participation levels. As a result of children's infrequent initiations and tendency to forfeit their turns, the caregivers increased their efforts and, therefore, control.

Bode (1997) explored the issue of the role of adults in interactions with children who use AAC. The adults engaged in conversations initiated by three preschool girls with cerebral palsy (ages 2–3 years) involved in an intensive early intervention program incorporating aided AAC (Porter & Kirkland, 1995). The adults were mothers and therapists working with the children according to the principles of Conductive Education, wherein the child is taught to be active in a holistic integrated program. Samples taken over a 6-month period of adult–child conversations, which were initiated by the child either independently or with prompting, were analyzed according to the functions of the adults' turns. These turns functioned most frequently to explicate the child's messages, thereby assisting the child in message formulation. In particular, the adults requested confirmations of their explications (e.g., speaking the children's symbol selections or verbally interpreting messages), and contributed to these messages, sometimes with instruction (e.g., modeling their own utterance with symbols). Less frequently, their turns had an instructional focus in the use of verbal and physical cues to emphasize the link between a symbol and its referent or meaning, such as selecting a symbol for a word that occurred in the conversation. The adults used metalinguistic functions also, such as identifying that a question was being asked.

The children in Bode's study fell along a continuum from least to most able, communicatively. The most able child initiated most turns in the samples independently, whereas the least able child did so only with assistance (according to Bode, these turns were responses to adult prompts, rather than true initiations). The third child initiated most turns independently but required prompting to extend the conversation. Bode found that the adults' turns were mostly their own contributions to conversations with the child who rarely initiated independently; in contrast, for the children who initiated independently, there was a larger ratio of didactic and metalinguistics functions. The pattern revealed by Bode's analysis was that of message co-construction when adults conversed with the two children who could initiate a turn, although for the child with few initiations, the adults placed more emphasis on instruction through modeling.

The style of adult interaction observed by Bode (1997) and also by Light and colleagues (1985a) suggests that their directiveness is used as a compensatory strategy in the face of poor or developing communication skills. This explanation is congruent with the transactional model (McLean & Snyder-McLean, 1978) and the hypotheses proposed by Marfo (1992) and others (as noted previously) for interactions involving children with developmental disability. Further support is found in a 15-year follow-up study of the children who participated in the study by Light and colleagues (1985a, 1985b, 1985c), which demonstrated the change in communication partner style according to more advanced discourse skills.

Lund and Light (2001) examined the interaction patterns of these participants, in addition to another individual experienced in the use of AAC, across three partners (i.e., a caregiver, an unfamiliar partner, and a peer). They found that, as in the original preschool study, the children who used AAC took fewer turns than did any of their partners. According to the researchers, these participants were far from passive, however, taking a mean of 42%–46% of turns across participants; in fact, two participants approximated reciprocity with their partners. They also found a significant increase over the preschool data in the taking of turn opportunities (an increase from a range of 29%–61% to 73%–77%), with a concomitant decrease in turns taken by communication partners. The individuals who used AAC tended to use "low-cost" turns to maintain their participation (i.e., they used strategies that required little physical effort, such as nodding). As with the preschool data, there were large individual differences across the individuals who used AAC, with two struggling to fulfill their turns with nonfamiliar partners.

The overall pattern observed by Lund and Light (2001) was one of greater participation by the individuals who used AAC across the different types of communication partners in comparison with the preschool data

(Light et al., 1985a). In addition, discussion on topics lasted longer, resulting in fewer topics being initiated. Despite these changes, three of the individuals who used AAC were still dependent on their partners to carry the burden of communication by determining the topics and course of the interaction. This dependence apparently resulted from their AAC systems being limited in generative capacity. Reliance on partners to initiate topics and infrequent requests for information by these now adults who used AAC reflected patterns seen in the preschool data (Light et al., 1985a).

Reliance on natural speakers in conversations involving AAC extends to co-construction of messages, especially with low-technology systems (e.g., partner-assisted scanning) and taking on a large part of the responsibility in repairing conversational breakdowns (Bode, 1997; Light, 1988; Lund & Light, 2001). Both message co-construction and repair appear to result in frequent requests for individuals who use AAC to confirm the communication partner's repeating of a message (Bode, 1997; Light et al., 1985a; Lund & Light, 2001). Conversational breakdowns occur frequently in AAC interactions (Kraat, 1985), with possible reasons including

1. Reliance on modes, such as gestures, vocalizations, and eye gaze (Bode, 1997; Harris, 1982; Heim & Baker-Mills, 1996; Hjelmquist & Dahlgren Sandberg, 1996; Light et al., 1985c; Lund & Light, 2001), which may be difficult to interpret (Hjelmquist & Dahlgren Sandberg, 1996; Light et al., 1985a)

2. Use of only single-word messages using the AAC system (Heim & Baker-Mills, 1996; Light et al., 1985a, 1985c)

3. Possible failure to reference a topic through joint attention (e.g., Cress, 1999; Light et al., 1985a)

These factors necessitate an often lengthy process of negotiation of meaning (Hjelmquist & Dahlgren Sandberg, 1996; Kraat, 1985).

The reliance on communication partners provides an impetus for interventions targeting facilitators (i.e., speaking conversational partners) (e.g., Basil, 1992; Light & Binger, 1998; Light et al., 1992; Lund & Light, 2001). Kaul (1999), however, demonstrated the benefit of a multifaceted intervention to enhance conversations for individuals who use AAC. The expansion of vocabulary and grammatical markers on the children's communication boards was followed by an increase in their use of the grammatical markers. These increases were associated with changes in the children's discourse patterns, changes that occurred prior to the facilitators receiving instruction in discourse strategies. In particular, there was an increase in the children's use of questions (suggesting increases in initiations), in giving more information and taking up more conversational space, and in the provision of reformulations. In addition, one child, who was the most linguistically competent at using AAC, increased his use of clarifications. Further changes were evident following facilitator instruction, and, as such, seemed attributable, to some extent, to strategies adopted by facilitators. According to the transactional model of communication development, changes in the children's communication would have assisted the facilitators further in engaging the children in conversation and in persevering in message construction.

Summary

Despite the heterogeneity amongst individuals with developmental disabilities who use AAC, common themes emerge in the literature relating to their pragmatic development. These themes are summarized in Table 10.1. Of concern has been their restricted range of communicative functions, evident early in development. Profiles of deficit in the use of prelinguistic means to signal joint attention or to regulate the behavior of others may relate to specific types of disabilities (e.g., the deficit in joint attention seen in children with autism and cerebral palsy). These early deficits may be associated with underlying difficulties with social cognition, or reflect the physical effort and sensory/motor coordination involved in emitting signals that are clear enough to elicit linguistic input from caregivers.

Disruptions to caregiver–child interactions appear to set up a cycle that places the child at risk of language delay and may contribute to a passive style in later conversational interactions. According to a growing body of evidence, individuals who use AAC have difficulty in taking more than a respondent role in interactions, but not all appear to be passive communicators. Motivation, the ability of interactants to take on a role of co-construction, differences in the physical effort required in relation to the individual's physical capability, the different goals in interactions (e.g., information sharing versus social closeness), and linguistic skills are likely factors contributing to individual differences in interaction patterns seen across individuals who use AAC. Recent research appears to address the specific roles of communication partners in attempting to engage the individual who uses AAC in a process of meaning negotiation, and the co-development of linguistic and pragmatic skills. In particular, an interaction between linguistic and social skills seen in typical development and argued to account for difficulties in both areas in children with communication deficits is evident in individuals who use AAC. Evidence for this interaction provides a strong argument for shifting the focus of pragmatic research in AAC to encompass linguistic domains.

CLINICAL IMPLICATIONS

Light (1989) noted the integration of linguistic, social, operational, and strategic skills required for individuals who use AAC to achieve communicative

Table 10.1. Themes emerging from the literature on pragmatic development in augmented communicators

Problems	Potential outcomes
Difficulty in acting on the environment	Disruption of cause–effect learning
Potentially communicative behaviors that are difficult to read and do not include indications of intentionality	Failure of adults to respond to potentially communicative behaviors Development of learned helplessness and passivity in interactions
Delays in developing prelinguistic pragmatic functions	Increased potential for later language delays
Access to limited modalities (e.g., few vocalizations, reliance on gestures, failure of gestures to develop beyond basic types)	Compromised readability of communication, resulting in reduced responses from interactants. Need for visual checking to ensure interactant participation
Nonresponsiveness because of limited communication and social-interaction skills	Controlling style adopted by conversational partners in interactions
Language delay or access to limited language	Restricted pragmatic repertoire Limited message content Reliance on partners in co-construction and repair of messages
Limitation in physical skills	Tendency to restrict conversational participation to "low-cost" responses

competence. The development of social skills has been the focus here, with the impact of linguistic skills highlighted, in particular through the work of Kaul (1999). Of relevance to gaining operational skills in using an AAC system (e.g., pointing to symbols on a display) and adopting relevant strategies (e.g., providing clarifications when communication breakdowns occur) is the motivation to communicate. Such motivation comes from an understanding of its role in obtaining needs and wants, sharing information, forming and maintaining relationships with others, and conforming to the social etiquette of one's culture (Light, 1988). Pragmatic intervention for individuals who use AAC, therefore, must address issues of motivation, in addition to the development of specific pragmatic skills at various levels of linguistic competency.

Establishing Motivation for Communication

Interventions to encourage conversational participation have included teaching specific strategies to the individuals who use AAC (Buzolich & Lunger, 1995; Light et al., 1999), peers (Hunt et al., 1991), and communication partners (Basil, 1992; Kaul, 1999; Light & Binger, 1998; Light et al., 1992; Lund &

Light, 2001). These interventions have met with some success (e.g., Buzolich & Lunger, 1995; Hunt et al., 1991; Kaul, 1999; Light et al., 1999; Light et al., 1992). There is some indication that attempts to teach conversational assertiveness may be impeded by an inherent passivity for some individuals who use AAC, however. As an example, Buzolich and Lunger (1995) attempted to empower a young adult who used AAC to identify the conversational patterns of four peers and to adopt regulatory phrases and strategies to manage turns in conversations. Although the participant, Vivian, learned to use these strategies with some success, she indicated a lack of concern if her speaking partner dominated all turns and would give up in the face of insufficient time to answer a question. In addition, Vivian preferred to use indirect rather than direct conversational control strategies. Buzolich and Lunger explained this preference in terms of Vivian's shy personality.

Basil (1992) also observed a pattern of passivity in four children with cerebral palsy in interactions with their mothers and teachers. She implemented an intervention designed to increase the children's conversational participation. The mothers and teachers learned to reduce their dominant role in the conversations, but the children maintained their role as responders, failing to increase initiations. Basil explained this pattern in terms of learned dependency, whereby "the children had not been taught to initiate and, moreover, they may have learned to expect someone else to initiate" (1992, p. 195). Unless appropriate intervention strategies are in place, learned dependency appears to follow learned helplessness, which results from repeated experiences of failure to exert control over the environment (Basil, 1992).

The potential that passivity may originate in early communication experiences argues for early interventions aimed at facilitating infants' experiences of control over their environments (Schweigert, 1989). Intervention using microtechnology, whereby motor behaviors are paired with nonsocial environmental consequences (e.g., turning on a cassette player allows the participant to hear music), has been found effective in teaching contingency awareness to individuals with severe disabilities (e.g., Brinker & Lewis, 1982; Hanson & Hanline, 1985). Schweigert (1989) and Schweigert and Rowland (1992) applied the principle of contingency awareness to teaching children with multiple disabilities, including dual sensory impairment, in the use of microtechnology to elicit a social response. The success of this intervention led to the development of both basic presymbolic communication and more formal symbolic systems.

The advantage of microtechnology over non–technology-based interventions is that the response to a behavior is both immediate and consistent. In addition, the use of microtechnology requires only minimal physical effort, providing children with disabilities an easy means of obtaining a response from the environment (Cress, 1999). For children with physical disabilities, this attention to the cost–benefit ratio may be crucial in encouraging acts of joint attention. Simple switches attached to single message systems, which function to obtain an adult's attention, might be sufficient to enable young children to realize their ability to initiate an interaction.

In addition to amplifying or clarifying a child's intent by access to basic AAC systems, teaching caregivers to respond to subtle and inconsistent signals, within nurturing interactions, also has been recommended (Cress, 1999; Siegel-Causey & Guess, 1989). Such strategies provide an alternative to microtechnology in teaching cause–effect, but rely on the caregivers being sensitized to potential communicative behaviors, which are often idiosyncratic, and responding to them consistently (Iacono, Carter, & Hook, 1998; Siegel-Causey & Guess, 1989).

Caregiver-based interventions might best begin with the identification and reinforcement of positive strategies already used (e.g., responding to the child's communication attempts). This type of strategy enables the intervention to begin with the caregiver's natural style and useful strategies already in his or her repertoire. Iacono, Chan, and Waring (1998) used this approach with a group of parents of children with Down syndrome in early intervention. Existing strategies were identified, with slight modifications introduced (e.g., use of pausing, modeling of vocabulary) according to each mother's style.

Specific strategies designed to encourage prelinguistic communication include imitation of a child's behavior, organizing the environment to create communication opportunities, following the child's attentional lead, providing models and inserting pauses into routine or ongoing activities (Mirenda & Iacono, 1988; Prizant & Wetherby, 1987; Warren et al., 1993). Although many of these strategies were not designed with AAC in mind, they can be adapted readily to incorporate various types of AAC systems (Kaiser, Ostrosky, & Alpert, 1993; Mirenda & Iacono, 1988).

Development of Form–Function Relationships

Communication development involves moving beyond simple requests and comments to include a larger range of pragmatic functions (e.g., requesting interactions, acknowledging, greeting, providing clarification). This pragmatic expansion is accompanied by replacement of prelinguistic signals (e.g., pointing and other gestures, vocalizations) with conventional symbols (words) and linguistic structures (e.g., grammatical morphemes) (Wetherby & Prizant, 1989). For children with a limited pragmatic repertoire and/or linguistic skills, a prerequisite to intervention is determining those forms already used (i.e., conventional and unconventional signals) and their communicative functions (Bloom & Lahey, 1978).

Identification of the forms and functions in a child's repertoire requires consideration of different communicative contexts and sampling conditions. Studies by Blackstone and Cassatt (1983), Light and colleagues (1985a, 1985b,

1985c), Wetherby and Rodriguez (1992), and Iacono and colleagues (1996) have demonstrated the differences in pragmatic functions and modality use sampled across different communicative contexts. Iacono and colleagues (1996), for example, found that structured sampling conditions, using Wetherby and colleagues' (1988) communicative temptations, resulted in more requests and comments than did free play with parents, which tended to elicit mostly responses. Sampling of communication skills, therefore, needs to occur in different contexts and across time. Of relevance to intervention planning is the caregiver's perceived role in interactions, such that they may see themselves as instructors when videotaped in a clinical context, resulting in a style that could contrast that used in their home environments (Bode, 1997).

Identification of a child's complete repertoire of pragmatic functions and the modalities with which these are expressed across contexts will facilitate intervention that builds on the child's current strengths. In addition, understanding how an individual child uses particular signals/modalities may inform the planning process. As an example, Cress (1999) identified two forms of gaze shift in her young children with cerebral palsy: 1) to reference joint attention, using a three-point shift between the partner and referent; and 2) a gaze that appeared to monitor the partner's reactions to the child's communication attempts. This latter use of gaze was associated with children at prelinguistic levels, whose intervention might best focus on developing other means to reference joint attention (e.g., pointing, vocalizations). Heim and Baker-Mills (1996), however, noticed a similar use of gaze by a young girl who successfully learned to use a communication board to engage in extended conversations. The gaze shift was used by the child in monitoring the partner's participation in the conversation, functioning as a means of controlling the rate of turn-taking. In this way, the same form may appear at different linguistic levels but serve similar functions.

Identification of functions communicated by informal or prelinguistic means enables adults to provide what Warren and colleagues (1993) referred to as a *linguistic map*. Warren and colleagues (1993) provided such linguistic maps by modeling a spoken word that conveyed the message produced by a child through prelinguistic means. Linguistic maps can also be provided using AAC modalities (e.g., pointing to an appropriate graphic symbol or producing a manual sign), thereby providing augmented language stimulation (Goossens', 1989).

Engaging in Conversational Discourse

Interventions at the discourse level for individuals with developmental disabilities who use AAC have focused on increasing active participation in conversations (e.g., Buzolich & Lunger, 1995; Crystal, Garman, & Fletcher, 1989; Dattilo & Camarata, 1991; Light et al., 1999; O'Keefe & Dattilo, 1992). In addition, facilitators, including adults (Light et al., 1992; McNaughton & Light, 1989) and peers (Carter & Maxwell, 1998; Hunt et al., 1991) have been taught to use strategies that provide opportunities for individuals who use AAC to engage in turn taking and initiations. Interventions that involve both the individuals who use AAC and facilitators, such as those described by Light and Binger (1998), could prove to be most effective.

In keeping with a principle of understanding the nature of interactions between individuals who use AAC and various partners, assessment protocols are needed that take into account the roles and priorities for each interactant. Certain interactions in classrooms, for example, by necessity of the teacher's aims, might be controlled by the teacher through questions, with the child's role being that of respondent. As a result of differences in demands across contexts, clinicians working in classrooms must differentiate for the individual who uses AAC and his or her peers situations that require high versus low levels of initiation. When working with parents, discussion of their perceptions of their role when interacting with the individual who uses AAC and siblings in different contexts is recommended as a first step in interventions aimed at changing interaction patterns. This discussion would facilitate both the parent's and clinician's understanding of the value in existing strategies, such as the use of turns to serve a didactic function in an early intervention environment, as opposed to more frequent pausing in naturalistic contexts (Basil, 1992). As a result, clinicians may gain a greater understanding of why some strategies work with some partners and not others, as occurred with a failure of increased use of pausing by parents to result in greater initiations by the children studied by Basil (1992).

The review of pragmatic development was presented here in the context of typical development. At the discourse level, such typical models are not always applicable. For individuals who use AAC, the co-construction of messages (Bode, 1997; Light & Binger, 1998) and negotiation of meaning (Hjelmquist & Dahlgren Sandberg, 1996; Kraat, 1985) takes on a more central and demanding role than in conversations between natural speaking partners. It would seem appropriate that interventions at the discourse level focus on assisting both partners to achieve their goals in the conversational interaction. According to Light (1988), the goal of communication will have implications for the skills required. In information transfer, therefore, negotiation of meaning will have greater importance than if the goal is social interaction or to maintain social etiquette, because of the importance of the content of the message; similarly, the independence of the communicator might be more important if the goal is information transfer than if it is social closeness. The effectiveness of a discourse level intervention is likely to be dependent on assisting communication partners to be sensitive to the changing goals of communication and learning a range of strategies to enable use of those most appropriate to the goal.

Research Directions

Longitudinal studies by Bode (1997), Cress (1999), and Kaul (1999) and the 15-year follow-up study of Lund and Light (2001) demonstrated the value in moving from a snapshot picture of communication interaction patterns to attempts to study the emergence of pragmatic skills over time and in relation to linguistic development. These studies, in addition to the growing research base in pragmatic development, provide pieces to a complex puzzle. In order to develop coherence of the emerging picture, future research must address the missing pieces. Also required, however, is a view of the gestalt so as to enable exploration of the whole dynamic and multifaceted nature of pragmatic development. Meeting these goals requires the identification of specific issues from literature that extends beyond individuals who use AAC, as well as extending the repertoire of tools, models, and methodologies suitable for this group.

Issues   Kaul's (1999) investigation into the relationship between pragmatic skills and linguistic development highlights the relevance of research that crosses domains. Researchers in AAC have focused on specific communication domains, with some arguing that there has been a strong focus on linguistic development (e.g., Todman et al., 1999). There have been attempts to investigate the multifaceted nature of communication, such as Light and colleagues' analyses of communication discourse, functions and the relationship between modalities and functions (Light et al., 1985a, 1985b, 1985c; Lund & Light, 2001). Such research provides the foundation from which to investigate 1) the rich connections amongst communication domains, in particular linguistic and pragmatic skills; 2) interrelationships across the domains of communication, motor development, and social development; and 3) how early skills and experiences predict later communication development.

There is also a need to address a more comprehensive notion of pragmatics: that is, extending beyond the expression of needs and wants, or conversational asymmetries. Light and Binger (1998) outlined pragmatic interventions that enable individuals who use AAC to fulfill different pragmatic needs (e.g., the use of introductions as a means of expanding social interactions). Research into the efficacy of these strategies has been limited (e.g., Buzolich & Lunger, 1995; Hunt et al., 1991; Light et al., 1999; Light et al., 1992), with no direct replication to determine the strength of effects or systematic replication to determine their generalizability. The focus of the few efficacy studies has been the use of specific strategies to encourage individuals who use AAC to have more control and participation in interactions, but research into strategies that are most relevant and useful to the goals of informing, forming social relationships, and conforming to social etiquette, as well as obtaining needs and wants, is lacking (Light, 1988). Similarly, research into characterizing and facilitating social interactions has failed to identify how both individuals who use AAC and partners perceive their roles in conversational interactions. These perceptions may change according to 1) stages of communication development, 2) contexts and goals of interactions, and 3) nature and timing of intervention. Addressing these issues will serve to socially validate research findings through the identification of the relevance and value of interventions for participants (Schlosser, 1999).

Of relevance to the clinical need to identify caregivers' perceptions of their roles in augmented conversations is the investigation of caregiver styles in interactions across different contexts. Sharing this identified style with caregivers and pointing out existing facilitatory strategies might assist in motivating them to make modifications. Caregivers are likely to perceive such modifications to be within their capability, in comparison to strategies outside their current repertoires. Research comparing this individual versus a more general approach would appear warranted as a means of exploring effective strategies for training facilitators.

An issue of particular relevance to individuals with autism who use AAC, and perhaps also to those with cerebral palsy, is how deficits in theory of mind may have an impact on pragmatic skills, from the emergence of functions to conversational interactions (Baron-Cohen, Leslie, & Frith, 1985; Dahlgren et al., 1998). According to Baron-Cohen and colleagues, a deficit in theory of mind results in an inability to attribute independent mental states to oneself and others. Such deficits are likely to affect the ability to engage appropriately in conversations by taking into account the communication partner's knowledge state and perspectives. Combined with linguistic delays, deficits in theory of mind are predicted to interfere with conversational interactions. Support for this hypothesis, or indeed for potential deficits in theory of mind amongst individuals who use AAC, awaits empirical investigation.

Despite the international nature of AAC, there has been a lack of investigation into cultural issues (Light, 1997). The cultural environment provides a communication context, requiring a specific set of vocabulary, syntactic structures, and social mores that will govern how conversations are conducted (Hetzroni & Harris, 1996). Research into cultural differences will enable the development of interventions that are culturally appropriate, thereby assisting families in taking on facilitator roles. In addition, research into cultural issues will inform models of social interaction involving AAC.

Assessment Tools   In order to profile the pragmatic skills of individuals who use AAC, taxonomies that accommodate use of prelinguistic and AAC modalities across developmental stages are required. Researchers have adapted existing taxonomies (e.g., Light et al., 1985a, 1985b, 1985c), although certain assessment protocols would appear suitable for children with developmental disabilities at particular stages (e.g., Wetherby & Prizant, 2003). Missing from the AAC literature are tools that have been validated with this population. Developing these tools requires a coherent model of pragmatic skills and development amongst individuals who use AAC.

Models   Comparison of pragmatic development in children with developmental disabilities with typically developing children provides a means of identifying and understanding potential relationships among variables that are often investigated in isolation. Models of typical development have their limitations in research into pragmatic skills of individuals who use AAC, however. As an example, the combined factors of possible linguistic delays, limitations inherent in current AAC systems and potential differences in how nonlinguistic modalities are used (e.g., gaze shifts) mean that AAC conversations will never have the same coordination of turns between speakers characteristic of fast-paced spoken conversations. Such differences argue for the development of new models of pragmatic development and conversational interactions of relevance to individuals who use AAC (Kraat, 1985). Some work towards this end is evident in the AAC literature (e.g., Gerber & Kraat, 1992; Light, 1997; Paul, 1997; Wolf Nelson, 1992). Future research will inform and develop these models, enabling them to direct further investigations into the pragmatic development of individuals with developmental disabilities who use AAC.

Methodologies   Longitudinal research may best serve the purpose of addressing many of the issues identified, in particular determining the relationships between 1) the caregivers' difficulties in reading prelinguistic signals of children with developmental disabilities and later pragmatic development, and 2) early and later linguistic and pragmatic development. This type of research allows investigation of the "dynamics of acquisition" (Plante, Swisher, Kiernan, & Restrepo, 1993, p. 775). Obstacles to longitudinal studies include cost, the need for relatively large samples, and potential participant attrition, significant problems when investigating low incidence and heterogeneous populations, such as individuals who use AAC (Light, 1999).

Alternatives to large group studies have included case studies, in which interventions are detailed (see von Tetzchner & Jensen, 1996). Case studies provide insight into potential developmental trends and the documentation of clinical strategies and insights that feed into empirical research. The efficacy of interventions appears best addressed through the use of controlled single-case designs, but on their own, these studies do not address questions about interactions amongst various communication domains across the developmental period (Light, 1999; Schlosser & Braun, 1994). Possible solutions include short-term descriptive studies that allow potential relationships to emerge (e.g., Chan & Iacono, 2001), periodic follow-up studies of participants in earlier studies (e.g., Lund & Light, 2001), and studies of children involved in prelinguistic and early AAC intervention (Bode, 1997). These methodologies call for rich data from varied sources, with detailed analyses. Chan and Iacono (2001), for example, obtained data from both structured informal assessments and repeated observations of natural interactions to develop a profile of developing communication skills in the children with Down syndrome. Similarly, Light and colleagues (1985a, 1985b, 1985c) and Lund and Light (2001) analyzed interaction samples along various dimensions, with Lund and Light supplementing this information with assessments of language, reading, self-determination, educational/vocational achievement, and quality of life.

These detailed descriptive methodologies provide a basis for qualitative studies. Qualitative methodology, comprising the gathering of rich and varied data sources and inductive analysis in a grounded theory approach (Denzin, 1989) has been under-utilized in the AAC literature. Data collection strategies, such as focus groups, allow researchers to obtain a range of perceptions of individuals who use AAC about conversations, their goals, and their perceived needs (Liamputtong Rice & Ezzy, 1999). Such data might enable the reformulation of conversation models based on speaking partners to better reflect those involving individuals who use AAC. Approaches such as the Delphi Technique (Jones & Hunter, 1996; Moore, 1994) would allow researchers to access individuals who use AAC, clinicians, and researchers from across the globe to identify research needs in pragmatic development and intervention. This approach requires that researchers pose two or three key questions to participants, who respond by mail or e-mail. The researcher summarizes responses and sends them back to participants for comment; this process is repeated until consensus is obtained. Another consensus approach, suitable for face-to-face discussions with groups of participants, is the Nominal Group Technique (Jones & Hunter, 1996; Moore, 1994). Participants are posed a key question, asked to make a list of "needs," and then asked to form a consensus as to those with the highest priority. This technique appears suitable for identifying issues of greatest concern to individuals who use AAC and potential strategies for successful conversational interactions, according to particular goals.

Although the research involving focus groups of individuals who use AAC has appeared in the literature (e.g., Iacono, Balandin, & Cupples, 2001), these and other qualitative methodologies have been rare in the AAC literature. These methods offer a means of including individuals who use AAC in the process of setting the agenda for research, including intervention strategies of relevance to them. In doing so, individuals who use AAC become more active participants in the research process, and the issues of social validation are addressed (Bersani, 1999; Krogh & Lindsay, 1999; Schlosser, 1999).

The appropriateness of a research methodology will depend on the questions posed. In AAC, however, concerns about heterogeneity amongst potential participants and the complexity of issues result in the favoring of single case designs, in particular for efficacy research (Calculator, 1999; Light,

1999). The addition of longitudinal descriptive studies and qualitative designs will allow the pieces to come together to deepen and extend understanding of the development of pragmatic skills amongst individuals who use AAC, and the most relevant, appropriate, and effective interventions to facilitate communication competency.

CONCLUSION

The complexity of pragmatic development in AAC arises from the nature of pragmatics itself and heterogeneity amongst individuals who use AAC. Information from literature on typical and atypical development has been drawn on in an attempt to understand how pragmatic skills develop in the face of disabilities that result in severe communication impairments. Overlaid on the emerging picture are the inherent characteristics of AAC and the skills required of both individuals who use AAC and interaction partners. During the relatively brief period of AAC clinical practice and research, many issues have been addressed in attempts to assist individuals who use AAC to become effective and efficient communicators. This journey has revealed the need for new models to represent the communication process in AAC, from which new directions for research and clinical interventions emerge.

REFERENCES

Akhtar, N., Dunham, F., & Dunham, P. (1991). Directive interactions and early vocabulary development: The role of joint attentional focus. *Journal of Child Language, 18,* 41–49.

Baron-Cohen, S., Leslie, A., & Frith, U. (1985). Does the autistic child have a "theory of mind?" *Cognition, 21,* 37–46.

Basil, C. (1992). Social interaction and learned helplessness in severely disabled children. *Augmentative and Alternative Communication, 8,* 188–199.

Bates, E., Begnini, L., Bretherton, I., Camaioni, L., & Volterra, V. (1977). From gesture to the first word: On cognitive and social prerequisites. In M. Lewis & L. Rosenblum (Eds.), *Interaction, conversation, and the development of language* (pp. 347–407). New York: John Wiley & Sons.

Bates, E., Begnini, L., Bretherton, I., Camaioni, L., & Volterra, V. (1979). *The emergence of symbols: Cognition and communication in infancy.* New York: Academic Press.

Bates, E., Camaioni, L., & Volterra, V. (1975). The acquisition of performatives prior to speech. *Merrill-Palmer Quarterly, 21,* 205–226.

Bersani, H., Jr. (1999). Nothing about me without me: A proposal for participatory action research. In F. Lonke, J. Clibbens, H. Arvidson, & L. Lloyd (Eds.), *Augmentative and alternative communication: New dimensions in research and practice* (pp. 262–277). London: Whurr Publishers.

Blackstone, S., & Cassatt, E.L. (1983). Interaction skills in children who use communication aids. In A. Kraat (Ed.), *Communication interactions between aided and natural speakers: An International Project on Communication Aids for the Speech-Impaired report.* Toronto: Canadian Rehabilitation Council for the Disabled.

Bloom, L., & Lahey, M. (1978). *Language development and language disorders.* New York: John Wiley & Sons.

Bode, T. (1997). *Overt co-construction: Speaking adult communication partners in interaction with young children who use AAC systems.* Unpublished master's thesis, University of Melbourne, Australia.

Brinker, R., & Lewis, M. (1982). Discovering the competent handicapped infant: A process approach to assessment and intervention. *Topics in Early Childhood Special Education, 2,* 1–16.

Bruner, J. (1974). The ontogenesis of speech acts. *Journal of Child Language, 2,* 1–19.

Bruner, J. (1981). The social context of language acquisition. *Language and Communication, 2,* 155–178.

Buzolich, M., & Lunger, J. (1995). Empowering system users in peer training. *Augmentative and Alternative Communication, 11,* 37–48.

Buzolich, M.J., & Wiemann, J. (1988). Turn taking in atypical conversations: The case of the speaker/augmented-communicator dyad. *Journal of Speech and Hearing Research, 31,* 3–18.

Calculator, S. (1999). AAC outcomes for children and youths with severe disabilities: When seeing is believing. *Augmentative and Alternative Communication, 15,* 4–12.

Calculator, S., & Dollaghan, C. (1982). The use of communication boards in a residential setting: An evaluation. *Journal of Speech and Hearing Disorders, 47,* 281–287.

Calculator, S., & Luchko, C. (1983). Evaluating the effectiveness of a communication board training program. *Journal of Speech and Hearing Disorders, 48,* 185–191.

Camaioni, L. (1992). Mind knowledge in infancy: The emergence of intentional communication. *Early Development & Parenting, 1,* 15–22.

Carr, E., & Kologinsky, E. (1983). Acquisition of sign language by autistic children: II. Spontaneity and generalization effects. *Journal of Applied Behavior Analysis, 16,* 297–314.

Carter, M., & Maxwell, K. (1998). Promoting interaction with children using augmentative and alternative communication through peer-mediated intervention. *International Journal of Disability, Development and Education, 45,* 75–96.

Chan, J., & Iacono, T. (2001). Gesture and word production in children with Down syndrome. *Augmentative and Alternative Communication, 17,* 73–87.

Chapman, R. (1981). Exploring children's communicative intents. In J. Miller (Ed.), *Assessing language production in children: Experimental procedures* (pp. 111–136). Baltimore: University Park Press.

Cirrin, R., & Rowland, C. (1985). Communicative assessment of nonverbal youths with severe/profound mental retardation. *Mental Retardation, 23,* 52–62.

Crawley, S., & Spiker, D. (1983). Mother–child interactions involving two-year-olds with Down Syndrome: A look at individual differences. *Child Development, 54,* 1312–1323.

Cress, C. (1999). *Joint attention and young children relying on AAC: Research implications for AAC interventions.* Paper presented at the Rehabilitation Engineering and Assistive Technology Society of North America Annual Conference, Long Beach, CA.

Cress, C., Shapley, K., Linke, M., Havelka, S., Deitrich, C., & Elliott, J. (1999). *Intentional communication patterns in young children with physical impairments.* Paper presented at the American Speech-Language-Hearing Association Annual Convention, San Francisco.

Crystal, D., Garman, M., & Fletcher, P. (1989). *Grammatical analysis of language disability* (2nd ed.). London: Whurr Publishers.

Dahlgren, S., Falkman, K., Dahlgren Sandberg, A., & Hjelmquist, E. (1998). *Theory of mind in children with communicative disabilities.* Paper presented at the International Society for Augmentative and Alternative Communication, Dublin, Ireland.

Damico, J. (1985). Clinical discourse analysis: A functional approach to language assessment. In C. Simon (Ed.), *Communication skills and classroom success: Assessment of language-learning disabled students* (pp. 165–206). San Diego: College-Hill Press.

Dattilo, J., & Camarata, S. (1991). Facilitating conversation through self-initiated augmentative communication treatment. *Journal of Applied Behavior Analysis, 24,* 369–378.

Denzin, N. (1989). *The research act: A theoretical introduction to sociological methods* (3rd ed.). Upper Saddle River, NJ: Prentice Hall.

Dewart, H., & Summers, S. (1988). *The pragmatics profile of early communication skills.* London: National Foundation for Educational Research.

Dore, J. (1974). A pragmatic description of early language development. *Journal of Psycholinguistic Research, 3,* 343–350.

Dunst, C. (1985). Communicative competence and deficits: Effects on early social interactions. In E. McDonald & D. Gallagher (Eds.), *Facilitating social-emotional development in multiply handicapped children* (pp. 93–140). Philadelphia: Michael C. Prestegord.

Farrier, L., Yorkston, K., Marriner, N., & Beukelman, D. (1985). Conversational control in nonimpaired speakers using an augmentative communication system. *Augmentative and Alternative Communication, 1,* 65–73.

Franco, F., & Wishart, J. (1995). Use of pointing and other gestures by young children with Down syndrome. *American Journal on Mental Retardation, 100,* 160–182.

Fujiki, M., & Brinton, B. (1994). Social competence and language impairment in children. In S.F. Warren & J. Reichle (Series Eds.) & R.V. Watkins & M.L. Rice (Vol. Eds.), *Communication and language intervention series: Vol. 4. Specific language impairments in children* (pp. 123–144). Baltimore: Paul H. Brookes Publishing Co.

Gallagher, T. (1981). Contingent query sequences within adult–child discourse. *Journal of Child Language, 8,* 51–61.

Gallagher, T. (1991). A retrospective look at clinical pragmatics. In T. Gallagher (Ed.), *Pragmatics of language: Clinical practice issues* (pp. 1–10). San Diego: Singular Publishing Group.

Garvey, C. (1977). The contingent query: A dependent act in conversation. In M. Lewis & L. Rosenblum (Eds.), *Interaction, conversation, and the development of language.* New York: John Wiley & Sons.

Gerber, S., & Kraat, A. (1992). Use of a developmental model of language acquisition: Applications to children using AAC systems. *Augmentative and Alternative Communication, 8,* 19–32.

Glennen, S., & Calculator, S. (1985). Training functional communication board use: A pragmatic approach. *Augmentative and Alternative Communication, 1,* 131–141.

Goossens', C. (1989). Aided communication intervention before assessment: A case study of a child with cerebral palsy. *Augmentative and Alternative Communication, 5,* 14–26.

Grove, N., & Walker, M. (1990). The Makaton vocabulary: Using manual signs and graphic symbols to develop interpersonal communication. *Augmentative and Alternative Communication, 6,* 15–28.

Halliday, M. (1975). *Learning how to mean.* London: Edward Arnold.

Hanson, M., & Hanline, M. (1985). An analysis of response-contingent learning experience of young children. *Journal of The Association for Persons with Severe Handicaps, 10,* 31–40.

Harris, D. (1982). Communicative interaction processes involving nonvocal physically handicapped children. *Topics in Language Disorders, 2,* 21–37.

Heim, M., & Baker-Mills, A. (1996). Early development of symbolic communication and linguistic complexity through augmentative and alternative communication. In S. von Tetzchner & M. Hygum Jensen (Eds.), *Augmentative and alternative communication: European perspectives* (pp. 232–248). London: Whurr Publishers.

Hemmeter, M.L., & Kaiser, A. (1994). Enhanced milieu teaching: Effects of parent-implemented language intervention. *Journal of Early Intervention, 18,* 269–289.

Hetzroni, O., & Harris, O. (1996). Cultural aspects in the development of AAC users. *Augmentative and Alternative Communication, 12,* 52–58.

Hjelmquist, E., & Dahlgren Sandberg, A. (1996). Sound and silence: Interaction in aided language use. In S. von Tetzchner & M. Hygum Jensen (Eds.), *Augmentative and alternative communication: European perspectives* (pp. 137–152). London: Whurr Publishers.

Hunt, P., Alwell, M., & Goetz, L. (1991). Interacting with peers through conversation turntaking with communication book adaptation. *Augmentative and Alternative Communication, 7,* 117–126.

Iacono, T., Balandin, S., & Cupples, L. (2001). Focus group discussions of literacy assessments and web-based reading interventions. *Augmentative and Alternative Communication, 17,* 27–36.

Iacono, T., Carter, M., & Hook, J. (1998). Identification of intentional communication in students with severe multiple disabilities. *Augmentative and Alternative Communication, 14,* 102–114.

Iacono, T., Chan, J., & Waring, R. (1998). Efficacy of a parent-implemented early language intervention based on collaborative consultation. *International Journal of Language and Communication Disorders, 33,* 281–304.

Iacono, T., Waring, R., & Chan, J. (1996). Sampling communicative behaviors in children with intellectual disability in structured and unstructured situations. *European Journal of Disorders of Communication, 31,* 417–431.

Jones, J., & Hunter, D. (1996). Consensus methods for medical and health services research. In N. Mays & C. Pope (Eds.), *Qualitative research in health care* (pp. 46–58). London: BMJ Publishing Group.

Kaiser, A., Ostrosky, M., & Alpert, C. (1993). Training teachers to use environmental arrangement and milieu teaching with nonvocal preschool children. *Journal of The Association for Persons with Severe Handicaps, 18,* 188–199.

Kaul, S. (1999). *A comparative study of language use and its effect on communication interaction patterns in two groups of children with cerebral palsy (speaking & nonspeaking) from Hindi speaking families in Calcutta.* Manchester England: Manchester Metropolitan University.

Kraat, A. (1985). *Communication interaction between aided and natural speakers: An International Project on Communication Aids for the Speech-Impaired study report.* Toronto: Canadian Rehabilitation Council for the Disabled.

Krogh, K., & Lindsay, P. (1999). Including people with disabilities in research: Implications for the field of augmentative and alternative communication. *Augmentative and Alternative Communication, 15,* 222–223.

Landry, S., Garner, P., Pirie, D., & Swank, P. (1994). Effects of social context and mothers' requesting strategies on Down's syndrome children's social responsiveness. *Developmental Psychology, 30,* 293–302.

Layton, T. (1988). Language training with autistic children using four different modes of presentation. *Journal of Communication Disorders, 21,* 333–350.

Liamputtong Rice, P., & Ezzy, D. (1999). *Qualitative research methods: A health focus.* London: Oxford University Press.

Light, J. (1988). Interaction involving individuals using augmentative and alternative communication systems: State of the art. *Augmentative and Alternative Communication, 4,* 66–82.

Light, J. (1989). Toward a definition of communicative competence for individuals using augmentative and alternative communication systems. *Augmentative and Alternative Communication, 5,* 137–144.

Light, J. (1997). "Let's go star fishing": Reflections on the contexts of language learning for children who used aided AAC. *Augmentative and Alternative Communication, 13,* 158–171.

Light, J. (1999). Do augmentative and alternative communication interventions really make a difference? *Augmentative and Alternative Communication, 15,* 13–24.

Light, J.C., & Binger, C. (1998). *Building communicative competence with individuals who use augmentative and alternative communication.* Baltimore: Paul H. Brookes Publishing Co.

Light, J., Binger, C., Agate, T., & Ramsay, K. (1999). Teaching partner-focused questions to individuals who use augmentative and alternative communication to enhance their communicative competence. *Journal of Speech, Language, and Hearing Research, 42,* 241–255.

Light, J., Collier, B., & Parnes, P. (1985a). Communicative interactions between young nonspeaking physically disabled children and their primary caregivers: Part 1. Discourse patterns. *Augmentative and Alternative Communication, 1,* 74–83.

Light, J., Collier, B., & Parnes, P. (1985b). Communicative interactions between young nonspeaking physically disabled children and their primary caregivers: Part II. *Augmentative and Alternative Communication, 1,* 98–107.

Light, J., Collier, B., & Parnes, P. (1985c). Communicative interactions between young nonspeaking physically disabled children and their primary caregivers: Part III. Modes of communication. *Augmentative and Alternative Communication, 1,* 125–133.

Light, J., Dattilo, J., English, J., Gutierrez, L., & Hartz, J. (1992). Instructing facilitators to support the communication of people who use augmentative communication systems. *Journal of Speech and Hearing Research, 35,* 865–875.

Locke, J. (1993). *The child's path to spoken language.* Cambridge: Harvard University Press.

Locke, P., & Mirenda, P. (1988). A computer-supported communication approach for a child with severe communication, visual, and cognitive impairments: A case study. *Augmentative and Alternative Communication, 4,* 15–22.

Loveland, K., Landry, S., Hughes, S., Hall, S., & McEvoy, R. (1988). Speech acts and the pragmatic deficits of autism. *Journal of Speech and Hearing Research, 31,* 593–604.

Lund, S., & Light, J. (2001). *Fifteen years later: An investigation of the long-term outcomes of augmentative and alternative communication interventions.* (Student-Initiated Research Grant HB24B990069). University Park: Pennsylvania State University.

Mahoney, G., Fors, S., & Wood, S. (1990). Maternal directive behavior revisited. *American Journal of Mental Retardation, 94,* 398–406.

Marfo, K. (1992). Correlates of maternal directiveness with children who are developmentally delayed. *American Journal of Orthopsychiatry, 62,* 219–233.

Mathy-Laikko, P., Iacono, T., Villarruel, F., Ratcliff, A., Yoder, D., & Vanderheiden, G. (1989). Teaching a deaf-blind multihandicapped child to use a tactile augmentative communication device. *Augmentative and Alternative Communication, 5,* 249–256.

McCathran, R., Yoder, P., & Warren, S. (1995). The role of directives in early language intervention. *Journal of Early Intervention, 19,* 91–101.

McCollum, J., & Hemmeter, M.L. (1997). Parent–child intervention when children have disabilities. In M.J. Guralnick (Ed.), *The effectiveness of early intervention* (pp. 549–576). Baltimore: Paul H. Brookes Publishing Co.

McConachie, H., & Ciccognani, A. (1995). "What's in the box?": Assessing physically disabled children's communication skills. *Child Language Teaching and Therapy, 11*, 253–262.

McLean, L., Brady, N., McLean, J., & Behrens, G.A. (1999). Communication forms and functions of children and adults with severe mental retardation in community institutional settings. *Journal of Speech, Language, and Hearing Research, 42*, 231–240.

McLean, J., McLean, L., Brady, N., & Etter, R. (1991). Communication profiles of two types of gesture using nonverbal persons with severe to profound mental retardation. *Journal of Speech and Hearing Research, 34*, 294–308.

McLean, J., & Snyder-McLean, L. (1978). *A transactional approach to early language training.* Columbus, OH: Merrill.

McLean, J., & Snyder-McLean, L. (1987). Form and function of communicative behavior among persons with severe developmental disabilities. *Australian and New Zealand Journal of Developmental Disabilities, 13*, 83–98.

McNaughton, D., & Light, J. (1989). Teaching facilitators to support the communication skills of an adult with severe cognitive disabilities: A case study. *Augmentative and Alternative Communication, 5*, 35–41.

McTear, M., & Conti-Ramsden, G. (1992). *Pragmatic disability in children.* London: Whurr Publishers.

Miller, J.F. (1987). Language and communication characteristics in children with Down syndrome. In S.M. Pueschel, C. Tingey, J.E. Rynders, A.C. Crocker, & D.M. Crutcher (Eds.), *New perspectives on Down syndrome* (pp. 233–262). Baltimore: Paul H. Brookes Publishing Co.

Miller, M., & Kraat, A. (1984). Hey you, I've got something to say: A study of the attention-getting ability of a nonspeaking, physically disabled pre-schooler. In A. Kraat (Ed.), *Communication interactions between aided and natural speakers: An International Project on Communication Aids for the Speech-Impaired report.* Toronto: Canadian Rehabilitation Council for the Disabled.

Mirenda, P., & Iacono, T. (1988). Strategies for promoting augmentative and alternative communication in natural contexts with students with autism. *Focus on Autistic Behavior, 3*, 1–16.

Mirenda, P., & Santogrossi, J. (1985). A prompt-free strategy to teach pictorial communication system use. *Augmentative and Alternative Communication, 1*, 143–150.

Moore, C.M. (1994). *Group techniques for idea building* (2nd ed.). Thousand Oaks, CA: Sage Publications.

Mundy, P., Kasari, C., Sigman, M., & Ruskin, E. (1995). Nonverbal communication and early language acquisition in children with Down syndrome. *Journal of Speech and Hearing Research, 38*, 157–167.

Mundy, P., Sigman, M., & Kasari, C. (1990). A longitudinal study of joint attention and language development in autistic children. *Journal of Autism and Developmental Disability, 20*, 115–128.

Mundy, P., Sigman, M., Kasari, C., & Yirmiya, N. (1988). Nonverbal communication skills in Down syndrome children. *Child Development, 59*, 235–249.

Ogletree, B., Wetherby, A., & Westling, D. (1992). Profile of the prelinguistic intentional communicative behaviors of children with profound mental retardation. *American Journal of Mental Retardation, 97*, 186–196.

O'Keefe, B., & Dattilo, J. (1992). Teaching response-recode form to adults with mental retardation using AAC systems. *Augmentative and Alternative Communication, 8*, 224–233.

Paul, R. (1997). Facilitating transitions in language development for children using AAC. *Augmentative and Alternative Communication, 13,* 141–148.

Plante, E., Swisher, L., Kiernan, B., & Restrepo, M. (1993). Language matches: Illuminating or confounding? *Journal of Speech and Hearing Research, 36,* 772–776.

Porter, G., & Kirkland, J. (1995). *Integrating augmentative and alternative communication into group programs: Utilising the principles of conductive education.* Melbourne, Australia: COA Press, the Spastic Society of Victoria.

Prizant, B., & Wetherby, A. (1985). Intentional communicative behavior of children with autism: Theoretical and practical issues. *Australian Journal of Human Communication Disorders, 13,* 25–59.

Prizant, B., & Wetherby, A. (1987). Communicative intent: A framework for understanding social-communicative behavior in autism. *Journal of the American Academy of Child Psychiatry, 26,* 472–479.

Prutting, C., & Kirchner, D. (1983). Applied pragmatics. In T. Gallagher & C. Prutting (Eds.), *Pragmatic assessment and intervention issues in language* (pp. 29–64). San Diego: College-Hill Press.

Reichle, J., & Johnston, S. (1999). Teaching the conditional use of communicative requests to two school-age children with severe developmental disabilities. *Language, Speech, and Hearing Services in Schools, 30,* 324–334.

Roach, M., Barratt, M., Miller, J., & Leavitt, L. (1998). The structure of mother–child play: Young children with Down syndrome and typically developing children. *Developmental Psychology, 34,* 77–87.

Rowland, C., & Schweigert, P. (2000). Tangible symbols, tangible outcomes. *Augmentative and Alternative Communication, 16,* 61–78.

Salvin, A., Routh, D., Foster, R., & Lovejoy, K. (1977). Acquisition of modified American Sign Language by a mute autistic child. *Journal of Autism and Childhood Schizophrenia, 7,* 359–371.

Sarria, E., Gomez, J., & Tamarit, J. (1996). Joint attention and alternative language intervention in autism: Implications of theory for practice. In S. von Tetzchner & M. Hygum Jensen (Eds.), *Augmentative and alternative communication: European perspectives* (pp. 65–88). London: Whurr Publications.

Schlosser, R. (1999). An introduction to consumer perspectives in AAC research: Approaches, techniques and their theoretical underpinnings. In F. Loncke, J. Clibbens, H. Arvidson, & L. Lloyd (Eds.), *Augmentative and alternative communication: New directions in research and practice* (pp. 257–261). London: Whurr Publishers.

Schlosser, R., & Braun, U. (1994). Efficacy of AAC interventions: Methodological issues in evaluating behavior change, generalization, and effects. *Augmentative and Alternative Communication, 10,* 207–223.

Schweigert, P. (1989). Use of microswitch technology to facilitate social contingency awareness as a basis for early communication skills. *Augmentative and Alternative Communication, 5,* 192–198.

Schweigert, P., & Rowland, C. (1992). Early communication and microtechnology: Instructional sequence and case studies of children with severe multiple disabilities. *Augmentative and Alternative Communication, 8,* 273–286.

Seligman, M. (1975). *Helplessness: On depression, development and death.* San Francisco: W.H. Freeman.

Siegel-Causey, E., & Guess, D. (1989). *Enhancing nonsymbolic communication interactions among learners with severe disabilities.* Baltimore: Paul H. Brookes Publishing Co.

Smith, L., & von Tetzchner, S. (1986). Communicative, sensorimotor, and language skills of young children with Down syndrome. *American Journal of Mental Deficiency, 91,* 57–66.

Stephenson, J., & Linfoot, K. (1995). Choice-making as a natural context for teaching early communication board use to a ten year old boy with no spoken language and severe intellectual disability. *Australia & New Zealand Journal of Developmental Disabilities, 20,* 263–286.

Sugarman, S. (1984). The development of preverbal communication: Its contribution and limits in promoting the development of language. In R. Schiefelbusch & J. Pickar (Eds.), *The acquisition of communicative competence* (Vol. VIII). Baltimore: University Park Press.

Todman, J., Rankin, D., & File, P. (1999). The use of stored text in computer-aided conversation: A single-case experiment. *Journal of Language and Social Psychology, 18,* 287–309.

Tomasello, M., & Camaioni, L. (1997). A comparison of the gestural communication of apes and human infants. *Human Development, 40,* 7–24.

Udwin, O., & Yule, W. (1990). Augmentative communication systems taught to cerebral palsied children: A longitudinal study: I. The acquisition of signs and symbols, and syntactic aspects of their use over time. *British Journal of Disorders of Communication, 25,* 295–309.

Udwin, O., & Yule, W. (1991). Augmentative communication systems taught to cerebral palsied children: A longitudinal study: II. Pragmatic features of sign and symbol use. *British Journal of Disorders of Communication, 26,* 149–162.

von Tetzchner, S., & Jensen, M. (Eds.). (1996). *Augmentative and alternative communication: European perspectives.* London: Whurr Publishers.

von Tetzchner, S., & Martinsen, H. (1996). Words and strategies: Conversations with young children who use aided language. In S. von Tetzchner & M. Hygum Jensen (Eds.), *Augmentative and alternative communication: European perspectives* (pp. 65–100). London: Whurr Publishers.

Wacker, D., Wiggins, B., Fowler, M., & Berg, W. (1988). Training students with profound or multiple handicaps to make requests via microswitches. *Journal of Applied Behavior Analysis, 21,* 331–343.

Warren, S. (1992). Facilitating basic vocabulary acquisition with milieu teaching procedures. *Journal of Early Intervention, 16,* 235–251.

Warren, S., & Bambara, L. (1989). An experimental analysis of milieu language intervention: Teaching the action–object form. *Journal of Speech and Hearing Disorders, 54,* 448–461.

Warren, S., & Yoder, P. (1998). Facilitating the transition from preintentional to intentional communication. In S.F. Warren & M.E. Fey (Series Eds.) & A.M. Wetherby, S.F. Warren, & J. Reichle (Vol. Eds.), *Transitions in prelinguistic communication* (pp. 365–384). Baltimore: Paul H. Brookes Publishing Co.

Warren, S., Yoder, P., Gazdag, G., Kim, K., & Jones, H. (1993). Facilitating prelinguisitc communication skills in young children with developmental delay. *Journal of Speech and Hearing Research, 36,* 83–97.

Watson, J. (1966). The development and generalization of "contingency awareness" in early infancy: Some hypotheses. *Merrill-Palmer Quarterly, 12,* 123–135.

Werner, H., & Kaplan, B. (1984). *Symbol formation.* Mahwah, NJ: Lawrence Erlbaum Associates.

Wetherby, A., Cain, D., Yonclas, D., & Walker, V. (1988). Analysis of intentional communication of normal children from prelinguisitic to the multiword stage. *Journal of Speech and Hearing Research, 31,* 240–252.

Wetherby, A., & Prizant, B. (1989). The expression of communicative intent: Assessment guidelines. *Seminars in Speech and Language, 10,* 77–91.

Wetherby, A.M., & Prizant, B.M. (2003). *Communication and Symbolic Behavior Scales manual: Normed edition.* Baltimore: Paul H. Brookes Publishing Co.

Wetherby, A., & Rodriguez, G. (1992). Measurement of communicative intentions in normally developing children during structured and unstructured contexts. *Journal of Speech and Hearing Research, 35,* 130–138.

Wetherby, A., Yonclas, D., & Bryan, A. (1989). Communicative profiles of preschool children with handicaps: Implications for early identification. *Journal of Speech and Hearing Disorders, 54,* 148–158.

Wolf Nelson, N. (1992). Performance is the prize: Language competence and performance among AAC users. *Augmentative and Alternative Communication, 8,* 3–18.

Yoder, P., & Feagans, L. (1988). Mothers' attributions of communication to prelinguistic behavior of developmentally delayed and mentally retarded infants. *American Journal of Mental Deficiency, 93,* 36–43.

Yoder, P., Warren, S., McCathren, R., & Leew, S. (1998). Does adult responsivity to child behavior facilitate communication development? In S.F. Warren & M.E. Fey (Series Eds.) & A.M. Wetherby, S.F. Warren, & J. Reichle (Vol. Eds.), *Transitions in prelinguistic communication* (pp. 39–58). Baltimore: Paul H. Brookes Publishing Co.

11

Finding a Place in the "Social Circle of Life"

The Development of Sociorelational Competence by Individuals Who Use AAC

Janice C. Light, Kara B. Arnold, and Elizabeth A. Clark

> I am alone in my thoughts. I am alone among other people. My identity is locked inside my mind. . . . The inability to speak, or the inability to communicate one's own words fluently, is the greatest disability a person can have in the social circle of life. (Diamanti, 2000, p. 98)

These words were written by a man with cerebral palsy who uses augmentative and alternative communication (AAC). They poignantly illustrate the human longing for meaningful social relationships as well as the powerful role of communication in fulfilling this longing. If individuals who require AAC are to connect with others in meaningful ways, if they are to touch other people and have their lives touched by others, they need to develop effective sociorelational skills. Sociorelational skills involve the *interpersonal* aspects of communication (e.g., demonstrating an interest in others, putting partners at ease, developing a positive rapport).

In 1989, Light proposed that the development of sociorelational skills is critical in the development of communicative competence by individuals who require AAC. She argued that communicative competence rests on the integration of knowledge, judgment, and skills in four interrelated domains: the linguistic domain, the operational domain, the social domain (including both sociolinguistic and sociorelational aspects), and the strategic domain (see Chapter 1 for further discussion). To date, research in the AAC field has focused primarily on issues related to the development of linguistic and sociolinguistic competencies (see Chapters 3, 5, 6, and 10). There has also been increased interest in the development of operational competence, especially as it relates to the learning of AAC technologies (e.g., see Beukelman & Ball, in press; Light & Drager, in press; see also Chapter 7). The sociorelational domain has largely been ignored within the AAC field despite its central importance to the development of meaningful social relationships and the attainment of communicative competence. Thus, the focus of this chapter is on the development of knowledge, judgment, and skills within the social domain, specifically in the sociorelational domain. (Readers are referred to Chapter 10 for further discussion of issues related to sociolinguistic or pragmatic development, another key area within the social domain.)

IMPORTANCE OF SOCIORELATIONAL SKILLS

According to Light (1989), the sociorelational domain includes knowledge, judgment, and skills in the *interpersonal* aspects of communication. Light (1988) proposed the following types of sociorelational skills that may further communicative competence: demonstrating an interest in others, participating in interactions actively, being responsive to partners, putting partners at ease, and projecting a positive self-image. The field of second-language learning has also emphasized the importance of sociorelational skills in the development of communicative competence in a second language. For example, Rubin (1975) argued that "good language learners" demonstrate a strong drive to communicate with others, a willingness to make mistakes in order to communicate, and a lack of inhibition. Savignon agreed that self-confidence is critical to the development of communicative competence: "It may be that communicative confidence leads to communicative competence" (1983, p. 45).

The development of sociorelational skills is of critical importance in meeting communication goals, especially in establishing, maintaining, and developing *social closeness* interactions. In these interactions, the focus is on the personal bond or relationship between the participants (Light, 1988). As the quote by Diamanti (2000) at the beginning of this chapter suggests, attaining and maintaining social closeness is frequently a priority for people. Unfortunately, many people with disabilities have limited social networks and very few friends (Fine, 1996). As a result, they may experience significant loneliness; this loneliness and social isolation may negatively impact overall health, mood, and behavior. O'Keefe concluded that, "Perhaps no prerequisite of a quality of life is placed more at risk by communicative disability than that of belonging" (1996, p. 227). If individuals who use AAC are to have opportunities to develop social closeness and achieve a high quality of life, they need to develop effective sociorelational skills.

Sociorelational skills may not be *as* critical to ensuring that individuals who use AAC are able to meet other communication goals such as expressing needs and wants and exchanging information effectively; however, socio-relational skills still play an important role in determining the ultimate effectiveness of these types of interactions. In interactions to express needs and wants, the focus is on obtaining the desired object or activity (or rejecting the undesired object or activity); in interactions for the purpose of information exchange, the focus is on the content of the information being shared (e.g., the curriculum at school, the agenda for a meeting at work; Light, 1988). These types of interactions do not focus specifically on the interpersonal relationship between the participants, so sociorelational skills may play a somewhat less critical role in these interactions than in interactions intended to build social closeness; however, interactions to express needs and wants and to share information may be more successful if individuals who require AAC have well-developed sociorelational skills. Communication partners such as teachers, aides, personal care attendants, classmates, and co-workers are more apt to communicate with people they enjoy than with people that they do not enjoy (e.g., McNaughton, Light, & Arnold, 2002; McNaughton, Light, & Gulla, 2002). If individuals who use AAC have well-developed sociorelational skills and are able to build positive relationships with others, they are more apt to be effective in meeting *all* of their communication goals—building social closeness, fulfilling needs and wants, and exchanging information with others.

Any consideration of sociorelational skills must focus on both sides of the communication process for communication is a transactional process. People influence each other in the course of their interactions and mutually determine the outcomes of the interactions. Thus, it is important to consider not only the sociorelational skills of the individual who uses AAC, but also the barriers and supports provided by partners in the environment. Therefore, the specific goals of this chapter are threefold:

1. To review what is known about the development of sociorelational skills by individuals with developmental disabilities who require AAC and to consider the implications for effective practice
2. To review what is known about the attitudes of others toward individuals who require AAC, to consider the influence of attitude barriers and other opportunity barriers on social relationships, and to discuss implications for intervention
3. To highlight what is *not* known and, thus, suggest directions for future research to advance understanding and practice in the field and improve outcomes for individuals who require AAC

DEVELOPMENT OF SOCIORELATIONAL SKILLS

In order to ensure that individuals who use AAC acquire the sociorelational skills that they need to develop communicative competence and establish meaningful social relationships, three issues must be considered: 1) the unique challenges that individuals who use AAC may experience acquiring socio-relational skills; 2) the specific sociorelational skills that should be targeted as goals for intervention; and 3) the components of effective interventions to teach these skills.

Challenges in Sociorelational Development

To date, we have limited empirical data on the development of sociorelational skills by individuals with developmental disabilities who use AAC. Warrick (1988) argued that individuals who use AAC frequently experience greater difficulty in the development of sociorelational skills than in the acquisition of other skills. Why might the acquisition of sociorelational skills be challenging for individuals who use AAC? There are four possible explanations to consider:

- Individuals who use AAC may lack the means to demonstrate socio-relational skills.
- They may lack the social experiences required to develop these skills.
- They may experience specific deficits in social development that impact their use of sociorelational skills.
- They may not receive appropriate intervention to facilitate their learning of these skills.

Lack of Means to Demonstrate Sociorelational Skills   Some in-dividuals who use AAC may have developed effective sociorelational skills but lack reliable means to demonstrate these skills within daily interactions. It is possible to communicate some sociorelational skills through nonlinguistic means. For example, people may communicate interest in their partners by smiling, making eye contact, and providing appropriate listener feedback in response to partner comments (e.g., head nod, facial expression); however, in-dividuals who require AAC and have significant motor impairments may have difficulty using these unaided modes and may produce signals (e.g., facial ex-pressions, vocalizations) that are unconventional and difficult for partners to interpret, thus impairing their sociorelational competence (Higginbotham & Yoder, 1982).

Other sociorelational skills (e.g., asking partner-focused questions) re-quire access to linguistic modes of communication. Many individuals with significant communication disabilities are dependent on others to provide them with access to appropriate vocabulary (Beukelman, McGinnis, & Mor-row, 1991). Because sociorelational issues have been neglected in the AAC field, many professionals fail to consider sociorelational skills a priority and fail to provide individuals who use AAC with the necessary vocabulary to fa-cilitate use of these skills. For example, Light, Binger, Agate, and Ramsay

(1999) reported on a research study designed to teach the use of partner-focused questions to six individuals who used AAC as a strategy for the participants to demonstrate an interest in their communication partners. At the start of the study, *none* of the six participants had access to appropriate partner-focused questions within their AAC systems; they lacked the means to demonstrate an interest in their partners. Intervention was two pronged. The individuals who used AAC were provided with 1) the vocabulary and means to express partner-focused questions; *and* 2) instruction in the use of this type of question. Given the design of the study, it was impossible to determine whether simply providing the necessary vocabulary would have resulted in increased use of partner-focused questions; however, it is clear that *without* access to the means to express sociorelational skills, individuals who require AAC will have limited success building meaningful social relationships.

Light used the case of Shawn, a woman in her mid-twenties who had significant speech and motor impairments resulting from a brain tumor, to illustrate the devastating impact when AAC systems fail to provide a means to express sociorelational skills and develop social closeness:

> The previous AAC interventions failed *not* because Shawn was unmotivated to communicate or because she was noncompliant, but rather the AAC interventions failed because they did not provide Shawn with a means to attain her most important communication goal: social closeness. (1997, p. 64)

If individuals who require AAC are to demonstrate effective sociorelational skills, they must have the means available to do so. Specifically, they must have access to appropriate AAC systems and vocabulary to support the use of sociorelational skills and strategies.

Lack of Social Experiences to Develop Sociorelational Skills

Sociorelational skills are learned over time through social interactions with others (Guralnick & Neville, 1997). As individuals engage in different social interactions, they have the opportunity to "read" a variety of social situations, generate sociorelational behaviors in response to these situations, observe the consequences of these behaviors on others, and determine the situations in which these behaviors are effective or not.

Unfortunately, many individuals who require AAC find themselves isolated socially and have few opportunities to build sociorelational skills through interactions with a wide range of partners. Light (1997) argued that the lack of meaningful opportunities to interact with others is a primary barrier in the development of communicative competence for many individuals who use AAC. She used the example of a 25-year-old man with cerebral palsy to illustrate the point. This man lived at home with his elderly mother; he had finished high school and was not employed. He typically interacted with only three people in a week: his mother, his speech-language pathologist, and a neighbor who provided technical support for his computer system. With so few opportunities for interactions within a week, this man obviously had a severely limited experiential base to allow him to develop effective socio-relational skills.

The already limited opportunities for social interaction experienced by individuals who use AAC may be further restricted by negative attitudes toward people with disabilities within society. As a result of these attitude barriers, prospective communication partners may avoid or limit meaningful interaction with individuals who use AAC. For example, an employer of an individual who used AAC described the reluctance of co-workers to interact with the individual: "I think probably 80% of the people that worked in that building would not set foot at the door to provide any social communication" (McNaughton, Light, & Gulla, 2002). (Further discussion of the problems associated with attitude barriers is provided in the section on Ensuring Meaningful Opportunities for Social Interaction.)

Specific Deficits in Social Development   Some individuals who require AAC may experience specific deficits that have an impact on their use of sociorelational skills. The development of sociorelational skills requires individuals to be able to take their partners' perspectives and to understand how their own communication and actions will affect their partners. Individuals must perceive, decode, and interpret social cues issued by others; select an appropriate social response from their repertoire; consider the perspectives of others and the potential consequences of the planned response; and then act. Doll, Sands, Wehmeyer, and Palmer (1996) referred to these skills as metarepresentation skills. Metarepresentation skills allow people to assess social situations and then decide what to do or say. If people do not have well-developed metarepresentation skills, they typically fail to take into account the perspectives of others. They assume that others see things as they themselves do and that others act as they would. This erroneous assumption is problematic in social situations because it leads people to misjudge the consequences of their communication and actions (Light & Gulens, 2000).

Individuals with significant communication impairments may be especially at risk in the development of metarepresentation skills, for they may have difficulty accessing essential information about others' feelings, intentions, and reactions due to their limited communicative interactions. Their lack of social experiences may be further aggravated when individuals who use AAC do not receive honest social feedback in response to their actions. For example, partners may not provide honest feedback when an individual who uses AAC behaves in a rude or inappropriate manner. Without realistic and appropriate feedback from others, it is extremely difficult for individuals who use AAC to learn to evaluate their own performance and to develop realistic perceptions of their own strengths and limitations. This problem is highlighted by the following comments from an employer who had hired an individual who used AAC: "I think a lot of [individuals who use AAC] have been told they have more . . . skills than they actually do. I think that's a real issue" (McNaughton, Light, & Gulla, 2002).

Many individuals who require AAC may also experience difficulties developing metarepresentation skills because they have limitations in their working memory capacity (Light & Lindsay, 1991). As a result, they may have difficulty holding in working memory the wide range of information required to demonstrate effective metarepresentation skills (e.g., their proposed action or message; the personalities, values, and priorities of each of the people involved in the situation; the anticipated reactions of these partners; the consequences of these reactions).

Deficits in the Development of "Theory of Mind"   There has been significant attention in the research literature to children's development of "theory of mind" (Tager-Flusberg, 1997). This research may have important implications for the development of metarepresentation skills by children who use AAC. The research on theory of mind has tracked children's cognitive and linguistic development as they learn that different people have different perspectives, beliefs, and understandings. Specifically, this research has investigated how children learn that the mind does not necessarily present a blueprint of reality, but rather a representation and interpretation of reality.

The development of theory of mind marks an important transition in social development. Once children understand that others have different understandings, beliefs, and perspectives, their social relationships are transformed for they begin to be able to consider the social consequences of their actions (Perner, 1988). Impairments in acquiring a theory of mind will clearly affect the development of sociorelational skills because without a theory of mind individuals will fail to accurately consider the perspectives of others. In fact, Tager-Flusberg argued that "Much of our everyday use of language involves understanding intentions and related mental states in other people. Impairments in a theory of mind lead to a highly restricted use of language" (1997, pp. 155–156).

There is a growing body of research that provides evidence that children with autism have a specific impairment in acquiring a theory of mind and that this deficit may account for many of the observed impairments in social interactions, communication, and symbolic play that are the hallmarks of autism (e.g., Baron-Cohen, Leslie, & Frith, 1985; Tager-Flusberg, 1997). Children with other disabilities who use AAC may also experience specific difficulties in the acquisition of theory of mind. Tager-Flusberg argued that the relationship between the development of a theory of mind and the development of language skills is not a unidirectional relationship, but rather it is a bi-directional relationship. The development of theory of mind supports the development of social interaction, communication, and the use of language. At the same time, language skills, especially syntactic knowledge, seem to influence the development of a theory of mind. If this is the case, then there is reason to believe that children who require AAC and experience significant challenges in language development may be at risk in the development of a theory of mind (see Chapter 3 for further discussion of the development of linguistic skills, including syntactic knowledge, by individuals who use AAC). For example, many individuals who use AAC may not have access in their AAC systems to the types of state verbs (e.g., believe, think, know, feel) that are critical to the development of theory of mind. It is unclear how lack of access to this type of vocabulary might influence the development of theory of mind.

Future research is clearly required to explore the development of theory of mind in children who require AAC; specifically, this research should investigate the effect of language skills on theory of mind and the effect of theory of mind on communication development and social relationships for children who require AAC. Should it be determined that children who use AAC are at risk for developing theory of mind, then future research should also consider how best to remediate this problem. For example, Tager-Flusberg (1997) proposed that syntactic training may be required to support individuals with autism in their capacity to understand the minds of others, to use language in more advanced ways, and to thus build improved social relationships. To date, there has been only limited attention to the development of effective interventions to remediate syntactic deficits in individuals who require AAC; however, research by Lund and Light (in press) suggests that, even as adults, individuals who use AAC can acquire new syntactic and morphological skills when provided with appropriate instruction.

Lack of Appropriate Instruction   Regardless of the source of the difficulties in acquiring sociorelational skills, many individuals who use AAC will require concerted intervention to ensure the development of knowledge, judgment, and skills in the sociorelational domain. Given the lack of attention to sociorelational skills in the AAC field, it is reasonable to assume that few individuals who use AAC actually receive concerted intervention to target sociorelational skills. Without appropriate instruction, it is not surprising that many individuals who use AAC fail to learn these skills successfully.

INTERVENTIONS TO BUILD SOCIORELATIONAL SKILLS

Intervention to build sociorelational competence must 1) target appropriate skills, and 2) implement effective practices to support the acquisition, generalization, and maintenance of these skills. The following sections consider each of these components of intervention in turn.

Sociorelational Skills to Target as Goals

Little is known about the specific sociorelational skills that support effective interpersonal relationships. It is by no means clear what factors determine whether an individual who uses AAC becomes "an accepted, valued, contributing member of a larger community" (Brinton & Fujiki, 1993, p. 10). Table 11.1 presents a summary of some examples of sociorelational skills that may be important for individuals who use AAC. It is important to note that, as of 2003, there is still only limited empirical evidence as to which of these skills actually contribute to effective social relationships and improved communicative competence.

Light (1997) argued that the specific constellation of skills required to build communicative competence will no doubt vary across individuals who use AAC, depending on numerous factors (see Chapter 1). Thus, it is dangerous to assume that there will be a single list of sociorelational skills that should be targeted for intervention with all individuals who use AAC regard-

Table 11.1.   Examples of target sociorelational skills and specific sociorelational behaviors to enhance interpersonal relationships

Examples of target sociorelational skills	Examples of specific sociorelational behaviors
Participate actively in interactions	Fulfill obligatory turns in interactions Fulfill nonobligatory turns in interactions Take turns reciprocally in interactions Contribute meaningfully in communicative turns
Be responsive to partners	Respond to partners' questions Respond to partners' comments Provide appropriate listener feedback (e.g., smile, eye contact)
Demonstrate interest in partners	Attend to partners; listen carefully Provide appropriate listener feedback (e.g., smile, eye contact) Ask partner-focused questions Express empathy as appropriate
Put partners at ease	Use an introduction strategy to describe means of communication and partner's role Use humor Display positive affect (e.g., smile) Provide positive feedback to partners
Project a positive, confident self image	Try to communicate with others even after making mistakes Demonstrate relaxed body posture Express enthusiasm Share personal thoughts and feelings as appropriate
Engage partners in interaction	Initiate interactions with others Select topics of mutual interest
Maintain a positive rapport with partner	Provide nonjudgmental responses; display respect Provide encouragement and positive feedback to partners Express affiliation Resolve conflicts using appropriate strategies

less of age, gender, personality, and other factors. Rather, various factors may influence the decision as to which sociorelational skills are priorities for which individuals at which points in time. Factors that might be expected to influence the selection of appropriate sociorelational skills as targets for intervention include factors intrinsic to the individual who uses AAC such as age, gender, culture, and personality, as well as extrinsic factors such as the context and partner.

Age   Different social strategies and skills are expected and required of communicators at different ages. Guralnick and Neville (1997) concluded that different social skills and behavior patterns emerge at different developmental stages in order to meet different social demands. The types of sociorelational skills required of preschool-age children who use AAC will differ from those required of adolescents or adults. For example, we may expect preschoolers to engage actively in social interactions with others; however, from a developmental perspective, we do not expect them to demonstrate well-developed other-orientation skills (i.e., a sensitivity to others' thoughts and feelings). In contrast, we expect adults not only to engage actively in social interactions, but also to demonstrate other-orientation skills to convey an interest in their partners.

Gender   Age is not the only factor that may influence the types of skills required of individuals who use AAC. Gender may also influence the selection of skills as priorities for instruction. For example, Stuart (1991) reviewed the literature on the differences between "male talk" and "female talk" and reported that men and women make connections in different ways within social interactions. According to Stuart, the literature suggests that women tend to talk more about people and interpersonal matters, whereas men tend to structure their interactions around work, sports, and so forth. These different types of interactions may require different types of sociorelational competencies. For example, other orientation skills (i.e., demonstrating an interest in the partner) may be valued more by women than men, whereas active participation in social interactions may be valued more by men than by women. Future research is required to determine how gender affects the value attached to different sociorelational skills, if it does at all.

Culture   Individuals who require AAC have diverse cultural backgrounds (Soto, Huer, & Taylor, 1997). Cultural history, practices, and orientation will influence the beliefs, values, communication styles, behaviors, and specific sociorelational skills that are valued by individuals who use AAC and their families. Bridges (2000) illustrated how the value attached to different skills varies across cultures through a case example of a young child who required AAC and was a Lumbee Indian. Within the Lumbee culture and in this child's church, significant value was attached to "making a joyful noise";

however, the same value was not attached to this communication skill in the child's music class at school, where he was discouraged from vocalizing loudly in class. In order to support this child's development of communicative competence and his participation in his social communities, it was critical for the AAC team to understand the cultural contexts of his communities.

Assessment of the cultural context of communication must be on an individual basis. Soto and colleagues cautioned that

> An individual's culture . . . is not a diagnostic category that necessarily explains how an individual thinks or acts. Change and variability are intrinsic to culture. First, cultural groups are constantly evolving as a result of contact with other groups. Second, individuals vary in the degree to which they identify themselves with a particular group. (1997, p. 406)

Care must be taken to avoid cultural stereotypes in targeting skills as priorities for intervention; rather, goal setting must focus on the individual values and priorities of the person who uses AAC and his or her family.

Personality   Individuals who use AAC each come to their social interactions with a unique personality (e.g., outgoing, quiet, humorous). These character traits will no doubt influence the types of sociorelational skills that will be an appropriate fit for each individual. For example, some individuals who use AAC may make effective use of humor as a strategy to put partners at ease and establish a positive social rapport (see Chapter 12). Others may be more serious in their demeanor and may prefer to establish social closeness by listening attentively to their partners and providing feedback (e.g., Blau, 1986; Higginbotham & Yoder, 1982). Little is known about the interaction between personality traits and the development of sociorelational competence; future research is warranted to better delineate this interaction.

Context and Partner   The specific sociorelational skills that are required of individuals who use AAC will vary, not only based on factors intrinsic to the individual who uses AAC and the broader cultural context of the interaction but also based on extrinsic factors such as the immediate social context and the partner(s). Light (1997) argued that different partners might value different types of communication skills that might be used by individuals who require AAC. For example, Light, Corbett, Gullapalli, and Lepkowski (1995) found that adults valued the use of partner-focused questions by individuals who used AAC and perceived the individuals who used AAC to be more competent communicators when they asked these types of questions than when they did not. In contrast, adolescents did not seem to value the use of partner-focused questions as much; the researchers concluded that the adolescents may have been more self-focused themselves and may have had fewer expectations that peers be other-oriented. As this example suggests, the need for specific sociorelational skills will depend not only on the characteristics of the individual who uses AAC but also on the characteristics of the partners and the context of the interaction.

Challenging Behaviors In addition to sociorelational skills that have a positive impact on social interactions, it is also important to consider maladaptive behaviors (e.g., screaming, biting) that may negatively impact an individual's social relationships (Brinton & Fujiki, 1993; see also Chapter 13). Interventions may need not only to target acquisition of new sociorelational skills but also to reduce challenging behaviors and replace them with socially acceptable communicative means. (It is beyond the scope of this chapter to provide a review of the literature on challenging behaviors and the use of communicative replacements; readers are referred to Mirenda, 1997, for a synthesis of the research literature on this topic and to Chapter 13 for discussion of effective intervention practices to reduce challenging behaviors.)

Summary Obviously, future research is urgently required to determine the specific types of knowledge, judgment, and skills in the sociorelational domain that are required to support individuals who use AAC in developing meaningful social relationships. Specifically, future research is required to explore which skills work best for whom in which situations with which partners. It is critical to ensure that the skills selected as goals for intervention are valid ones that serve to increase the communication and social interaction of the participants (Light, 1999). Too often, target skills are selected as goals for intervention with limited understanding of the potential impact of these skills on daily interactions and with limited empirical evidence to support the validity of these skills as intervention goals (Calculator, 1999). For example, much has been written in the AAC literature about increasing the conversational control of individuals who use AAC, yet little is known about the potential impact of conversational control on social interaction. Does conversational control by individuals who use AAC result in enhanced communication and social interaction? Or does it in fact impede the development of positive social relationships when individuals who use AAC attempt to "control" the conversation? Calculator cautioned,

> Let us be certain that the same outcomes that cause us to rejoice (as statistically significant and publishable findings) are of use to the persons necessitating the studies to begin with. These are the AAC users, their families, and the broader social network of educators and professionals. (1999, p. 31)

Instruction to Teach Sociorelational Skills

As of 2003, there have been few documented interventions that focus on the acquisition of sociorelational skills by individuals with developmental disabilities who require AAC (e.g., Light, Binger, Bailey, & Millar, 1997; Light & Mc-

Naughton, 2002; Light et al., 1999; Light, McNaughton, Krezman, & Williams, 2002). Light and colleagues (1997) focused on the development of early socio-relational skills by teaching beginning communicators who required AAC to participate actively in interactions; Light and colleagues (1999, 2002) focused on the development of more sophisticated sociorelational skills with individuals who used AAC (e.g., the development of other-orientation skills).

Intervention with Beginning Communicators One strategy to demonstrate an interest in a communicative partner is to participate actively in the interaction and to respond to the partner's comments and questions, providing regular feedback to the partner. The research literature suggests that many individuals who use AAC are typically not active participants in social interactions; instead, partners frequently dominate interactions, and individuals who use AAC participate infrequently (e.g., Light, 1988; Light, Binger, & Kelford Smith, 1994; Light, Collier, & Parnes, 1985). The research further suggests that individuals who use AAC tend to fulfill obligatory turns following specific questions but forfeit nonobligatory turns that provide feedback following partners' comments (Light et al., 1985). Without regular feedback and active participation from individuals who use AAC, partners must carry the burden of the conversation. The interaction will lack the reciprocity and cooperative interdependence that is considered a foundation to the development of meaningful social relationships (Yuker, 1994). One approach to increase active participation in social interactions is to teach individuals who use AAC to fulfill not only their obligatory turns, but also their nonobligatory turns. One way to fulfill nonobligatory turns is through social interjections such as "cool," "yeah," "no way," and "uh-huh." These social interjections impose minimal linguistic demands for individuals who require AAC, but they provide important social feedback that demonstrates responsivity to the partner and encourages social interaction.

Research by Light and colleagues (1997) investigated the effect of nonobligatory turns on others' perceptions of the communicative competence of individuals who use AAC. They found that adults and adolescents who had no prior experience in AAC and professionals with experience in AAC valued the use of nonobligatory turns and felt that these turns contributed positively to perceived communicative competence for individuals who used AAC who had relatively efficient rates of turn transfer. Therefore, Light and colleagues used a single subject research design to evaluate the impact of instruction on the use of social interjections to fulfill nonobligatory turns by six individuals who used AAC. The participants included

1. A 4-year-old girl with cerebral palsy
2. A 9-year-old girl with a moderate developmental delay
3. A 12-year-old girl with a moderate developmental delay
4. A 14-year-old boy with autism

5.   A 21-year-old woman with severe mental retardation and cerebral palsy
6.   A 5-year-old boy with cerebral palsy

The participants used a variety of means to communicate including some speech approximations, gestures, signs, communication boards with line drawings, and simple voice output communication aids (VOCAs). The 12-year-old girl had an expressive vocabulary of several hundred spoken words, signs, and graphic symbols and was able to engage in displaced talk about events outside the immediate context. The other participants had expressive vocabularies of between 50 and 200 items and performed best when language input was concrete and related to the immediate context. All of the participants could understand simple *wh-* questions and follow one-step commands.

Prior to intervention, the participants fulfilled fewer than 30% of their nonobligatory turns in social interactions. They were not perceived as competent communicators; parents, teachers, and aides noted that it was often difficult to interact with the participants because they provided minimal feedback. The intervention to increase the use of nonobligatory turns by the participants included three key components: 1) identification of appropriate shared activities as a focus for social interactions (e.g., play activities, looking at magazines or photo albums); 2) provision of appropriate vocabulary to promote the use of social interjections as nonobligatory turns that provided feedback to the partner (e.g., "cool," "yeah," "no way"); and 3) guided practice in the use of nonobligatory turns in naturally occurring shared activities using a least to most prompting hierarchy (Light & Binger, 1998). The prompting hierarchy consisted of the following: 1) the occurrence of a natural cue signaling the opportunity to take a nonobligatory turn (i.e., a comment by the partner or a pause in the interaction); 2) an expectant delay clearly signaling the opportunity for a nonobligatory turn (an extended pause during which the partner maintained eye contact and an expectant body posture and facial expression); 3) a pointing prompt (i.e., pointing to the individual and/or AAC system); and 4) a model (i.e., production of an appropriate nonobligatory turn using the individual's AAC systems; see Light & Binger, 1998, for further details).

Five of the six participants acquired the targeted skill successfully following intervention; the sixth participant did not complete the instructional program. He made good progress during the first eight instructional sessions; at that time, his speech-language pathologist made significant revisions to his VOCA, changing from use of one-symbol selection to two-symbol sequences to access vocabulary. With the increased operational demands of his AAC system, his use of nonobligatory turns decreased significantly. He did not complete the instructional program; his speech-language pathologist chose to focus on teaching the new operational demands of his AAC system instead. The other participants required approximately 4–6 hours of instruction to demonstrate significant gains in social participation (i.e., gains from less than

30% use of nonobligatory turns at baseline to greater than 80% use after intervention). Four of the five participants generalized the skill to new partners and situations; the fourth participant (the 14-year-old boy with autism) required additional instruction with different partners to facilitate generalization. All five participants demonstrated maintenance of the skill in probes up to 2 months postinstruction.

Facilitators (i.e., family members, teachers, aides) reported that, as a result of intervention, the participants interacted more frequently at home and school and that the interactions were "easier" for them because the individuals who used AAC provided more feedback. Adults with no prior experience in AAC (who were blind to the goals of the study and the experimental conditions) viewed randomly selected videotapes of the participants before and after intervention. For four of the five participants, the observers indicated that the participant was a "more competent communicator" in the videotape recorded after intervention. For the third participant, the majority of the observers indicated that there was no significant difference in her communication skills between the two videotapes.

In summary, the study by Light and colleagues (1997) suggests that intervention using guided practice in the natural environment with a least-to-most prompting hierarchy resulted in the successful acquisition, generalization, and maintenance of nonobligatory turns by all participants who completed the intervention program. The acquisition of this skill resulted in increased quantity and quality of social interactions and in enhanced communicative competence for the majority of the participants. This study focused on the development of a basic sociorelational skill by beginning communicators. As individuals who use AAC successfully attain basic communication skills, they will be ready to learn more advanced sociorelational skills to further their communicative competence. The next two intervention studies to be discussed focus on the development of more complex sociorelational skills, specifically the development of other-orientation skills and the development of effective interpersonal communication skills such as reflective listening.

Intervention to Promote Other-Orientation   Spitzburg and Cupach (1984) argued that individuals who are competent communicators are "other-oriented"; they demonstrate an interest in others, rather than a self-focus. Ironically, many AAC interventions focus only on the individual who requires AAC. For example, the speech-language pathologist may use conversations about the individual who uses AAC and his or her interests and daily activities as a focus for instruction. Seldom do these interactions consider the perspectives, feelings, or interests of the communicative partner. These interventions may unintentionally promote a self-focus by individuals who require AAC. In essence, individuals who use AAC are taught to talk about themselves in response to questions from the speech-language pathologist, teacher, or educational assistant. Ultimately, this approach to intervention may be counter-productive for it fails to support the development of other-orientation skills.

Randy Kitch, a disability rights advocate and an expert at using AAC, emphasized the importance of other-orientation in the following e-mail message that he sent, as a mentor, to an adolescent experiencing difficulties with her peers at school:

> I know what you're going through. When I was in high school I was called names and made fun of. And all I had was a letter board to communicate with. So you think you don't have any friends in school . . . Do you ask other students questions about themselves, about the homework assignments, and school activities?? Sometimes you need to focus on them first before they will focus on you. (R. Kitch, personal communication, September 24, 2000)

In this message, Kitch proposes that one way to demonstrate other-orientation is to ask partner-focused questions, that is, questions that focus on partners and their experiences, interests, and feelings.

Light, Corbett, Gullapalli, and Lepkowski (1995) investigated the impact of partner-focused questions on the perceived communicative competence of individuals who use AAC. They found that adults who had no prior experience in AAC perceived individuals who used AAC to be more competent communicators when they asked partner-focused questions than when they did not. Therefore, Light, Binger, Agate, and Ramsay (1999) instructed six individuals who used AAC in the use of partner-focused questions and then evaluated the impact of this instruction. The participants included

1. A 44-year-old woman with cerebral palsy
2. A 25-year-old man with cerebral palsy
3. A 33-year-old man with moderate mental retardation
4. A 35-year-old man with severe speech and motor impairments, resulting from a traumatic brain injury 15 years prior
5. A 13-year-old boy with moderate mental retardation
6. A 10-year-old girl with cerebral palsy

The participants used various means to communicate including speech, speech approximations, gestures, pointing, communication boards, and VOCAs. They all understood simple *wh-* questions and were able to participate in basic social conversations that involved displaced talk.

Prior to intervention, the participants asked partner-focused questions in less than 30% of the opportunities that they had to do so (range 0%–30%). Approximately 5–10 partner-focused questions were selected individually for the participants based on their needs and skills (e.g., How was your weekend? What did you do last night? What's up?); these questions were pre-stored in their VOCAs or added to their communication boards. The participants were taught to use these partner-focused questions in their daily interactions through the instructional procedures described by Light and Binger (1998): 1) identification of contexts to promote social interaction; 2) provision of appropriate vocabulary and AAC systems to express partner-focused questions; and 3) guided practice in the use of partner-focused questions in the natural environment (supplemented with role plays) using a least-to-most prompting hierarchy (i.e., natural cue, expectant delay, point, model). All of the participants successfully learned to ask partner-focused questions spontaneously during real-world interactions (i.e., they spontaneously asked appropriate partner-focused questions in at least 80% of the opportunities that they had). They required between 3 and 11 hours of instruction before they reached criterion.

All of the participants also generalized use of partner-focused questions to new partners and new situations encountered in their daily lives. Two of the participants learned to generate their own novel partner-focused questions as well. Five of the six participants maintained their use of partner-focused questions as measured by probes up to 2 months postinstruction; Participant 6 (the 10-year-old girl) required booster instructional sessions to ensure long-term maintenance of the skill.

Social validation interviews were conducted with the participants and their facilitators to determine the real-world value of the intervention; results indicated that the use of partner-focused questions enhanced the quantity and quality of the participants' social interactions. After intervention, participants interacted with others more frequently and sustained these interactions for longer. One of the facilitators summarized the impact of the intervention as follows: "It was surprising to note the reaction of communicative partners when [the individual] asked a question. They showed pleasure and surprise. They seemed happy to share in the conversation." This observation was further supported by comments from adults with no prior experience with individuals who used AAC who observed videotapes of interactions involving the participants taken before and after intervention. The adults were blind to the goals of the study and to the experimental conditions. For most of the participants, the observers indicated that the participants seemed more competent, more interactive, more involved, and more interested in the partner and the conversation in the videotapes recorded after instruction compared to those recorded before instruction.

Web-Based Intervention to Build Sociorelational Skills   Light and colleagues (2002) expanded on the research by Light and colleagues (1999) and focused on teaching adults who used AAC a series of sociorelational skills, including the use of partner-focused questions, reflective listening, and positive encouragement. Light and colleagues (Light & McNaughton, 2002; Light et al., 2002) explored a different approach to intervention to build these sociorelational skills. Specifically, they developed a web-based leadership training program to teach adults who used AAC and demonstrated functional language and literacy skills to be effective mentors of adolescents and young adults who also used AAC. The web-based training program targeted skills in three domains: 1) effective sociorelational skills to foster positive reciprocal interactions with the adolescents or young adults who used AAC (their protégés); 2) collaborative problem-solving and goal-setting skills to support their protégés in overcoming challenges; and 3) strategies to access relevant disability-related information and services. Of relevance is the first of these domains—the instructional module designed to teach effective sociorelational skills. (For further discussion of the other two instructional modules, readers are referred to Light and McNaughton, 2002, and Light et al., 2002.)

Specifically, the instructional module used the acronym LAF to teach participants three important sociorelational skills:

L = Listen and communicate respect for their partners
A = Ask questions to demonstrate interest in their partners and to find out more
F = Focus on what their partners are saying and provide positive encouragement

The instructional module also cautioned the participants to avoid behaviors that would affect their social interactions negatively. Specifically, the instructional module used the acronym CRY and cautioned the participants "not to CRY," specifically:

C = Not to criticize their partners
R = Not to react hastily without considering the consequences of what they were going to say and do
Y = Not to "yakkity yak" (i.e., talk excessively) about themselves

The module used the following steps of effective strategy instruction adapted from Van Reusen, Bos, Schumaker, and Deshler (1994) to teach the targeted sociorelational skills:

1. Demonstrate the benefits of using the LAF strategy by giving examples of what happens when individuals use this strategy and what happens when they do not.
2. Outline the specific strategy steps by describing and giving examples of the *L, A,* and *F* steps.
3. Model strategy use in situations relevant to the participants.
4. Check that the participants can describe the three target sociorelational skills (i.e., the steps in the LAF strategy—Listen and communicate respect, Ask partner-focused questions, and Focus on what the partner is saying).

5. Provide opportunities for the participants to recognize appropriate use of the LAF strategy in role-play examples and to recognize opportunities when this strategy was not used but should have been; give feedback for the participants' responses.
6. Provide the participants with opportunities to use the target sociorelational skills (the LAF strategy) themselves in a variety of meaningful role-play situations; encourage them to self-check their use of the strategy.
7. Give feedback as to the participants' use of the target sociorelational skills in the role-plays.
8. Provide opportunities for the participants to use the skills in new situations to ensure generalization and maintenance.

Although this intervention could have been implemented in traditional one-on-one face-to-face instructional sessions, Light and colleagues explored the use of the world wide web as a vehicle to deliver this instruction (Light & McNaughton, 2002; Light et al., 2002). Using the guidelines for Internet accessibility for people with disabilities,[1] the researchers developed a web site that provided participants with the opportunity for self-paced instruction.

A total of 31 adults with cerebral palsy who used AAC participated in the full leadership-training program. Of these participants, 20 demonstrated effective sociorelational skills, specifically use of the LAF strategy, at baseline prior to the leadership training. The remaining 11 participants who did not demonstrate use of the LAF strategy at baseline ranged in age from 20 to 48 years (mean of 32 years) and had levels of educational achievement ranging from high school graduation to 4-year undergraduate degrees. They used a variety of means to communicate, including natural speech, gestures, signs, alphabet boards, word boards, and various types of VOCAs.

All of the 11 participants (100%) successfully demonstrated acquisition of the LAF strategy in role-plays after completion of the web-based instruction. Furthermore, the participants demonstrated generalization of the LAF strategy to use within the actual mentoring relationships with their protégés via e-mail over many months postinstruction. All of the 11 mentors reported high levels of satisfaction with the web-based training on the LAF strategy. Furthermore, all but one of the protégés of these mentors expressed satisfaction with the relationships that the mentors developed with them and indicated that they would continue to keep in touch with their mentor at the end of the mentoring program.

Future Research   Although these interventions provide important first steps in documenting effective approaches to teaching sociorelational skills to individuals who use AAC, future research is urgently required to ex-

---

[1]Readers are referred to the following web site for information on the guidelines for Internet accessibility for people with disabilities http://www.w3.org/WAI/.

tend these interventions to teach other important sociorelational skills (see Table 11.1). Future research is also required to explore the effectiveness of a range of instructional approaches and to determine the relative effectiveness of these different instructional techniques. The AAC population is a heterogeneous one. Therefore, careful attention should be given to the unique needs and skills of individuals who require AAC and to determining which interventions are most successful with which individuals who require AAC.

Key Components of Effective Intervention   Ultimately, the following factors must be considered if interventions are to be effective in developing sociorelational skills:

- The interventions must target appropriate sociorelational skills that will serve to enhance the development of meaningful and positive social relationships.
- They must provide access to appropriate AAC systems and vocabulary so that individuals who require AAC have the tools to participate successfully in social interactions.
- They must provide effective instruction to ensure successful acquisition, generalization, and maintenance of the target skills
- They must ensure meaningful opportunities for individuals who require AAC to interact with others within their natural environments to build positive social relationships.

The first three factors ensure that the individual who uses AAC has the means, knowledge, judgment, and skills to develop valued social relationships; however, having the means, knowledge, judgment, and skills is not enough. Individuals who use AAC frequently confront significant opportunity barriers imposed by others in the environment that limit their attempts to develop meaningful social relationships. Intervention may be required to overcome these barriers and ensure that individuals who use AAC have opportunities for meaningful social interactions within their daily lives.

ENSURING MEANINGFUL OPPORTUNITIES FOR SOCIAL INTERACTIONS

"Why [are] some people scared of people who are in a wheelchair?" (e-mail message sent by Marlon Christie, a young adult with cerebral palsy who uses AAC, to his mentor)

"Why are people scared of people in wheelchairs? GOOD QUESTION Pal. I have always thought it was because those other people just don't understand that we [people with cerebral palsy and other similar disabilities] are as smart, caring, funny, and loving as THEY are, underneath these bodies of ours which don't walk, talk, or work for US as well as their bodies do, you know? To me the people who are scared of folks in wheelchairs are just DUMB about what [people with disabilities] can do, you know? At least that's what I have thought always about that!" (Response sent via e-mail to Marlon by his mentor, Bill Richards, a man with cerebral palsy who uses AAC)

This e-mail exchange clearly highlights the challenges that individuals who use AAC regularly confront in finding opportunities to interact with others in their schools, places of work, and broader social communities. Beukelman and Mirenda (1998) referred to these restrictions as opportunity barriers, that is, barriers that are imposed by others in the environment. They cited five types of opportunity barriers: policy, practice, knowledge, skill, and attitude barriers.

Policy and Practice Barriers

Policy and practice barriers refer to barriers resulting from legislation, policies, and practices that limit opportunities for individuals who use AAC to engage in social interactions. For example, in the United States prior to the Education for All Handicapped Children Act of 1975, PL 94-142, some students with significant disabilities were excluded from an appropriate education. When children who use AAC do not attend school with their peers and when adults who use AAC are segregated in institutions, they are limited in their access to social interactions and have few opportunities to develop meaningful relationships with others (Mirenda, 1993). Fortunately, in many countries, many policy barriers have been removed with the passage of disability rights legislation. Unfortunately eliminating policy barriers has not ensured that all opportunity barriers are removed; rather, many knowledge, skill, and attitude barriers continue to restrict the full social participation of individuals who use AAC.

Knowledge and Skill Barriers   Knowledge and skill barriers refer to partners' lack of knowledge and skill with AAC systems and interaction strategies. As a result of this lack of knowledge and skill, partners may experience difficulty interacting socially with individuals who use AAC and may be hesitant to do so. For example, Light, Seligson, and Lund (1998) observed three children who used AAC in play contexts with other children. At baseline, prior to intervention, there was minimal, if any, social interaction between the children who used AAC and their peers without disabilities. When asked, the peers without disabilities reported that it was difficult to talk to the children who used AAC. After a series of sessions designed to teach the peers strategies to interact effectively with the children who used AAC (e.g., waiting for the child who used AAC to respond; modeling AAC use), the frequency of interaction between the children increased significantly.

Hunt and colleagues found similar results in a series of studies in which they taught children with significant disabilities and peer facilitators without disabilities to interact with the use of conversation books (e.g., Hunt, Alwell, & Goetz, 1988; 1991; Hunt, Alwell, Goetz, & Sailor, 1990). Results of this line of research demonstrated increases in conversational initiations and turn taking and decreases in challenging behaviors by the children with significant disabilities as a result of the intervention. Results did not generalize to untrained peers, however, suggesting the critical importance of facilitator instruction for peers to support opportunities for social interaction with children with significant disabilities.

In subsequent studies, Hunt and colleagues (e.g., Hunt, Alwell, Farron-Davis, & Goetz, 1996; Hunt, Farron-Davis, Wrenn, Hirose-Hatae, & Goetz, 1997) evaluated the effects of interventions that trained networks of peer facilitators that were linked to individual students with significant disabilities. The interventions were customized to meet the needs of individual students, but each intervention included the following components:

1. AAC systems were provided to facilitate interactions
2. Information was provided to the peers about appropriate activities, communication systems, and adaptive equipment for the target students
3. School staff established a buddy system matching the target students with peers and implemented interactive activities throughout the day
4. Staff facilitated social interactions between the target students and the peers by prompting and interpreting communication as required

Results suggested that there were more frequent reciprocal interactions between the target students and their peers after intervention and that there was less need for staff assistance and support in these interactions. Furthermore, teachers and peer facilitators reported that friendships were formed between target students and their peer facilitators as a result of the intervention program.

Carter and Maxwell (1998) also examined the effects of a peer intervention program on social interactions between children who used AAC and peers. The peer intervention highlighted the difficulties encountered when communicating without speech and then taught the peers procedures for using the students' AAC systems as well as the following interaction strategies: establish eye contact, ask a question, wait 5 seconds for a response, and respond to communicative attempts. Results of the study demonstrated an increase in the frequency of social interactions between the students who used

AAC and their peers after intervention; these changes were maintained at least 10 weeks after intervention.

The studies by Carter and Maxwell (1998), Hunt and colleagues, and Light and colleagues (1998) all suggest that intervention with peers without disabilities can serve to reduce knowledge and skill barriers and increase opportunities for positive social interactions with individuals who use AAC. It is interesting to note that in these studies, the instruction of the peer partners was conducted by school staff or other professionals. To date, there has been minimal attention to involving individuals who use AAC in the training of their peers and other partners. Interventions conducted by individuals who use AAC are of particular importance because these interventions would increase the independence of individuals who use AAC and empower them to overcome their partners' knowledge and skill barriers themselves.

Partner Instruction Conducted by Individuals Who Use AAC

Light, Binger, Dilg, and Livelsberger (1996) investigated the use of an introduction strategy by individuals who use AAC as a strategy to reduce knowledge and skill barriers and increase partner comfort and confidence. According to Light and Binger (1998), an introduction strategy is a message used when meeting new communication partners. It is intended to put new partners at ease and facilitate interaction; it empowers individuals who use AAC to teach their partners themselves. An introduction strategy has two essential components: information about the individual's means of communication (e.g., I look up to say "yes"; I shake my head to say "no"); and information about what the partner should do to facilitate the interaction (e.g., Please repeat my message back to check that you have understood correctly; please wait for me to type my message; Light & Binger, 1998). The introduction strategy may also include an attention-getting phrase, a greeting, the name of the individual who uses AAC, a joke, or other components depending on the personal preferences of the individual who uses AAC, the partner, the demands of the situation, and the anticipated length of the relationship (Light & Binger, 1998).

Research by Light, Binger, and colleagues (1996) found that adults and adolescents with no prior experience in AAC judged individuals who used AAC to be more competent communicators when they used an introduction strategy when they met new people than when they did not. In a follow-up study, Light and colleagues provided instruction in the use of an introduction strategy to five individuals who used AAC:

1. A 16-year-old boy with cerebral palsy
2. A 44-year-old woman with cerebral palsy
3. A 12-year-old girl with a developmental delay

4. A 28-year-old man with autism
5. A 35-year-old man with significant speech and physical impairments resulting from a traumatic brain injury 15 years earlier

Prior to instruction, none of the individuals made use of an introduction strategy; all of the individuals experienced significant difficulties meeting new people and communicating with them effectively. The instruction was based on the procedures described by Light and Binger (1998). The skill was taught in the context of meaningful interactions in the real world; this instruction was supplemented by role-plays of real-world situations because most of the participants only encountered new people in their daily lives several times a week. Within the role-plays and naturally occurring interactions, a least-to-most prompting hierarchy was used to ensure that the participants successfully used an introduction strategy as required. In these situations, a variety of natural cues signaled the need to use an introduction strategy (e.g., approaching an unfamiliar person, being introduced to someone new). If the participant did not use an introduction strategy spontaneously following the natural cue, the prompting hierarchy was as follows: expectant delay (i.e., the instructor makes eye contact, uses an expectant body posture, and waits an extended period to mark the opportunity for an introduction strategy); point (i.e., the instructor points to the individual's communication system to mark the opportunity for an introduction strategy and waits expectantly); and model (i.e., the instructor demonstrates use of an introduction strategy for the participant) (see Light & Binger, 1998).

All of the participants learned to use an introduction strategy spontaneously. Most of the participants required five or fewer instructional sessions to acquire the skill (range 3–13). All of the participants generalized use of an introduction strategy to new partners, new environments, and new communication tasks. All of the participants maintained use of an introduction strategy at least 2 months postinstruction.

The five participants and their facilitators all reported high levels of satisfaction with the instruction and its outcomes, and indicated that the participants experienced fewer difficulties with new partners. Furthermore, people with no prior experience in AAC, blind to the conditions and goals of the study, rated four of the five participants to be more competent communicators in their interactions after instruction in the use of an introduction strategy than in interactions that occurred prior to instruction. This study suggests that use of an introduction strategy by individuals who use AAC may positively influence the attitudes and behaviors of unfamiliar people meeting individuals who use AAC for the first time; however, neither the attitudes of the unfamiliar partners nor their resulting behaviors were measured directly. Future research is required to investigate the effect of an introduction strategy and other consumer-driven interventions on interactions with children and adults.

Attitude Barriers

Although policy, practice, knowledge, and skill barriers can negatively affect opportunities for individuals who use AAC to develop meaningful social relationships, attitude barriers probably have the most devastating effect. According to Yuker, there is a "fundamental negative bias" in the attitudes of people toward individuals with disabilities (1988, p. xii). Negative social attitudes within a group or community form a significant barrier to true membership in school classes, communities, and places of work for individuals who use AAC. Mirenda (1993) emphasized that membership in a community can only be achieved when there is acceptance by everyone—the individual who uses AAC and the other members of the group:

> I am talking about community living situations that help people become members of, not just residents in, communities. I am talking about programs in which a lot of emphasis is placed on helping people get to know and connect with their neighbors and their local shopkeepers . . . .(M)embership is different than joining or living next door to or affiliating with—you can do all of those things on your own. But you have not achieved membership in a group until the group says you have; it is mutual, it is consensual. That is what we want—membership in communities. (Mirenda, 1993, p. 6)

Negative social attitudes limit the opportunities for individuals who use AAC to meet people and to develop friendships. These negative attitudes also limit the enjoyment individuals who use AAC may experience in social interactions. O'Keefe explained, "It is difficult to find satisfaction in personal interactions when the speaker experiences constant anxiety over the reactions of communicative partners" (1996, p. 233).

Triandis defined an attitude as "an idea charged with emotion which predisposes a class of actions to a particular class of social situations" (1971, p. 2). According to Triandis, attitudes consist of a cognitive component, an emotional component, and a behavioral component. The cognitive component refers to the information that the individual has about the person or event; this information serves to form a foundation for the beliefs held. The emotional aspect of an attitude refers to the feelings that are connected to the beliefs that are held. Finally, the behavior component refers to the tendency to respond to the person or event in a specific way. The relationship between attitudes and actual behaviors toward individuals who use AAC is not well understood. In general, it is assumed that attitudes predispose certain behaviors, although the relationship is probably not unidimensional. Other factors besides attitudes most certainly influence individuals in their behaviors toward individuals who use AAC (e.g., social norms, peer expectations).

Attitude barriers result from the negative attitudes of others that lead to behaviors that limit or preclude meaningful social interaction. It has been well documented that many people demonstrate a negative bias in their attitudes toward people with disabilities (Yuker, 1988). This negative bias may be even more pronounced in people's attitudes toward individuals who require AAC for these individuals often have significant disabilities and therefore stand out (Wright, 1988). Furthermore, judgments of a person's competence or value are frequently based on the person's ability to express ideas, thoughts, and opinions effectively; individuals who require AAC frequently experience significant challenges in communication (Light & Gulens, 2000).

Attitudes toward individuals who use AAC may be influenced by three sets of factors: those related to the partner or potential partner; those related to the individual who uses AAC; and those related to the AAC systems (see Table 11.2).

Factors Related to the Partner or Potential Partner

Characteristics such as gender, age, education, and experience with people with disabilities influence peoples' attitudes toward individuals with disabilities.

Gender   The research suggests that females tend to have more positive attitudes toward individuals with disabilities than males (e.g., Rosenbaum, Armstrong, & King, 1986a, 1986b). These results have been replicated in some of the research on attitudes toward individuals who use AAC (e.g., Beck & Dennis, 1996; Blockberger, Armstrong, O'Connor, & Freeman, 1993; Gorenflo, Gorenflo, & Santer, 1994).

Age   It is also believed that age influences attitudes, although the relationship between age and attitudes is not simple. Ryan (1981) noted that people's attitudes toward individuals with disabilities change across the life span; he proposed that attitudes might become more positive from early childhood through early adolescence; more negative through later adolescence; then more positive through adulthood; and finally more negative again with

Table 11.2.   Factors that may affect attitudes toward individuals who use AAC

Type of factor	Specific factor
Factors related to the partner or potential partner	Gender of the partner Age of the partner Education of the partner Partner's experience with people with disabilities Relationship with the individual who uses AAC Perceived similarity to the individual who uses AAC
Factors related to individuals who use AAC	Appearance Age Competence Sociorelational skills
Factors related to AAC systems	Type of AAC system

late adulthood. Beck, Fritz, Keller, and Dennis (2000) studied the attitudes of children without disabilities toward children who use AAC and concluded that children's attitudes do not improve steadily across the elementary grades, rather they seem to fluctuate. Beck and colleagues further proposed that gender and age may interact to influence attitudes.

Education   Level of education has also been found to affect attitudes toward people with disabilities in general, with higher levels of education being associated with more favorable attitudes and lower levels of education being associated with less favorable attitudes (e.g., English, 1971). In the AAC field, Blockberger and colleagues (1993) found that children with higher levels of reading comprehension demonstrated more positive attitudes toward children who used AAC than did children with lower levels of reading comprehension.

Experience with People with Disabilities   The research literature suggests that prior experience with people with disabilities also affects attitudes. Blockberger and colleagues (1993) found that children who reported experience with children with disabilities had more positive attitudes than those who reported no such experience. In two separate studies, Beck and colleagues compared the attitudes of children attending schools that integrated children with disabilities to those of children attending schools without integration and found that the children from integrated schools had more positive attitudes than those in nonintegrated schools (Beck & Dennis, 1996; Beck, Kingsbury, Neff, & Dennis, 2000); however, gender and age may interact with experience (Beck & Dennis, 1996).

Relationship with the Individual Who Uses AAC   The disability literature also suggests that attitudes may vary across people depending on their relationship with the individual with disabilities (e.g., family, professional, educator, stranger; e.g., Wright, 1988; Yuker, 1994). To date, the effect of type of relationship on attitudes has not been investigated in the AAC field, although it seems reasonable to assume that this factor would be influential.

Perceived Similarity to the Individual Who Uses AAC   Attitudes may also be influenced by the observers' perceived similarity to the individual who uses AAC. For example, Gorenflo and Gorenflo (1997) found that observers had more positive attitudes toward individuals of the same gender who used AAC and were perceived to be similar to them in values and activities of daily living than toward those of the same gender who were not perceived to be similar.

In summary, the research suggests that people's attitudes may be affected by their gender, age, education, experience with individuals with disabilities, roles, and perceived similarity to the individual who uses AAC. The influences of these variables may not be simple; rather there may be interactions across variables that influence attitudes toward individuals who use AAC.

Factors Related to Individuals Who Use AAC

Numerous factors related to individuals who use AAC may also influence others' attitudes toward them including appearance, age, competence, and sociorelational competence.

Appearance   Wright (1988) noted that the more a person with disabilities stands out as "different," the more apt others are to hold negative attitudes toward the person. To date, there has been no research in the AAC field to investigate the effects of appearance and severity of disability on others' attitudes.

Age   There has been some suggestion that people may be more accepting of young children with disabilities than of adults. Only one study has investigated the effect of age of the individual who uses AAC on others' attitudes. This study found that there were no differences in the attitudes of undergraduate students based on the age of the individual who uses AAC (child versus adolescent; Macke, 1992).

Competence   Light and Gulens (2000) argued that individuals who use AAC may be especially vulnerable to negative attitudes because judgments of a person's competence or value are frequently based on the person's ability to express ideas, thoughts, and opinions effectively. Beck and colleagues (2001) attempted to investigate the effect on attitudes of "competence" (as defined by the length of time and number of prompts required for the individual who used AAC to respond). Results of their study suggested that observers showed more positive scores toward the individual who demonstrated high competence than the low-competence condition, at least on the cognitive subscale of the Assessment of Attitudes Toward Augmentative/Alternative Communication. Future research is required to explore the effects of competence on attitudes because competence is a multidimensional construct that involves many more factors than response time and prompting (cf. Light, 1989).

Sociorelational Skills   It has been argued in the first part of this chapter that the sociorelational skills of individuals who use AAC are important determinants of others' attitudes toward them. It is for this reason that it is critical that individuals who use AAC acquire appropriate sociorelational skills. To date, there has been no research to investigate the effect of sociorelational skills on the attitudes of others toward individuals who use AAC. This area is a priority for future research. If this research establishes that others are more apt to have positive attitudes toward individuals with well-developed sociorelational skills, then there would be clear evidence of the social validity of this goal as a priority for future intervention.

As of 2003, there has been only minimal research in the AAC field to investigate factors intrinsic to individuals who use AAC that may influence attitudes. Potential factors include attribute variables such as age and appearance or severity of disability. Although these variables are of interest to identify situations where specific individuals who use AAC may be especially vulnerable to attitude barriers, for the most part, these variables are not amenable to intervention. However, some variables related to individuals who use AAC are amenable to intervention, such as the sociorelational competence of the individual who uses AAC. Future research should consider the effect of the latter variables on others' attitudes and willingness to interact socially with individuals who use AAC.

Factors Related to AAC Systems

Many of the research studies on attitudes toward individuals who use AAC have focused on the impact of AAC systems on people's attitudes toward individuals who use AAC (e.g., Beck & Dennis, 1996; Beck, Fritz, et al., 2000; Beck et al., 2001; Blockberger et al., 1993; Gorenflo & Gorenflo, 1991; O'Keefe, 1992). Blockberger and colleagues suggested that attitudes toward individuals who use AAC are particularly intriguing "because of the possibility that attitudes toward an individual may be affected by physical or design characteristics of the AAC system" (1993, p. 243). Most of these studies have compared the effect of light-technology AAC systems (e.g., alphabet board) to high-technology systems (e.g., VOCA) with some studies also investigating the effect of unaided systems (e.g., sign, gesture). Results of the studies have been mixed: most studies reported no statistically significant differences in attitudes based on the type of AAC system used (e.g., Beck, Fritz, et al., 2000; Beck et al., 2001; Blockberger, et al., 1993); one study by Gorenflo and Gorenflo (1991) found that participants (undergraduate students) had more positive attitudes when a VOCA was used than when an alphabet board was used.

The research to date in the AAC field has focused on identifying factors that influence attitudes positively or negatively, including factors related to the partner or potential partner (e.g., gender, age, education, experience with people with disabilities, and perceived similarity to the individual who uses AAC), factors related to the individual who uses AAC (e.g., age, competence), and factors related to the AAC systems used. Results of this research provide individuals who use AAC, their families, and professionals in the field with information about groups of people who may be at risk for forming negative attitudes toward individuals who require AAC, and situations in which individuals who use AAC may be most vulnerable to negative attitudes. Future research is critical to evaluate the efficacy of interventions to affect attitude and behavior change, especially with these "at risk" groups and in these vulnerable situations.

Interventions to Address Attitude Barriers

As of 2003, there is limited published research that has evaluated the efficacy of interventions to change attitudes and behaviors toward individuals who use AAC. There are a number of techniques that have been proposed to affect attitude change toward people with disabilities that may have relevance to the AAC field. These include provision of information, contact with people with disabilities, use of an introduction strategy, vicarious experience, persuasive messages, positive reinforcement, and systematic desensitization (e.g., Gorenflo & Gorenflo, 1991; Light & Binger, 1998; Rosenbaum et al., 1986b; Shaver, Curtis, & Strong, 1989). Table 11.3 provides descriptions of these different interventions.

Shaver, Curtis, and Strong (1989) conducted a meta-analysis of intervention studies to change attitudes toward individuals with disabilities. Results of the meta-analysis found that persuasive messages, provision of information plus personal contact, personal contact alone, and vicarious experience had the largest effects on attitude change. In the AAC field, research has investigated the effectiveness of information and contact as mechanisms to change attitudes.

Provision of Information   Provision of information is one avenue for producing change in people's attitudes toward individuals with disabilities. In general, this approach has involved providing accurate background information regarding disabilities in order to change negative stereotypes (Barrett & Pullo, 1993). For example, Gorenflo and Gorenflo (1991) found that people reported more positive attitudes when they were provided with information about the person who used AAC than when they were not provided with information. Information may serve to enrich the context in which the person is observed; Wright (1988) posited that people are more apt to have positive attitudes when the individual with disabilities is viewed in a meaningful context.

Contact with People with Disabilities   Personal contact is another mechanism to effect positive attitude change toward individuals who use AAC. The literature suggests that in order to be effective, contact with individuals with disabilities should be interactive and should occur over an extended period of time (Rosenbaum et al., 1986b). Donaldson (1980) further argued that individuals with disabilities should have equal status in these interactions. Rosenbaum and colleagues (1986b) investigated the impact of a buddy program on attitudes of children without disabilities toward children with disabilities. The buddy program matched students without disabilities (ages 9–13) with children with disabilities (ages 6–17), including some children who used AAC. The children were required to meet at least once a week during a 3-month period with opportunities for interaction. Results suggested

Table 11.3. Techniques that may be used to change attitudes

Technique	Description
Provision of information	Provision of accurate information about disability or provision of individual background about the person with a disability
Personal contact	Contact with individuals with disabilities in a supportive, reciprocal interaction, ideally over an extended period of time
Introduction strategy	Provision of information by the individual who uses AAC about his or her means of communication and about strategies for the partner to facilitate interaction
Vicarious experience	Role-play or simulation experience designed to replicate the experience of disability, ideally with the opportunity to observe others' reactions
Persuasive message	Messages (e.g., television commercials) that challenge negative stereotypes held by people toward individuals with disabilities; messages intended to force people to rethink their assumptions and beliefs
Positive reinforcement	Positive reinforcement for actions that demonstrate acceptance of individuals with disabilities
Systematic desensitization	Gradual exposure to individuals with disabilities; use of nonthreatening situations to think about disabilities

Sources: Gorenflo & Gorenflo, 1991; Light & Binger, 1998; Rosenbaum, Armstrong, & King, 1986b; and Shaver, Curtis, & Strong, 1989.

that this weekly contact had a positive effect on the attitudes of the peers without disabilities.

Future research is required to determine the specific parameters of personal contact associated with positive attitude change (e.g., type of contact, length of contact, roles). Barrett and Pullo (1993) emphasized that the interactions should occur in settings that emphasize the capabilities of the individual who uses AAC. McCarthy and Light (2001) suggested that theater activities may provide a rich venue for facilitating collaborative, positive, equal-status, regular interactions between children who require AAC and their peers without disabilities.

Strategies Used by Individuals Who Use AAC to Effect Attitude Change   All of the studies conducted to date have focused on interventions implemented by educators or other professionals to effect attitude change. Although these types of interventions are important, it is also of paramount interest to explore the techniques to overcome attitude barriers utilized by individuals who use AAC themselves. Randy Kitch, a disability advocate and expert user of AAC, points out that individuals who use AAC need to play a role in educating others in order to change their attitudes; he wrote the following e-mail message as part of a mentoring program to an adolescent who uses AAC who reported significant problems with her peers in high school:

> So you're giving up on your peers huh??? Well this is when I may make you mad . . . You can't give up on your peers because you need to educate them. Get real . . . You're only 16 and they are too . . . They are human. Humans need someone to teach them that people with disabilities are just like anyone else. I went through the same thing you are going through. Only I had a letter board and not a device, which was a heck of a lot harder. Giving up is the easy way out. Of course, it's your decision. (R. Kitch, personal communication, October 15, 2001)

Mirenda and Bopp (see Chapter 12) reviewed the writings of individuals who used AAC and identified the following strategies used to overcome partner discomfort and social constraints resulting from attitude barriers: ensuring well-kept appearance to overcome stereotypes about people with disabilities; use of an icebreaker or joke to place the partner at ease; and use of an introduction strategy to provide the partner with information to facilitate interaction. Future studies should investigate the effectiveness of these and other consumer-driven techniques in overcoming attitude barriers and promoting positive social interactions.

FUTURE DIRECTIONS

It is clear from this chapter that we are still in the early stages of understanding the development of sociorelational competence by individuals who use AAC. Future research is urgently required to

- Delineate the specific skills that enhance the sociorelational competence of individuals who use AAC and allow them to develop meaningful social relationships
- Investigate which of these skills work best for whom in which situations
- Determine effective instructional techniques to ensure that individuals who use AAC acquire, generalize, and maintain these skills successfully in their daily lives
- Identify barriers that limit opportunities for individuals who use AAC to participate meaningfully in social interactions at school, work, and the broader social community
- Investigate interventions to overcome these opportunity barriers and change the attitudes and behaviors of others toward individuals who use AAC, especially interventions that are consumer driven

This research will lay the empirical foundation to ensure that individuals who use AAC have the tools, knowledge, judgment, and skills, as well as the opportunity to attain sociorelational competence, to build meaningful social relationships with others, and ultimately to "find a place in the social circle of life" (Diamanti, 2000, p. 98).

REFERENCES

Baron-Cohen, S., Leslie, A.M., & Frith, U. (1985). Does the autistic child have a "theory of mind"? *Cognition, 21,* 113–125.

Barrett, K.E., & Pullo, R.E. (1993). Attitudinal change in undergraduate rehabilitation students as measured by the Attitudes Toward Disabled Persons Scale. *Rehabilitation Education, 7,* 119–126.

Beck, A.R., & Dennis, M. (1996). Attitudes of children toward a similar-aged child who uses augmentative communication. *Augmentative and Alternative Communication, 12,* 78–87.

Beck, A.R., Fritz, H., Keller, A., & Dennis, M. (2000). Attitudes of school-aged children toward their peers who use augmentative and alternative communication. *Augmentative and Alternative Communication, 16,* 13–26.

Beck, A., Kingsbury, K., Neff, A., & Dennis, M. (2000). Influence of length of augmented message on children's attitudes toward peers who use augmentative and alternative communication. *Augmentative and Alternative Communication, 16,* 239–249.

Beck, A., Thompson, J., Clay, S., Hutchins, M., Vogt, W. P., Romaniak, B., & Sokolowski, B. (2001). Preservice professionals' attitudes toward children who use augmentative/alternative communication. *Education and Training in Mental Retardation and Developmental Disabilities, 36,* 255–271.

Beukelman, D.R., & Ball, L.J. (in press). Improving AAC use for persons with acquired neurogenic disorders: Understanding human and engineering factors. *Assistive Technology.*

Beukelman, D., McGinnis, J., & Morrow, D. (1991). Vocabulary selection in augmentative and alternative communication. *Augmentative and Alternative Communication, 7,* 171–185.

Beukelman, D.R., & Mirenda, P. (1998). *Augmentative and alternative communication: Management of severe communication disorders in children and adults* (2nd ed.). Baltimore: Paul H. Brookes Publishing Co.

Blau, A. (1986). *Communication in the backchannel: Social structural analyses of nonspeech/speech conversations.* Unpublished doctoral dissertation, City University of New York.

Blockberger, S., Armstrong, R.W., O'Connor, A., & Freeman, R. (1993). Children's attitudes toward a nonspeaking child using various augmentative and alternative communication techniques. *Augmentative and Alternative Communication, 9,* 243–250.

Bridges, S. (2000). Delivery of AAC services to a rural American Indian community. *Augmentative and Alternative Communication, ASHA Special Interest Division 12 Newsletter, 9*(2), 6–9.

Brinton, B., & Fujiki, M. (1993). Communication skills and community integration in adults with mild to moderate retardation. *Topics in Language Disorders, 13*(3), 9–19.

Calculator, S. (1999). AAC outcomes for children and youths with severe disabilities: When seeing is believing. *Augmentative and Alternative Communication, 15,* 4–12.

Carter, M., & Maxwell, K. (1998). Promoting interaction with children using augmentative communication through peer-directed intervention. *International Journal of Disability, Development, and Education, 45,* 75–96.

Diamanti, T. (2000). Get to know me. In M.B. Williams & C.J. Krezman (Eds.), *Beneath the surface: Creative expressions of augmented communicators* (pp. 98–99). Toronto, Canada: ISAAC Press.

Doll, B., Sands, D.J., Wehmeyer, M.L., & Palmer, S. (1996). Promoting the development and acquisition of self-determined behavior. In D.J. Sands & M.L. Wehmeyer (Eds.), *Self-determination across the life span: Independence and choice for people with disabilities* (pp. 65–90). Baltimore: Paul H. Brookes Publishing Co.

Donaldson, J. (1980). Changing attitudes toward handicapped persons: A review and analysis of research. *Exceptional Children, 46,* 504–514.

Education for All Handicapped Children Act of 1975, PL 94-142, 20 U.S.C. §§1400 *et seq.*

English, R.W. (1971). Correlates of stigma toward physically disabled persons. *Rehabilitation Research and Practice Review, 2,* 1–17.

Fine, A.H. (1996). Leisure, living, and quality of life. In R. Renwick, I. Brown, & M. Nagler (Eds.), *Quality of life in health promotion and rehabilitation: Conceptual approaches, issues, and applications* (pp. 342–354). Thousand Oaks, CA: Sage Publications

Gorenflo, C.W., & Gorenflo, D.W. (1991). The effects of information and augmentative communication technique on attitudes toward nonspeaking individuals. *Journal of Speech and Hearing Research, 34,* 19–26.

Gorenflo, C.W., & Gorenflo, D.W. (1997). Effects of synthetic speech, gender, and perceived similarity on attitudes toward the augmented communicator. *Augmentative and Alternative Communication, 13,* 87–91.

Gorenflo, C.W., Gorenflo, D.W., & Santer, S.A. (1994). Effects of synthetic voice output on attitudes toward the augmented communicator. *Journal of Speech and Hearing Research, 37,* 64–68.

Guralnick, M.J., & Neville, B. (1997). Designing early intervention programs to promote children's social competence. In M.J. Guralnick (Ed.), *The effectiveness of early intervention* (pp. 579–610). Baltimore: Paul H. Brookes Publishing Co.

Higginbotham, D.J., & Yoder, D. (1982). Communication within natural conversational interaction: Implications for severe communicatively impaired persons. *Topics in Language Disorders, 2*(2), 1–19.

Hunt, P., Alwell, M., Farron-Davis, F., & Goetz, L. (1996). Creating socially supportive environments for fully included students who experience disabilities. *Journal of The Association for Persons with Severe Handicaps, 21,* 53–71.

Hunt, P., Alwell, M., & Goetz, L. (1988). Acquisition of conversation skills and the reduction of inappropriate social interaction behaviors. *Journal of The Association for Persons with Severe Handicaps, 13,* 20–27.

Hunt, P., Alwell, M., & Goetz, L. (1991). Interacting with peers through conversation turntaking with a communication book adaptation. *Augmentative and Alternative Communication, 7,* 117–126.

Hunt, P., Alwell, M., Goetz, L., & Sailor, W. (1990). Generalized effects of conversation skill training. *Journal of The Association for Persons with Severe Handicaps, 15,* 250–260.

Hunt, P., Farron-Davis, F., Wrenn, M., Hirose-Hatae, A., & Goetz, L. (1997). Promoting interactive partnerships in inclusive educational settings. *Journal of The Association for Persons with Severe Handicaps, 22,* 127–137.

Light, J. (1988). Interaction involving individuals using augmentative and alternative communication systems: State of the art and future directions for research. *Augmentative and Alternative Communication, 4,* 66–82.

Light, J. (1989). Toward a definition of communicative competence for individuals using augmentative and alternative communication systems. *Augmentative and Alternative Communication, 5,* 137–144.

Light, J. (1997). "Communication is the essence of human life": Reflections on communicative competence. *Augmentative and Alternative Communication, 13,* 61–70.

Light, J. (1999). Do augmentative and alternative communication interventions really make a difference?: The challenges of efficacy research. *Augmentative and Alternative Communication, 15,* 13–24.

Light, J.C., & Binger, C. (1998). *Building communicative competence with individuals who use augmentative and alternative communication.* Baltimore: Paul H. Brookes Publishing Co.

Light, J., Binger, C., Agate, T.L., & Ramsay, K.N. (1999). Teaching partner-focused questions to individuals who use augmentative and alternative communication to enhance their communicative competence. *Journal of Speech, Language, and Hearing Research, 42,* 241–255.

Light, J., Binger, C., Bailey, M., & Millar, D. (1997, November). *Increasing turn taking by individuals who use AAC to enhance communicative competence.* Miniseminar presented at the annual convention of the American Speech-Language-Hearing Association, Boston.

Light, J., Binger, C., Dilg, H., & Livelsberger, B. (1996, August). *Use of an introduction strategy to enhance communicative competence.* Miniseminar presented at the biennial conference of the International Society for Augmentative and Alternative Communication, Vancouver, British Columbia.

Light, J., Binger, C., & Kelford Smith, A. (1994). The story reading interactions of preschoolers who use augmentative and alternative communication and their mothers. *Augmentative and Alternative Communication, 10,* 255–268.

Light, J., Collier, B., & Parnes, P. (1985). Communicative interaction between young nonspeaking physically disabled children and their primary caregivers: Part I. Discourse patterns. *Augmentative and Alternative Communication, 1,* 74–83.

Light, J., Corbett, M.B., Gullapalli, G., & Lepkowski, S. (1995, December). *Other orientation and the communicative competence of AAC users.* Poster presented at the annual convention of the American Speech-Language-Hearing Association, Orlando, FL.

Light, J., & Drager, K. (in press). Improving the design of augmentative and alternative communication technologies for young children. *Assistive Technology.*

Light, J.C., & Gulens, M. (2000). Rebuilding communicative competence and self-determination for adults with acquired disabilities who require augmentative and alternative communication. In D.R. Beukelman & J. Reichle (Series Eds.) & D.R. Beukelman, K.M. Yorkston, & J. Reichle (Vol. Eds.), *Augmentative and alternative communication series: Augmentative and alternative communication for adults with acquired neurologic disorders* (pp. 137–182). Baltimore: Paul H. Brookes Publishing Co.

Light, J., & Lindsay, P. (1991). Cognitive science and augmentative and alternative communication. *Augmentative and Alternative Communication, 7,* 186–203.

Light, J., & McNaughton, D. (2002). *The AAC Mentor Project: Exemplary practices for developing supportive mentor–protégé relationships via the Internet for people with significant physical and speech disabilities who require augmentative and alternative communication.* Final grant report, National Institute on Disability and Rehabilitation Research, Washington, DC.

Light, J., McNaughton, D., Krezman, C., & Williams, M. (November 2002). *The AAC Mentor Project: Sharing the expertise of AAC users.* Miniseminar presented at the annual convention of the American Speech-Language-Hearing Association, Atlanta, GA.

Light, J., Seligson, L., & Lund, S. (1998, August). *Teaching nondisabled peers to interact with children who use AAC.* Paper presented at the biennial conference of the International Society for Augmentative and Alternative Communication, Dublin, Ireland.

Lund, S.K., & Light, J. (in press). The effectiveness of grammar instruction for individuals who use augmentative and alternative communication systems: A preliminary study. *Journal of Speech, Language and Hearing Research.*

Macke, R. (1992). *Preservice teacher attitudes towards nonvocal individuals using high-technology augmentative and alternative communication devices versus low-technology communication boards.* Unpublished dissertation, University of North Texas, Denton.

McCarthy, J., & Light, J. (2001). Instructional effectiveness of an integrated theater arts program for children using augmentative and alternative communication and nondisabled peers: A preliminary study. *Augmentative and Alternative Communication, 17,* 88–98.

McNaughton, D., Light, J., & Arnold, K. (2002). "Getting your wheel in the door": The full-time employment experiences of individuals with cerebral palsy who use AAC. *Augmentative and Alternative Communication, 18,* 59–76.

McNaughton, D., Light, J., & Gulla, S. (2002). *Opening up "a whole new world": Employer and co-worker perspectives on working with individuals who use augmentative and alternative communication.* Manuscript submitted for publication.

Mirenda, P. (1993). AAC: Bonding the uncertain mosaic. *Augmentative and Alternative Communication, 9,* 3–9.

Mirenda, P. (1997). Supporting individuals with challenging behavior through functional communication training and AAC: Research review. *Augmentative and Alternative Communication, 13,* 207–225.

O'Keefe, B.M. (1992). *Effects of communication aid outputs on attitudes toward individuals who use augmentative communication and on output preferences.* Unpublished doctoral dissertation, The Pennsylvania State University, University Park.

O'Keefe, B. (1996). Communication disorders: Just minor inconveniences? In R. Renwick, I. Brown, & M. Nagler (Eds.), *Quality of life in health promotion and rehabilitation: Conceptual approaches, issues, and applications* (pp. 219–236). Thousand Oaks, CA: Sage Publications.

Perner, J. (1988). Higher order beliefs and intentions in children's understanding of social interaction. In J.W. Astington, P.L. Harris, & D.R. Olson (Eds.), *Developing theories of mind* (pp. 217–239). New York: Cambridge University Press.

Rosenbaum, P.L., Armstrong, R.W., & King, S.M. (1986a). Children's attitudes toward disabled peers: A self-report measure. *Journal of Pediatric Psychology, 11,* 517–530.

Rosenbaum, P.L., Armstrong, R., & King, S. (1986b). Improving attitudes toward the disabled: A randomized controlled trial of direct contact versus Kids-on-the-Block. *Developmental and Behavioral Pediatrics, 7,* 302–307.

Rubin, J. (1975). What the "good" language learner can teach us. *TESOL Quarterly, 9,* 41–50.

Ryan, K.M. (1981). Developmental differences in reactions to the physically disabled. *Human Development, 24,* 240–256.

Savignon, S. (1983). *Communicative competence: Theory and classroom practice.* Reading, MA: Addison-Wesley.

Shaver, J., Curtis, C., & Strong C. (1989). The modification of attitudes toward persons with disabilities: Is there a best way? *International Journal of Special Education, 4,* 33–57.

Soto, G., Huer, M.B., & Taylor, O. (1997). Multicultural issues. In L.L. Lloyd, D.R. Fuller, & H.H. Arvidson (Eds.), *Augmentative and alternative communication: A handbook of principles and practices* (pp. 406–413). Needham Heights, MA: Allyn & Bacon.

Spitzburg, B., & Cupach, W. (1984). *Interpersonal communication competence.* Thousand Oaks, CA: Sage Publications.

Stuart, S. (1991). *Topic and vocabulary use patterns of elderly men and women in two age cohorts.* Unpublished doctoral dissertation, University of Nebraska–Lincoln.

Tager-Flusberg, H. (1997). Language acquisition and theory of mind: Contributions from the study of autism. In L.B. Adamson & M.A. Romski (Eds.), *Communication and language acquisition: Discoveries from atypical development* (pp. 135–160). Baltimore: Paul H. Brookes Publishing Co.

Triandis, H.C. (1971). *Attitudes and attitude change*. New York: John Wiley & Sons.

Van Reusen, A.K., Bos, C.S., Schumaker, J.B., & Deshler, D.D. (1994). *The self-advocacy strategy*. Lawrence, KS: Edge Press.

Warrick, A. (1988). Socio-communicative considerations within augmentative communication. *Augmentative and Alternative Communication, 4*, 45–51.

Wright, B. (1998). Attitudes and the fundamental negative bias: Conditions and corrections. In H.E. Yuker (Ed.), *Attitudes toward persons with disabilities*. New York: Springer.

Yuker, H.E. (1988). *Attitudes toward persons with disabilities*. New York: Springer.

Yuker, H.E. (1994). Variables that influence attitudes toward people with disabilities: Conclusions from the data. *Journal of Social Behavior and Personality, 9*, 3–22.

V

Strategic Competence

12

"Playing the Game"

Strategic Competence in AAC

Pat Mirenda and Karen D. Bopp

Despite important advances since the 1980s in the availability of user- and partner-friendly augmented and alternative communication (AAC) strategies, technologies, and instructional techniques, there is simply no doubt that individuals who use AAC are often in the position of not being able to say "what they want to, when they want, and how they want to" (Yoder & Kraat, 1983, p. 32). This may occur for a variety of reasons, including limitations that lie within the individuals themselves, their communicative partners, or the AAC techniques they use. In order to overcome such limitations, individuals who use AAC must have at their disposal a variety of "compensatory strategies [that] allow them to communicate effectively within restrictions" (Light, 1989, p. 141). Individuals who are able to use strategies effectively to overcome the limitations imposed by AAC use can be said to demonstrate strategic competence.

Because the skills that are needed for strategic competence are often seen as the icing on the cake—that is, helpful to the communication enterprise but not essential to it (which is, of course, erroneous)—very little has been written about them to date. Thus, in writing this chapter, we relied heavily on the experiences of the people who know the most about strategic competence in AAC—individuals who use AAC (primarily with cerebral palsy) who have written about how they "play the game" of communication. We read the books, essays, and poems they have written, as well as published accounts by AAC clinicians and researchers, to learn about strategic competence as it is required regularly in day-to-day interactions. In February 2001, we also interviewed a group of AAC specialists (teachers and speech-language pathologists) in British Columbia and asked them to tell us about the skills related to strategic competence that they have observed in the children and adults they support.[1] We organized what both individuals who use AAC and AAC professionals had to say into three categories—strategies to compensate for operational constraints, strategies to compensate for linguistic constraints, and strategies to compensate for social constraints—and also interspersed what we know from the professional literature across those three areas. Our purpose in this chapter is twofold: 1) to discuss the components of strategic competence and give examples of how individuals who use AAC demonstrate it in a variety of contexts; and 2) to identify issues related to strategic competence for future research.

WHAT IS STRATEGIC COMPETENCE?

As noted previously, strategic competence refers to a collection of adaptive skills that enable individuals who use AAC to compensate for 1) inherent linguistic, cognitive, motoric, sensory perceptual, or social limitations; or for 2) limitations that are imposed on them by external factors such as partner constraints or a specific AAC modality or device (e.g., because of the slow rate of communication, relative to natural speech, that is inherent in AAC use). When faced with such limitations, the "effective use of coping strategies is important for communicative competence . . . and distinguishes highly competent communicators from those who are less so" (Savignon, 1983, p. 43). The extent to which an individual has and is able to use the required "coping strategies" is a measure of his or her strategic competence.

Strategic competence is influenced by many factors, including a person's metacognitive skills (which, in turn, may be related to age, cognitive ability, and/or amount of experience with AAC), personality, and culture. The first of these, metacognitive skills, is actually comprised of several subcomponents, including an awareness of one's own abilities to plan, evaluate, and problem-solve as well as to regulate and understand the learning of others. First, the individual who uses AAC must be able to identify that a communication breakdown either has occurred or (ideally) might be prevented through the use of some type of strategy. Second, the person must be able to select an appropriate strategy that "matches" the problem, the context, and the communication partner's ability. Of course, the level of decision-making and problem-solving ability required for the second component can be reduced considerably if the individual who uses AAC is provided with and taught to use broad-based strategies that apply to a wide variety of situations and partners. Third, the person must know how to employ the strategy accurately and in a timely manner.

---

[1]We are grateful to our friends and colleagues for providing numerous examples of strategic competence that are reflected in the examples used in this chapter. The AAC specialists we interviewed included (in alphabetical order): Susan Blockberger, Patty Dixon, Christy Farahar-Amidon, Brenda Fossett, Jean Fowler, Sydney Hook, Lorraine Kamp, Katherine Munro, Sharon O'Dornan, Dave Platt, and Kathy Ryan.

Most children who use AAC, like most young children who use natural speech to communicate, have limited metacognitive abilities and this, in turn, limits their ability to either know that they need to use an adaptive strategy or to have one readily available. Similar problems may also be seen in individuals with cognitive impairments related to, for example, an acquired brain injury, mental retardation, or autism. Adults with acquired disabilities who begin to use AAC after a lifetime of speaking may also need assistance to develop and use appropriate strategies, depending on the extent to which their metacognitive and problem-solving abilities are affected. Of course, when more than one factor affects problem-solving ability (e.g., age and cognitive impairment, cognitive impairment and lack of experience with AAC), the difficulties are compounded.

Added to this is the issue of personality, which greatly influences the strategies that someone might choose to use. This was evidenced in a study that involved a 12-year-old girl named Vivian, who had severe speech and physical impairments and communicated via a Light Talker with an infrared sensor secured to her eyeglass frame (Buzolich & Lunger, 1995). Vivian was taught to use preprogrammed phrases to regulate her communicative partner's behavior in four types of situations that call for strategic competence:

1. When her partner was not positioned correctly for communication, relative to Vivian and her device
2. When her partner was unfamiliar with her device and how she used it
3. When her partner dominated the conversation
4. When a communication breakdown occurred

Vivian was taught to use a variety of preprogrammed regulatory messages that corresponded to each of these situations, such as, *"Can you come over here where I can see you?,"*[2] *"Say each letter as I point to it,"* *"Just a minute; I have something to say,"* and *"Wait, let me say it differently."* She was also taught to use several indirect strategies such as answering a question and then asking another one if the speaker was dominating the conversation, or making a repair when a communication breakdown occurred. In practice situations where the speech-language pathologist coached Vivian to use the preprogrammed phrases with speaking peers without disabilities, she did so quite successfully; however, Vivian's use of the regulatory messages during uncoached conversations with peers did not increase over baseline; instead, she used several of the indirect strategies she had been taught, to manage interactions more successfully. The authors noted that, given Vivian's shy personality, her selection of the less intrusive strategies might have been predicted from the outset and concluded

---

[2]In this chapter, we adopted the conventions used by the *Augmentative and Alternative Communication* journal for transcribing interaction modalities of individuals who use AAC and natural speakers. These conventions were originally described by Stephen von Tetzchner and Mogens Hygum Jensen (1996) in their book, *Augmentative and Alternative Communication: European Perspectives.*

that "matching the strategies taught to the needs, preferences, priorities, and personalities of AAC users is an important consideration" (p. 44).

It is also critical to consider the skills needed by communication partners who are the "recipients" of the strategies employed by individuals who use AAC. Some rate enhancement strategies, such as teaching a partner to guess the content of a message while it is being constructed, are unlikely to be successful with young children or individuals with limited cognitive or linguistic skills. Other strategies, such as those that are used to compensate for the semantic limitations of a communication display, may require that a partner be able to read a printed message, guess a rhyming or associated word, interpret gestures or facial expressions, and so forth. Some strategies may require the partner to understand synthetic speech or sign language, while others may require aided symbol or literacy skills. In virtually all situations in which strategies are used, communicative partners require the sensory (i.e., hearing and vision), linguistic, and social-pragmatic skills that are needed for effective communication in general.

A final consideration that is often overlooked is the effect of culture on the selection of adaptive strategies. Hetzroni and Harris (1996) noted that three issues are important to consider in this regard. First, individuals who use AAC may behave quite differently in settings populated by people from cultures other than their own, rendering brief observational assessments in such contexts invalid. Second, cultural norms may not be readily identified by individuals who use AAC due to language barriers or traditions of privacy. Finally, there are no exact formulas for determining the cultural appropriateness of various strategies. Thus, professionals seeking to encourage the development of strategic competence may be at a distinct disadvantage when supporting individuals from different cultural backgrounds and need to be aware of the impact of culture on the selection of strategies. For example, specific gestures (e.g., thumbs down for "no good") or error correction strategies (e.g., giving prolonged eye contact to signal that a listener has misunderstood) might be either misunderstood or unacceptable within some cultural contexts. Similarly, asking a communication partner to guess the content of message while it is being spelled may be perceived as impolite by the members of some cultural groups. In such situations, individuals who use AAC require adaptive strategies that are both culturally appropriate and successful.

From this brief discussion, it should be clear that strategic competence is not simply a collection of "tricks" that can be taught uniformly to all individuals who use AAC. Rather, individuals tend to develop strategies that work for them and their typical communication partners over time—resulting in a collection of "different strokes for different folks." In the sections that follow, we will attempt to provide examples of adaptive strategies that have been documented by individuals who use AAC themselves or the professionals who support them. We have summarized the strategies discussed in the sections that follow in Table 12.1. We have also indicated in Table 12.1 which strategies

Table 12.1. Summary of constraints and associated strategies

Constraint	Adaptive strategy	Temp[1]	Perm[2]
I. Operational constraints			
Rate of communication is too slow	Boot up computerized device or open communication book before it is needed		X
	Have a Personal Care Assistant (PCA) take notes in class		X
	Teach new communicative partners to guess message content as it is being constructed (e.g., by using a PLEASE GUESS WHAT I AM TRYING TO SAY symbol)	X	
	Involve a PCA to elaborate verbally on familiar topics on behalf of the augmented communicator	X	
Communication partner interrupts during message construction	Turn on electronic activation feedback beep or click to signal that message construction is occurring		X
	Use a pre-stored PLEASE WAIT or PLEASE DON'T INTERRUPT message		X
Natural or synthetic speech is difficult to understand	Substitute words that are difficult to understand with those that are more easily/accurately articulated		X
	Use short, unambiguous statements		X
Voice or printed output is not available when needed (e.g., filling out a form, in a classroom)	Have a communicative partner/PCA transcribe written responses onto appropriate form	X	X
	Prepare oral reports in advance and have a communicative partner/PCA read them out loud	X	X
Telephone conversations present numerous challenges	Have a PCA repeat or elaborate on telephone messages	X	X
	Use a speaker phone, write the message, and have a PCA read the message on the computer screen out loud	X	X
	Use a PCA as an interpreter or negotiator during telephone conversations	X	X
	Use a pre-stored message such as "I am using a communication device so please be patient and listen carefully."		X
	Use e-mail instead of the telephone	X	X

(continued)

405

Table 12.1. *(continued)*

Constraint	Adaptive strategy	Temp[1]	Perm[2]
II. Linguistic Constraints			
Augmented communicator has difficulty understanding the communication partner	Ask the communication partner to speak at a slower rate	X	
	Ask the communication partner to write or point to symbols in addition to speaking	X	
Word or phrase is not available on communication display	Use a SOUNDS LIKE or SOUNDS SORT OF LIKE symbol in combination with a word that is available on the display (e.g., SOUNDS LIKE + CAT = fat)		X
	For Blissymbols, use marker symbols combined with regular Blissymbols to change word meanings (e.g., RHYME MARKER + COLD = sold)		X
	Use gestures or facial expressions to change the meaning of an available word (e.g., FAST + turn hand over for "opposite" = slow)		X
	Use available symbols or phrases in novel ways (e.g., TOMORROW TOMORROW TOMORROW = 3 days from now; LONG + MORE = sounds like lawnmower)		X
	Use pre-stored phrases that are "close to" the desired message (e.g., "I like cats" + "I feel sick" = I'm allergic to cats)		X
	Direct the communication partner to ASK A MULTIPLE CHOICE QUESTION or ASK YES/NO QUESTIONS		X
Syntactic or grammatical markers are not available on the communication display	Paraphrase or use alternative word order to convey a message		X
	Use gestures in combination with symbols (e.g., EAT CAKE + waving a hand backwards to indicate past tense = ate cake)		X
	Use existing symbols in novel ways (e.g., point to a symbol multiple times to indicate the plural form)		X
Difficulty expressing emotions or nuances with electronic or low-tech communication display	Use a PCA to communicate emotional messages using speech	X	X
	Point to a symbol many times to indicate emphasis		X
	Change the synthesized voice on a VOCA to increase loudness, whisper, and so forth	X	X
III. Social Constraints			
Communication partner is unfamiliar or uncomfortable with AAC	Ensure good grooming and well-kept appearance to overcome stereotypes about people with disabilities		X
	Use an introductory message explaining AAC system and how to use it	X	X
	Use an icebreaker or joke to place a new communication partner at ease	X	
	Teach the PCA to always direct conversation back to the augmented communicator		X

Strategy	Temp[1]	Perm[2]
Conversational partner dominates the conversation		
Respond to yes/no questions and immediately add additional information or ask a question	X	X
Use a preprogrammed phrase (e.g., "Do you know what?") to introduce a new topic		
Use a preprogrammed phrase (e.g., "Just a minute") to act as a place holder for a turn in the conversation	X	X
Conversational partner guesses during message construction when augmented communicator prefers otherwise		
Use a preprogrammed phrase to ask the communicative partner not to guess		
Deliberately change a message mid-way through construction to prevent the communicative partner from guessing	X	
Communication partner misinterprets or has difficulty understanding the augmented communicator's message		
Use a preprogrammed phrase to indicate sarcasm (e.g., THAT WAS A JOKE) or to get interpretation assistance from another person (e.g., ASK MY MOM)	X	X
Repeat and/or rephrase the message		X
Use a symbol or phrase to signal a repair (e.g., "Wait, let me say it differently")		
Switch to a communication "backup" mode if the communication partner is unfamiliar with the primary mode of communication (e.g., manual signing) or does not understand it	X	
Switch the mode of communication to overcome unanticipated vision, literacy, or language limitations of the communication partner	X	
IV. Environmental Constraints		
Busy environment does not allow time for message construction — Use personalized preprogrammed messages stored under individuals' names for rapid recall		X
Environment is unusually quiet or noisy — Turn the volume on a VOCA down or up, depending on noise level	X	X
Communication is difficult in formal environments because of time constraints — Switch to an unaided or low-technology mode of communication	X	X
Provide a letter of introduction that includes relevant history and current concerns	X	
E-mail or fax a letter of introduction in advance	X	
People eavesdrop during message construction by reading a VOCA's computer screen — Change the display angle on the screen so that it is unreadable to onlookers		X

[1]Temp = strategy may be used to overcome communication difficulties that are temporary in nature (i.e., occasional)

[2]Perm = strategy may be used to overcome communication difficulties that are permanent (i.e., regularly occurring)

are likely to be used to overcome communication difficulties that are temporary in nature (i.e., they may occur in a specific context or situation) and that are more permanent (i.e., they may occur regularly, across many contexts and situations).

STRATEGIES TO COMPENSATE FOR OPERATIONAL CONSTRAINTS

Operational skills refer to the skills required for the technical operation of AAC systems. Light and Binger (1998) listed a number of operational skills, including producing the correct hand shapes, positions, orientations, and movements required within a manual sign system; selecting symbols accurately from a display by using an appropriate access technique; producing messages that are intelligible to a partner; formulating messages at an acceptable rate; delivering messages with appropriate timing; and maintaining the smooth flow of a conversation. In ideal situations, most individuals who use appropriately individualized AAC systems are unlikely to experience difficulties with most of these skills. But what happens when the room in which conversation takes place is quite noisy, or when the synthetic speech produced by a device is difficult to understand? What happens when the individual who uses AAC is a student in a fast-paced classroom, or is an executive participating in an overseas conference call? Can an individual who uses AAC order a pizza over the phone or answer a phone call made to his or her home? These "ordinarily unusual" situations are part of daily life for many people who use AAC and often require adaptive strategies in order to be managed successfully. The main operational constraints that may require strategic competence are the slow rate of AAC message production, the use of communicative output that may be difficult to understand, and the difficulties that may arise during telephone conversations.

Communication Rate

Perhaps the most common operational constraint faced by individuals who use AAC is related to the slow rate of communication. Even in the best of circumstances, using electronic AAC devices with the most sophisticated rate enhancement features available, communication via AAC is substantially slower than natural speech. Because no single strategy will suit every person or every situation, most individuals who use AAC develop and/or learn a variety of strategies for speeding up the rate of communication beyond that which can be achieved by their AAC systems alone. Some of these strategies may be quite simple, such as turning on a computerized AAC device a few minutes before it is needed, so that it has time to boot up; opening a communication book to the appropriate page before initiating a conversation, if page turning takes too much time; or having an assistant take notes during a class or meeting, if letter-by-letter writing is slow and laborious (McMillen, 2000). Other strategies may be more elaborate, such as teaching a communication partner to indicate his or her understanding of a message and/or guess the contents of a message while it is being constructed. Peg Johnson commented on the use of such strategies:

> When I am speaking or using my VOCA, it is essential that my communication partner indicate in some manner that they are receiving and understanding the message . . . Giving my communication partner the subject matter of the exchange oftentimes facilitates efficient interaction. It also speeds up the communication process. To save time and energy, I prefer to allow my communication partner to finish my sentences, as long as she is in tune with what I am attempting to say. In order to speed up the process, I need to clarify, deny, or confirm the accuracy of their interpretation. . . .However, some augmentative communicators want to finish their own words or sentences whether their partner can predict the message or not. It's up to the individual. (Johnson, 2000, p. 52)

One of the most commonly used strategies for teaching a partner to guess is the use of a *PLEASE GUESS WHAT I AM TRYING TO SAY* symbol or message (Buzolich & Lunger, 1995; Light & Binger, 1998). Alternatively, many individuals who use AAC prefer to use nonverbal modes such as facial expressions to encourage guessing (e.g., spelling out the first few letters of a word and then looking at the partner expectantly) and hand gestures or head shakes to indicate that a guessing error has been made.

Another common speed enhancement strategy is to involve a personal care assistant (PCA) or another person in communication interactions. Peg Johnson noted that she expects her PCAs to be involved with interactions "so they can readily expand or offer background information when necessary. Ideally, my assistants and I develop an understanding that there will be specific times when . . . I will need them to expound on what I'm saying. . . .Some kind of signal or cue needs to be in place" (Johnson, 2000, pp. 52–53). Tara McMillen defended her use of this strategy for communication speed enhancement:

> When I am out in public where people are concerned with time, I use my assistant. Some people think that I shouldn't because they think people should wait and listen to me. Heck, if I wanted to do that I could go home and write them a 10-page essay. The fact is, I don't want to make them wait and I don't want to wait, not when I have an assistant . . . [What I have to say is] more important than the vehicle I use to say it. To me, my assistant . . . just functions as a higher-level communication device, . . . communicating my exact ideas, only faster than I can type. (McMillen, 2000, pp. 81, 83)

McMillen also described how she and her PCA worked together to prepare for and communicate during an important meeting:

> My assistant and I spent hours to make sure that she knew what I had to say. We were prepared. She was going to talk, and I was going to nod my head showing them that they were my words. . . .I made a note saying that although it might seem like she's talking for herself, she's really talking for me . . . [At the meeting], my assistant said, "Tara would like to say . . . " before she started talking. She always does this. . . . (McMillen, 2000, p. 82)

Of course, individuals are likely to have differing opinions about the appropriateness of this strategy and the extent to which they wish to use it, so it is important to establish a clear understanding about when "translating" is acceptable. Michael Williams noted that his PCAs are not allowed to speak for him "unless they are authorized to do so," and he teaches them "to redirect any question asked of them about me back to me" (Williams, 2000, p. 235). Jim Prentice emphasized that, although "I don't mind if [my assistant finishes] my sentence because. . . it's faster," he does not use his assistant while having a conversation because he does not feel "that there is any time that is appropriate for an assistant to speak on my behalf" (Prentice, 2000, p. 212). As noted previously, such choices about the use of specific strategies are usually driven by factors such as personality, culture, and experience.

Another common problem for individuals who use AAC is being interrupted during message construction, especially when letter-by-letter spelling is used, because of the slow speed with which they communicate. Two useful strategies in this regard include turning on the activation feedback beep or click provided in many electronic AAC devices, so the communication partner is aware that message construction is taking place and using a pre-stored *PLEASE WAIT* or *PLEASE DON'T INTERRUPT* message (Light & Binger, 1998). David Chapple, an engineer at a small software company named Cyber-Access, described his unique use of activation feedback during message construction:

> I think it would be ludicrous to think that while I am in meetings with a lot of people, like project meetings, department meetings, or company meetings, everybody should wait in silence while I type what I have to say. The employees at CyberAccess realize that when they hear my clicking, I am going to say something, but the meeting doesn't come to a halt. The discussion continues until they don't hear the clicking. At that time, they acknowledge me, and I speak what is on my mind. (Chapple, 2000, p. 159)

Chapple's strategy of using feedback clicks to signal message construction during meetings serves to emphasize the importance of using individualized strategies that "match" specific communicative contexts. In this case, the same strategy that might be used in one situation to signal, "I'm typing; please wait" may be used in another situation to signal "I'm typing; please listen for me to finish and then give me the floor," depending on the preferences of the individual involved. It is clear that a wide variety of strategies are likely to be used by individuals who use AAC to compensate for their relatively slow rates of interaction.

Communicative Output

Strategies related to communicative output may be necessary if the mode of output (e.g., natural speech, synthetic speech, print) is likely to result in either a communication breakdown or unusual difficulty with message transmission. For example, many individuals who use AAC are able to use natural speech or speech approximations to say specific words or phrases and often prefer to speak whenever possible. Mick Joyce shared a strategy that he has developed so that he can use his speech most effectively and minimize the likelihood of being misunderstood:

> I anticipate words that are not easily understood before I say them and fill in the appropriate substitution almost automatically. For example, words starting with "v" or "f" are usually difficult for me. The word "fish" usually comes out "pish" and the word "various" will come out "berries." When I see these words coming, I usually substitute them before they leave my mouth. Some words just can't be substituted. That's when I need my computer or voice synthesizer. (Joyce, 2000, pp. 93–94)

Similarly, the synthetic speech produced by some AAC devices may be difficult to understand, either in general or in specific situations. Toby Churchill suggested that, when using a voice output communication aid (VOCA), "short, unambiguous statements are best for most people—a bus driver or shop assistant doesn't need the user's life story. One idea is ideal ('Let's do this'). Two ideas are all that most people can manage ('If this then this, if not then that'). Three ideas usually confuse . . ." (Churchill, 2000, p. 133)

Classroom situations often present special challenges with respect to output, which require unique solutions. Gordon Cardona (2000) developed several strategies to compensate for the lack of voice output and conventional print output produced by the Canon Communicator he used while attending a university. In order to take tests or exams, he first enlisted the assistance of a test proctor to transfer his responses from the long strip of paper printed by the Canon to the "official" answer form. Then, the proctor put the exam, the official form, and the strip of paper in an envelope and sealed it, so that Cardona could take the package to the instructor to grade. When he had to make a presentation to an entire class, Cardona used an "advance preparation" strategy (Beukelman & Mirenda, 1998) and typed his speech at home on a typewriter so that it could be read out loud to the class by the instructor; he then used his Canon to type brief answers to questions after the "oral" presentation. This strategy solved two problems simultaneously: the slow speed of letter-by-letter typing and the fact that voice output was not available in the Canon Communicator. Individualized strategies such as these are critical in order for individuals who use AAC to be able to participate fully in elementary, secondary, and postsecondary school classrooms.

Telephone Conversations

One of the books that was invaluable to us as we wrote this chapter was *Speaking Up and Spelling It Out* (Fried-Oken & Bersani, 2000), a collection of essays by individuals who use AAC about various aspects of the AAC experience. As we searched the essays for examples of strategic competence, we were struck by the fact that the constraining situation that was mentioned most often throughout the book was use of the telephone. Mick Joyce, who described himself as feeling like a "fish out of water" (p. 89) in some types of communication situations, explained the difficulty he experiences with telephone use, even when using his VOCA:

> I have trouble with this wonderful trinket of technology. . . .For me, a telephone is a constricting device. . . .Most [people] fuss and fume, put you on hold several times, and then expect you to say who you want, why, and where you can be reached, all in five seconds. (Joyce, 2000, p. 94)

Individuals who use AAC employ a variety of operational strategies when telephone interactions are necessary. Joyce uses "whatever works for the individual caller" (p. 94) and noted that

> When possible, I prefer my [PCA] to stand by to repeat what I say, at least in the initial stages of the conversation. Then I phase them out after I get the person I want or the topic of the conversation is established . . . Many times I use my voice output device, as well. This sometimes works . . . [And] sometimes it's just faster to have [someone] make calls for me themselves, like for ordering a computer part. (Joyce, 2000, p. 94)

With regard to the latter strategy, Toby Churchill noted that he prefers to use a speaker phone and have his PCA

> [Read] out the words on my computer screen. This means that I can be silently typing the next thought while the person at the other end is talking, and my assistant can reply almost immediately. The conversation is thus more fluid (and quicker, cheaper, less tiring, and more productive). (Churchill, 2000, p. 134)

Of course, Churchill's strategy of using his PCA as an "interpreter" can also be used to assist individuals who use symbols and/or unaided communication modes during telephone conversations. Collier (1998) noted that, when telephone interpretation is used, it is important for the interpreter to

1. Introduce him- or herself by first name or not at all
2. Explain that he or she is there to relay the messages of the individual who uses AAC, and provide the full name of the individual who uses AAC
3. Explain that the listener may need to wait while the individual who uses AAC constructs each message

4. Relay the message as it is constructed so that the meaning is intact and understandable

5. Stay out of the discussion otherwise

Collier also described two variations of the interpretation strategy. One is to have a second party simply deliver a message over the telephone, without the individual who uses AAC present to co-construct it. This might be appropriate when the message is quite straightforward, such as canceling an appointment or asking about the times a movie is being screened. The second is to have someone else negotiate a decision on behalf of the individual who uses AAC during a telephone call, such as might occur if an appointment needs to be made. In this case, the individual who uses AAC typically provides options (e.g., potential dates and times for an appointment) that are then conveyed over the telephone, and the listener chooses from among them. If none of the options are acceptable, the "negotiator" goes back to the individual who uses AAC, relays this message, gets more options, and calls again.

In addition, specific telephone situations may call for specialized telephone strategies, such as the one used by an executive whose PCA regularly functioned as his "voice" during conference calls. He instructs his PCA to expand on a topic on his behalf (*Tell him about...*) and then uses the buzzer on his device to signal "I have something to say" during the call. This is similar to the strategy described previously by David Chapple for use during face-to-face business meetings.

Because some individuals who use AAC find second-party strategies unacceptable, additional strategies may also be needed. Jim Prentice commented,

> I am a very independent person; therefore, I do not feel that I need my assistant to make telephone calls for me. In order to avoid having the other party on the line hang up on me, especially when they answer and it takes me a minute to get started, I have preprogrammed an explanation. As soon as they say *Hello*, I press the icon where I have stored the message that says, *"I am using a communicating device so please be patient and listen carefully."* It's amazing how that message can bring about such good results. They inevitably answer, *Thank you, I will, and you just take your time.* (Prentice, 2000, p. 212)

Other individuals, such as Gordon Cardona, find yet other solutions: "There are many people to whom I only e-mail instead of picking up the phone and calling them. I feel e-mail is the most efficient way to communicate" (Cardona, 2000, p. 244).

It is clear that telephone use remains a major challenge for some individuals, and a range of strategies is likely to be needed in this area, depending on the situation and the people involved. Overall, it seems that much work remains with regard to the development of increasingly user-friendly technologies that preclude the need for the wide array of operational strategies that are currently needed by individuals who use AAC. In particular, innovations related to improving the rate of communication with electronic devices as well as the interface between such devices and conventional telephone technology appear to be top priorities.

STRATEGIES TO COMPENSATE FOR LINGUISTIC CONSTRAINTS

In general, linguistic skills refer to the ability to understand and express information in one's native language and, in the case of individuals who use AAC, in the "linguistic code" of the AAC system (Light & Binger, 1998). Linguistic skills include demonstrating an understanding of the meaning of spoken words or sentences (e.g., yes/no questions, *wh-* questions, comments) and using appropriate words or grammatical forms. In general, the "linguistic code" is broken into four areas: semantic skills; morphosyntactic skills; prosodic skills; and pragmatic skills, which are related to the use of language in social contexts and will be addressed in a subsequent section focused on "social limitations." Semantic skills enable people to understand and produce a variety of word meanings. Morphosyntactic skills refer to understanding and use of the rules that govern grammar and sentence construction, such as appropriate word order (e.g., *I went to the store* versus *The store to I went*) or language forms such as possessives (e.g., boy/boy's), past tense (e.g., walk/walked), and plural endings (e.g., cat/cats). Finally, prosodic skills enable people to add stress and intonation to their spoken words by making changes in pitch or loudness level, in order to convey a variety of meanings.

Many individuals who use AAC have no difficulty understanding the unaided (e.g., gestured, spoken, signed) or aided (e.g., written) messages communicated to them by others, but adequate language comprehension is certainly not universal in this population. Competent communication for many individuals with both developmental disabilities (e.g., mental retardation, autism, deafblindness) and acquired disabilities (e.g., traumatic brain injury, severe aphasia, Huntington's disease) is often impeded by their receptive language deficits. Individuals who use AAC and are aware of their need for supports in this area require strategies for signaling their communication partners to revise, restate, or recode their messages so that they can be better understood.

Similarly, many individuals who use AAC have the ability to utilize specific semantic, morphosyntactic, or prosodic skills through their individual AAC systems; however, most AAC devices are not capable of accommodating language production in all of these areas, all of the time. For example, what if a desired word or phrase is not programmed into a device, or what if a person wishes to emphasize a point or express a specific emotion through pitch or loudness level? In addition, Light (1997) noted that a majority of the AAC symbol sets in current use (e.g., Picture Communication Symbols, Picsyms, Minspeak icons, key word signing) lack many of the basic parameters of language and are limited with regard to the range of word meanings and/or morphosyntactic components that they can convey (e.g., tense or plural forms). Thus, it is almost inevitable that individuals who use AAC, especially those who rely on symbols rather than orthography to communicate, will at least occasionally find themselves needing to express a word meaning, concept, or specific language form or wanting to emphasize a point or use their device to speak with emotion, only to discover that the options they require are not readily available. It is in these situations that individuals using AAC must rely on their strategic competence.

Comprehension Skills

As noted previously, language comprehension is often problematic for individuals who use AAC because they experience either developmental or acquired disorders that affect this area of linguistic ability. In addition, comprehension problems may occur because of a second-language barrier or because of a communication partner's unfamiliar speech pattern or accent. Sometimes, the solution is as simple as asking a partner to speak more slowly or with less affect. In other situations, a technique for "augmented comprehension" may be used by the communication partner (see, for example, Wood, Lasker, Siegel-Causey, Beukelman, & Ball, 1998). Relevant to the issue of strategic competence is the question, Does the individual who uses AAC have a strategy for cueing his or her communication partner to use one or more augmented comprehension techniques when comprehension difficulty occurs?

Several authors have described the use of augmented comprehension cueing strategies, especially with adults who use AAC. For example, Cress and King (1999) described "CE," a 60-year-old man with severely impaired comprehension as a result of primary progressive aphasia. With the support of an AAC interventionist, CE and his family developed symbol communication displays that they used, along with speech, to give him information about upcoming events. CE himself learned to use symbols such as *TELL ME AGAIN, SHOW ME,* and *I DON'T UNDERSTAND* to let his communication partners know that a misunderstanding had occurred and that they needed to use his display for clarification. Similarly, Garrett and Beukelman provided an example of an "augmented input explanation card" that individuals with severe aphasia could use to request various comprehension enhancement techniques. Among other things, the card contained the following written information:

> If I look puzzled, *don't* talk louder. *Do* use this notebook to: 1) Write down important words you say; 2) Write down what you think I said—that way I can change it if it's wrong; and 3) Write down the name of the topic (especially if you change it fast). Seeing our conversation in print really helps. Thanks for taking the time. (1992, p. 301)

Although the previous examples both involved adults with aphasia, similar strategies are also appropriate for use by children or adolescents with a wide variety of disabilities. For example, Darcy, an adolescent with Down syndrome, immigrated with her family to North America from Israel. Although Darcy had used PCS symbols (with printed word labels in Hebrew) to communicate with others for several years, her English comprehension skills were minimal. Unfortunately, she soon began to engage in aggressive behavior toward others (e.g., hitting, kicking, pinching) whenever she became frustrated with her inability to understand spoken directions or explanations from others. Darcy learned to hand her PCS symbol book to her communication partner whenever she did not understand a spoken message; on the front of the book was a large red card that read: "If I give you this book, please try to find a symbol that means what you are trying to say, and point to it so I will understand. If you can't find a symbol, try acting it out." Use of this strategy resulted in a dramatic reduction in Darcy's aggressive behavior and, in addition, enhanced her ability to learn to understand English because she had frequent opportunities to associate spoken English words with already-familiar PCSs. While Darcy's story may be somewhat unusual, her predicament—that of being an individual who uses AAC with a different language background than those in the majority culture—is certainly not. It is also important to note that the strategy Darcy learned to use could be applied to a wide variety of situations in which comprehension breakdowns may occur.

Semantic Limitations

Semantic skills refer to a person's ability to understand and use a variety of word meanings. Unfortunately, many AAC systems include only core vocabulary words and lack the fringe vocabulary that is needed for true individualization (Beukelman & Mirenda, 1998). Semantic limitations arise primarily when a word or a phrase is not available in the AAC system or when questions are asked in a confusing format that cannot be readily answered.

Many strategies are used by individuals who use AAC to overcome limitations in vocabulary. Not uncommonly, various combinations of facial expressions, gestures, and symbols are used to communicate novel messages. Some individuals use a *SOUNDS LIKE* or *SOUNDS SORT OF LIKE* symbol and then relate it to an existing word that is available in their system. For example, when Tracy wanted to describe Santa Claus to her classmates, she activated the *SOUNDS LIKE* symbol on her VOCA, followed by the symbol for *CAT* to communicate the word *fat*.

Individuals who use Blissymbols (Hehner, 1980) are quite familiar with the use of such strategies through the use of marker symbols that can be combined with regular Blissymbols to change their conventional meanings. For example, Audra used the *OPPOSITE MEANING* Blissymbol combined with the Blissymbol for *MANY* to tell her friends that she only got a *few* gifts for her birthday. However, she assured them that she was happy with her gifts because they consisted of a brand new set of *BEDROOM FURNITURE* (the latter word was constructed by combining the *GENERALIZATION MARKER + CHAIR + TABLE = FURNITURE*). Blissymbol markers are also available to create new "negative meaning" words (e.g., *MINUS MARKER + SOUND = SILENCE*), homonyms (e.g., *SIMILAR SOUND MARKER + THERE = THEIR*), rhyming words (e.g., *RHYME MARKER + COLD = SOLD*), and group words (e.g., *GROUP MARKER + TREE = FOREST*), among others. The system of Blissymbolics, which is one of the first widely available symbol systems used in AAC (Bliss, 1965), was also the first to incorporate such strategies to bypass semantic constraints.

Another semantic strategy is to combine gestures and available symbols, as Jonathan did when he turned his hand over (indicating "opposite of") and then selected the symbol *FAST* to communicate the word *slow*. Light (1997) provided an excellent example of how a young boy demonstrated his ability to use a multimodality compensatory strategy to communicate a unique message to his mother:

> Tim vocalized to get his mother's attention, then looked at his mom, looked at his dinner, looked back at his mom, frowned, then selected the line drawing of the dog from his computer-based AAC system (thus retrieving the preprogrammed message *"My dog's name is Skippy"*). After numerous attempts, Tim's mother eventually determined that Tim intended to communicate the intrinsic message "dog," not the extrinsic message produced by the speech synthesizer, and that he was trying to tell her to give his dinner to his dog because he didn't like it. (Light, 1997, p. 165)

Yet another strategy is to use only the symbols available on an AAC display, but use them in novel ways. For example, on Monday, Julio wanted to tell his friend that he would be going to see a movie the following Saturday. Unfortunately, his display did not have symbols for the days of the week, but it did have symbols for *YESTERDAY, TODAY,* and *TOMORROW*. Julio simply pointed to the *TOMORROW* symbol five times to indicate that he would be going to the movie in five "tomorrows," or on Saturday.

Two other individuals who use AAC were also inventive in overcoming the semantic limitations of their AAC systems. Melissa, a first-grade student, wished to tell her teacher that she needed to get something from her cubby. The word *cubby* was not available on her symbol display, so Melissa pointed to the symbols *LITTLE* and *BEAR* (a little bear is called a *cub*) and gestured towards the cubby area. Similarly, Ken, a third-grade boy, wanted to tell his friend to look out of the classroom window at the lawnmower, a word that was not available on his display. Ken combined the symbols for *LONG* and *MORE* (say it fast: sounds like *lawnmower*) and gestured toward the window. Clearly, these students have all developed strategies for communicating unique messages, even when the exact symbols they need are unavailable. Although they were all limited semantically by their AAC symbol displays, they were still able to communicate their messages using individualized approaches that demonstrated excellent strategic competence.

Some of the difficulties encountered with regard to semantics are not limited to the meanings of single words. Many individuals use AAC displays that contain primarily phrases and sentences and may find themselves constrained in conversations that are not well represented in the messages available. A common solution to this dilemma is to use one or more phrases or sentences that are close in meaning to the desired message. For example, when Sara wanted to tell her friend that she had gone shopping over the weekend at Zeller's department store, she used the preprogrammed phrase *"I want to go to Zeller's,"* and her friend was able to figure out the correct meaning. Another teenager, Elaine, was having a conversation with some friends about cats and combined the phrases *"I like cats"* and *"I feel sick"* to indicate that she was allergic to cats. Another strategy when the desired message is not available is to use a pre-stored message directing the communication partner to, for example, *ASK A MULTIPLE CHOICE QUESTION* or *ASK YES/NO QUESTIONS*, so that the individual who uses AAC can participate accurately in the interaction.

Morphosyntactic Limitations

Morphosyntactic skills refer to the use of the rules that govern the formation of grammatical phrases, such as appropriate word combinations. They also include the use of morphological language forms such as plural or past tense endings. Limitations requiring strategic competence may occur in one or both of these areas if the necessary language forms are not available in the AAC system. Syntactic or grammatical limitations may result if the "little words" that are so important for correct grammatical construction (e.g., *the, and, of,* prepositions) are omitted from an AAC display. Morphological limitations often occur as a result of the lack of availability of markers such as the *'s* for possessives or the *–ed* ending for past tense.

One strategy that is often used to compensate for missing syntactic or grammatical markers is paraphrasing or alternating the word order in a message. Van Balkom and Welle Donker-Gimbrère (1996) offered a number of excellent examples of this strategy in their description of the communication of four adolescents who used aided symbol displays. For example, one child used the sequence *BOY WILL PUSH TO STORE GIRL* to mean "The boy will push the girl to the store" (p. 165). Another student communicated *CLEAN GIRL MUMMY DESK,* meaning "They (the girl and her mummy) clean the desk" (p. 165). Even more creative were the multiple position deviations seen in the message *TWO BED SLEEP BOY ONE GIRL WHITE BED BROWN BED,* meaning "The boy and the girl are sleeping in two beds, one in a white bed and one in a brown bed" (p. 165). All of these are excellent examples of individuals who use AAC "mak[ing] the best of what they . . . know and can do," to compensate for syntactic elements that are missing from their symbol displays (Light, 1989, p. 141).

Sometimes, the appropriate words are available on a communication display, but the morphological markers are not. Often, gestures can be used effectively to substitute for markers for past or future tense. For example, when Mark wanted to indicate to his brother that he had eaten some birthday cake during the lunch hour, he combined the symbols *EAT CAKE* with a gesture of waving his hand back over his shoulder to indicate the past tense. Using existing symbols in novel ways is also a useful strategy that is particularly applicable to plural nouns, as demonstrated by Graeme when he wanted to buy several cookies from the bakery. He communicated this to the store clerk by activating his VOCA to say *"I want cookie, cookie, cookie, cookie, cookie, cookie,"* meaning "I want a half dozen cookies." It is important to both teach the use of strategies such as these and to encourage individuals who use AAC to develop their own strategies for overcoming morphosyntactic limitations that may arise in specific situations.

Prosodic Limitations

Think for a moment about a recent discussion that you may have had, in which you were defending a belief or position. Did you find yourself raising your voice or changing your voice pitch to make your point? Think as well about how many times each day you use one- or two-word phrases to ask questions. You accomplish this quite simply, by using a rising intonation at the end of a word or phrase—for instance, by asking *Apple?* to mean "Do you want an apple?" Finally, think about how most natural speakers express emotions such as happiness or sadness; again, much of the message is in the tone of voice that is used. For an individuals who use AAC, the limitation of being unable to use prosodic features such as pitch, volume, tone, or emotion to communicate is one that is most likely faced every day. As Toby Churchill wrote, "(t)he human voice can give my words intonation, spontaneity, humor, and wit. Machines can't do that (yet)" (Churchill, 2000 p. 134).

Individuals who use AAC often develop or learn numerous strategies to overcome this limitation. Tara McMillen described her solution:

> One thing that an assistant can do that a machine cannot do is show emotions. . . . A machine can do only so much; you can turn the volume up or down, but that's about it. When I am really happy or concerned with something, my assistant can show that emotion because she is with me most of the time. I grab her attention to show her that I want to interject on an issue. She reads me and knows how to act to show what I am feeling. (McMillen, 2000, p. 82)

Clearly, McMillen's use of her PCA to express emotion is a solution that works well for her. Use of a human voice is not the only answer, however. Often, existing messages on an AAC device can be used in novel ways, for example, to emphasize a point. For example, Tricia, a university student, was speaking with a friend and wanted to make it perfectly clear that she did not agree with a specific political stance the friend was taking. To emphasize her point, Tricia pointed to the *NO* symbol on her communication display over and over again, because she could not raise her voice volume or adjust her pitch.

Some individuals with sophisticated VOCAs may learn to adjust the volume, pitch, or baud rate of their devices to vary the speech output, especially when preprogrammed messages are used. For example, Martha was not feeling well one day and wanted to make this point clear to her mother. She programmed the message *"I have a sore throat"* into her AAC device and then changed its synthesized voice to one called "Rough Rita," a female voice that is deep and husky. Upon arriving home, Martha activated the appropriate icon sequence and told her mother *"I have a sore throat,"* complete with raspy, scratchy voice, sounding just like anyone with a sore throat might! Martha has clearly mastered the intricacies of her AAC device and makes maximum use of its ability to communicate the prosodic features of communication.

To conclude, it is clear that linguistic limitations related to semantics, morphosyntax, and prosody remain a challenge to persons using AAC systems; however, it is also evident that numerous strategies are available to enable individuals who use AAC to overcome these limitations.

STRATEGIES TO COMPENSATE FOR SOCIAL CONSTRAINTS

Sociocommunicative skills or pragmatic skills, as they were referred to in the previous section, include how we initiate, maintain, develop, and terminate interactions (Light & Binger, 1998). They are skills that we use to "develop positive relationships and interactions with others . . . [and they allow us to] express a full range of communicative functions (e.g., requests for objects, protests, requests for information, etc.)" (Light & Binger, 1998, p. 2). Think for a moment about the numerous sociocommunicative skills that you use everyday during interactions with others. You use various verbal and nonverbal behaviors to gain attention, take your turn when conversing, respond appropriately to questions that are asked, make comments about what others are saying, seek clarification when necessary, and demonstrate your interest in the interaction.

Generally, interactions flow smoothly between two or more individuals who use natural speech to communicate because all of the parties involved have had considerable experience interacting according to social and cultural conventions; however, individuals who use AAC may face difficulties in social interactions because of the unique challenges presented by the form of their communication. Some people may be uncomfortable around individuals who use AAC and may be reluctant to interact with them at all. Because of the relative slowness of AAC compared with natural speech, communication partners may dominate or control conversations by not allowing individuals who use AAC time to initiate topics, make comments, or ask questions. And, even when communication control is shared, it is inevitable that communication breakdowns will occur and will require repair strategies. In addition, environmental constraints such as noisy, busy, or unusually quiet environments can also lead to social breakdowns. Finally, the need for privacy in conversations or other types of interactions may be difficult for individuals who use AAC to achieve in some contexts. Each of these situations is likely to require specific strategies for overcoming social constraints.

Unfamiliar Communication Partners

It is not at all uncommon for social breakdowns to occur during interactions between individuals who use AAC and unfamiliar communication partners such as shopkeepers, waitpersons, or people encountered in casual social contexts. Some individuals are simply not comfortable around people with disabilities in general, and thus may avoid interactions with individuals who use AAC. Others may have never encountered a specific AAC device or technique before and may be unsure how to interact with someone who uses it. Still others may not understand the role of a PCA and may address comments and questions to him or her instead of to the individual who uses AAC.

Other people's discomfort around people with disabilities is not a constraint that can be easily overcome because it can have many sources. Often, the assumption is made that people with disabilities who cannot speak are also cognitively impaired. This, in turn, can lead to increased fear and avoidance because even today, many people associate cognitive impairments with unpredictability, lack of control, and even violent behavior. Peg Johnson wrote about her experience in this regard and the strategy she uses to overcome the stereotype:

> Due to my poor speech, people automatically assume that I am retarded and treat me accordingly. In order to overcome this, I consider my appearance to be extremely important. . . . I have found that when I am dressed in proper suits, it is easier for people to interact on an equal basis. It is expected that the assistant that gets me dressed in the morning will do her best to make sure my hair is styled, my makeup is applied neatly, and that my clothes and jewelry are put on correctly. Other assistants that come throughout the day are expected to help me maintain this appearance. . . . My nonverbal message or statement opens doors which can turn into verbal interchange. (Johnson, 2000, pp. 53–54)

Less extreme is the reluctance of many natural speakers to interact with individuals who use AAC, not because of negative attitudes about specific disabilities but because they are unfamiliar with AAC in general. As Light and Binger

(1998) noted, "Communication is a two-way process; the success of any interaction depends on both participants" (p. 46). A large body of research studies has focused on the impact of AAC on the attitudes of communication partners. In these studies, participants without disabilities typically view videotapes of individuals who use AAC or actors without disabilities using various AAC techniques and then respond to statements designed to assess their attitudes (e.g., "I would be comfortable interacting with this person at work") using Likert-type scales (e.g., 1 = strongly disagree; 5 = strongly agree).

In general, children's attitudes appear to be less influenced than adults' by the type of AAC technique used. For example, studies conducted in the United States and Canada compared VOCAs to nonelectronic communication displays and/or manual signs with children in elementary school (grades 1–5) and found no significant effect of AAC modality on children's attitudes (Beck & Dennis, 1996; Beck, Fritz, Keller, & Dennis, 2000; Blockberger, Armstrong, O'Connor, & Freeman, 1993). However, a recent South African study found that children 11–13 years of age (grades 6–7) responded more positively to videotapes of a child who spelled messages using a VOCA than one who used a nonelectronic alphabet display (Lilienfeld & Alant, 2002).

Similarly, studies with adult participants have shown consistently more positive attitudes about and/or increased interactions with individuals who use VOCAs compared to those who use alphabet displays (e.g., Gorenflo & Gorenflo, 1991; Lasker, 2000; Schepis & Reid, 1995). Attitudes about VOCAs may be enhanced by high-quality speech output (Gorenflo & Gorenflo, 1994), and attitudes about alphabet displays may be improved by the inclusion of common words and phrases in addition to single letters (Raney & Silverman, 1992).

Because it appears that age may be a significant factor in determining attitudes about individuals who use AAC, strategies to overcome attitudinal barriers may be more important with adolescent and adult communication partners than with those who are children. Regardless, it is important for individuals who use AAC to develop strategies for putting potential communication partners at ease and instructing them how to interact effectively using their AAC systems. To meet this goal, many individuals who use AAC have an introduction strategy when meeting new people. For example, Ann has this typed message on the cover of her communication book:

> Please read these instructions to learn how to communicate with me. Please stand on my right side when you talk to me; I see best on my right side. I understand everything so speak to me as you would anyone else. I shake my head to say "no." I nod my head to say "yes." I communicate by pointing to words in this book with the knuckle of my right index finger. When I point to a word, please say the word and check with me to make sure you are right. It takes me a while to make a selection. Please wait patiently; give me lots of time. Thanks a lot! (Light & Binger, 1998, p. 46)

Marty, a man with apraxia and aphasia following a stroke, used a message stored in his VOCA to introduce himself to unfamiliar partners in the community: *"I had a stroke, and this machine helps me to talk"* (Lasker & Bedrosian, 2001). In contrast, Stuart, a 15-year-old, deals with this issue in typical teenage fashion by having a preprogrammed message on his VOCA that says, *"Hi, I'm not a robot, I'm Stuart! I talk with this machine. You don't have to do anything different. Just chill out so I have time to compose my messages."*

Another type of introductory strategy that can be quite effective when the AAC system itself requires little explanation is to use a simple icebreaker message such as a joke. For example, Meghan, age 6, uses various knock-knock jokes as a strategy to put new classmates at ease; she points to symbols on her communication display to tell each joke as her new acquaintances take their prescribed turns. Of course, it is also important to note that some individuals who use AAC do not wish to use introductory strategies at all. As Michael Williams wrote,

> Some people believe it is a good idea to explain how their communication systems work. I don't share this view. On the contrary, I believe in total immersion . . . I just really think the best way to explain my communication techniques to people is to communicate with them. (Williams, 2000, p. 234)

Overall, each of these approaches solves the "unfamiliarity problem" in different ways while also reflecting the personalities and preferences of the individuals who use them.

People unfamiliar with individuals who use AAC may also misunderstand the role of the PCA and may, as a result, direct conversation toward the PCA instead of toward the individual who uses AAC. Peg Johnson's strategy in this situation has been to teach her PCA to direct the conversation back to her: "She can simply turn her head and eyes my way and wait for me to generate a response" (Johnson, 2000, p. 53). Michael Williams (2000) instructs his PCAs in a similar manner and wrote that, "if he [a PCA] wants to keep working for me . . . [he will] quickly learn to redirect any question asked of [him] about me back to me. This is how I quickly establish with strangers who's really in charge of the communication process" (Williams, 2000, p. 235). Clearly, Johnson's and Williams' targeted training of their PCAs is a reflection of their strategic competence in social situations.

Conversational Control

Buzolich and Lunger noted that "natural speakers typically are in a position of conversational control in their interactions with aided speakers" (1995, p. 37). Often, this means that natural speakers determine what to talk about, ask most of the questions, and do most of the talking, whereas individuals who use AAC answer questions and otherwise remain quite passive. This was certainly the case for Vivian, the 12-year-old girl who was introduced previously. Her conversational partners often asked her yes/no questions and thus limited her to one-word responses (Buzolich & Lunger, 1995). To overcome this social constraint, Vivian learned to respond to her partners' questions with either a "yes" or a "no" and then to add additional information immediately. For example, if a friend asked her, *Did you see the new Star Wars movie?* she might respond *"Yes, I saw Star Wars, and I loved it."* She also learned to respond to a yes/no question and then to ask her friend a question in return, such as, *"No, I didn't. What movie did you see?"* By using these two strategies, Vivian was able to exert more conversational control during interactions.

A second type of social constraint that is often encountered by individuals who use AAC is a tendency toward topic control or conversational dominance by the communicative partner. In part, this may occur because of the slowness of AAC relative to natural speech, making it difficult for individuals who use AAC to get a word in edgewise. Vivian encountered this barrier regularly during conversations, so she learned to use the preprogrammed phrase, *"Do you know what?,"* to let her friends know that she wanted to introduce a new topic when they had finished talking about the previous one. Similarly, some individuals who use AAC may prefer to use preprogrammed "placeholder" phrases such as *"Just a minute," "Wait a second,"* or *"I need more time"* to signal that they want to take a turn during a conversation.

A third conversational control issue for some individuals who use AAC is related to the guessing issue discussed in Strategies to Compensate for Operational Constraints. Although many individuals who use AAC prefer to teach their partners to guess and expand their messages for the sake of speed, some have strong preferences to the contrary—that is, they prefer that their partners *not* guess the content of a message while it is being constructed. Such individuals may use a *PLEASE DON'T GUESS WHILE I AM SPELLING* symbol or a pre-stored *PLEASE WAIT* message to discourage this practice (Light & Binger, 1998). A more complex strategy was developed by Spencer, a 16-year-old who used AAC and felt quite strongly that his communication partners should wait until he had spelled out or constructed an entire message before responding. Spencer's strategy was simple yet devious: he would deliberately change his message midway through a phrase or word if his partner was guessing, so that he or she would guess incorrectly. For example, on one occasion, Spencer was telling his friend Roy about a movie he had seen recently, and Roy guessed *movie* after Spencer had spelled *"I saw the m-o-v."* Spencer's teacher reported that she could "almost see the wheels turning in his head" as Spencer searched for another word that began with the letters, m-o-v, until he finally continued with "e-m-e-n-t" to spell "movement." After some confusion, the conversation continued, and Roy continued to attempt to guess Spencer's messages several more times. In each instance, Spencer switched his intended message to derail Roy's attempts until, finally, Roy lost confidence in his guessing ability and ceased guessing altogether. Spencer's persistent use of this strategy for teaching "un-guessing" was a indication of both his level of strategic competence and the extent to which he perceived partner guessing as both rude and frustrating.

Communication Breakdowns

It should not be surprising to note that, at least occasionally, individuals who use AAC need strategies for repairing communication breakdowns because such breakdowns are inevitable in *all* communication—spoken or augmented! For individuals who use AAC, breakdowns may occur for three primary reasons: 1) linguistic limitations in the communication display or device that result in misunderstandings, 2) environmental barriers, and 3) partner variables that interfere with effective communication. Strategies that enable individuals who use AAC to respond quickly and effectively to these issues are critical for communicative competence.

Linguistic limitations that may lead to communication breakdowns can be related to prosodic, semantic, and/or morphosyntactic limitations of a communication display or device. Prosodic breakdowns occur primarily because of the uninflected synthetic speech in most VOCAs, which can lead to message misinterpretation. For example, Manuel, who likes to joke around with his family and friends, made a big mistake when he teased his wife by telling her (with his VOCA) that he had not missed her when she went away for the weekend with a friend because he had *"more time to watch football and sleep."* Manuel now has preprogrammed messages in his VOCA that enable him to say *"I was just kidding!"* and *"That was a joke!"* if someone is accidentally offended by his remarks.

One of the most important repair strategies for breakdowns that occur because of semantic and morphosyntactic limitations is rephrasing or paraphrasing. For example, Linda, a young person who uses AAC, went to a country fair that many of her classmates also attended over the weekend. On the following Monday, her teacher held a short discussion with the class about their weekend activities, and Linda produced the message *FUN HAT CLOWN GIVE BALLOON* using the symbols that were available on her display, meaning "A clown who was wearing a funny hat gave me a balloon." Her teacher did not understand her message, so Linda repeated it verbatim, but to no avail. Finally, Linda rephrased her message as *CLOWN HAT*, and then looked at her teacher, who said, "Oh, the clown wore a hat?," to which Linda replied "yes" with a head nod. She then proceeded with *HAT FUN*, which her teacher understood to mean "the hat was funny." Finally, Linda pointed to the symbols *GIVE BALLOON* and her teacher exclaimed, "Oh, the clown with the funny hat gave you a balloon!" If the teacher had continued to have difficulty,

Linda might have used her *ASK MY MOM* symbol as a last-resort backup strategy, because she had been taught to "repeat, rephrase, and then get help" when breakdowns such as this occurred. Regulatory phrases such as "Do you know what I mean?" "I'll say it again" or "Wait, let me say it differently" can also be used to signal the need for a repair strategy in such situations (Buzolich & Lunger, 1995).

Environmental and partner barriers may also lead to communication breakdowns. Unusually noisy environments may make it difficult for a communication partner to hear synthetic speech output, requiring a repair strategy such as directing the partner's attention to the word display on the VOCA instead. Unusually dark environments (such as a movie theatre) may render nonelectronic communication displays useless because they cannot be seen; the same problem can occur for electronic devices without back-lit screens when there is too much light available (such as in a park on a sunny day). Repair strategies in such situations usually involve "mode switching" by the individual who uses AAC, who then attempts to get the message across using contact gestures, body language, vocalizations, or some other unaided strategy that is less affected by ambient light.

Mode switching can also be used to repair some breakdowns that are partner-related, such as might occur when a partner is unfamiliar with the primary output modality of the individual who uses AAC (e.g., Reichle & Ward, 1985) or does not have the skills needed to understand the modality. For example, Ming, who is deaf and has autism, uses manual signing as his primary communication mode and a small typing communication device as a backup. He has learned that if he begins signing and his partner does not respond, he should point to the message "Do you use sign language?" that is affixed to his typing device. If his partner answers no, Ming switches to his typing device for all subsequent communication. In this situation, communication breakdowns may occur because of an incompatibility between Ming's and his partner's knowledge of manual sign language.

In other cases, breakdowns may occur because of a partner's sensory-perceptual or linguistic limitations. For example, Marty, the man with apraxia and aphasia referred to previously, used the preprogrammed message in his VOCA to introduce himself to an elderly man whose job it was to greet and assist customers when they entered a large chain store in the town where Marty lived; however, the greeter did not understand the message because he himself was hearing impaired! Following instruction, Marty learned to simply turn up the volume on his VOCA when such breakdowns occurred (Lasker & Bedrosian, 2001). Similarly, Klasner and Yorkston (2001) taught WD, a man with Huntington Disease, to point to written descriptions of household repair tasks if tradespeople had difficulty understanding his verbal instructions. Repair strategies may also be required for communication breakdowns that occur because of unanticipated vision, literacy, or language limitations of partners.

Environmental Constraints

Conversations can begin almost anywhere, anytime: in the hallway at school, in a checkout line at the grocery store, at a rock concert, in church, in a doctor's office waiting room, and so forth. For most people, initiating conversations in noisy or busy environments can be challenging at the best of times, but for individuals who use AAC, the challenge can be even greater because of the unusually high speed and/or volume requirements in such settings. There just isn't time in the high school hallway between classes to compose a personalized message, and it may not be easy to attract someone's attention in a noisy store if you can't simply call their name in a loud voice. Of course, VOCA users can turn up the volume on their devices and use preprogrammed, generic "small talk" messages in such situations, but individuals who use AAC and want to initiate personalized messages on the fly need to develop a strategy for doing so (Beukelman & Mirenda, 1998).

Joanne faced this limitation almost every day as she silently passed her friends by in the hallway at school. As a solution, she placed each of her friends' names on dedicated buttons on her VOCA, and each evening, she programmed short, personalized messages under each of the names. For instance, after the school music concert, she preprogrammed the message, *"What did you think of the jazz band?"* under her friend Jessica's name because Jessica was a jazz fan. This enabled Joanne to initiate quick, personalized exchanges with her friends in the busy environment of her large high school.

Initiating and maintaining conversations in quiet or unusually formal environments can also present unique social challenges. For example, after several embarrassing experiences at church, Edith learned to turn down the volume of her VOCA when she wanted to make a brief comment to her friend during the service. Formal settings such as doctors' offices may be quite intimidating and/or busy, thus requiring specific strategies related to topic initiation and maintenance. For example, some individuals who use AAC provide a written letter of introduction that includes relevant medical history and current needs when they meet a new physician or other health care provider for the first time. Stan, a 67-year-old who uses AAC, found that faxing or e-mailing a brief letter to his doctor before each appointment enabled him to get his needs met and his questions answered efficiently. Individualized strategies such as these can help to overcome some of the environmental barriers that may otherwise limit communication.

Privacy

Many social interactions are private in nature and are not meant to be shared widely; however, AAC is often a very public enterprise in that an observer may be able to peer over the shoulder of an individual who uses AAC during message construction or read the completed message from the display screen. One strategy for dealing with eavesdroppers was developed by Elaine, an eleventh-grade student whose VOCA included a large display screen that could easily be seen by anyone sitting close by or standing behind her. Elaine's strategy was simple but effective: she used the "change display angle" button on her electronic device to adjust the display so that it was unreadable whenever she encountered curious onlookers.

FUTURE RESEARCH

It is probably clear by now that many challenges remain when it comes to strategic competence in AAC. Because one of the purposes of this chapter is to foster research to advance the field, we conclude this chapter with a brief outline of a research agenda in this area, focusing on: 1) the key questions or issues that remain to be addressed and 2) the challenges that are likely to be confronted by this research and appropriate methodologies for overcoming them.

Key Questions and Issues

This section is organized around three goals: 1) to develop a strategic competence curriculum, 2) to identify effective instructional techniques for teaching strategy use, and 3) to design AAC systems in ways that preclude the need for compensatory strategies.

Strategic Competence Curricula   There is clearly a need for a flexible assessment and curricular process designed to enable identification and instruction of skills for strategic competence to individuals with a wide array of disabilities who use AAC; however, it is important to note that most of the examples in this chapter were based on the experiences of individuals with cerebral palsy and little or no cognitive impairment. The fact is that we know very little about the strategies used by individuals with other types of disabilities, primarily because they often lack the literacy skills required to report on strategy use. In order to develop a robust curriculum designed to enhance strategic competence, research is sorely needed to identify the constraints that may be faced by individuals with, for example, cognitive impairments secondary to intellectual disabilities, autism, acquired brain injury, aphasia, dementia, and other disorders, as well as those with visual and dual sensory impairments. Research is needed to address questions such as

- What (if any) "prerequisite skills" are needed for successful strategy learning, in general?
- How do we facilitate the development of such prerequisite skills?

- Are specific constraints particularly relevant to individuals with specific disabilities?
- What strategies can be used most successfully by individuals across the range of problem-solving, metacognitive, and/or social interaction skills?

Questions such as these must be addressed to guide the development of a well-articulated, comprehensive curriculum.

Similarly, we know very little about the impact of personality and culture on strategic competence.

- Are certain strategies more likely to be used by individuals with specific temperaments and/or from specific cultures who use AAC?
- What personality or cultural variables affect the acceptability of strategy use, both for individuals who use AAC and for their communication partners (e.g., O'Keefe, Brown, & Schuller, 1998)?
- How do we assess the cultural acceptability of potential strategies prior to teaching them?
- What assessment techniques can be used to identify both the prerequisites and the strategies that will be required by individuals who use AAC?
- How can such assessment techniques lead to the development of individualized curricula in this area?

These and many other questions related to individuals who use AAC and their communication partners are critical.

Instructional Issues   Closely related to the issue of a strategic competence curriculum (i.e., what to teach) is the issue of instruction (i.e., how to teach). Unfortunately, we know no more about this than we do about curricular issues; in fact, most of the examples used in this chapter involve strategies that were invented by their users rather than taught to them by others. The general instructional model that has been used to teach skills related to communicative competence was adapted by Light and Binger (1998) from the work of Deshler and Schumaker (1988) and involves the following primary steps:

1. *Introduction:* Define the target skill for the individual who uses AAC and explain why it is important. Demonstrate how to use the skill or have the individual who uses AAC observe another person using it, accompanied by think-aloud statements explaining when to use it. Ask the individual to think of situations in which he or she should use the skill.
2. *Instruction:* Set up situations for the individual who uses AAC to practice the skill, either during natural interactions or during a combination of role plays and actual interactions. Use several different settings, partners, and sets of materials during instruction. Provide guided practice for the person to use the skill and prompt only as required using a "least to most" cueing hierarchy (natural cue, expectant delay, general point and pause,

and model). Provide feedback on both appropriate use of the skill and problem areas after each instructional session.

3. *Follow-up:* Evaluate progress regularly to measure the effects of instruction, and practice until the individual uses the skill spontaneously in the majority of opportunities during instructional sessions. Conduct probes in novel settings with novel partners, to evaluate the generalized effects of instruction, and offer "booster sessions" of role-playing and practice as needed to facilitate generalization.

Although this general instructional model has been used successfully in a few published reports to teach specific communication strategies (e.g., Buzolich & Lunger, 1995; Lasker & Bedrosian, 2001; Light & Binger, 1998), very little empirical research exists with regard to its effective use. Thus, research is needed to answer questions such as:

- How are compensatory strategies best taught to individuals without cognitive impairments who have intact problem-solving and metacognitive abilities (e.g., those with cerebral palsy, spinal cord injury) and use AAC?
- What instructional techniques are most effective with individuals who have limited problem-solving skills and metacognitive skills (e.g., those with intellectual disabilities, autism, acquired brain injuries, and degenerative disorders such as Huntington Disease and dementia)?
- Which instructional techniques are most likely to result in generalized outcomes, rather than in context-specific learning?

In addition, some strategies require individuals who use AAC to teach specific skills, such as guessing or paraphrasing messages, to others (e.g., PCAs, unfamiliar partners).

- What partner prerequisites may be needed for effective strategy learning?
- How do individuals who use AAC best learn the skills they need for teaching others?
- What instructional strategies can be used successfully by individuals who use AAC in this regard?

These and many other instructional issues remain to be resolved.

A related issue is the need for advance planning related to outcome evaluation of both curricular goals and instructional procedures. Light (1999) noted that three questions are relevant in this regard: 1) What is the immediate effect of the intervention? (e.g., can the individual who uses AAC use the target strategy in the teaching setting, following instruction?), 2) Is there evidence of generalization and maintenance of this effect? (e.g., when faced by a problem situation in the "real world," does the person use the strategy?) and 3) Is the effect valued by the individual who uses AAC, his or her communication partner(s), and society in general (e.g., does use of the strategy effectively "solve" the problem or limitation for which it was designed?). In the past, the limited outcome research in AAC has primarily focused on the first of these questions, rather than on the latter two, and it is important that this error not be repeated in research designed to facilitate strategic competence (Schlosser & Lee, 2000). Thus, we need to develop ecologically valid ways for measuring outcomes by addressing questions such as:

- How do we define and measure "effective strategy use"?
- How do we measure it in ways that are reliable and valid (i.e., useful) and that facilitate future research?
- How do we measure the social validity of target strategies across stakeholder groups such as individuals who use AAC, family members/friends, and unfamiliar communication partners?

AAC System Design Issues   There is no doubt that, since the 1990s, enormous strides have been made in the area of AAC system design of both nonelectronic and electronic systems. The robotic-sounding and largely unintelligible synthetic speech of past VOCAs has been replaced with digitized and synthetic speech that is understandable as well as age- and gender-specific (e.g., Mirenda & Beukelman, 1987; Mirenda, Eicher, & Beukelman, 1989). For many individuals who use AAC, dynamic display screens now preclude the need for third-party assistance for changing paper symbol displays on electronic devices, and numerous techniques are now available in such devices for rate enhancement (Beukelman & Mirenda, 1998). Techniques for increasing vocabulary size and efficiency of use now are in common use (e.g., Goossens', Crain, & Elder, 1992; Porter, 2001), and symbol sets representing concepts and words specific to a variety of cultural and linguistic groups are widely available (Beukelman & Mirenda, 1998).

Despite such advances, it should be obvious from the examples in this chapter that many of the strategies developed by individuals who use AAC are designed to compensate for inadequacies in the communication systems they use. Continued research and development is needed to overcome limitations such as those related to communication rate, poorly inflected synthetic speech, limited vocabulary capacity, and the lack of morphosyntactic flexibility in most systems. As advances continue to be made in the area of improved design and customization of AAC systems, the need for strategy use to compensate for current limitations is likely to be reduced substantially.

Challenges and Methodologies

Such an ambitious agenda presents numerous challenges at each step of the research process because of the heterogeneity of the AAC population, the complexities of AAC systems and interventions, and the "transactional and dynamic nature of the communication process" itself (Light, 1999, p. 13).

Challenges related to defining a research question and measuring outcomes were discussed previously. Thus, in this section, we focus on some of the most important methodologies that will be required to answer the proposed research questions in reliable and valid ways.

Social Validity Establishing the social validity of strategies to be taught should be a critical prerequisite to research in this area; numerous techniques can be used in this regard (Schlosser, 1999). Light and Binger (1998) based their general communicative competence curriculum on a series of research studies designed to identify and validate the target skills to be taught. First, they held extensive discussions with individuals who were experts at using AAC and experienced AAC professionals, with the goal of identifying skills that these consultants believed were critical for communicative competence. Participatory qualitative research methods such as focus groups may be particularly suited to this type of inquiry (Krogh & Lindsay, 1999; Krueger, 1994) and have been used successfully in previous AAC research to gather information from both individuals who use AAC (Iacono, Balandin, & Cupples, 2000) and professionals (Soto, Müller, Hunt, & Goetz, 2001). The current widespread availability of Internet technology also allows the formation of on-line focus groups that can be used to interview and gather information from individuals who use AAC and others around the world (e.g., McNaughton, Light, & Groszyk, 2001). Less interactive qualitative methods such as surveys and questionnaires can also be used to identify potential strategies for instruction.

The second phase of Light and Binger's (1998) process was to conduct a series of research studies to evaluate the extent to which the "nominated" skills actually affected others' perceptions of the communicative competence of individuals who use AAC. In order to accomplish this, a series of videotapes was constructed in which individuals who use AAC interacted in a variety of social situations with a range of partners. In some of the videotapes, the individuals who use AAC used one of the nominated skills and in others, they did not. Judgments (i.e., ratings) of their communicative competence were elicited from professionals without disabilities with AAC experience as well as from adults and adolescents without such experience. From the ratings, a final curriculum of target skills was developed, representing those that the evaluators agreed were most important for communicative competence.

A similar process could be used to identify socially valid strategies across evaluators of different ages, cultural/linguistic groups, and levels of experience with AAC (e.g., familiar/unfamiliar), by having evaluators view videotapes of individuals who use AAC using strategies that are applicable to specific constraints. Of course, the evaluators should include both individuals who use AAC and participants without disabilities because the opinions of both "users" and "consumers" of such strategies are equally relevant. For example, the difficulties caused by the slow rate of output in AAC might be amenable to strategies such as using key word phrases (i.e., telegraphic grammar) rather than complete sentences, teaching a partner to guess as messages are constructed, and so forth. Evaluators could be asked to rate both the effectiveness and the acceptability of such strategies after viewing videotapes of their use. The resulting curriculum would then be comprised of those strategies that are rated most highly with regard to both effectiveness and acceptability by evaluators from a range of backgrounds and experiences. These would constitute the dependent variables for investigation.

Equally important, but often overlooked, is validation of the independent variable(s) in a research study. In the case of research on strategic competence, the independent variables are the intervention procedures under investigation—that is, the techniques used for strategy instruction (Schlosser & Lee, 2000). If, as is most desirable, strategies are taught in ecologically valid ways in real-world contexts (rather than in laboratory settings), measures of procedural integrity are needed to insure that the procedures specified were actually the procedures used (Peterson, Homer, & Wonderlich, 1982). This can be accomplished in a variety of ways, such as by conducting regular procedural reliability checks to ensure that (in this case) instruction is delivered accurately across various interventionists (e.g., Light, Binger, Agate, & Ramsay, 1999).

Research Design   Research related to the identification of critical strategic skills (as described previously) can be conducted using repeated measures or randomized group experimental designs, in which groups of evaluators view one or more videotapes of individuals who use AAC using various strategies and the rate their perceptions using some type of ordinal response scale (e.g., a Likert-type scale). Such group designs are appropriate here because the procedures required (i.e., watching videotapes and rating responses) can be performed in an identical manner across all participants. However, research investigating the efficacy of strategy instruction is more amenable to single-subject experimental designs such as those used in previous research on communicative competence (see Light & Binger, 1998), because of the need to individualize instruction for the specific individuals who use AAC who participate. Of course, decisions with regard to the selection of an appropriate research design are complex and thus cannot be covered adequately here. Readers are referred to the tutorials on this topic provided in the March 1999 issue of *Augmentative and Alternative Communication* for extensive discussions of specific designs that can be used.

SUMMARY

It should be clear from this discussion that sociocommunicative interactions are a two-way street in which breakdowns can occur at any level. Thus, AAC strategies must reflect the needs of both individuals who use AAC and their communicative partners. Sometimes, strategies are required to overcome the fears or misconceptions of unfamiliar listeners, to regain conversational control, to adjust interaction styles in different environments, or to maintain privacy. Other strategies may be required to overcome linguistic constraints that reflect the semantic, morphosyntactic, or prosodic limitations of AAC systems or to deal with operational constraints such as the slow rate of augmentative communication, output limitations, or unique situations such as telephone conversations. Whatever the situation, the solutions should always reflect the diversity and uniqueness of the individuals who use AAC who develop and use them. It is only through the development of strategic competence that individuals who use AAC will be truly able to use their AAC systems in ways that enable them to "play the game" and achieve a level of communicative competence that is equal to that of their naturally speaking peers.

REFERENCES

Beck, A., & Dennis, M. (1996). Attitudes of children toward a similar-aged child who uses augmentative and alternative communication. *Augmentative and Alternative Communication, 12,* 78–87.

Beck, A., Fritz, H., Keller, A., & Dennis, M. (2000). Attitudes of school-aged children toward their peers who use AAC. *Augmentative and Alternative Communication, 16,* 13–26.

Beukelman, D.R., & Mirenda, P. (1998). *Augmentative and alternative communication: Management of severe communication disorders in children and adults* (2nd ed.). Baltimore: Paul H. Brookes Publishing Co.

Bliss, C. (1965). *Semantography.* Sydney, Australia: Semantography Publications.

Blockberger, S., Armstrong, R., O'Connor, A., & Freeman, R. (1993). Children's attitudes toward a nonspeaking child using various augmentative and alternative communication techniques. *Augmentative and Alternative Communication, 9,* 243–250.

Buzolich, M., & Lunger, J. (1995). Empowering system users in peer training. *Augmentative and Alternative Communication, 11,* 37–48.

Cardona, G.W. (2000). Spaghetti talk. In M. Fried-Oken & H.A. Bersani, Jr. (Eds.), *Speaking up and spelling it out: Personal essays on augmentative and alternative communication* (pp. 237–243). Baltimore: Paul H. Brookes Publishing Co.

Chapple, D. (2000). Empowerment. In M. Fried-Oken & H.A. Bersani, Jr. (Eds.), *Speaking up and spelling it out: Personal essays on augmentative and alternative communication* (pp. 153–159). Baltimore: Paul H. Brookes Publishing Co.

Churchill, T. (2000). The AAC manufacturer's tale. In M. Fried-Oken & H.A. Bersani, Jr. (Eds.), *Speaking up and spelling it out: Personal essays on augmentative and alternative communication* (pp. 127–133). Baltimore: Paul H. Brookes Publishing Co.

Collier, B. (1998). *Communicating matters: A training guide for personal attendants working with consumers who have enhanced communication needs* [Videotape]. Baltimore: Paul H. Brookes Publishing Co.

Cress, C., & King, J. (1999). AAC strategies for people with primary progressive aphasia without dementia: Two case studies. *Augmentative and Alternative Communication, 15,* 248–259.

Deshler, K., & Schumaker, J. (1988). An instructional model for teaching students how to learn. In J. Graden, J. Zins, & M. Curtis (Eds.), *Alternative educational delivery systems: Enhancing instructional options for all students* (pp. 391–411). Washington, DC: National Association of School Psychologists.

Fried-Oken, M., & Bersani, Jr., H.A. (Eds.). (2000). *Speaking up and spelling it out: Personal essays on augmentative and alternative communication.* Baltimore: Paul H. Brookes Publishing Co.

Garrett, K., & Beukelman, D. (1992). Augmentative communication approaches for persons with severe aphasia. In K. Yorkston (Ed.), *Augmentative communication in the medical setting* (pp. 245–338). Tucson, AZ: Communication Skill Builders.

Goossens', C., Crain, S., & Elder, P. (1992). *Engineering the preschool environment for interactive, symbolic communication.* Birmingham, AL: Southeast Augmentative Communication Conference Publications.

Gorenflo, C., & Gorenflo, D. (1991). The effects of information and augmentative communication technique on attitudes toward nonspeaking individuals. *Journal of Speech and Hearing Research, 34,* 19–26.

Gorenflo, C., & Gorenflo, D. (1994). Effects of synthetic voice output on attitudes toward the augmented communicator. *Journal of Speech and Hearing Research, 37,* 64–68.

Hehner, B. (1980). *Blissymbols for use.* Toronto: Blissymbolics Communication Institute.

Hetzroni, R., & Harris, O. (1996). Cultural aspects in the development of AAC users. *Augmentative and Alternative Communication, 12,* 52–58.

Iacono, T., Balandin, S., & Cupples, L. (2001). Focus group discussions of literacy assessment and World Wide Web-based reading intervention. *Augmentative and Alternative Communication, 17,* 27–36.

Johnson, P.L. (2000). If I do say so myself! In M. Fried-Oken & H.A. Bersani, Jr. (Eds.), *Speaking up and spelling it out: Personal essays on augmentative and alternative communication* (pp. 47–55). Baltimore: Paul H. Brookes Publishing Co.

Joyce, M. (2000). A fish story. In M. Fried-Oken & H.A. Bersani, Jr. (Eds.), *Speaking up and spelling it out: Personal essays on augmentative and alternative communication* (pp. 87–95). Baltimore: Paul H. Brookes Publishing Co.

Klasner, E., & Yorkston, K. (2001). Linguistic and cognitive supplementation strategies as AAC techniques in Huntington Disease: A case report. *Augmentative and Alternative Communication, 17,* 154–160.

Krogh, K., & Lindsay, P. (1999). Including people with disabilities in research: Implications for the field of augmentative and alternative communication. *Augmentative and Alternative Communication, 15,* 222–233.

Krueger, R. (1994). *Focus groups: A practical guide for applied research.* Newbury Park, CA: Sage Publications.

Lasker, J. (2000). *Attitudes of people with aphasia, peers, family members, and speech-language pathologists to AAC.* Retrieved November 18, 2002, from http://aac.unl.edu/drb/lskr2000/

Lasker, J., & Bedrosian, J. (2001). Promoting acceptance of AAC by adults with acquired communication disorders. *Augmentative and Alternative Communication, 17,* 141–153.

Light, J. (1989). Toward a definition of communicative competence for individuals using augmentative and alternative communication systems. *Augmentative and Alternative Communication, 5,* 137–144.

Light, J. (1997). "Let's go star fishing": Reflections on the contexts of language learning for children who use aided AAC. *Augmentative and Alternative Communication, 13,* 158–171.

Light, J. (1999). Do augmentative and alternative communication interventions really make a difference?: The challenges of efficacy research. *Augmentative and Alternative Communication, 15,* 13–24.

Light, J.C., & Binger, C. (1998). *Building communicative competence with individuals who use augmentative and alternative communication.* Baltimore: Paul H. Brookes Publishing Co.

Light, J., Binger, C., Agate, T., & Ramsay, K. (1999). Teaching partner-focused questions to enhance the communicative competence of individuals who use AAC. *Journal of Speech, Language, and Hearing Research, 42,* 241–255.

Lilienfeld, M., & Alant, E. (2002). The attitudes of children to unfamiliar peers using augmentative and alternative communication devices. *Augmentative and Alternative Communication, 18,* 91–101.

McMillen, T.M. (2000). Communication my way. In M. Fried-Oken & H.A. Bersani, Jr. (Eds.), *Speaking up and spelling it out: Personal essays on augmentative and alternative communciation* (pp. 77–85). Baltimore: Paul H. Brookes Publishing Co.

McNaughton, D., Light, J., & Groszyk, L. (2001). "Don't give up": The employment experiences of individuals with amyotrophic lateral sclerosis who use AAC. *Augmentative and Alternative Communication, 17,* 179–195.

Mirenda, P., & Beukelman, D. (1987). A comparison of speech synthesis intelligibility with listeners from three age groups. *Augmentative and Alternative Communication, 3,* 120–128.

Mirenda, P., Eicher, D., & Beukelman, D. (1989). Synthetic and natural speech preferences of male and female listeners in four age groups. *Journal of Speech and Hearing Research, 32,* 175–183, 703.

O'Keefe, B., Brown, L., & Schuller, R. (1998). Identification and rankings of communication aid features by five groups. *Augmentative and Alternative Communication, 14,* 37–50.

Peterson, L., Homer, A., & Wonderlich, S. (1982). The integrity of independent variables in behavior analysis. *Journal of Applied Behavior Analysis, 15,* 477–492.

Porter, G. (2001). "Low tech" dynamic displays: User-friendly multi-level communication books. In *Proceedings of the 9th Biennial Conference of the International Society for Augmentative and Alternative Communication* (pp. 587–590). Washington, DC: International Society for Augmentative and Alternative Communication (ISAAC).

Prentice, J. (2000). With communication, anything is possible. In M. Fried-Oken & H.A. Bersani, Jr. (Eds.), *Speaking up and spelling it out: Personal essays on augmentative and alternative communication* (pp. 207–213). Baltimore: Paul H. Brookes Publishing Co.

Raney, C., & Silverman, F. (1992). Attitudes toward nonspeaking individuals who use communication boards. *Journal of Speech and Hearing Research, 35,* 1269–1271.

Reichle, J., & Ward, M. (1985). Teaching discriminative use of an encoding electronic communication device and Signing Exact English to a moderately handicapped child. *Language, Speech, and Hearing Services in Schools, 16,* 58–63.

Savignon, S. (1983). *Communicative competence: Theory and classroom practice.* Reading, MA: Addison-Wesley.

Schepis, M., & Reid, D. (1995). Effects of a voice output communication aid on interactions between support personnel and an individual with multiple disabilities. *Journal of Applied Behavior Analysis, 28,* 73–77.

Schlosser, R. (1999). Social validation of interventions in augmentative and alternative communication. *Augmentative and Alternative Communication, 15,* 234–247.

Schlosser, R., & Lee, D. (2000). Promoting generalization and maintenance in augmentative and alternative communication: A meta-analysis of 20 years of intervention research. *Augmentative and Alternative Communication, 16,* 208–226.

Soto, G., Müller, E., Hunt, P., & Goetz, L. (2001). Critical issues in the inclusion of students who use augmentative and alternative communication: An educational team perspective. *Augmentative and Alternative Communication, 17,* 62–72.

Van Balkom, H., & Welle Donker-Gimbrère, M. (1996). A psycholinguistic approach to graphic language use. In S. von Tetzchner & M. Hygum Jensen (Eds.), *Augmentative and alternative communication: European perspectives* (pp. 153–170). London: Whurr Publishers.

Williams, M.B. (2000). Just an independent guy who leads a busy life. In M. Fried-Oken & H.A. Bersani, Jr. (Eds.), *Speaking up and spelling it out: Personal essays on augmentative and alternative communication* (pp. 231–235). Baltimore: Paul H. Brookes Publishing Co.

Wood, L., Lasker, J., Siegel-Causey, E., Beukelman, D., & Ball, L. (1998). Input framework for augmentative and alternative communication. *Augmentative and Alternative Communication, 14,* 261–267.

Yoder, D., & Kraat, A. (1983). Intervention issues in nonspeech communication. In J. Miller, D. Yoder, & R. Schiefelbusch (Eds.), *Contemporary issues in language intervention* (pp. 27–51). Rockville, MD: American Speech-Language-Hearing Association.

VI

Interventions to Build Communicative
Competence

13

Intervention Strategies for Communication

Using Aided Augmentative Communication Systems

Joe Reichle, Mary Jo Cooley Hidecker,
Nancy C. Brady, and Nancy Terry

Because the primary communicative mode in our society is vocal, the bulk of communication intervention efforts have addressed establishing spoken language. In the early 1980s, as a result of proposed decision rules, interventionists tended to pursue speech intervention until they were certain that speech would not result in a sufficiently functional system before an augmentative communication system was considered (Chapman & Miller, 1980; Shane & Bashir, 1980). Since the 1980s, our knowledge of communication intervention has expanded dramatically. We no longer consider failure to acquire intelligible speech as a precondition to the implementation of an augmentative communication system (Lloyd, Fuller, & Arvidson, 1998; Reichle & Karlan, 1985). Communication interventionists now recognize the value of relying on a combination of communication modes to maximize communicative efficiency; however, an increasing reliance on multiple modes of communication has increased the number and complexity of variables that a communication interventionist must consider in implementing an augmentative communication system.

An important aspect of intervention strategies is establishing a well-discriminated, yet appropriately generalized, use of communicative behavior. In this chapter, we review a range of intervention options that focus on establishing initial symbol use. We address a range of procedures used to establish semantic/pragmatic communication skills as well as strategies that address selected operational skills that may be required to operate an aided augmentative communication system. Many of the intervention strategies that we address are relevant to users of both graphic and gestural modes; however, the primary focus of this chapter is on aided communication systems.

OVERVIEW OF INTERVENTION STRATEGIES
TO ESTABLISH COMMUNICATIVE SYMBOL USE

Early efforts at teaching communicative behavior focused on ensuring that the intervention procedures (rather than uncontrolled variables) were actually influencing the acquisition of communicative behavior. Consequently, great emphasis was placed on the internal validity of the instructional procedures (e.g., Guess, Sailor, & Baer, 1974). Typically, the setting, the specific arrangement of materials, and the absence of distracting people or activities were tightly controlled. In addition, most procedures explicitly specified instructional cues, correction procedures, and continuous schedules of reinforcement associated with the instructional procedure. Consequently, procedures tended to be replicated easily, resulting in superb internal validity. Unfortunately, the excellent procedural clarity often sacrificed the opportunity for intervention to occur in a sufficient range of contexts to ensure generalization. A common outcome of these interventions was that generalization exhibited by learners was extremely limited and was considered only after an acquisition criterion had been met. The social validity of intervention outcomes was often also somewhat suspect. For example, frequently learners mastered vocabulary that was selected by interventionists with limited consideration of the number of opportunities that learners might have to use the vocabulary functionally.

Beginning in the early 1980s, interventionists became more sensitive to the external validity of intervention strategies. Increasingly, researchers and interventionists began to more carefully consider the learner's communicative interests as well as the listeners' needs. Additionally, many interventionists began to address how existing social behavior interacted with the selection of new vocabulary to be taught (e.g., Carr, 1977; Carr & Durand, 1985a, 1985b; Durand & Carr, 1987). Instead of viewing generalization as a cognitively driven phenomenon that occurred only after acquisition, interventionists started to plan for generalization by considering the range of stimuli that should exert control over the communicative skill being taught.

The critical question facing a prospective interventionist is how to best design an effective strategy that is the least intrusive to the learner (and the interventionists) but, at the same time, employs cues and prompts sufficiently overt to result in the acquisition of new communicative behavior. We have selected a sample of potential intervention strategies that span a continuum of interventionist involvement from very limited (fast mapping) to substantial involvement (direct instruction). The strategies vary greatly in the extent to which they have been empirically validated; however, all seem potentially applicable to a wide range of learners who could benefit from augmentative and alternative communication (AAC).

Fast Mapping

Among strategies that involve the least amount of overt interventionist involvement is fast mapping. Fast mapping requires that learners make inferences about unknown referents through a process of elimination. Fast mapping has been reported among both typically developing children and some individuals with developmental disabilities (Chapman, Kay-Raining Bird, & Schwartz, 1990; Kay-Raining Bird & Chapman, 1998). An example may best illustrate a fast mapping opportunity. Suppose that there are four items on a snack table and the learner's communicative partner names one of the items. Although the learner does not comprehend the spoken word, she does comprehend the spoken names that correspond to each of the other snack items. Consequently, the learner observes that because she does not comprehend the word spoken, it must go with the referent for which she has not previously learned a name.

Mervis and Bertram (1993) provided empirical analyses that supported a correlative relationship between fast mapping and the onset of a vocabulary spurt that emerges in typically developing children. The implication is that children who begin to fast map are better able to take advantage of natural teaching opportunities that do not always present totally unambiguous prompts. In spite of the apparent value of fast mapping, little information exists describing intervention strategies to facilitate young communicators' use of fast mapping. Although fast mapping may be a strategy that has promise with some candidates for augmentative communication systems, more information is needed with respect to skills that may be helpful in predicting the emergence or the ability to utilize this subtle strategy. If these areas can be delineated, strategies to teach learners skills that place them in a position to fast map may be possible.

Wilkinson and McIlvane (2002) discussed similarities between fast mapping and learning by exclusion. In learning by exclusion, the learner recognizes one or more members of a choice array as known elements. If the vocabulary item (or other sample stimulus) presented cannot be associated with known responses and a novel response is available, the learner may select the novel response. If this response results in a history of reinforcement, the learner is more likely to select the novel response in the future when presented with the previously unknown vocabulary item and thereby exhibit fast mapping.

Fast mapping may come into play in areas important in graphic mode instruction that are not typically considered in the speech/auditory communication modes. For example, some people use communication wallets. In this application, a learner can manually locate a desired symbol. Learning by exclusion may come into play when a learner examines a choice array of symbols on a page. If he or she does not see a symbol that matches the referent of interest, he or she may turn to a page(s) to locate the desired symbol. In this context, skills associated with fast mapping may provide a mechanism for an individual to learn to search for a novel symbol when presented with an unknown referent (in an intervention context that minimizes response prompting). It should be noted, however, that learners who utilize fast mapping will benefit from responsive feedback to locating new symbols.

Responsive Communication Intervention

In our culture, adults respond to both linguistic and nonlinguistic acts produced by children (Hart & Risley, 1995; Warren & Yoder, 1998). In their seminal work on early language development, Hart and Risley found that the most advanced child communicators had parents who were the most responsive to child-produced communicative acts. Wilcox (1992) and Wilcox, Shannon, and Bacon (1992) examined responsive teaching strategies implemented by parents of children who were just beginning to use intentional communication. Parents were taught to comply to child communicative acts and to request clarification when they did not understand child productions. Children who received responsive intervention made greater gains than those who did not receive the intervention. Other investigators have also reported the successful implementation of responsive intervention strategies (Girolametto, 1988; Girolametto, Verbey, & Tannock, 1994; MacDonald, 1989). In delineating responsive intervention strategies, specific communicative behaviors can be targeted for intervention. Alternatively, the interventionists (in this case, parents) may choose to be responsive to each viable socially acceptable communicative act without such specification.

For people who rely on graphic augmentative communication systems, increasing communicative partners' propensity to engage in responsive intervention strategies may be extremely important. Often, communication partners are not responsive to the communicative overtures of people with moderate to severe developmental disabilities who use AAC (Linfoot, 1994). Across a range of populations using AAC, investigators have noted limitations in partner responsivity. Kaiser and colleagues (1997) suggested that although responsive intervention strategies are well suited to people who are beginning to communicate, responsivity may not be the most efficient strategy for teaching first words. They proposed that for children learning first words, additional intervention strategies might be useful in directing a child's attention to specific linguistic information. Two options that have received significant attention include augmented communication input and milieu communication intervention.

Augmented Communicative Input

Several investigators have discussed the specific application of partner use of augmentative communication forms (Goossens', 1989; Romski & Sevcik, 1996; Romski et al., 1999). Augmented communicative input requires teaching caregivers to use the learner's augmentative communication device. Subsequently, augmented communication input encourages the communicative partners of individuals who use AAC to supplement their speech with the use of the learner's primary communicative mode (see Chapter 5). The limited available literature suggests that the frequency of interactive communication, language comprehension (Light, Roberts, Dimarco, & Greiner, 1998; Peterson, Bondy, Vincent & Finnegan, 1995), complexity of speech output (Light et al., 1998), and spontaneous production can be enhanced by augmenting communicative input. The available literature supporting augmented language is summarized by Romski and Sevcik (Chapter 5).

In the gestural mode literature, key word signing appears to share some of the same characteristics of augmented language. In key word signing, the communicative partner signs the most relevant content words that are included in spoken utterances (Lloyd et al., 1998). Often, key word signing is viewed as an assist to a learner's comprehension of spoken words. Makaton, for example, uses a core manual vocabulary of 350 signs to provide conceptual support for spoken language. Key word signing has been demonstrated to alter a partner's speaking rate and pause time; these alterations may enhance comprehensibility (Windsor & Fristoe, 1991).

To date, intervention protocols have not provided great specificity in identifying strategies that partners should use in selecting message components to augment. Milieu communication intervention suggests specific types of partner communicative acts that can be produced via speech or augmented input to facilitate the acquisition of specific communicative forms and functions.

Milieu Communication Intervention

A package of naturalistic teaching strategies originally described by Hart (1985) has been referred to as "milieu instruction" (Kaiser, Yoder, & Keetz, 1992). Milieu teaching strategies involve optimizing arrangement of the environment as well as selecting specific intervention targets and offering specific prompting strategies to interventionists. Warren and Yoder (1998) described prelinguistic milieu teaching procedures that focus on people transitioning into initial vocabulary production. Milieu procedures articulated by Hart (1985) include three distinct components: incidental teaching, mand–model instruction, and time delay.

In *incidental teaching*, the learner initiates a communicative utterance, and the communication partner then expands or otherwise elaborates to provide a subtle model for the child. For example, the child might approach a television set and produce the symbol TV. The partner contingently touches WATCH and TV symbols to model the relevant action vocabulary that could be combined to produce a request. During incidental teaching episodes, the interventionist may not have direct control over specific communicative forms being taught. Incidental teaching is very similar to some applications of responsive teaching techniques that have a prescribed intervention target identified prior to a specific teaching opportunity. An intervention target may focus on a specific communicative form or communicative function. An episode of incidental teaching can occur only after the learner has produced some communicative act. Consequently, some learners may lack the spontaneity required to benefit from the exclusive use of incidental teaching. With individuals who have a low rate of communicative acts, mand–model instruction may represent a viable alternative or supplemental strategy.

Mand–model instruction requires that the learner be able to imitate a model of a communicative act produced by another person. Initially, the interventionist produces a mand (e.g., "What do you want?" or "What is this?"). If the learner produces the targeted response after the mand, the interventionist contingently responds (i.e., provides the requested object or comments about the child's label). If the learner does not respond to the mand, the teacher produces a model for the child to imitate. The goal in mand–model instruction is to evoke a learner-produced communicative act by systematically lessening the learner's reliance on an interventionist's model.

Mand–model is a teacher-initiated intervention strategy, whereas incidental teaching is child initiated. Both instructional strategies embed teaching opportunities within naturally occurring interactions. In mand–model instruction, the teacher delivers tightly specified cues, for example, "What do you want?" (associated with behavioral regulation) and "What's that?" (associated with joint attention). The challenge in implementing mand–model instruction is ensuring that the learner does not become overly dependent on spoken cues provided by the interventionist.

Time delay represents a strategy that can serve as a bridge between mand–model and incidental teaching. It is an intervention that systematically delays the delivery of a response prompt. When successful, the context of the situation is a sufficient natural prompt for the learner's communicative act. For example, if a history of successfully responding to a mand prompt has been established, the interventionist, in the context of a predictable situation, would look expectantly at the learner but wait a fixed number of seconds before delivering the mand prompt (e.g., Hart, 1985, reported using a 15-second delay). The goal of the time-delay prompt is to transfer the evoking property of the mand prompt to the context of the situation.

In traditional mand–model instruction, the learner's ability to comprehend interventionist produced communicative acts may be an important component of a successful intervention. Because mands are usually utterances directed to the learner, failing to comprehend the utterance may compromise its effectiveness. If the child does not comprehend the mand, he or she must be able to act on modeled behavior. When a learner is not able to take advantage of response prompts and natural cues associated with communicative opportunities, interventionists may turn to more direct instructional strategies, such as interrupted chain training.

Interrupted Chain Training

Hunt, Goetz, Alwell, and Sailor (1986) described an intervention procedure that met many of the characteristics of the time delay component of milieu language instruction, yet provided much of the structure and interventionist intrusion that one considers in implementing more direct instructional strategies. They termed their intervention procedure *interrupted chain training*. This procedure has been successfully implemented in establishing an initial repertoire of requesting behavior among people with moderate and severe developmental disabilities who may not be able to take full advantage of the prompting strategies used in traditional milieu communication intervention.

In an interrupted chain, the interventionist interrupts a learner's ongoing activity and waits for the production of a communication act to restore or resume the activity. Because in this situation the referent and communicative partner have been clearly established, the coordination between referent, partner, and communicative symbols may be simplified. In implementing interrupted chain training, the interventionist wishes to identify an activity that is extremely familiar and of interest to the learner. Next, the interventionist must determine a point within the activity when the learner will become moderately upset if the activity is interrupted (this provides the motivation to request continuation of the activity). After interrupting the routine at this predetermined point, the interventionist delivers the least intrusive prompt that is required to obtain a communicative act signaling a desire to re-engage in the activity. For example, the learner might be prompted to touch a symbol or produce a sign representing an item needed to continue the activity. This strategy has been demonstrated to result in the acquisition of generalized requesting with learners who experience moderate/severe mental retardation.

One limitation of the interrupted behavior chain strategy, however, is that it is not amenable to teaching other communication functions such as joint attention. One critical aspect that appears to facilitate the successful application of less intrusive strategies is the predictability of the context in which a communicative exchange takes place. More predictable exchanges may allow individuals who use AAC to maximize their speed and fluency in producing messages, thereby increasing their confidence in using their commu-

nicative system. Next, we discuss a teaching strategy that capitalizes on predictability, specifically joint activity routines.

Joint Activity Routines

One key to establishing less effortful communication may lie in the emergence
of predictable social exchanges that have come to be called *joint activity routines*.
Joint activity routines may provide predictable and well-rehearsed contexts
for learners to fluently practice elements of their communicative repertoire. In
this section, we will explore the emergence and possible importance of these
interactive sequences in the communication intervention process.

Snyder-McLean, Solomonson, McLean, and Sack defined joint activity
routines as activities involving,

> A ritualized interaction pattern; involving joint action; unified by a specific theme or goal.
> They follow a logical sequence; including a clear beginning point; and in which each par-
> ticipant plays a recognized role, with specific response expectancies, that is essential to the
> successful completion of that sequence. (1984, p. 214)

Eight critical elements characterize joint activity routines:

1. Obvious unifying theme or purpose
2. Requirement for joint focus and interaction
3. Limited number of clearly delineated roles
4. Exchangeable roles
5. Logical, nonarbitrary sequence
6. Structure for turn-taking in predictable sequence
7. Planned repetition
8. Plan for controlled variation

Three major types of joint activity routines include creation of a product, acting out a story, and a turn-taking game. Some have suggested that established
routines may require fewer memory resources, thus allowing for more resources to be available for learning new goals (Shatz, 1983).

Joint activity routines can be effective contexts for teaching both behavior regulation and joint attention communicative functions. Behavior regulation acts can be taught in much the same way described in the preceding
section on interrupted behavior chains. Joint attention acts can be taught by
violating the predictability of the routine. Once a predictable routine is established, unexpected events may be embedded as salient cues for communicative acts.

Designing joint activity routines for children with severe physical impairments can be challenging. Children with severe physical impairments may be

limited to observing, rather than participating in, certain aspects of routines. Little is known about the difference between observing and participating in a joint-activity routine and what effect this may have on the world and word knowledge of the child (Nelson, 1986). Cress (2002) studied parent interaction with young children with physical impairments. She proposed that many early routines (i.e., Peekaboo or Pat-a-cake) require physical and/or vocal skills. She observed that parents must either adapt these or develop routines that allow for the child to interact.

Designing age-appropriate joint activity routines for adults with developmental disabilities may also create some challenges for the interventionist. Much of the available literature discusses joint activity routines in the context of activities that are most appropriate for preschoolers. Simple activities such as playing catch, tossing a Frisbie, and engaging in a simple meal preparation can be arranged to organize the criteria inherent in a joint activity routine.

When naturally occurring cues do not result in the increased propensity to produce communicative behavior, it is possible that they are too subtle for the discriminations that are required to learn functional communication. When learners have a history of failing to acquire more conventional communicative skills implemented in the context of naturally occurring activities, interventionists often consider increasing the clarity of the discriminations that must be made. The goal of direct instruction is to maximize the learner's ability to acquire those discriminations.

Direct Instruction

Direct instruction represents an alternative or a supplement to some of the intervention strategies that we have described. In implementing direct instruction, the interventionist presumes that more natural cues may not be sufficiently clear, or sufficiently dense, to set the occasion for discriminations that are required in acquiring communication skills. As a result, direct instruction seeks to make cues associated with responses extremely discriminable and to provide extensive distraction-free intervention opportunities. As the learner begins producing correct responses, steps are taken to "loosen" instructional control to more closely approximate environments in which the learner is apt to need or want to communicate. Direct instruction is characterized by

1. Massing of instructional opportunities
2. Very tight definition of the behavior being taught
3. Careful defining of the discriminative stimuli that are associated with an opportunity to use the behavior being taught
4. Careful delineation of consequences to be provided for correct and incorrect responses

Often, direct instruction occurs in environments different from or in addition to environments in which the target behavior will be used in order to achieve large numbers of highly discriminable instructional opportunities. In addition, during the early phases of intervention, it is probable that teaching opportunities are interventionist initiated. A number of studies with children and adults who experience significant developmental disabilities have demonstrated the successful implementation of graphic and gestural communication modes using direct instruction (Carr & Durand, 1985a; Durand & Carr, 1991; Peterson et al., 1995; Richman, Wacker, & Winborn, 2001; Shirley, Iwata, Kahng, Mazaleski, & Lerman, 1997; Wacker et al., 1990; Worsdell, Iwata, Hanley, Thompson, & Kahng, 2000).

Two sequences of response prompts have been most commonly reported in direct instructional strategies. In a *most-to-least prompt hierarchy,* the interventionist begins with the least intrusive prompt that guarantees a response approximation. Then, systematically this response prompt is reduced (faded). The objective in a most-to-least prompt hierarchy is to minimize errors. Across teaching opportunities, the interventionist strives to maintain response approximations under increasingly less intrusively prompted conditions. Several situations may be associated with the use of most-to-least prompt hierarchies. With some learners who engage in problem behavior, a more intrusive prompt at the outset may result in the learner more quickly being able to obtain the reinforcer associated with the communicative act. Among learners who mildly dislike physical contact, the use of a more intrusive prompt may create additional incentive for the learner to become more independent. Finally, most-to-least prompt hierarchies usually result in fewer errors during the initial phase of intervention.

Several disadvantages may be associated with a most-to-least prompt hierarchy. First, some learners may enjoy the attention that occurs when more intrusive prompts are delivered. If this occurs, prompts can be difficult to fade. In addition, interventionists implementing a most-to-least prompt hierarchy must be sufficiently disciplined to fade prompts quickly to avoid prompt dependency.

In *least-to-most prompt hierarchies,* the interventionist implements the natural cue available in the learner's environment that should eventually serve as a cue signaling the opportunity for a communicative act. If the learner does not respond within a specified period, the interventionist supplements the natural prompt with a slightly more intrusive prompt. Increasingly, prompts become more intrusive until the learner responds (taking for granted that the learner does not simply learn to wait for the more intrusive prompts). Assuming that the learner is highly motivated to get the outcome associated with the communicative behavior, there is less of a risk of overprompting in this sequencing strategy; however, using a least-to-most hierarchy may result in a longer delay from the point of the initial cue until a communicative act is produced.

As mentioned previously, aided communication systems may create the additional challenge to the interventionist of requiring a prompting system to select a symbol and to coordinate symbol selection with directing the listener's attention to the symbol being selected. Consequently, individuals who are beginning to use aided communication must concurrently establish joint attention with the listener and choose a symbol from a menu. Bondy and Frost (1994) suggested a direct instructional strategy (Picture Exchange Communication System) that teaches the learner a chain that includes selecting a symbol and seeking a listener for the communicative message. One interventionist serves as the recipient of the learner's communicative act. A second interventionist physically prompts the child to pick up a symbol representing the object and hand it to the recipient of the communicative act (sitting across from the child). In addition to locating a listener at the point of initiating a communicative act, a beginning communicator must be able to discriminate between symbol choices. Research using direct instructional strategies has yielded a wealth of information regarding efficient stimulus prompting (Carr & Carlson, 1993; Carr & Durand, 1985a, 1985b; Durand & Carr, 1991; Hinderscheit & Reichle, 1987; Reichle & Brown, 1986; Reichle, Rogers, & Barrett, 1984; Reichle & Ward, 1985; Reichle & Yoder, 1985; Wacker et al., 1990).

Unlike response prompts, stimulus prompts involve a manipulation of the materials to which the learner responds. The goal is to establish a pattern of correct responding with no or minimal response prompts. Subsequently, the stimuli are made less discriminable. A primary advantage of stimulus prompting is that it permits prompting in the absence of having to physically contact the learner. When implemented well, stimulus prompts serve to minimize error patterns that may emerge in other instructional prompting strategies. Two types of stimulus prompts include stimulus shaping and stimulus fading.

In stimulus shaping, the physical features of a symbol are progressively altered across successive teaching opportunities by enhancing symbol features. For example, initially, distracters are made to look very dissimilar from target symbols, as is shown in Figure 13.1. Across successive correct responses, features are added to the distracter to provide a greater challenge to the learner's emerging symbol discrimination skill. During stimulus fading, the enhancement of a symbol is gradually reduced during successive successful teaching opportunities, as is depicted in Figure 13.2. Both stimulus shaping and stimulus prompting can be implemented concurrently. Wilkinson and McIlvane (2002) provided a discussion of stimulus prompting parameters as they apply to graphic mode communication.

Although an excellent instructional tool, stimulus prompting can create instructional problems when it is not executed carefully. For some learners, an enhancement that was designed to facilitate discriminability can become the sole basis for the discrimination. Thus, when this enhancement is eliminated, the child may not discriminate between symbols. For example, a symbol

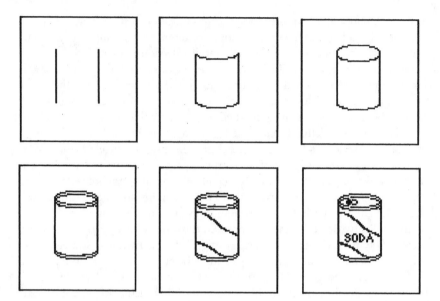

Figure 13.1.   Example of stimulus building.

could be enhanced by making it larger than other symbols in an array of symbol choices. If not introduced carefully, the learner may focus exclusively on the size difference. If this occurs, the learner will no longer discriminate between symbols when the size difference is eliminated. Research has indicated that stimulus shaping and fading are more successful when the enhancement capitalizes on exaggerating critical features of choice items that should be used to make the discrimination. Stimulus prompting can be labor intensive, although a number of commercially available software programs have greatly reduced the effort required to create these stimuli.

There appears to be widespread and growing consensus that direct instruction may be very helpful as a supplement to some of the less intrusive intervention strategies. When implementing direct instruction, it is important to fade prompts that will not be available in environments where the new behavior being taught will be used very quickly. It is also important to ensure that there are natural maintaining contingencies in the natural environments where the target behavior is to be used. A frequent criticism of more structured intervention strategies is that there is a tendency for learners to become dependent on particular contexts that may have been emphasized during intervention. This is particularly dangerous with individuals who have a propensity to respond more than initiate. Consequently, interventionists must take care to ensure that newly established communicative behavior can serve a full range of topic-initiating and continuing functions.

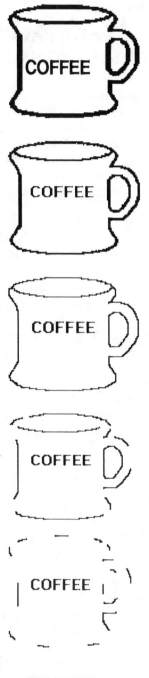

COFFEE

Figure 13.2. Example of stimulus fading. (From Sigafoos, J., Mustonen, T., DePaepe, P., Reichle, J., & York, J. [1991]. Defining the array of instructional prompts for teaching communication skills. In J. Reichle, J. York, & J. Sigafoos [Eds.], *Implementing augmentative and alternative communication: Strategies for learners with severe disabilities* [p. 186]. Baltimore: Paul H. Brookes Publishing Co; reprinted by permission.)

ENSURING A FULL RANGE OF COMMUNICATIVE ACTS TO INITIATE AND CONTINUE EXCHANGES

Regardless of the intervention strategies selected, it is critical to decide who will implement the communicative event that provides the teaching opportunity: the learner or the interventionist. Responsive intervention strategies are learner initiated. This approach focuses on initiations that, traditionally, have been a weak aspect of an augmentative communication system user's conversational repertoire. By acting contingently on a learner's communicative production, the interventionist also ensures that the topic of the exchange will be motivating to the learner.

One challenge associated with a learner-initiated approach is the propensity for many individuals who use augmentative communication systems to produce communicative acts primarily as responses to obligatory overtures to their partners' requests (e.g., Light, Collier, & Parnes, 1985, 1985b). Second, when an initiated act does occur, communicative partners may not respond contingently because they cannot decipher the purpose of the learner's communicative act (see Reichle, Halle, & Drasgow, 1998). However, there is a growing base of compelling evidence suggesting that listener responsivity provides the basis for increases in intentional communicative acts (Yoder, Warren, McCathren, & Leew, 1998).

An important area for future research involves an examination of variables in the natural environment that may increase contexts of highly discriminable routines that include the individual who uses AAC as both initiator and responder in communicative exchanges.

Initiating Communicative Acts

Coordinated visual attention between learner, communication partner, and referent is a key component to intentional communication for most learners. It is important because it provides evidence that learners are directing their communication to their partners. For the individual who uses a graphic AAC system, coordinating eye gaze may be significantly more effortful. Eye gaze must be coordinated between the graphic symbol, the referent, and the partner (whereas for a speaking or signing individual, eye gaze must be coordinated between the referent and the listener). We know very little about the importance of coordinating eye gaze for an individual using graphic symbols; however, there may be strategies to identify the directionality of the learner's communication act that do not necessitate the triangulation of eye gaze just described.

For example, Bondy and Frost's (1994) Picture Exchange Communication System separates the act of finding a listener from selecting the symbol. This strategy requires the learner first to select the desired symbol, and then to locate a listener and offer the symbol that he or she wishes to communicate. This strategy may directly influence operational competence because after the learner has focused on symbol selection, he can then focus exclusively on locating and directing the communicative utterance to a listener.

Responding to the Communicative Acts of an Individual Who Uses AAC

As discussed previously, evidence suggests that partners of communicators with developmental disabilities often miss a significant number of opportunities to respond to communicative overtures. One reason for limited responsivity may involve the listener's inability to identify relatively idiosyncratic behavior as a possible communicative overture. Consequently, examining the criteria that are used for listeners to make judgments about intentional communicative acts requires consideration.

Wetherby and Prizant (1989) described a number of phenomena that may be associated with intentional communicative acts:

1. Shifting one's gaze between referent and listener
2. Increasing the vehemence of an act until a contingent partner action is provided
3. Directing the communicative act to other individuals until an action is provided
4. Ceasing a behavior contingent on an adult contingent action
5. Continuing to repeat an act until a predictable consequence is provided

Applying these criteria to individuals who use AAC may create some challenges.

For an individual who uses a graphic AAC system, increasing the vehemence of a communicative symbol presents a formidable challenge. Directing an utterance to a different listener contingent on communicative failure may require significantly greater physical effort for a learner who uses gestural or graphic modes. In these instances, the individual who uses AAC may be less apt to repair his or her original communicative act unless it was very important. It is also possible that because of the slowness of message production, being persistent is made more difficult (see Chapter 12).

A critical area for future exploration involves examining strategies that may increase the responsivity of communicative partners to behaviors produced by individuals beginning to use AAC systems. Being responsive to initial communicative overtures is likely to lessen the need for the learner to resort to less socially acceptable communicative behaviors. Furthermore, increasing partner responsivity is also apt to decrease the propensity for learned helplessness to emerge. In learned helplessness, learners experience so few responses to their overtures that their initiations gradually decelerate. If a learner is already producing a repertoire of socially marginal communicative behavior, applied research must focus on validating carefully conceived strategies to identify the most efficient conventional communicative alternatives that suit both the learner and his prospective communicative partners. At the most basic level, the interventionist can implement a gestural dictionary. This dictionary provides a careful description of communicative overtures that a learner is apt to produce. By familiarizing oneself with this dictionary, learners' communicative partners have a greater probability of being responsive to a learner-initiated communicative overture.

With less familiar listeners, individuals who use AAC may benefit from being able to briefly describe their system and its use for a prospective communication partner. Light and Binger (1998) described strategies that focused on providing the learner with symbols and corresponding messages that could be used to explain strategies that could be used to optimize the communicative exchange. Once interacting with a less familiar listener, the individual who uses AAC can use strategies that may increase his or her partner's awareness of a topic change. Prompts can be given to a partner explaining preference for interrupting message formulation to guess the utterance being constructed. Mirenda and Bopp (Chapter 12) observed that individuals who use AAC are not in agreement regarding their preference for interruption to speed interaction. When partners are participating in message construction, users of augmented systems can clearly communicate to their partners when the partners have guessed incorrectly (so that the miscommunication is not perpetuated further). By clarifying rules of interaction from the outset, a prospective partner may more comfortably respond to the communicative acts of an individual who uses AAC.

Taking advantage of a wide variety of communicative opportunities requires the efficient use of one's communicative repertoire. Individuals who use AAC face a more challenging task in referencing their listener, the referent, and the communicative symbol than their speaking counterparts. Because many listeners are not familiar with graphic AAC modes, listeners must exert greater effort in attending to the subtleties of an individual who uses AAC; however, the individual can lessen this listener responsibility by providing clear descriptions of strategies that can result in greater communicative efficiency. The ability to produce well-discriminated communicative utterances for which the user has a well-generalized command represents a critical characteristic of efficient communication.

Repairing Communication Breakdowns

Communicative exchanges often involve breakdowns. Breakdowns occur for several reasons, including misunderstanding. When conversational partners do not understand the other participant's message, they frequently request clarification. Successful responding to the request for clarification can "repair" the breakdown, enabling a continuation of the conversation. A few studies have expressly looked at communication breakdowns and repair between speakers and AAC communicators; this research is reviewed in Brady and Halle (2002). Brady and Halle concluded that successful repair of communication breakdowns is essential for competent conversation with AAC communicators and is an area in need of more research.

ENSURING WELL-DISCRIMINATED, YET HIGHLY GENERALIZED, COMMUNICATIVE SKILLS

Maximizing the Conditional Use of Communicative Acts

DePaepe, Reichle, and O'Neill (1993) discussed the importance of selecting teaching opportunities that include situations where the new communicative behavior should be used as well as those that require the learner to refrain from using the new response (or that require the use of a different member of the learner's communicative repertoire). Attending to these parameters is possible, at some level, for each of the intervention strategies previously described. Positive teaching opportunities sample a range of important stimuli that the interventionist wishes to be associated with the communicative act to be taught. For example, in teaching requesting assistance, the interventionist might choose to include opportunities to 1) obtain desired items/activities that the learner can select, but not open or effectively activate, and 2) receive help with difficult, less preferred activities. In addition, opportunities might involve each of several primary interventionists who are apt to come in contact with the learner and a range of environments and activities. In the case of the same communicative act, an interventionist could identify negative teaching examples that include preferred and less preferred activities that the learner could perform independently.

Often, interventionists do not consider contexts in which the learner should refrain from using the communicative act being taught (negative teaching examples) when planning intervention contexts (Reichle et al., 1998). A common intervention strategy is to reinforce a new communicative act at a high rate (i.e., reinforcing symbol use whenever it occurs). Initially, this means that its use may be reinforced in contexts that eventually would be considered unacceptable (negative teaching examples). If a history develops where the new communicative behavior is reinforced during what will eventually become negative teaching examples, when the interventionist stops reinforcing the symbol selection, it is likely that the learner will become frustrated. One strategy to prevent this outcome is to arrange both positive and negative teaching examples from the outset of intervention.

Sometimes, events that constitute positive teaching examples at the outset of intervention become negative teaching examples as learners become increasingly competent. For example, when requests for assistance are taught, the learner is concurrently being taught to more independently perform the task associated with the assistance request. That is, a request for assistance results in the delivery of a response prompt aimed at teaching the learner to independently act. As independent requests for assistance are mastered, a potential generalization dilemma is created. The learner must be able to discriminate that requests for assistance should be used only when the learner cannot perform a task independently. Consequently, some learners may continue to produce requests for assistance when they no longer actually need the assistance (Reichle & Dahl, 2000). For these individuals, reinforcement associated with independent work may need to be made greater than the reinforcement associated with assistance requests.

Issues regarding when to conditionally use new communicative acts often involve the content of the communicative message (as in the preceding example); however, individuals who use multiple modes of communication must also make conditional decisions regarding which mode to emphasize in any given communicative context. People who sign but also have learned to use a graphic AAC system may match the communicative mode to their listener. For example, at home with significant others who sign, the individual will use signs because of their relative speed and portability, but when communicating with a salesperson in the community, the same person may use symbols housed in a communicative wallet because the salesperson will most likely not understand sign.

Using a communicative utterance conditionally represents an extremely important area of competence that interventionists are only beginning to address systematically. Being able to communicate conditionally, paired with well-generalized use of communicative behavior, represent two areas that differentiate individuals with truly functional communication from those who have a more limited communicative repertoire.

Maximizing Generalization of Communicative Acts

Typically, discussions of generalization focus on specific vocabulary (e.g., Can a learner use the symbol APPLE to refer to red, green, and yellow apples?); however, generalized use of pragmatic functions represents a critical area that is often overlooked. If the learner fails to recognize the range of situations for the use of symbols associated with a particular pragmatic function, subsequent vocabulary taught to serve the same function is also apt to be limited in generalizability.

Sophisticated communicators realize that a single communicative function can be used in a variety of very different social situations. For example, a learner can "protest" to avoid an offer of a nonpreferred food item, but he or she can use that same protest in the presence of a preferred food item for which they have satiated (e.g., a third cup of coffee). Although these two situations call for the same communicative function and vocabulary ("no thanks"), some learners may not recognize these two situations as communicatively equivalent (Reichle, Drager, & Davis, 2001). Several years ago, an intervention strategy was implemented with an adult with severe developmental disabilities who engaged in throwing tantrums and aggression to use a rejecting gesture when offered nonpreferred snack items (Reichle, 1999). After mastery, the learner generalized the use of his gesture to a number of items that he did not like; however, when he became satiated on preferred items such as coffee, he continued to use problem behavior rather than his newly established communicative gesture. In identifying positive teaching examples with some vocabulary, it is important to consider uses that are not static and locked to particular social functions. If teaching examples do not sample a range of conditions, use of this communicative function may be compromised.

Previously, we discussed the range of teaching examples used to teach requesting assistance. This pragmatic function provides an example in which a single pragmatic function can be used in two very different social situations. Requests for assistance can be used to gain access to desired items (e.g., child who cannot open a candy wrapper); however, requests for assistance can also be used to gain release from aversive situations (e.g., the zipper is stuck on a child's coat). There is some evidence to suggest that this full range of examples may need to be addressed to establish fully generalized use (Reichle et al., 2001).

Finally, an individual word can be used across pragmatic functions. *Spoon* can be used to provide information but can also be used as a request (e.g., a child needs a spoon to eat ice cream). Few interventionists have examined whether generalization of this type must be systematically addressed in intervention (see Reichle et al., 1984).

For the most part, our discussion has focused on more general procedural aspects of a variety of strategies that can influence the acquisition of a communicative repertoire; however, for an individual who may prospectively use AAC, some more idiosyncratic forms are often being used at the point of beginning communication intervention. Consequently, interventionists encounter critical questions regarding how an existing communicative repertoire is either integrated with or replaced by augmentative communication modes.

USING MULTIPLE COMMUNICATION MODES

Regardless of the instructional approach taken, the interventionist must consider the communicative forms that will be established if the planned communication intervention is effective. Many of the intervention strategies (with the exception of the Picture Exchange Communication System and augmented language input) that we have discussed do not specifically address the communication modes that were considered in designing the intervention strategy. A particularly important consideration prior to choosing targets for augmentative communication intervention is considering the portion of an individual's existing communicative repertoire that needs to be supplemented or replaced. Many decisions regarding mode selection and implementation appear to be based on interventionist convenience. Reichle (1991) asked special educators and speech-language pathologists serving young children with severe disabilities how they selected augmentative communication modes. The most common response was they selected a single mode with which they (as interventionists) were most familiar.

Wetherby, Reichle, and Pierce (1998) reviewed development of graphic, gestural, and vocal mode skills in typically developing children. They concluded that children use multiple communication modes throughout their development; children appear to most quickly learn the least effortful form that has the greatest chance of achieving the desired outcome in any given situation. The most basic decisions facing an interventionist, regardless of a learner's chronological age or developmental status, are what part of an existing repertoire is functional and should be maintained and/or strengthened and, conversely what portion of a learner's existing repertoire should be replaced with more socially acceptable communicative means.

Building on Existing Communicative Means

Examining an individual's existing communicative acts may be important for several reasons. First, if socially unacceptable communicative acts are being used, it is important to implement communicative replacement intervention. If the intentional communicative act is not part of a conventional communication system but is functional, interventionists can consider how to incorporate the act into the communication system being designed.

In considering the selection of augmentative communication modes, a common fear among parents has been that the introduction of AAC will result in a diminished use of (or propensity to use) the vocal mode (Romski & Sevcik, 1996; Schepis, Reid, Behrman, & Sutton, 1998). Fortunately, this concern does not appear to be warranted. To the contrary, Romski and Sevcik (1996) reported that individuals with mental retardation who participated in their longitudinal study of the acquisition of AAC use did not unilaterally adopt a graphic AAC system when it was introduced. Instead, participants incorporated it into their existing communicative repertoire. Graphic symbols were used during approximately 37% of communicative exchanges whereas natural vocalizations were included in a large proportion of utterances. Romski and Sevcik (1996) reported increases in both the numbers of spoken words and the intelligibility of spoken words among their participants. Seven of their thirteen participants demonstrated improved speech intelligibility subsequent to the introduction of voice output devices. Schepis, Reid, Behrmann, and Sutton (1998) reported no decrement in spoken communication after the implementation of a graphic AAC system among participants with significant developmental disabilities. Instead, there was a slight increase in other communicative responses that included gestures, spoken words, and vocalizations. A number of other investigators have reported increases in speech output subsequent to the implementation of a graphic AAC system (Goossens', 1989; Iacono & Duncum, 1995; Iacono, Mirenda, & Beukelman, 1993; Schepis et al., 1998).

A careful examination of the existing literature suggests that augmentative communication modes, when implemented carefully, do not work at cross-purposes with the enhancement of natural speech production. Millar, Light, and Schlosser (2002) examined the effect of AAC intervention on natural speech production. The results support the conclusion that AAC intervention did not impede speech production. Few participants demonstrated declines in speech production and most showed modest gains in speech following AAC intervention. Although there are limited available empirical data addressing the use of augmentative communication modes to supplement spoken output in children, there is a growing literature addressing speech supplementation (see Chapter 2). The available literature suggests that individuals with reduced intelligibility can significantly improve their partners' ability to decipher spoken messages when speech supplementation is used.

In summary, there appears to be a growing evidentiary base supporting the use of multiple communication modes to enhance communicative ability without a deteriorating effect on speech production; however, the area of multimodal communicative intervention warrants continued investigation with an emphasis on dependent measures that examine the effects of multimode production on qualitative aspects of speech output.

Replacing Socially Unacceptable Acts with Conventional Communicative Forms

There is a growing literature suggesting that listeners' responsivity to child actions directly influences the emergence of intentional communicative acts (Harwood, Warren, & Yoder, 2002; Warren & Yoder, 1998). Often, responses produced by listeners are reinforcing. Reinforcing a behavior increases the probability that it will occur in the future. Sometimes, socially inappropriate acts are reinforced by adults. For example, an individual who throws a tantrum at a restaurant (because he wishes to leave) may be reinforced by being removed from the setting. Once socially unacceptable behavior gets established as a mechanism to obtain reinforcement, it can be very difficult to replace with a competing socially acceptable form. To do so requires that the new form be made more efficient than the problem behavior. Replacing socially marginal behavior represents a high priority during the early phases of communication intervention.

A growing compendium of intervention strategies to replace problem behavior with socially acceptable communicative alternatives exists (e.g., Carr & Carlson, 1993; Carr & Durand, 1985a, 1985b; Day, Horner, & O'Neill, 1994; Derby et al., 1997; Durand, 1999; Durand & Carr, 1991, 1992; Hagopian, Fisher, Sullivan, Acquisito, & LeBlanc, 1998; Hanley, Iwata, & Thompson, 2001; Kahng, Hendrickson, & Vu, 2000; Lalli, Casey, & Kates, 1995; Peck et al., 1996; Richman et al., 2001; Shirley, Iwata, Kahng, Mazaleski, & Lerman, 1997; Shukla & Albin, 1996; Wacker et al., 1990). Many of these successful reports share certain commonalities in their intervention approach that can be summarized as best practices that have been experimentally validated.

Do Not Continue to Reinforce the Problem Behavior
Wacker and colleagues (1990) compared the effectiveness of implementing functional communication training alone with a second intervention in which functional communication training was paired with a procedure designed to extinguish *problem* behavior. In a series of reversals, they demonstrated that the combined procedure was more effective. The logic to this approach is clear. Make the new communicative behavior as efficient as possible and, at the same time, make the problem behavior as inefficient as possible.

Implement Communicative Replacement Prior to the Emission of Problem Behavior
There is a propensity for interventionists to react to socially unacceptable behavior. If problem behavior is used as a cue to implement a communicative replacement strategy, it is possible that a response chain will be established. In a response chain, first the learner engages in problem behavior. Subsequently, he engages in the more socially acceptable response when the problem behavior does not result in the desired outcome (Reichle et al., 1998). In order to avoid chained behavior, the interventionist must identify situations that are likely to be associated with problem behavior. During these situations, the interventionist should make it as easy as possible for the new communicative behavior to be produced. For example, during an early phase of intervention, if a learner tends to predictably throw a tantrum 15–20 minutes into a task, the interventionist may wish to prompt "Let's take a break" just after 14 minutes.

Match the Communicative Behavior Taught to the Function of the Problem Behavior
A variety of subtle variables may contribute to the emergence of a problem behavior that serves a communicative function; however, experts are in agreement that there are several social functions that ac-

count for a significant portion of problem behavior. Many learners engage in problem behavior to escape undesirable situations (e.g., throwing a tantrum to get out of completing a math worksheet). Others produce problem behavior to obtain or maintain the attention of others (e.g., spilling food to obtain attention associated with providing assistance). In still other situations, problem behavior may occur to gain access to desired objects or activities (e.g., screaming until a snack is provided). New communicative forms taught must be carefully matched to the function of the problem behavior. For example, with a learner who attempts to escape a school activity, several plausible but subtly different communicative functions may be available. Suppose that a learner struggled with a difficult task. The interventionist might consider teaching a request for assistance to decrease problem behavior; however, prior to implementing an intervention procedure, the interventionist could determine whether assistance functions as a reinforcer. During one condition, she could provide assistance as soon as difficult work is provided. During other opportunities, no assistance would be offered. If less problem behavior occurs in the former condition, there is reason to proceed.

In other situations, a learner may be perfectly competent in performing a task but may habituate because the task is lengthy. In this situation, a request for a break may be the most plausible replacement because, after the break, the learner will be able to complete the task. In still a third escape scenario, a learner may wish to avoid eating green beans. In this situation (assuming that green beans are not vital to the learner's diet), using a protest/reject "no" may be the most reasonable communicative alternative to problem behavior.

Make Communicative Replacement Maximally Efficient In applying an intervention strategy, it is important to consider the response efficiency of alternative responses available to the learner. Most learners have a repertoire of several actions that they can exercise during any given communicative opportunity. For example, a 3-year-old wants a slice of pie. He could produce any or a combination of behaviors that include 1) vocalizing unintelligibly, 2) using a graphic symbol representing pie, 3) climbing on the table and grabbing the pie, and 4) throwing a tantrum until pie is offered. Each of these options represents a member of the same response class. Even though each is a different form, they all represent functionally equivalent responses in that they result in the same outcome. Because a learner is likely to first use a behavior that has been most successful in the past, functionally equivalent responses may not be equally efficient in any given context.

Several investigators have examined how learners may operationalize response efficiency. Generally, four parameters are discussed that include 1) immediacy of reinforcement, 2) rate of reinforcement, 3) quality of reinforcement, and 4) physical/cognitive effort required. In any given situation, the specific behavior that a learner chooses to produce is apt to be the one that provides the greatest overall efficiency.

As a result of investigations addressing response efficiency, intervention-ists have begun rethinking "generalization failure." It is possible that some learners may choose not to use a newly taught behavior in favor of one that was already part of their repertoire. Drasgow, Halle, and Ostrosky (1998) exam-ined this issue as they taught each of three learners with severe developmen-tal disabilities to request desired activities using socially acceptable requests rather than reaching, grabbing, or leading that they used during baseline. Ini-tially, all participants learned to request desired items in their classrooms. Subsequently, probes conducted in a generalization setting demonstrated that the communicative requesting originally taught was not being used. Instead, learners continued to use their original, more idiosyncratic forms to obtain ac-cess to desired activities. After ensuring that the old communicative forms were no longer reinforced (placed on extinction), two of the learners showed a substantial increase in use of their new socially acceptable communicative behavior, whereas the third learner showed a moderate increase. It appeared that prior to extinction, participants continued to use existing old behavioral forms because they were more efficient than the newly taught socially accept-able communicative behavior; however, once problem behavior was made less efficient, the newly established behavior became a more attractive com-municative option.

Typically, communicative replacement is an option where the function associated with problem behavior can be reinforced; however, there are nu-merous situations in which the function (or desired outcome from the learn-er's perspective) cannot be reinforced. For example, a learner may wish to avoid taking seizure control medication but doing so could be injurious to his or her health. In this situation, the intervention plan may call for strategies that make taking the medication as palatable as possible but may not include communicative replacement. For example, the learner might be allowed to choose when he or she takes the medication, how the medication is taken (e.g., mixed in peanut butter and jelly), or what activity will occur immediately after medication. These strategies are geared at altering conditions of engagement to enhance self-regulatory skills. Combining communication replacement with strategies such as those just described requires a carefully coordinated intervention plan that may require the collaboration of several disciplines.

In considering intervention options, many intervention strategies focus primarily on the content of what is to be taught rather than considering how the specific augmentative communication mode being used may force addi-tional intervention issues for parents and educators. For many individuals who use aided augmentative communication, communicative content will not result in an efficient communication system without equal effort being allo-cated to the procedures required to efficiently select and construct a message in multiple contexts. Next, we focus on several important operational vari-ables that are exemplary of the challenges that some individuals face in ac-quiring functional communication.

CONSIDERING VARIABLES IN
OPERATING AIDED COMMUNICATION SYSTEMS

The advent of an increasingly sophisticated array of graphic AAC systems requires that interventionists consider intervention that may be required to teach the learner to competently operate an augmentative communication system. In this section, we discuss the selection of a display format (fixed/dynamic) and considerations in the implementation of a scanning selection technique as two of the more challenging considerations that interventionists face because of the limited research on which to base intervention decisions.

Selection of Symbol Display Formats

Increasingly, electronic communication devices are incorporating dynamic display options. In a dynamic display, a variety of pages (each containing an array of symbols) are available to the user. Pages may be electronically linked. Dynamic displays can also be constructed in nonelectronic applications in the form of a communication wallet or communication notebook. In this application, the user must manually navigate between pages of a communication display. One advantage of a dynamic display is that a large repertoire of symbols can be organized so that relatively few symbols need to be displayed on any single page. This is a distinct advantage for individuals whose performance deteriorates when they are required to search larger symbol arrays to formulate a message. A second advantage of dynamic displays is the decreased need to execute encoding techniques. Because symbols on a main page can be directly linked to symbols on a related page, the need to chain memorized symbol sequences to retrieve a stored message or message component can be minimized.

For some learners, it may be challenging to move from a fixed display to a dynamic display. They may need to be taught to search for symbols that are dispersed across multiple pages of a display housed in a communication wallet or notebook. Few intervention procedures have been validated to teach a searching skill. Reichle (2000) described a procedure to teach searching. If the target symbol was not on the first page of a display, the learner was reinforced for waiting and being prompted to the next page. If the target symbol was on the first page, the learner was reinforced for selecting it. Across opportunities, instructional prompts to wait and turn a page were faded.

Of course, the hypothesized advantages cited for a dynamic display may pose disadvantages for some individuals. First, efficiently using a dynamic symbol display may require that an individual be able to engage in a reasonably sophisticated nonidentity matching skill. For example, assume that a learner wanted a Big Mac sandwich. A plausible search path might require that the learner select a symbol corresponding to "places I like to dine." Selecting this symbol might link to a page containing the logos of a number of fast-food restaurants. After selecting a McDonald's logo, the learner would be offered a "pop-up" containing items that could be ordered. To follow this search path efficiently, the individual would need to be able to match Big Mac (the end point of the search) with the "places I like to dine" symbol (the entry point for the search). To date, very little effort has been made to scrutinize how being able to engage in this level of matching influences learner performance in becoming functionally competent in using a dynamic display.

In teaching learners to use dynamic page displays, it may be helpful to teach a hierarchical matching skill. For example, an interventionist could teach a learner to match a BIG MAC symbol to a McDonald's logo. Concurrently, the interventionist could teach the learner to match a McDonald's logo with a symbol signifying "places I like to eat." After learning these two matches, the learner may be better able to create a chain of responses that results in the selection of a chain of three selections (places I like to eat, McDonald's, and Big Mac).

One of the most pressing areas for applied research involves a careful examination of the skills that are necessary to create messages using each of these display techniques. An equally important area of scrutiny needs to address establishing viable sequences of instruction.

Strategies to Teach Participation in Scanning Selection Techniques

There are two primary selection techniques: direct selection and scanning. Each technique has advantages and disadvantages that affect a user's communication rate, effort, fatigue, and accuracy. Most often, scanning techniques are used when a person is unable to directly select the vocabulary item he or she desires due to a motor impairment. There are two types of scanning modes: auditory and visual. In auditory scanning, the selected item's label is stated either by the facilitator or in electronic communication aids by a synthetic voice. The user hears the items as they are being menued and makes a selection once the desired item is heard (see Chapter 9 for an extensive discussion of auditory scanning). In visual scanning, a cursor selects the vocabulary items by highlighting them. Once the desired item is highlighted, the user must select that item using a response of some type. These two scanning types can be used individually or together to meet the needs of the user.

Several experiments have compared direct selection and several types of visual scanning that include linear, circular, and row–column (Horn & Jones, 1996; Petersen, Reichle, & Johnston, 2000; Ratcliff, 1994; Szeto, Allen, & Littrell, 1993). Consistently, research has shown that direct selection is the most accurate and quickest selection technique (although the difference may not have been statistically significant; Petersen et al., 2000; Ratcliff, 1994; Szeto et al., 1993).

Of the common scanning patterns (linear, circular, row–column, group–item, and directed scanning), linear scanning is among the simpler scanning patterns (Reichle, Sigafoos, & Remington, 1991). When using linear scanning, the cursor moves from left to right across each row in the display until the individual selects a symbol. Linear scanning only requires one motor response to activate or deactivate the cursor. In linear scanning, the learner need not engage in significant advanced planning. If the cursor is moving slowly, the learner can respond as it menus the symbol without any anticipatory planning. Although very slow, linear scanning may be a good choice for individuals who need time to plan and carry out their motor response.

Row–column scanning may be more cognitively challenging than linear or circular scanning because a chain of at least two responses is required to select a symbol (Mizuko, Reichle, Ratcliff, & Esser, 1994). First, the user must control a switch to stop the cursor when it is on the row that contains the desired symbol. Once that has been done, the cursor menus each symbol in that row. Again, the user must activate a switch to stop the cursor on the desired symbol (Beukelman & Mirenda, 1998). Because this technique highlights several symbols at one time, fewer cursor movements are required to reach the desired symbol. This causes the time needed to make a selection to decrease, allowing the rate of communication to increase (Reichle et al., 1991). Most agree, however, that row–column may be more cognitively demanding than linear scanning because once a group is selected, the user must decide immediately whether the desired symbol is in that group. The user must emit a response if the symbol is in the group or allow the next group of symbols to be menued. Generally, when row–column scanning has been compared with direct selection, the results have revealed that using row–column scanning results in more errors (Ratcliff, 1994).

Directed scanning has been suggested as a scanning selection technique that best maximizes rate of selecting symbol choices. To use directed scanning, an individual must be able to use a multifunction switch to control cursor movement. In directed scanning, the cursor starts in either the top left corner or in the center of the display. The user then uses the multifunction switch to direct the cursor to the desired symbol. To efficiently utilize directed scanning, an individual must be able to locate the symbol before activating the switch and use the cursor to move the switch to the desired symbol.

Szeto and colleagues (1993) examined college students' ability to use row–column, directed scanning, and direct selection with various communication devices. They found that direct selection was the fastest and most accurate selection technique. Directed scanning was the second most efficient selection technique but was not significantly more accurate than row–column scanning.

In spite of few specific experimentally validated intervention procedures, there are some reasonable applications of validated general instructional techniques that can be applied to scanning instruction. Reichle and colleagues

(1991) described several aspects of direct instructional strategies that could be implemented to teach scanning that did not require an electronic communication device during the early phases of intervention.

When learners use a scanning selection technique, they must engage in the same discriminations between symbols that are required of a direct selection technique. When one considers simple linear scanning, there are two presentation arrangements to consider. In both, there is an array of two symbol locations presented. One of the locations functions as a distracter; the other is the target symbol. If the cursor moves to the distracter, the learner should refrain from responding. If the cursor moves to the target symbol, the learner must contingently activate the switch. The positions of the target symbol and the distracter are randomized across opportunities to avoid a position-biased pattern of responding.

Reichle (2001) implemented this procedure with a 3-year-old learner with severe cerebral palsy and a moderate intellectual delay to teach symbol discrimination using simple linear scanning. A most-to-least prompting hierarchy was implemented. The positive teaching examples included the location of a HUG ME symbol placed randomly in each of four symbol locations. Initially, the remaining three symbol locations remained blank (contained no graphic symbol). Negative teaching examples occurred when the cursor offered a blank symbol location. In other words, a cursor touching the target symbol was a discriminative stimulus for a signaling response. The cursor touching a blank symbol location was a discriminative stimulus for "no signaling response" to be produced. Initially, full physical guidance was used to prompt a response to the target symbol and correspondingly to prompt the learner to refrain from responding to the blank symbol location. Once the response prompts had been completely faded, graphics were gradually introduced to the blank symbol locations (stimulus shaping/building) to make the discrimination more challenging. Finally, new target symbols were introduced.

A particularly challenging intervention procedure involves teaching a learner to participate in directed scanning. Piché and Reichle (1991) described a procedure that relied on a matrix training strategy to teach the learner to search for a target in a directed scanning array. The procedure assumes that the learner can engage in simple linear scanning. The initial phase of intervention places the cursor in the upper left hand corner of the display. A joystick is made available that only permits movement to the right and down. The interventionist verifies that the learner can select a target that is placed at any location on the uppermost horizontal row and leftmost vertical column of the array as depicted in Cell A of Figure 13.3. When the learner meets this objective, locations are identified along a diagonal depicted in Cell B of Figure 13.3. In this step, the learner is taught to chain two consecutive movements to locate a target. Once this is mastered, probes are arranged at random locations as depicted in Cell C of Figure 13.3. If the learner does not correctly

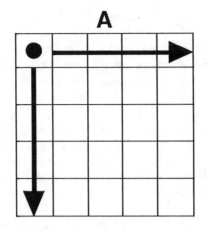

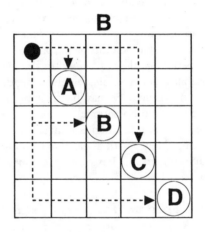

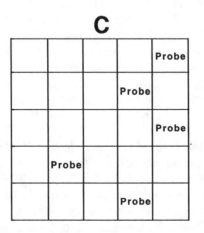

Figure 13.3. A matrix training approach applied to directed scanning.

identify these probe targets, additional intervention is required. During subsequent intervention activities, quadrants are systematically added to the array. Training within newly added quadrants may be necessary. As a new quadrant is added, an additional direction of switch movement is made available to the learner.

Little research has been conducted to advance the field's ability to systematically teach the operational use of aided communication systems. It is likely that with greater attention to systematic intervention strategies, we can dramatically lessen the time required for an individual to become competent at using an aided AAC system.

When Should New Selection Techniques Be Introduced?

Clinicians often wait for the individual to deteriorate before they consider introducing alternative selection techniques (e.g., introducing directed scanning with an individual who uses direct selection). Our bias is that the potential techniques that may be next steps should be introduced early so that the individual can achieve operational fluency before the dramatic deterioration of his or her physical disability. For example, initially using directed scanning in the context of a recreational activity may be an appropriate option. Only when individuals have achieved operational competence should they be expected to use their new selection technique. Currently, we know little about the effect that establishing fluency with a selection technique prior to using it as a primary communicative means has on user competence, and user and communicative partner attitude.

Using Different Selection Techniques for Different Communicative Partners

Although unfortunate, it is often the case that the fastest, most efficient selection techniques require the greatest amount of physical effort. It is possible that an individual might be able to conserve energy using a scanning technique with extremely familiar listeners who are more apt to use context and participate accurately in the co-construction of messages. With less familiar listeners, a direct selection technique may be more useful. Once again, few researchers have tackled the range of variables that must be addressed to determine whether the conditional use of selection techniques would increase overall communicative efficiency.

Considering the Hybrid Use of Selection Techniques

Some individuals with deteriorating physical disabilities may be able to directly select relatively large symbol groupings but lack the precision to directly select smaller symbol targets within the group. These individuals may benefit from hybrid selection techniques that allow the interactive use of direct selection and scanning (see Chapter 7). Using hybrid techniques will require that interventionists rethink the placement of symbols on a communication display.

Considering Strategic Factors in Message Creation   Obviously, using letter encoding or spelling to create messages offers the greatest flexibility in creating messages that are topically appropriate. The obvious disadvantage is that letter encoding is slow. Although listener prediction of the message being encoded may dramatically increase the rate of utterance production during a communicative exchange, it is likely that the individual who uses AAC will have to consider larger units of combination. Controversy exists regarding message access strategies. Individuals have options that include single symbols, each of which corresponds to a complete message. Alternatively, the learner can engage in rule-based combinations of two or more symbols (e.g., icons, letters) to access a vocabulary item, message fragment, or message unit. Semantic compaction is an example of icon encoding. Among competent communicators who use fixed display devices, the limited available literature suggests that icon encoding is the most frequently used strategy (Romich & Hill, personal communication). Considering the range of communicative contexts that an individual encounters, however, it seems likely that a variety of encoding strategies is more apt to be helpful. The type of message formulation used may well depend on the explicitness of the message required, the range of plausible messages that might be required, and the immediacy required to take advantage of the communicative opportunity.

For example, Beukelman (personal communication, Nov. 2001) made a compelling argument for preprogrammed stories that can be segmented into units that allow fluent participation in conversational exchanges. In addition, preprogramming utterances that represent "small talk" (e.g., simple comments and queries designed to maintain a conversational exchange) may be very important socially. These types of communicative utterances appear to be prevalent in the conversational exchanges of adults (King, Spoenemen, Stuart, & Beukelman, 1995). As a field, we are at a very rudimentary level in describing decision strategies to guide the mix of message formulation strategies for individuals who may prospectively use AAC systems.

SUMMARY

Designing and implementing AAC systems for people with developmental disabilities represents a relatively new undertaking for the research community. Since the 1970s, skilled practitioners and engineers have challenged researchers. For the most part, this has been a comfortable and productive relationship. With increasing funding streams being made available for the procurement of augmentative communication technology, it becomes increasingly critical to have well-documented and experimentally validated protocols to guide many of the decisions that interventionists must make in designing the most efficient options. These validated protocols must address all of the stakeholders in the communicative process. By continuing a well-coordinated relationship between research and practice, the field has an opportunity to establish the accountability that consumers, service providers, and policymakers should demand.

The bulk of well-articulated intervention strategies were designed to be implemented in the vocal mode with individuals who experience developmental disabilities. Although many of these strategies seem to be highly applicable to individuals who may prospectively use augmentative communication, there is limited supporting empirical literature. This creates a significant need for collaboration between interventionists and applied researchers to work carefully to identify special considerations that must be addressed in customizing intervention protocols. Doing so will provide the solid foundation required to continue to expand the scope of applicability of augmentative communication services.

Perhaps the greatest challenge facing interventionists is how to create intervention protocols that are sufficiently subtle to be used in a range of natural environments. These options should provide opportunities for participants to both initiate and continue communicative exchanges fluently. They must also have a mechanism to ensure that well-discriminated yet sufficiently generalized use of communicative utterances occurs. Considering future needs of individuals who use AAC requires the full attention of applied researchers. For the individual with significant developmental disabilities who has never had a conventional communication repertoire, researchers need to carefully examine the quantitative and qualitative effects of AAC on spoken language comprehension and production.

REFERENCES

Beukelman, D.R., & Mirenda, P. (1998). *Augmentative and alternative communication: Management of severe communication disorders in children and adults* (2nd ed.). Baltimore: Paul H. Brookes Publishing Co.

Bondy, A., & Frost, L. (1994). The Picture Exchange Communication System. *Focus on Autistic Behavior, 9,* 1–19.

Brady, N., & Halle, J. (2002). Breakdowns and repairs in conversations between beginning AAC users and their partners. In D.R. Beukelman & J. Reichle (Series Eds.) & J. Reichle, D.R. Beukelman, & J.C. Light (Vol. Eds.), *Augmentative and alternative communication series: Exemplary practices for beginning communicators: Implications for AAC* (pp. 323–352). Baltimore: Paul H. Brookes Publishing Co.

Carr, E.G. (1977). The motivation of self-injurious behavior: A review of some hypotheses. *Psychological Bulletin, 84,* 800–816.

Carr, E.G., & Carlson, J.I. (1993). Reduction of severe behavior problems in the community using a multicomponent treatment approach. *Journal of Applied Behavior Analysis, 26,* 157–172.

Carr, E.G., & Durand, V.M. (1985a). Reducing behavior problems through functional communication training. *Journal of Applied Behavior Analysis, 18,* 111–126.

Carr, E.G., & Durand, V.M. (1985b). The social-communicative basis of severe behavior problems in children. In J. Reiss & R.R. Bootzin (Eds.), *Theoretical issues in behavior therapy* (pp. 219–254). San Diego: Academic Press.

Chapman, R., Kay-Raining Bird, E., & Schwartz, S.E. (1990). Fast mapping of words in event contexts by children with Downs syndrome. *Journal of Speech and Hearing Disorders, 55,* 761–770.

Chapman, R.S., & Miller, J.F. (1980). Analyzing language and communication in the child. In R.L. Schiefelbusch (Ed.), *Nonspeech language and communication* (pp. 159–196). Baltimore: University Park Press.

Cress, C. (2002). Expanding children's early augmented behaviors to support symbolic development. In D.R. Beukelman & J. Reichle (Series Eds.) & J. Reichle, D.R. Beukelman, & J.C. Light (Vol. Eds.), *Augmentative and alternative communication series: Exemplary practices for beginning communicators: Implications for AAC* (pp. 219–272). Baltimore: Paul H. Brookes Publishing Co.

Day, H.M., Horner, R.H., & O'Neill, R.E. (1994). Multiple functions of problem behaviors: Assessment and intervention. *Journal of Applied Behavior Analysis, 27,* 279–289.

DePaepe, P., Reichle, J., & O'Neill, R. (1993). Applying general case instructional strategies when teaching communicative alternatives to challenging behavior. In J. Reichle & D. Wacker (Eds.), *Communicative alternatives to challenging behavior: Integrating functional assessment and intervention strategies* (pp. 237–262). Baltimore: Paul H. Brookes Publishing Co.

Derby, K.M., Wacker, D.P., Berg, W., DeRaad, A., Ulrich, S., Asmus, J., Harding, J., Prouty, A., Laffey, P., & Stoner, E.A. (1997). The long-term effects of functional communication training in home settings. *Journal of Applied Behavior Analysis, 30,* 507–531.

Drasgow, E., Halle, J., & Ostrosky, M. (1998). Effects of differential reinforcement on the generalization of a replacement mand in three children with severe language delays. *Journal of Applied Behavior Analysis, 31,* 357–374.

Durand, V.M. (1999). Functional communication training using assistive devices: Recruiting natural communities of reinforcement. *Journal of Applied Behavior Analysis, 32,* 247–267.

Durand, V.M., & Carr, E. (1987). Social influences on "self stimulator" behavior: Analysis and treatment application. *Journal of Applied Behavior Analysis, 20,* 119–132.

Durand, V.M., & Carr, E. (1991). Functional communication training to reduce challenging behavior: Maintenance and application in new settings. *Journal of Applied Behavior Analysis, 24,* 251–264.

Durand, V.M., & Carr, E. (1992). An analysis of maintenance following functional communication training. *Journal of Applied Behavior Analysis, 25,* 777–794.

Girolametto, L. (1988). Improving the social-conversational skills of developmentally delayed children: An intervention study. *Journal of Speech and Hearing Disorders, 53,* 156–167.

Girolametto, L., Verbey, M., & Tannock, R. (1994). Improving joint engagement in parent–child interaction: An intervention study. *Journal of Early Intervention, 18,* 155–167.

Goossens', C. (1989). Aided communication intervention before assessment: A case study of a child with cerebral palsy. *Augmentative and Alternative Communication, 5,* 14–26.

Guess, D., Sailor, W., & Baer, D. (1974). To teach language to retarded children. In R.L. Schiefelbusch & L.L. Lloyd (Eds.), *Language perspectives: Acquisition, retardation and intervention* (pp. 529–563). Baltimore: University Park Press.

Hagopian, L.P., Fisher, W.W., Sullivan, M.T., Acquisto, J., & LeBlanc, L.A. (1998). Effectiveness of functional communication training with and without extinction and punishment: A summary of 21 inpatient cases. *Journal of Applied Behavior Analysis, 31,* 211–235.

Hanley, G.P., Iwata, B.A., & Thompson, R.H. (2001). Reinforcement schedule thinning following treatment with functional communication training. *Journal of Applied Behavior Analysis, 34,* 17–38.

Hart, B. (1985). Naturalistic language training techniques. In S. Warren & A. Rogers-Warren (Eds.), *Teaching functional language* (pp. 63–88). Austin, TX: PRO-ED.

Hart, B., & Risley, T.R. (1995). *Meaningful differences in the everyday experience of young American children.* Baltimore: Paul H. Brookes Publishing Co.

Harwood, K., Warren, S., & Yoder, P. (2002). The importance of responsivity in developing contingent exchanges with beginning communicators. In D.R. Beukelman & J. Reichle (Series Eds.) & J. Reichle, D.R. Beukelman, & J.C. Light (Vol. Eds.), *Augmentative and alternative communication series: Exemplary practices for beginning communicators: Implications for AAC* (pp. 59–96). Baltimore: Paul H. Brookes Publishing Co.

Hinderscheit, L.R., & Reichle, J. (1987). Teaching direct select color encoding to an adolescent with multiple handicaps. *Augmentative and Alternative Communication, 3,* 137–142.

Horn, E., & Jones, H. (1996). Comparison of two selection techniques used in augmentative and alternative communication. *Augmentative and Alternative Communication, 12,* 23–31.

Hunt, P., Goetz, L., Alwell, M., & Sailor, W. (1986). Using an interrupted behavior chain strategy to teach generalized communication responses. *Journal of The Association for Persons with Severe Handicaps, 11,* 196–204.

Iacono, T.A., & Duncum, J.E. (1995). Comparison of sign alone and in combination with an electronic communication device in early language intervention: Case study. *Augmentative and Alternative Communication, 11,* 249–254.

Iacono, T., Mirenda, P., & Beukelman, D. (1993). Comparison of unimodal and multi-modal AAC techniques for children with intellectual disabilities. *Augmentative and Alternative Communication, 9,* 83–94.

Kahng, S., Hendrickson, D.J., & Vu, C.P. (2000). Comparison of single and multiple functional communication training responses for the treatment of problem behavior. *Journal of Applied Behavior Analysis, 33,* 321–324.

Kaiser, A.P., Yoder, P.J., Fischer, R., Keefer, M., Hemmeter, M.L., & Ostrosky, M.M. (1997). *A comparison of milieu teaching and responsive interaction implemented by parents.* Unpublished manuscript.

Kaiser, A., Yoder, D., & Keetz, A. (1992). Evaluating milieu teaching. In S. Warren & J. Reichle (Series and Vol. Eds.), *Communication and language intervention series: Vol. 1. Causes and effects in communication and language intervention* (pp. 9–48). Baltimore: Paul H. Brookes Publishing Co.

Kay-Raining Bird, E., & Chapman, R. (1998). Partial representation and phonological selectivity in comprehension of 13–16 month olds. *First Language, 18,* 105–127.

King, J., Spoeneman, T., Stuart, S., & Beukelman, D. (1995). Small talk in adult conversations. *Augmentative and Alternative Communication, 11,* 244–248.

Lalli, J.S., Casey, S., & Kates, K. (1995). Reducing escape behavior and increasing task completion with functional communication training, extinction, and response chaining. *Journal of Applied Behavior Analysis, 28,* 261–268.

Light, J.C., & Binger, C. (1998). *Building communicative competence with individuals who use augmentative and alternative communication.* Baltimore: Paul H. Brookes Publishing Co.

Light, J., Collier, B., & Parnes, P. (1985a). Communicative interaction between young nonspeaking physically disabled children and their primary caregivers: Part 1. Discourse patterns. *Augmentative and Alternative Communication, 1,* 74–83.

Light, J., Collier, B., & Parnes, P. (1985b). Communicative interaction between young nonspeaking physically disabled children and their primary caregivers: Part 2. Communicative functions. *Augmentative and Alternative Communication, 1,* 98–107.

Light, J.C., Roberts, B., Dimarco, R., & Greiner, N. (1998). Augmentative and alternative communication to support receptive and expressive communication for people with autism. *Journal of Communication Disorders, 31,* 153–180.

Linfoot, K. (1994). *Communication strategies for people with developmental disabilities: Issues from theory to practice.* Baltimore: Paul H. Brookes Publishing Co.

Lloyd, L.L., Fuller, D.R., & Arvidson, H.H. (1998). *Augmentative and alternative communication: A handbook of principles and practices.* Needham Heights, MA: Allyn & Bacon.

MacDonald, J. (1989). *Becoming partners with children: From play to conversation.* San Antonio, TX: Special Press.

Mervis, C., & Bertram, J. (1993). Acquisition of early object labels: The roles of operating principles and input. In S.F. Warren & J. Reichle (Series Eds.) & A. Kaiser & D.B. Gray (Vol. Eds.), *Communication and language intervention series: Vol. 2. Enhancing children's communication: Research foundations for intervention* (pp. 287–316). Baltimore: Paul H. Brookes Publishing Co.

Millar, D., Light, J., & Schlosser, R. (2002). *The impact of augmentative and alternative communication on speech development: A research review.* Manuscript submitted for publication.

Mizuko, M., Reichle, J., Ratcliff, A., & Esser, J. (1994). Effects of selection techniques and array sizes on short-term visual memory. *Augmentative and Alternative Communication, 10,* 237–244.

Nelson, K. (1986). Event knowledge and cognitive development. In K. Nelson (Ed.), *Event knowledge: Structure and function in development* (pp. 125–141). Mahwah, NJ: Lawrence Erlbaum Associates.

Peck, S.M., Wacker, D.P., Berg, W.K., Cooper, L.J., Brown, K.A., Richman, D., McComas, J.J., Frischmeyer, P., & Millard, T. (1996). Choice-making treatment of young children's severe behavior problems. *Journal of Applied Behavior Analysis, 29,* 263–290.

Peterson, S., Bondy, A., Vincent, Y, & Finnegan, C. (1995). Effects of altering communicative input for students with autism and no speech: Two case studies. *Augmentative and Alternative Communication, 11,* 93–100.

Peterson, K., Reichle, J., & Johnston, S. (2000). Examining preschoolers' performance in linear and row–column scanning techniques. *Augmentative and Alternative Communication, 16,* 27–36.

Piché, L., & Reichle, J. (1991). Teaching scanning selection techniques. In J. Reichle, J. York, & J. Sigafoos (Eds.), *Implementing augmentative and alternative communication: Strategies for learners with severe disabilities* (pp. 257–274). Baltimore: Paul H. Brookes Publishing Co.

Ratcliff, A. (1994). Comparison of relative demands implicated in direct selection and scanning: Considerations from normal children. *Augmentative and Alternative Communication, 10,* 67–74.

Reichle, J. (1991). *A survey of speech-language pathologists who serve clients using AAC.* Unpublished manuscript, University of Minnesota, Minneapolis.

Reichle, J. (1999). *Examining the generality of the rejecting communicative function for an individual with severe developmental disabilities.* Unpublished manuscript, University of Minnesota, Minneapolis.

Reichle, J. (2000). *Teaching symbol searching.* Unpublished manuscript, University of Minnesota, Minneapolis.

Reichle, J. (2001). *Teaching simple linear scanning to a child with a significant physical disability.* Unpublished manuscript, University of Minnesota, Minneapolis.

Reichle, J., & Brown, L. (1986). Teaching the use of a multipage direct selection communication board to an adult with autism. *Journal of The Association for Persons with Severe Handicaps, 11,* 68–73.

Reichle, J., & Dahl, N. (2000). *Discriminated use of a request assistance response during skill acquisition training.* Unpublished manuscript, University of Minnesota, Minneapolis.

Reichle, J., Drager, K., & Davis, C. (2001). *Using requests for assistance to obtain desired items and to gain release from non-preferred activities: Implications for assessment and intervention.* Unpublished manuscript, University of Minnesota, Minneapolis.

Reichle, J., Halle, J., & Drasgow, E. (1998). Implementing augmentative communication systems. In S.F. Warren & M.E. Fey (Series Eds.) & A.M. Wetherby, S.F. Warren, & J. Reichle (Vol. Eds.), *Communication and language intervention series: Vol. 7. Transitions in prelinguistic communication* (pp. 417–436). Baltimore: Paul H. Brookes Publishing Co.

Reichle, J., & Karlan, G. (1985). The selection of an augmentative system in communication intervention: A criteria of decision rules. *Journal of The Association for Persons with Severe Handicaps, 10,* 146–156.

Reichle, J., Rogers, N., & Barrett, C. (1984). Establishing pragmatic discriminations among the communicative functions of requesting, rejecting, and commenting in an adolescent. *Journal of The Association for Persons with Severe Handicaps, 9,* 31–36.

Reichle, J., Sigafoos, J., & Remington, R. (1991). Beginning an augmentative communication system with individuals with severe disabilities. In B. Remington (Ed.), *The challenge of severe mental handicap* (pp. 189–213). New York: John Wiley & Sons.

Reichle, J., & Ward, M. (1985). Teaching discriminative use of an encoding electronic communication device and signing exact English to a moderately handicapped child. *Language, Speech and Hearing Services in Schools, 16*(1), 58–63.

Reichle, J., & Yoder, D.E. (1985). Communication board use in severely handicapped learners. *Language, Speech and Hearing Services in Schools, 16,* 146–157.

Richman, D.M., Wacker, D.P., & Winborn, L. (2001). Response efficiency during functional communication training: Effects of effort on response allocation. *Journal of Applied Behavior Analysis, 34,* 73–76.

Romski, M.A., & Sevcik, R.A. (1996). *Breaking the speech barrier: Language development through augmented means.* Baltimore: Paul H. Brookes Publishing Co.

Romski, M., Sevcik, R., Adamson, L., Browning, J., Williams, S., & Colbert, N. (1999, November). *Augmented communication input for toddlers: A pilot study.* Poster presented at the Annual Meeting of the American Speech-Language-Hearing Association, San Francisco.

Schepis, M., Reid, D., Behrmann, M., & Sutton, K. (1998). Increasing communicative interactions of young children with autism using a voice output communication aid and naturalistic teaching. *Journal of Applied Behavior Analysis, 31,* 561–578.

Shane, H.C., & Bashir, A.S. (1980). Election criteria for the adoption of an augmentative language. In W.C. McCormack & S.A. Wurm (Eds.), *Language and society: Anthropological issues* (pp. 408–414). The Hague and Paris: Mouton de Gruyter.

Shatz, M. (1983). Communication. In P.H. Mussen (Ed.), *Handbook of child psychology: Cognitive development* (pp. 841–889). New York: John Wiley & Sons.

Shirley, M.J., Iwata, B.A., Kahng, S., Mazaleski, J.L., & Lerman, D.C. (1997). Does functional communication training compete with ongoing contingencies of reinforcement? An analysis during response acquisition and maintenance. *Journal of Applied Behavior Analysis, 30,* 93–104.

Shukla, S., & Albin, R.W. (1996). Effects of extinction alone and extinction plus functional communication training on covariation of problem behaviors. *Journal of Applied Behavior Analysis, 29,* 565–568.

Sigafoos, J., Mustonen, T., DePaepe, P., Reichle, J., & York, J. (1991). Defining the array of instructional prompts for teaching communication skills. In J. Reichle, J. York, & J. Sigafoos (Eds.), *Implementing augmentative and alternative communication: Strategies for learners with severe disabilities* (pp. 173–192). Baltimore: Paul H. Brookes Publishing Co.

Snyder-McLean, L., Solomonson, B., McLean, J., & Sack, S. (1984). Structuring joint action routines: A strategy for facilitating communication and language development in the classroom. *Seminars in Speech and Language, 5,* 213–228.

Szeto, A., Allen, E., & Littrell, M. (1993). Comparison of speed and accuracy for selected electronic communication devices and input methods. *Augmentative and Alternative Communication, 9,* 229–242.

Wacker, D.P., Steege, M.W., Northup, J., Sasso, G., Berg, W., Reimers, T., Cooper, L., Cigrand, K., & Donn, L. (1990). A component analysis of functional communication training across three topographies of severe behavior problems. *Journal of Applied Behavior Analysis, 23,* 417–429.

Warren, S.F., & Yoder, P.J. (1998). Facilitating the transition from preintentional to intentional communication. In S.F. Warren & M.E. Fey (Series Eds.) & A.M. Wetherby, S.F. Warren, & J. Reichle (Vol. Eds.), *Communication and language intervention series: Vol. 7. Transitions in prelinguistic communication* (pp. 365–384). Baltimore: Paul H. Brookes Publishing Co.

Wetherby, A., & Prizant, B. (1989). The expression of communicative intent: Assessment guidelines. *Seminars in Speech and Language, 10,* 77–91.

Wetherby, A., Reichle, J., & Pierce, P. (1998). The transition to symbolic communication. In S.F. Warren & M.E. Fey (Series Eds.) & A.M. Wetherby, S.F. Warren, & J. Reichle (Vol. Eds.), *Communication and language intervention series: Vol. 7. Transitions in prelinguistic communication* (pp. 197–232). Baltimore: Paul H. Brookes Publishing Co.

Wilcox, M.J. (1992). Enhancing initial communication skills in young children with developmental disabilities through partner programming. *Seminars in Speech and Language, 13,* 194–212.

Wilcox, M.J., Shannon, M., & Bacon, C. (1992, December). *From prelinguistic to linguistic behavior: Outcomes for young children with developmental disabilities.* Paper presented to the International Early Childhood Conference on Children with Special Needs, Washington, DC.

Wilkinson, K.M., & McIlvane, W.J. (2002). Considerations in teaching graphic symbols to beginning communicators. In D.R. Beukelman & J. Reichle (Series Eds.) & J. Reichle, D. Beukelman, & J. Light (Vol. Eds.), *Augmentative and alternative communication series: Exemplary practices for beginning communicators: Implications for AAC* (pp. 273–322). Baltimore: Paul H. Brookes Publishing Co.

Windsor, J., & Fristoe, M. (1991). Key word signing: Perceived and acoustic differences between signed and spoken narratives. *Journal of Speech and Hearing Research, 24,* 260–268.

Worsdell, A.S., Iwata, B.A., Hanley, G.P., Thompson, R.H., & Kahng, S. (2000). Effects of continuous and intermittent reinforcement for problem behavior during functional communication training. *Journal of Applied Behavior Analysis, 33,* 167–179.

Yoder, P., Warren, S., McCathren, R., & Leew, S. (1998). Does adult responsivity to child behavior facilitate communication development? In S.F. Warren & M.E. Fey (Series Eds.) & A.M. Wetherby, S.F. Warren, & J. Reichle (Vol. Eds.), *Communication and language intervention series: Vol. 7. Transitions in prelinguistic communication* (pp. 39–58). Baltimore: Paul H. Brookes Publishing Co.

14

Outcomes Measurement in AAC

Ralf W. Schlosser

Do our interventions and services really make a difference? This question not only plagues clinicians and educators of many service-providing agencies in AAC but also occupies funding agencies and families of people who potentially or currently use AAC. The purpose of this chapter is to synthesize our knowledge base related to three approaches to outcomes measurement in AAC (goal attainment scaling [GAS], participation, and quality of life [QOL]) and to derive directions for future practice and research. The chapter is arranged as follows: First, definition of key terms and proposition of a multidimensional approach to outcomes measurement in AAC. Next, synthesis of the knowledge base on the methodology and application of GAS and directions as to how this technique may be applied in AAC. Then, the state of what is known about participation as a potential outcome of AAC intervention and recommendations for future research. Finally, issues related to the measurement of QOL and directions for studying QOL as a potential outcome of AAC intervention.

DEFINITIONS

Outcomes may be defined in a number of ways. For the purposes of this chapter, *outcomes* will be defined as changes attributed to an AAC intervention. These changes may be positive (i.e., in the desired direction), negative (i.e., in a direction opposite to the one desired), or unplanned (i.e., not anticipated; Schlosser, 1999; Wolf, 1978). *Efficacy* has been used as an umbrella term including effectiveness, efficiency, and effects[1] in communication disorders and related fields (Calculator, 1991; Kendall & Norton-Ford, 1982; Olswang, 1990; Schlosser & Braun, 1994). *Effectiveness* has been defined as the demonstration

---

[1]Schlosser (2003a) engaged in a critical analysis of existing definitions of efficacy research, outcomes research, and outcomes measurement. Readers who wish to follow the derivation of these definitions may consult the original reference.

of behavior change as a direct result of intervention. *Efficiency* refers to the demonstration of comparative effectiveness of at least two interventions in terms of one or more criteria such as time, cost, error rate, and so forth. A comparison in terms of efficiency requires that the effectiveness of each intervention be already established. *Effects* refers to the determination of intervention components that are relevant and the demonstration of links of components to specific changes.

The efficacy of an AAC intervention is demonstrated under ideal or optimal conditions (Office of Technology Assessment, 1978; Robey & Schultz, 1998). *Efficacy research in AAC* may thus be defined as the process of demonstrating 1) behavior change as a direct result of intervention, 2) comparative effectiveness of at least two interventions, and/or 3) intervention components that are relevant and links of components to specific changes under ideal conditions.

Robey and Schultz (1998) defined *outcomes research* as a process designed to index differences between observations made prior to an intervention and observations made after an intervention. Differences may also be indexed between observations made prior to an intervention and observations made *during* an intervention, as would be the case when data are collected in time-series format.

Moreover, it is important to point out that outcomes research typically indexes differences of *everyday* AAC interventions; that is, interventions that occur under average conditions or below-average conditions (Granlund & Blackstone, 1999; Office of Technology Assessment, 1978; Robey & Schultz, 1998). Outcomes research under average conditions may involve typically selected and trained clinicians, typically selected clients who receive treatment delivered in an average manner, typically structured conditions for delivering treatment, and typical measures or indices of change, and so forth. The results of outcomes research are then used to change the way interventions are provided (Blackstone, 1995). Thus, *outcomes research in AAC* may be defined as a process designed to index differences between observations made prior to an everyday intervention and observations made during or after an everyday intervention; everyday interventions may be applied under average or below-average conditions. Borrowing from the definition of the Office of Technology Assessment (1978), the results of outcomes research speak to the probability of benefit to individuals in a defined population from AAC intervention applied for a given communication problem under typical or sub-average conditions of use.

Outcomes measurement represents a suitable umbrella term for both efficacy research and outcomes research as they are defined here because both are concerned with the measurement of outcomes (Frattali, 1999). Schlosser (2003a) views the relation between efficacy research and outcomes research on a continuum of outcomes measurement (see Figure 14.1). As one moves along the continuum from ideal conditions to more typical (average) conditions and marginal conditions, this type of research may be referred to as outcomes research.

Efficacy	Outcomes measurement: A continuum of conditions		
	Efficacy research	Outcomes research	
	Ideal conditions	*Average conditions*	*Marginal conditions*
Effectiveness			
Efficiency			
Effects			

Figure 14.1. A schematic conceptualization of outcomes measurement in AAC. (From Schlosser, R.W. [2003a]. *The efficacy of augmentative and alternative communication: Towards evidence-based practice.* New York: Academic Press; reprinted by permission.)

MULTIDIMENSIONAL APPROACH TO EVALUATING OUTCOMES

Outcomes research in AAC may benefit from taking a multidimensional approach. In addition to the obvious need for gathering objective hard data, such an approach involves the perspective of evaluation, the focus of evaluation, and the level of evaluation (Light & Schlosser, 2003). This multidimensional model is illustrated in Figure 14.2.

Perspective of Evaluation

Stakeholders who directly or indirectly control the feasibility of the intervention should be included in outcomes measurement efforts (Fawcett, 1991). Based on the work of Schwartz and Baer (1991), Schlosser (1999) distinguished four types of stakeholder groups in AAC: 1) direct, 2) indirect, 3) immediate community, and 4) extended community.

 Direct Stakeholders Individuals who use AAC will be the direct stakeholders in many cases because they tend to be the primary recipients of the intervention. In some instances, however, communication partners and peers may be considered direct stakeholders if they participate in communication partner training or facilitator training programs.

 Indirect Stakeholders Indirect stakeholders are strongly affected by the change in communicative behavior of the direct stakeholder and may thus

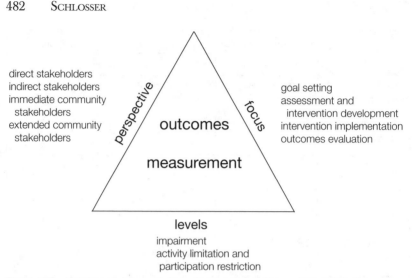

Figure 14.2. Multidimensional model. (From Light, J.C., & Schlosser, R.W. [2003]. *Outcomes research in augmentative and alternative communication: A multimodal approach.* Manuscript in preparation. Copyright © 2003 R.W. Schlosser; reprinted by permission.)

indirectly influence the feasibility of interventions. Family members of individuals who use AAC and are receiving intervention often are considered indirect stakeholders. Other indirect stakeholders involved in social validation may include caregivers and friends.

Immediate Community Stakeholders   Immediate community stakeholders may influence the feasibility of interventions indirectly through regular professional or social interactions (or lack thereof) with direct and indirect stakeholders. Unlike indirect stakeholders, immediate community stakeholders are not as strongly affected by targeted change. Examples include supervisors of individuals who use AAC in supported employment situations who have been targeted for intervention (e.g., requesting assistance), prospective regular education teachers, and peers without disabilities.

Extended Community Stakeholders   Extended community stakeholders do not interact with direct or indirect stakeholders on a regular basis and probably do not even know them; they may be drawn from two groups with possibly quite distinct perspectives: experts in the field of study and laypersons (J. Light, personal communication, June 25, 2001). Experts may not necessarily interact with the targeted participants on a regular basis, but they may have some degree of familiarity with the population from which the participants are drawn and/or they may be knowledgeable about AAC and its application relative to the intervention. Although the perspectives of experts can add important perspectives to the measurement of outcomes in AAC, it is the extended community stakeholder group of laypersons that has been heralded as the ultimate judges of communicative competence (Light, 1989).

Focus of Evaluation

The focus of evaluation perspective proposes that outcomes measurement should consider all key stages of service delivery or intervention, from goal setting, to assessment and intervention development, to intervention implementation, to the evaluation of outcomes. For an in-depth discussion and examples of social validation of goals, methods, and outcomes, the reader may consult Schlosser (1999).

Goal Setting The social validation of goals involves the validation of the topography of the behavior and the level of the behavior that should be achieved before terminating intervention (Fuqua & Schwade, 1986). In terms of goals, the goal levels may be scaled from "worst expected outcome" to "best expected outcome" as it would be done when using GAS (an extensive discussion is presented later in the chapter).

Assessment and Intervention Development The social validation of methods includes the validation of materials (Schlosser, 1999) and procedures (type and form; Kazdin, 1980). In addition to the process of social validation, one may want to evaluate whether the chosen treatments are based on the principles of evidence-based practice. One may examine the documentation to what extent the best research evidence has been integrated with the other considerations in selecting a certain treatment for an individual.

Intervention Implementation Regarding the implementation of treatment, perhaps the most crucial aspect is that of treatment integrity, defined as the degree to which the treatment (independent variable) is implemented as intended (see Schlosser, 2002). The monitoring of the outcome variable alone will allow unambiguous conclusions about changes in the outcome variable, but it will not permit conclusions about the source of these changes (Billingsley, White, & Munson, 1980).

Outcomes Evaluation Outcomes evaluation may occur at the individual level, the program or service level, and the system level (Granlund & Blackstone, 1999). At the individual level, data are collected concerning the success of an intervention or service to a given direct stakeholder such as a learner using AAC or communication partners. At the program or service level, outcomes evaluation is aimed at determining the outcomes of AAC interventions across direct stakeholders served by the program. This requires data that lend themselves to be aggregated across individual direct stakeholders. At the system level, further aggregation of program or service data is required across programs/services, centers, agencies, school systems, and assistive technology teams.

In addition to these various levels at which outcomes may be evaluated, outcomes may be socially validated depending on their role in the treatment process (i.e., immediate effects, instrumental effects, and ultimate effects) by various stakeholder groups as described previously (Fawcett, 1991; Schlosser, 1999).

Levels of Evaluation

Outcomes can be evaluated at each of the levels of the International Classification of Functioning, Disability, and Handicap (ICF): body functions, body structures, activities and participation, and environmental factors (World Health Organization, 1980, 2001). The constructs of the ICF and related terms are defined as follows

> Body functions are the physiological functions of body systems (including psychological functions).
>
> Body structures are anatomic parts of the body such as organs, limbs, and their components.
>
> Impairments are problems in body function or structure such as a significant deviation or loss.
>
> Activity is the execution of a task or action by an individual.
>
> Participation is involvement in a life situation.
>
> Activity limitations are difficulties an individual may have in executing activities.
>
> Participation restrictions are problems an individual may experience in involvement in life situations.
>
> Environmental factors make up the physical, social, and attitudinal environment in which people live and conduct their lives. (World Health Organization, 2001, p. 8)

For each construct (e.g., body functions, body structures, activities and participation), domains are identified that represent the units of classification. For example, the construct of "body functions" includes mental functions; sensory functions; and pain, voice, and speech functions. The construct of "activities and participation" includes learning and applying knowledge; general tasks and demands; communication; movement; self-care; domestic life areas; interpersonal interactions; major life areas; and community, social, and civic life. The construct of "environmental factors" includes products and technology (including assistive AAC devices); natural environment and human-made changes to environment; support and relationships; and attitudes, services, systems, and policies.

A generic qualifier scale is then used to denote health states or the degree to which a problem exists relative to the construct. The scale ranges from 0 to 4:

- 0 No problem (none, absent, negligible) 0%–4%
- 1 Mild problem (slight, low) 5%–24%
- 2 Moderate problem (medium, fair) 25%–49%
- 3 Severe problem (high, extreme) 50%–95%
- 4 Complete problem (total) 96%–100%

This scale can be used to assess outcomes or a trajectory over time as a result of intervention or services.

Lund and Light (2001) applied the ICF model to the AAC field when they revisited participants of an earlier study (Light, Collier, & Parnes, 1985a, 1985b, 1985c) 15 years later to assess impairments, activity limitations, and participation restrictions. Table 14.1 provides an overview of domains, positive aspects, negative aspects, areas of measurement, and methods of measurement evaluated by Lund and Light (2001).

GOAL ATTAINMENT SCALING (GAS)

Level-independent measurement approaches are versatile in that they permit the measurement of outcomes regardless of the ICF level of evaluation. GAS is such a method in that the attainment of goals may be evaluated at any of the four levels: body functions, body structures, activities and participation, and environmental factors.

GAS, first brought to the attention of the AAC field by Calculator (1991), is a simple and precise method for evaluating individual progress toward unique goals (Kiresuk & Sherman, 1968; Kiresuk, Smith, & Cardillo, 1994). Since it was first brought to our attention, however, a critical engagement with this technique, including a discussion of strengths and weaknesses along with a review of clinical trials using GAS, has not yet occurred. See Schlosser, 2003b, for a critical engagement of GAS as it pertains to the field of speech-language pathology.

Seven Steps

GAS involves the following seven steps (Kiresuk & Sherman, 1968):

1. Specify a set of goals.
2. Assign a weight for each goal according to priority.
3. Specify a continuum of possible outcomes (worst expected outcome [−2], less than expected outcome [−1], expected outcome [0], more than expected outcome [+1], and best expected outcome [+2]).
4. Determine current or initial performance.
5. Intervene for a specified period.
6. Determine performance attained on each objective.
7. Evaluate extent of attainment.

Table 14.1. Measurement approaches based on the ICF

Domain	Positive aspect	Negative aspect	Areas of measurement	Method of measurement
Body function and structures	Functional and structural integrity	Impairment	Motor function	From medical and therapy reports
			Sensory functions (vision, hearing)	From medical and therapy reports
Activities and participation	Activity and participation	Activity limitation; participation restriction	Receptive language skills	Peabody Picture Vocabulary Test Revised (Dunn & Dunn, 1981)
				Test of Auditory Comprehension of Language, Revised (Carrow-Woolfolk, 1985)
			Reading comprehension	Gray Silent Reading Test (Wiederholt & Bialock, 2000)
			Discourse skills, communicative functions, modes of communication	Conversational samples with caregiver, peer, student investigator
			Functional communication	Functional Assessment of Communication Skills for Adults (ASHA FACS) (Frattali et al., 1995)
			Educational/vocational achievement	Interviews with participants and therapy reports
			Participation	Activity Standards Inventory (Beukelman & Mirenda, 1998)
			Self-determination	The Arc's Self-Determination Scale (Wehmeyer & Kelchner, 1995)
			Quality of life	Quality of Life Profile for People with Physical and Sensory Disabilities (Renwick, Brown, & Raphael, 1998)
Contextual factors (environmental)	Facilitators	Barriers/hindrances	Products and technology	Interviews with participants and professionals
			Support and relationships	Interviews with participants and professionals
			Services	Interviews with participants and professionals

From Lund, S., & Light, J. (2001). *Fifteen years later: An investigation of long-term outcomes of augmentative and alternative interventions. Final grant report* (p. 35). University Park: The Pennsylvania State University; adapted by permission.

Note: Participation as an outcome was evaluated by Schlosser and colleagues (2000) rather than Lund and Light (2001). It is an appropriate area of measurement of "activities and participation."

The extent to which goals are attained is evaluated through simple visual analysis or through statistical analysis. Visual analysis allows one to compare the initial performance with the level of attainment per goal and across goals for an individual. Statistical analyses (via either a standardized T score [mean $= 50, SD = 10$] or a weighted percentage improvement score) permit an analysis of attainment across all goals for a given individual and also allow for aggregation across individuals. The p value reflects the estimated average intercorrelation of attainment scores; Kiresuk and Sherman (1968) argued that it can be safely assumed that this value is .30 and safely used as a constant in this formula.

Applying the Model

Consider this method of outcomes evaluation for student Josh. I used as a departure point some of the annual goals and short-term objectives developed for Josh by Jorgenson (1994, p. 71; see Table 14.2). Then, I assigned weights to the respective goals according to priority (see Table 14.3). Processes described by Jorgensen (1994) such as the MacGill Action Planning System (Vandercook, York, & Forest, 1989), Personal Futures Planning (Mount, 1987), and Choosing Outcomes and Accommodations for Children (Giangreco, Cloninger, & Iverson, 1998) were helpful in deriving the weights for each goal.

Table 14.2. Goals for Josh

1. Goal: When talking with a responsive peer, Josh will take three conversational turns using his communication book or natural gestures. (Weight = .4)

    Objective: During informal conversation or buddy-reading in the classroom, Josh will maintain his interest in a book or a picture from home by answering at least three questions posed by a peer. The SLP will interview Josh's buddies and observe in the classroom once a week in different settings to evaluate progress.

2. Goal: Within real-life situations such as choosing food in the lunchroom, selecting books in the library, or picking friends to be on his team in physical education, Josh will make a choice among three offerings. (Weight = .3)

    Objective: When presented with a natural cue and a gestural prompt across various settings (e.g., the server asking him what he wants for hot lunch and if he doesn't choose, the server will point to the various choices). Josh will point to a choice (from among three) within the time limit given other students. This will be measured by observations across at least three settings and by interviewing peers and teachers.

3. Goal: Josh will demonstrate an understanding of one-to-one correspondence by passing out materials such as books, milk cartons, or art supplies to peers in class. (Weight = .1)

    Objective: When accompanied by a peer who cues Josh by counting, "One, two, three, four," Josh will pass out materials to peers in class, with accuracy up to 10. This objective will be evaluated by interviewing peers and observing Josh in class.

Table 14.3.   Example of Josh's goals along with goal attainment levels

Goal attainment levels	Goal 1: Conversational turns (Weight = 4)	Goal 2: Choice making (Weight = 4)	Goal 3: One-to-one correspondence (Weight = 1)
Best expected outcome (+2)	Answers at least four questions during buddy-reading and informal conversation	Chooses within a typical time frame after natural prompts in four or more settings	Shows correspondence with accuracy of at least 15 while handing out 3 materials based on gestural cues
More than expected outcome (+1)	Answers three questions during buddy-reading and informal conversation	Chooses within a typical time frame after natural prompts in three settings (A)	Shows correspondence with accuracy up to 15 while handing out 3 materials based on spoken cues
Expected outcome (0)	Answers three questions during buddy-reading or informal conversation (A)	Chooses within a typical time frame after natural and gestural prompts in three settings	Shows correspondence with accuracy up to 10 while handing out 3 materials based on spoken cues
Less than expected outcome (−1)	Answers two questions during buddy-reading or informal conversation	Chooses within a typical time frame after natural and gestural prompts in two or fewer settings	Shows correspondence with accuracy up to five while handing out three materials based on spoken cues (A)
Worst expected outcome (−2)	Answers one or no questions during buddy-reading or informal conversation (I)	Chooses using more time than typical after modeling and/or physical prompts in two or fewer settings (I)	Shows correspondence with accuracy up to five while handing out two or fewer materials based on spoken cues (I)

Key: I = Initial performance, A = Attained performance.
Copyright © 2003 R.W. Schlosser.

Next, I determined the levels of attainment (see Table 14.3). In determining the levels, it is best to first set the expected level followed by the two mid-levels (i.e., more than expected outcome, less than expected outcome) and to conclude with the two extremes (i.e., best expected outcome, worst expected outcome).

The next step involves the determination of current or initial performance (see Table 14.3 for initial performance [I]). The initial performance usually will be at the level of the "worst expected outcome." Exceptions are goals that target the maintenance rather than the acquisition of skills (e.g., direct stakeholders with progressive disorders); here, it may be best to set the initial performance at "–1" in order to not only leave room for betterment but also for a worsening in performance.

Intervention then takes place for a specified period of time, which should be individualized for each goal. According to Smith (1994), the timing has to do with the purpose of the evaluation of measurement, not with the technique of GAS itself. I intervened for 6, 5, and 3 months for Goals 1, 2, and 3, respectively. Once the times had elapsed, I revisited the goals to evaluate the level of attainment (see Table 14.3 for level of attainment [A]). For a given individual, the extent of attainment can be determined visually by examining scale attainment levels for each of the goals. Should the AAC application of GAS call for an aggregation of attainment within and across individuals (as it may be the case for an entire AAC service), statistical analyses may be necessary.

Strengths of Goal Attainment Scaling

Although its primary strength is the ability to evaluate individualized longitudinal change (Kiresuk & Sherman, 1968; Ottenbacher & Cusick, 1993), GAS has several other strengths relative to the multidimensional model, including the following: GAS 1) permits aggregation across levels of outcomes evaluation; 2) is adaptable to any ICF level, categories within a level, and population; 3) is conducive to the evaluation of everyday interventions; 4) encourages multiple perspectives of evaluation, and 5) focuses team energies from goal-setting to outcomes evaluation.

Permits Aggregation Across Levels of Outcomes Evaluation   A crucial strength of GAS is that it facilitates comparisons across goals, individuals, service and programs, and systems. At the individual level, the attainment levels for each of Josh's goals, for example, can be aggregated to get an overall sense of outcomes for Josh. At the service level, GAS scores can be aggregated across clients. At the system level, GAS would allow aggregation across agencies, school systems, assistive technology teams, and so forth.

Adaptable to ICF Levels, Categories within Levels, and Populations   GAS is independent of and adaptable to virtually any of the levels specified by ICF and any domain within these levels. That is, GAS may be used to evaluate goal attainment at the levels of impairment, activity limitation, and participation restriction and domains within each of these levels such as voice and speech functions, community activities, and community participation. This flexibility is essential for AAC, given that the domains targeted in AAC vary considerably, including the four aspects of communicative competence plus the projected spin-off changes in participation, QOL, and self-determination (Light & Binger, 1998). GAS is also flexible in terms of being applicable to any population. In fact, GAS has been used in various fields such as intellectual disabilities (Bailey & Simeonsson, 1988), cognitive rehabilitation (Rockwood, Joyce, & Stolee, 1993), early intervention (Simeonsson, Bailey, Huntington, & Brandon, 1991), geriatrics (Rockwood & Stolee, 1993; Stolee, Stadnyk, Myers, & Rockwood, 1999), and physical and occupational therapy (Stephens & Haley, 1991). Adaptability to any population is critical for AAC because the people who may benefit from AAC may present with a variety of conditions such as developmental disabilities, acquired disabilities, progressive disorders, and temporary conditions (Kangas & Lloyd, 1998).

Conducive to the Evaluation of Everyday Interventions   Outcomes research focuses on the evaluation of everyday interventions carried out by practitioners. GAS appears to be enthusiastically accepted by clinicians and other practitioners (Bailey & Simeonsson, 1988; Burgee, 1996; Lewis, Spencer, Haas, & DiVittis, 1987), possibly because it " . . . reproduces the typical clinician's thinking as he or she judges actual outcome against what he or she would have predicted at the time treatment was started" (Lewis et al., 1987, p. 408).

Encourages Multiple Perspectives of Evaluation   GAS encourages an evaluation from multiple perspectives. Ideally, goal-setting should occur through a consensus-building process involving clinicians and all relevant stakeholders, including but not limited to the direct stakeholder (e.g., Kiresuk et al., 1994; Ottenbacher & Cusick, 1993; Simeonsson et al., 1991). This approach is highly consistent with the consensus-building process to be utilized as part of an AAC assessment and a family-centered service-delivery model (Beukelman & Mirenda, 1998).

Focuses Team Energies from Goal-Setting to Outcomes Evaluation   One of the premises of the multidimensional model is that the focus of evaluation should not solely rest on the outcomes to be evaluated. Rather, other stages of service/intervention delivery, including goal setting, assessment and intervention development, and intervention implementation provide the necessary context that helps people to understand the outcomes yielded. It has been postulated that clearly specified goals generated by a client and his or her treatment system can mobilize staff energies into a more coherent pursuit of relevant, feasible outcomes, perhaps by focusing assessment and intervention development, and intervention implementation (Smith, 1994).

Along a similar vein, Smith (1994) hypothesized that the goal-setting process itself may have a positive impact on treatment outcomes. This hypothesis has received support from two studies, one on a teacher support consultation team model and the other on the self-efficacy of college students (Burgee, 1996; Parilis, 1996). These studies seem to suggest that GAS is not only a technique for measuring outcomes but perhaps also a facilitator of existing treatments.

GAS has a number of strengths as a potential technique for outcomes research based on the multidimensional model proposed in this chapter. For a discussion of other strengths the reader is referred to Schlosser (2003b), including GAS 1) minimizes problems of other measures, 2) is tied to expected outcomes, 3) affords validity and reliability, and 4) is responsive to change.

Weaknesses and Possible Safeguards

GAS is not without potential weaknesses, however, including 1) outcomes may reflect the biases of those who construct the guides, 2) the computation and statistical analyses of GAS scores may not be appropriate, and 3) the interpretation of GAS scores may not be appropriate.

Outcomes May Reflect Biases   One of the concerns with GAS is whether an outcome is more a function of the team's ability to make accurate and reliable predictions rather than an indication of client progress or intervention effectiveness (Cytrynbaum, Birdwell, Birdwell, & Brandt, 1979). Adequate team training is likely to reduce biases, and with that prediction, accuracy can be increased over time (Bailey & Simeonsson, 1988). Furthermore, the extent of bias may depend on what source of information is used as the underlying basis for arriving at the attainment scores. If, for example, the opinions of the team are used as the sole source of information, GAS scores are subjective (Schlosser, 1999). Such perspectives are more useful when they supplement more objective data but not by themselves. Thus, GAS scores need to be based not only on subjective data such as interviews and progress notes in client files but also on direct data such as observations that are objective.

Ottenbacher and Cusick (1993) provided several safeguards to minimize bias. First, they called for operational definitions of the outcome criteria. Related to our example, what is a "typical time frame" and what qualifies as "natural prompts?" Second, the examiner must be able to record accurately and reliably the levels of attainment before using GAS. Third, they encourage the determination of attainment by an independent examiner without previous involvement in the treatment or the goal setting process. Fourth, inter-observer agreement data need to be collected on the assessment of performance for each distinct goal similar to recording agreement with other evaluative procedures with an individual focus such as single-subject experimental designs. Here, GAS fares fairly well (e.g., Stolee, Rockwood, Fox, & Streiner, 1992).

Inappropriate Computation and Statistical Analyses of Scores
MacKay, Somerville, and Lundie (1996) argued that outcomes scores of −2 to +2 are treated as if they were interval data, when in fact they may be ordinal (rankings on perceived continuum of achievement) or even nominal ("used simply to classify an object, person or characteristic"; Siegel, 1956, p. 23). Regardless of these properties, GAS typically transforms them into standard

scores, which may cause distortions in the data and shed doubt about the conclusion drawn from any test. Thus, GAS does not fulfill its claim to be a parametric expression of nonparametric information.

As a solution, MacKay and colleagues (1996) advocate the use of nonparametric methods for inferential analyses involving GAS scores. To do so, they suggested ways by which –2 to +2 may become stages in a sequence so that they may describe ordinal data or categories in a particular sequence so that they may describe nominal data. This would be accomplished by detailing how frequently each score occurs for each direct stakeholder or by categorizing the scores dichotomously (e.g., below goal, at or above goal), respectively. Either approach would then allow the researcher to apply nonparametric statistics to determine differences between the experimental group and the control group.

Inappropriate Interpretation of Goal Attainment Scaling Scores   GAS is not a research methodology for establishing causal inferences between independent and dependent variables. Nonetheless, procedures associated with GAS can be folded into a traditional research design by ensuring the internal validity of the treatment (Ottenbacher & Cusick, 1993). In fact, only when GAS is used in the context of an (quasi-) experimental design can some of the criticisms be ruled out. Simeonsson and colleagues (1991), for example, raised the possibility that a lack of attaining expected levels may not be due to the lack of effectiveness of the treatment but the underestimation or overestimation of goals. This threat can be minimized by using control goals or a control group with random allocation of goals to experimental goals or control goals or subjects to the respective group. There is no reason to believe that overestimation or underestimation would occur differently for experimental goals/subjects than for control goals/subjects. Another explanation for the lack of attaining expected outcomes could be the lack of adequate treatment integrity (Simeonsson et al., 1991). Here, the procedures described by Schlosser (2002) may be useful.

Future of Goal Attainment Scaling in AAC

The features of GAS make it very conducive to evaluating outcomes of AAC interventions within the proposed multidimensional model. Except for a Swedish project by Granlund and Steénson (1998), the AAC field has no applications of this methodology. We are in the beginning stages of evaluating its utility. In order to evaluate whether GAS can live up to its potential, studies need to be conducted that examine its validity, reliability, and responsiveness at various 1) levels of outcomes evaluation (e.g., individual, service, system), 2) service delivery systems (e.g., center-based, private-practice, consultation), and 3) populations (e.g., people with developmental disabilities).

In terms of validity, researchers need to focus primarily on construct validity. Single-subject experimental designs, an accepted method for evaluating individualized longitudinal change, may be used to evaluate the effectiveness of an intervention while using GAS. Changes in single-subject designs should coincide with changes in GAS scores. In terms of reliability, researchers need to treat GAS no differently from methods to evaluate intervention effectiveness, which require inter-observer agreement for dependent measures and treatment integrity. Directing efforts into the reliability of goal construction itself is, for these reasons, largely counterproductive given the nature of the GAS process. In absence of a commonly accepted single method for measuring responsiveness, it becomes crucial to use multiple methods to assess responsiveness (Stolee et al., 1999). If researchers are to evaluate whether GAS is truly responsive to changes due to AAC intervention, they need to conduct studies that also apply GAS to control goals (i.e., goals that are not targeted for treatment) or control groups (i.e., participants with goals that do not receive treatment). They can expect to see changes only in goals or subjects that are treated.

In summary, GAS has considerable potential for outcomes research in AAC. Some of the priority questions that could be answered through GAS and that are being studied include (Schlosser & Kovach, 2002):

- Do changes observed in GAS scores coincide with changes observed through other individualized measures of change in AAC?
- What is the social validity of GAS (process and outcomes) among practitioners and other stakeholders in AAC?
- Is GAS responsive to change in individuals, services, and systems?
- What is the extent of goal attainment nationwide for individuals receiving service from center-based service delivery systems?
- What is the extent of goal attainment nationwide for students receiving AAC services in the schools?

GAS is a methodology that accommodates measurement at any ICF level. In fact, it depends entirely on the level at which the goals are anchored. GAS does not dictate what measure to use in order to arrive at a judgment of degree of attainment. Therefore, it becomes necessary to discuss some of the measurement approaches that are tied to specific ICF levels.

LEVEL-DEPENDENT MEASUREMENT APPROACHES AND ISSUES

Level-dependent measurement approaches permit the measurement of outcomes at only one specific level of the ICF classification. The first level-dependent measurement approach is concerned with participation as an outcome of AAC interventions and services. The second level-dependent measurement approach addresses QOL issues. Both participation and QOL find themselves at the heart of the "activities and participation" domain of ICF.

Participation

Ferguson concluded that the real point of communication intervention efforts should be membership in society, "specifically participatory, socially valued, image-enhancing membership" (1994, p. 10). The Participation Assessment Framework was developed as a process to guide decision making and intervention in AAC (Beukelman & Mirenda, 1998). The framework provides four variables that can be manipulated to achieve a participation pattern that is appropriate to the needs and capabilities of the student who uses AAC. These include three levels of overall integration (i.e., fully, selective, and none). The framework then becomes specific with regard to the levels of academic and social participation (i.e., competitive, active, involved, and none). Finally, the student's level of independence is noted. Each of these levels of participation can be charted along a continuum.

Participation Matrix and Activity Standards Inventory The Participation Matrix allows a team to come to a consensus about the student's level of integration and participation and provides a baseline from which the team can agree on goals and expectations. The Activity Standards Inventory is used to document and analyze the student's actual participation in classroom activities. The team can use it to determine whether the student's actual participation reflects the agreed-on goals. Following is a summary of findings from a recent study that employed the Activity Standards Inventory to evaluate the outcomes of an AAC intervention (Schlosser et al., 2000).

The Evaluating Participation Outcomes of an AAC Intervention study aimed at evaluating the effectiveness of training a school team in using the Participation Assessment Framework along with various technologies (via adult learning strategies) on the participation of a student during literacy and math activities in an inclusive classroom. Participants included a multidisciplinary school team and one student supported by this team. The school team consisted of a general education teacher, two educational assistants, a program support teacher, a speech-language pathologist, an occupational therapist, a library resource teacher, and the student's mother. The target student, Nick, was 10 years old with cerebral palsy and no functional speech. He used a powered wheelchair for mobility. At the time of this study, his face-to-face communication system included a nonelectronic communication display, a yes-and-no option placed on opposite armrests of his wheelchair, and gestures. His communication display included Picture Communication Symbols (Johnson, 1992) and words. For written communication, Nick used Write

Away without speech feedback on a standard IBM-compatible desktop computer with a track ball.

A multiple-probe design across instructional formats was used to evaluate the effects of training the team on the percentage of barriers, percentage of participation, and the percentage of peer participation. "Nick was given credit for participating if he was involved in the performance of the activity step, even if assistance was provided by the teacher, educational assistant, or a peer in setting-up the technology or materials, providing AAC or other assistive technology device, or changing Nick's physical position" (Schlosser et al., 2000, p. 33). Two trained research assistants derived the dependent measures from coded videotape segments. Training was sequentially introduced across the instructional formats, beginning with the group format, individual format (i.e., one-to-one), and small group format (i.e., less than five students). Intervention, applied over a 4-month period, involved a Participation Assessment Framework workshop (including the use of the Activity Standards Inventory), several technology workshops, and ongoing coaching. After completing the project, the team members were asked to evaluate the social validity of the project via postintervention focus groups and individually through questionnaires.

Results indicated substantial decreases in the percentage of barriers across instructional formats for Nick. At the same time, a notable increase in the percentage of participation occurred across the instructional formats. The subjective evaluation results are in support of these objective outcome data. The team strongly agreed that Nick was provided with more opportunities, participated more, and experienced fewer barriers due to intervention. Also, the team rated the support provided as either very useful or useful, depending on the type of support. Focus group results were also in support of the objective findings and the subjective evaluation obtained from questionnaires. In summary, this preliminary study offers suggestive evidence that the Activity Standard Inventory may be sensitive to changes in participation.

Future of Participation and Beyond   Researchers are clearly in the early stages when it comes to understanding the role of AAC in fostering participation. They need to study how different instructional formats have an impact on the participation patterns in inclusive classrooms and how conducive the respective formats are to changes in participation patterns.

In addition, it would be desirable to explore whether school teams can be taught to use the Activity Standards Inventory as an outcomes measurement tool. This would permit the team to monitor themselves the outcomes of their own efforts in reducing barriers to participation. Studies need to be conducted to examine the effects of AAC interventions directed at the learner (e.g., introducing an AAC system, teaching of strategies to enhance communicative competence) on participation patterns of this learner. The Schlosser and colleagues (2000) study took a facilitator-training approach and did not monitor the learner's communicative performance. Such research would shed light on the relationship between AAC intervention, functional communication (possibly communicative competence), and participation.

It is essential to have pre- and postintervention measures in order to evaluate whether intervention had an effect. Thus, the question arises to what extent researchers should rely solely on the Activity Standards Inventory to measure participation changes in inclusive settings. Unlike self-contained classrooms, inclusive classrooms are known for rapidly changing activities, making it difficult to evaluate whether a barrier for a given step *within* an activity has been removed. Perhaps, researchers need to also examine those specific steps involving barriers *across* activities. Finally, it may be worthwhile to consider modifications to the Activity Standards Inventory that permit direct linkages between participation and communicative competence.

At a conceptual level, the Participation Assessment Framework and the Activity Standards Inventory offer several important contributions to the understanding and measurement of participation outcomes of AAC intervention. The field, however, should not limit itself to this framework and inventory.

Membership

The concepts of "participation" and "membership" are different, and it is precisely these differences that make it so worthwhile to consider membership as an essential outcome of AAC intervention. Participation is perhaps but one ingredient for "conferring" membership under the right circumstances. It seems that participation must be *active* and *socially valued* in order to confer membership. Membership should also be characterized by status in the group. The question arises how to measure changes in membership as a result of changes in participation patterns.

Calculator (1994, 1999) offered several useful suggestions along these lines that are worth considering when examining changes in membership. Sociometric ratings (e.g., Asher & Taylor, 1981) might be used to evaluate changes in status and acceptance by peers. Peers might be asked questions such as "Which three children would you most/least like to sit next to you?" Semantic differentials might be another viable avenue; here, peers use a Likert-type scale to indicate the extent to which various adjectives, presented as polar opposites, describe a particular student (Lass, Ruscello, & Lakawicz, 1988). Whether these ratings are sensitive to changes resulting from AAC intervention and participation patterns should be explored in future research. Given the complexity of membership, however, researchers should also begin exploring the use of mixed methodology in AAC outcomes measurement (e.g., Tashakkori & Teddlie, 1998).

The complexity of membership would lend itself to the use of qualitative methods (e.g., participant observation and structured interviews; see also Ferguson, 1994) along with the quantitative methods just described. Ferguson

(1994) noted that "membership" is a community concept that conveys a certain sense of "belonging" that is the hallmark of membership. This is where membership and QOL are possibly related as conceptualized in some of the scales. It would be worthwhile to extend participation as an outcomes measurement area from school to community activities and settings (e.g., leisure).

Researchers may want to begin exploring what *learning* outcomes (if any) might be associated with increases in participation. It would seem that participation is a necessary but not sufficient precondition to learning. Data to evaluate learning outcomes would be highly desirable.

Future Research   In summary, participation is an important area of measurement in AAC. In fact, the field has the tools (i.e., the Activity Standards Inventory), definitions (e.g., barriers), and processes (e.g., selecting a comparison standard) to serve as a leader in providing specific meaning to the ICF construct of "activity and participation." Research into this area should receive high priority in the field. Some priority questions that should be addressed are

- What are the effects of facilitator training in the Participation Assessment Framework, the Activity Standards Inventory, and technologies on student participation under ideal conditions?
- What are the effects of facilitator training in the Participation Assessment Framework, the Activity Standards Inventory, and technologies on student participation under typical conditions?
    Can typical practitioners use the Activity Standards Inventory reliably as an outcomes measure?
    Which instructional formats are more susceptible to participation and interventions aimed at enhancing participation?
- What are the effects of learner-directed AAC interventions on functional communication and participation?
    How are communicative competence and participation related?
- How does enhanced participation lead to enhanced membership?
- Do changes in participation affect social and academic learning and, if so, how?

Participation and membership are two important outcome measures of AAC intervention in the "activities and participation" domain of the ICF. QOL is another important outcome measure that is at the heart of this domain.

Quality of Life

The QOL construct is complex, so it is not surprising that there is no agreed-on definition with well over 100 instruments that purport to measure some aspect of QOL (Cummins, 1997). This chapter relies on the following definition:

> Quality of life is both objective and subjective, each axis being the aggregate of seven domains: material well-being, health, productivity, intimacy, safety, community, and emotional well-being. Objective domains comprise culturally-relevant measures of objective well-being. Subjective domains comprise domain satisfaction weighted by their importance to the individual. (Cummins, 1997, p. 6)

The status of communication has a significant influence on people's QOL. This hypothesis is anecdotally substantiated by the lived experiences of many individuals using AAC. Robert Segelman, for example, wrote in a proposal for a professional conference "that finally obtaining a satisfactory method to communicate was one of the most important events in my life—right up there with getting married and earning my Ph.D." (Segalman, 2001, p. 5).

Taking this notion further, techniques that aim to improve one's ability to communicate may thus be viewed as enhancing a person's QOL—a so-called "quality enhancement technique" (Schalock, 1994). AAC should be recognized as a potential *direct* quality enhancement technique that also serves as an *indirect* quality enhancement technique. For instance, a child who learns to use an AAC system to communicate basic needs and wants is more likely able to make choices and decisions and to exert control over his or her environment.

To date, only a few studies have assessed the QOL status of individuals with developmental disabilities using AAC (Lund, Light, & Schlosser, 2000; Slesaransky-Poe, 1997). Slesaransky-Poe (1997) asked whether people with significant speech disabilities who use VOCAs have a better QOL than people who do not use VOCAs. Sixty-five adults (20 in the non-VOCA group and 45 in the VOCA group) were administered the Quality of Life Questionnaire (QOLQ; Schalock & Keith, 1994). Findings indicated that the QOL of individuals who use VOCAs was somewhat better than the QOL of those who did not; however, the difference was not statistically significant.

The retrospective study of seven individuals who used AAC and originally participated in descriptive studies by Light and colleagues (1985a, 1985b, 1985c) raised some interesting issues pertaining to QOL (Lund & Light, 2001). First, all participants reported a positive QOL, but there was significant variation across individuals with respect to global QOL scores. Second, the factors that contributed positively or negatively to QOL varied across individuals. That is, individuals who used AAC could achieve a positive QOL through different avenues. Finally, QOL did not seem to be directly related to educational achievement or communicative competence. In other words some of the young men with higher levels of educational achievement and communicative competence reported lower QOL than others who had lower levels of educational achievement, community involvement, and so forth. Lund and Light (2001) attributed this finding to the key role of individual expectations.

There appear to have been only a few published studies that examine QOL as an outcome of AAC services or interventions (Hass, Anderson, Brodin, & Persson, 1997; Tolley et al., 1995). Hass and colleagues (1997) studied the impact of computer-aided assistive technology on goal fulfillment, cost, and health-related QOL in 74 clients recruited from regional assistive technology centers in Sweden. The clients ranged in age from 5 to 74 years (mean = 24 years) with the majority in the range from 5 to 20 years (64%). Goal fulfillment measures included an estimation of degree of goal fulfillment based on a visual-analogue scale, with the endpoints "not fulfilled" corresponding to the score of 0 and "completely" corresponding to 10. Results indicated various levels of goal fulfillment, but no differences in terms of pre- and post-QOL measures. Furthermore, the clients fared lower in terms of QOL compared to the typical population both prior to and after implementation of computer-aided assistive technology.

Tolley and colleagues (1995) studied QOL outcomes of assessment programs provided by Specialist Communication Aids Centres (CACs) in the United Kingdom. In order to assess the QOL impact of the prescription of a communication aid, a modified version of the Rosser Classification of Disability/Distress States was used (Kind, Rosser, & Williams, 1982). The disability rating scale ranges from I (no disability, normal conversation) to VII (no mobility or no communication ability). The distress rating scale ranges from A (no distress) to D (severe distress).

Tolley and colleagues (1995) aimed at testing the "reliability" of the instrument used by using a second simple measure of QOL change based on clients' own self-perception. Specifically, clients were asked to assess the effect of the communication aid on their QOL in terms of "much better," "slightly better," "no change," "slightly worse," or "much worse." Results of the study indicated that 38% of clients demonstrated a gain in their disability/distress ratings using the Rosser system. Using the self-perception measure, nearly four fifths of clients perceived some improvements and less than one third claimed that their QOL was "much better." These results need to be viewed with extreme caution given the numerous methodological and conceptual problems with this study.

Priorities for Future Research   Improvement in QOL is perhaps the ultimate desired outcome of AAC services and interventions. Great strides have been made in assessing QOL of people with intellectual disabilities (Goode, 1994); however, relatively little attention has been directed toward the assessment of QOL of people with little or no functional speech. Table 14.4 provides a comparative overview of five QOL scales in terms of QOL definition, evaluation domains and subdomains, evaluation method, population targeted, and strengths and weaknesses. These measures were selected due to their focus on developmental disabilities and frequent citation in QOL articles and other texts.

A good QOL scale

• Has adequate psychometric properties
• Is normed for the population targeted

Table 14.4. Comparison of selected quality of life scales

Instrument (reference)	Quality of life (QOL) definition	Evaluation domains and subdomains	Evaluation method	Population targeted	Strengths	Weaknesses
Quality of Life Profile: People with Physical and Sensory Disabilities (Renwick, Brown, & Raphael, 1998)	The degree to which a person enjoys the important possibilities of his or her life	Being—"who one is" (physical, psychological, spiritual) Belonging—person's fit with his or her environment (physical, social, community) Becoming—purposeful activities carried out to achieve personal goals, hopes, and wishes (practical, leisure, growth)	92-item self-report questionnaire 5-level scale defined by written and visual descriptors Rated in terms of self-perceived levels of satisfaction, importance, control, and opportunity Rated also in terms of the quality of the environment in which a person lives Scores more reflective of individual client's perception of QOL; allow for preferential weighting as part of final score calculation A basic QOL score is determined by the interaction between importance and enjoyment scores	Adults with physical disabilities of unknown age	Based on an individual concept of QOL (weighting in terms of satisfaction, importance, control, and opportunity) Adequate psychometric properties (Renwick, Brown, & Nagler, 1995) Available in parallel form for populations without disabilities	Responsiveness for outcomes evaluation is unknown Unclear whether any of the respondents used any form of AAC Pretesting for necessary skills to complete questionnaire not available
Quality of Life Profile: Instrument Package for Persons with Developmental Disabilities (Raphael, Brown, Renwick, & Rootman, 1996)	The degree to which a person enjoys the important possibilities of his or her life	Being—"who one is" (physical, psychological, spiritual) Belonging—person's fit with environment (physical, social, community)	1. Participant interview (of person with developmental disabilities); Semi-structured interview 54 key questions (6 for each of 9 subdomains) Examines importance and enjoyment Information provided is used by interviewer for ratings Importance and enjoyment ratings lead to Basic QOL score	Adults with developmental disabilities. Participants were able to understand and respond to the demands of the participant interview and self-ratings	Based on an individual concept of QOL (weighting in terms of satisfaction, and importance)	Responsiveness for outcomes evaluation is unknown Time-consuming to do all instruments

500

		measure. Some individuals who used AAC were included (I. Brown, personal communication, February 12, 1998)	For outcomes evaluation purposes, it is unclear what the interview would add to the self-report
Becoming—purposeful activities carried out to achieve personal goals, hopes, and wishes (practical, leisure, growth)	2. Self-ratings (by person with developmental disabilities): 36-item self-report measure (four for each subdomain) 5-point continual scale Examines self-perceived importance, enjoyment, control, and opportunities	Ratings on control, and opportunity provide contextual/ environmental information for interpretation	Not normed for children
	3. Who decides questionnaire (by person with developmental disabilities): 16-item self-report measure Examines who makes decisions about daily living Two sections: life decisions and daily routine decisions	Satisfactory reliability and validity (see Raphael et al., 1996)	Objective pretesting not available (people judged to have sufficient communicative ability took part in the interview, and others did not; (I. Brown, personal communication, February 12, 1998)
	4. Other questionnaire (by close other person): 216-items (6 concepts x 9 subdomains x 4 rating types) Examines importance, enjoyment, control, and opportunity	Use of multiple instruments and sources	
	5. Who decides questionnaire (by close other person)	Available in parallel form for populations without disabilities	
	6. Assessor checklist (by an expert assessor): 27-item checklist (four per subdomain, except for "becoming") Examines commonly held expectations of people's QOL Based on observations, results of the interview, informal conversations with close others		

(continued)

501

Table 14.4. Continued

Instrument (reference)	Quality of life (QOL) definition	Evaluation domains and subdomains	Evaluation method	Population targeted	Strengths	Weaknesses
Quality of Life Questionnaire (Schalock, 1990, 1991; Schalock & Keith, 1994)	A person's desired conditions of living related to home and community living, employment, and health functioning (Schalock, 1994)	Domains: satisfaction, competence/ productivity, empowerment/ independence, social belonging/community integration Core dimensions: emotional well-being, interpersonal relations, material well-being, personal development, physical well-being, self-determination, social inclusion, rights	Questionnaire: 3-level scale defined by written descriptors Verbal clients: Use self-report Nonspeaking clients: Use proxies	Adults with mild to moderate intellectual disabilities	Validated through cross-cultural studies with populations with mental and developmental disabilities in five countries (Schalock, 1994) Adequate reliability and validity (Schalock, Keith, & Hoffman, 1990).	Unknown responsiveness 3-level scale rather than 5- or 7-level scale Pretesting for skills not available Nomothetic (only available for adults with intellectual and developmental disabilities) Pictographic differentials are not provided
Quality of Life Interview Schedule (QUOLIS) (Ouellette-Kuntz & McCreary, 1995)	Provides no exact definition but states that QOL and quality of care are inseparable	Health services, family guardianship, income maintenance, education–employment, housing and safety, transportation,	Semi-structured interview Proxies as respondents 72 QOL indicators Rated in terms of four dimensions: support (available, not available), access (7-point scale), participation, and contentment (7-point scale)	People with severe to profound intellectual disabilities (IQ < 35) and severe communication disorders	Some psychometric properties are available for the contentment scale (Ouellette-Kuntz, 1989, 1990)	Unknown responsiveness Only few psychometric properties are available Semi-structured interviews are time-consuming

502

		social-recreational, religious-cultural, case management, advocacy, counseling, aesthetics	Scores are combined with narrative responses to summarize QOL			Research has shown that proxy reports do not correlate with client reports of subjective QOL
						Nomothetic definition of QOL and measure
Comprehensive Quality of Life Scale—Intellectual Disability (Cummins, 1993; Cummins, McCabe, Romeo, Reid, & Waters, 1997)	QOL is both objective and subjective, each axis being the aggregate of seven domains: material well-being, health, productivity, intimacy, safety, place in community, and emotional well-being. Objective domains comprise culturally-relevant measures of objective well-being. Subjective domains comprise domain satisfaction weighted by their importance to the individual.	Material well-being, health, productivity, intimacy, safety, community, emotional well-being Two axes: objective and subjective	Questionnaire: *Objective axis:* 21-items on a 5-point scale (three items per domain) *Subjective axis:* importance (5-point scale), satisfaction (7-point scale) *Pretesting protocol:* determines whether the person is able to validly complete the subjective axis including three tasks: size ordering of five wooden cubes, matching cube size to a printed scale of importance, and ranking an item known to be personally valued on an importance scale, thereby demonstrating the ability to use this scale in an abstract manner. The first two tasks commence with a binary choice, moving gradually to a 3- and 5-point choice. The highest level of scale complexity that was used successfully is adopted for responding to the scale (simplest = binary response mode) *Pictographic differentials:* Replacement of the Likert scale of satisfaction with a series of outline faces, from happy to very sad. *Parallel scale for proxies:* To provide vicarious subjective responses on behalf of the person with a disability. This scale is used when client is unable to complete subjective scale or for experimental inquiry in the process of vicarious responding.	59 people living in group homes were randomly selected. Age (range: 17–63 years; mean = 37.2). Slosson mean age equivalent was 5.4 years (range: 2.7 to 9.3). Comparative student data were derived from 69 university students. Age (range 17–44 years; mean = 21.4).	Designed for individuals with communication disorders and severe intellectual disabilities Provides guidelines for interviewer preparation and proxy use Psychometric properties are satisfactory Provides objective pretesting Provides pictographic differentials Provides a parallel version for people without disabilities Less time-consuming and demanding in terms of communicative competence than semi-structured interviews	Responsiveness of outcomes evaluation is unknown Pretesting does not include a test of participants' understanding of the concept of satisfaction The source of the pictographic differentials is unclear Does not assess the dimensions of control and opportunity (see Raphael et al., 1996 entry)

- Is grounded in current QOL theory (QOL construct is the same as for population without disabilities)
- Permits first-hand reports
- Has adequate pretesting protocols to determine necessary skills
- Includes objective and subjective domains and provides personalized domain-weighting for subjective QOL
- Is time-efficient and easily quantifiable.

Psychometric properties include the scales' reliability, validity, and sensitivity. The greatest weakness in terms of psychometric properties, however, rests with the sensitivity of the measures reviewed.

To be appropriate for use as an outcomes measure in AAC, the scale should be normed on individuals who use AAC. None of the instruments reviewed were specifically normed for individuals with severe communication impairments. Each instrument included some individuals who were nonspeaking more or less accidentally through random selection of a larger population. The exact number of participants and their specific characteristics (e.g., communicative competence), however, have not been reported. Furthermore, all instruments reviewed were normed for adults, although some of them included parallel forms for adolescents without disabilities (Cummins et al., 1997; Raphael, Brown, Renwick, & Rootman, 1996; Renwick, Brown, & Raphael, 1998). There is a dearth of measures that are intended for use with children with developmental disabilities, in general, and individuals who use AAC in particular.

QOL theory suggests that the measure should *also* be normed on the population at large. To consider the QOL domains measured as specific to people with disabilities rather than the population at large is consistent with a monothetic conceptualization of QOL. This is counterproductive, prevents normative comparisons of life quality, and may even bear dangerous consequences:

> The QOL of people with an intellectual disability may be judged by a standard which would be personally unacceptable to most people in the community; . . . if the criteria for a high quality of life do not rise above the attainment of basic needs and normative living, then these people may have a low QOL in relation to the general population, but this fact will be masked. (Cummins et al., 1997, p. 9)

Research has shown that proxy reports, defined as reports from someone else on behalf of the direct stakeholder, do not necessarily correspond with first-hand reports and are thus of questionable validity (Cummins et al., 1997; Heal & Sigelman, 1990; Sigelman et al., 1983; Woodend, Nair, & Tang, 1997). Among the instruments reviewed here, only QUOLIS is based on the assumption that client responses cannot be obtained and therefore proxy responses are considered the only possible solution. All other measures have some mechanism in place to determine whether first-hand responses are possible, and if not, use proxy reports.

QOL theory suggests that there are objective and subjective domains to someone's QOL (e.g., Cummins, 1997). Most measures incorporate only *subjective QOL*. Only the ComQol-I provides both subjective and objective aspects to QOL. Once one acknowledges that many aspects of QOL are essentially subjective, the next logical step is to provide for respondents the opportunity to make their preferences known—a process referred to as "personalized domain weighting." For example, an individual who watches television all weekend long may be considered to have a poor QOL given that this person does not seem to interact with other human beings. Perhaps, one may even go as far as to say that this person does not have any friends. Personalized domain weighting would allow this individual to indicate how important it is to him to have friends. As a result one may come to different conclusions concerning the individual's subjective QOL. The following three measures include personalized domain weighting: the QOLP-PD, the QOLP-DD, and the ComQol-I.

When aiming to use QOL instruments as outcomes measures it is important that they can be used within the time constraints of daily practice. Most of the instruments are relatively time-efficient. To be useful in outcomes measurement, the scales need to lend themselves to easy quantification. All of the measures are easily quantifiable, including the semi-structured interviews (the interviewer assigns a rating based on the responses of the interviewees). The complexity of quantification varies somewhat among instruments. Instruments that incorporate some form of personalized domain weighting tend to be somewhat more complex. This small amount of added complexity is justified for obtaining a score that is based on recent QOL theory.

What would it take to evaluate the effects of AAC interventions or services on the QOL of an individual using AAC? In addition to the selection of an appropriate scale, the following constitutes a list of essential principles. First, the goals (or expected outcomes) across the participants in terms of AAC and QOL need to be comparable. In other words, one would not want to mix participants with progressive disorders with individuals with developmental disorders due to differing expectations in terms of QOL. Second, both pre-intervention and post-intervention measures of QOL need to be collected in real time. Third, there needs to be documentation that the AAC intervention did indeed yield its expected outcomes. Fourth, in order to rule out that extraneous variables may have caused QOL changes, it is essential to have a control group if the group design strategy is employed. The experimental group is expected to demonstrate goal attainment for AAC and improvement in QOL. The control group, which does not receive AAC services or interventions, however, is expected to show no goal attainment and no comparable changes in QOL. Alternatively, researchers should explore how QOL measurements can be mapped onto intervention studies using single-subject experimental designs. Studies that incorporate these principles would move this field forward both in research and practice.

Clearly, the field of QOL has made considerable strides in terms of measuring QOL. Yet, little of this knowledge appears to have been consulted by AAC researchers. QOL researchers have not consulted with AAC researchers in terms of specific issues pertaining to the assessment of QOL in people with little or no functional speech. The time is right for collaborative undertakings among researchers in the field of QOL and AAC. The mutual benefits are numerous. QOL researchers, for example, have yet to consider AAC as a potential quality enhancement technique in their deliberations (Schalock, 1994). We need to study not only how AAC might function as a quality enhancement technique itself but also how it might facilitate other quality enhancement techniques (e.g., self-determination). Moreover, some of the developers of QOL instruments need to revise their procedures for determining whether or not to rely on proxy reports. It is very clear to us in the AAC field that the lack of functional speech does not automatically translate into the need to use proxy reports. After all, speaking is not one of the necessary skills for completing a QOL instrument.

QOL researchers may also benefit from collaboration by improving pretesting protocols through AAC research. The use of "pictographic differentials" as alternate response formats in the ComQol-I certainly has considerable potential and is a noteworthy attempt to increase the yield of first-hand reports. The source of the pictographs, however, is unknown, and perhaps there are other line drawings available that are more iconic. In the current pretesting protocol, an individual who does not pass a certain level of scale difficulty (say a three-level scale) moves on to a less difficult scale (a two-level scale). This assumes that the individual is unable to handle the complexity of the scale. It may also be that the individual has difficulties with graphic representations, not with the referents themselves. Studies into the comparative iconicity of various graphic symbols (drawn from various symbol sets) that are used to anchor the various Likert scales (satisfaction, importance, opportunity) may assist us in maximizing first-hand reports yielded from the existing scales. It may also be worthwhile exploring whether the individual's existing graphic symbol set can represent a better source for the "pictographic differentials" rather than the standard set that comes with the scale. In other words, a person with experience using Picture Communication Symbols may be familiar with the graphic representations of some of the scale values and therefore do better with these symbols than with the standard pictographic differentials.

Some AAC users are sufficiently literate to read the questions on QOL instruments, but may have motoric difficulties responding to the questionnaire. Here, research may help identify whether alternate response formats such as scanning (or partner-assisted scanning) may be appropriate to yield the same results that would have been obtained through standard means.

AAC clinicians and researchers can learn from the QOL literature concerning the construct of QOL, with all its domains both subjective and objective, and its ratings such as satisfaction, importance, and opportunity. Secondly, AAC clinicians and researchers can benefit from the many measurement issues discussed here and apply them to the selection of QOL instruments in their own research.

Priority Questions

Following are some of the priorities important for the field to address in order to enhance understanding of AAC and its role in shaping QOL. Efficacy research should precede outcomes research (the same specific questions could be repeated under everyday interventions), and research into conceptual and methodological issues should take precedence over other work.

- What are the effects of *controlled* AAC interventions on the QOL of individuals using AAC?
     What are the effects of teaching a beginning communicator to use symbolic means to request and reject on their QOL?
     What are the effects of changes in communicative competence as perceived by proxies on QOL?
     What are the effects of changes in self-perceived communicative competence on QOL?
- What are the effects of *everyday* AAC interventions on the QOL of individuals using AAC?
- What are the effects of AAC intervention as an *indirect* quality enhancement technique?
- What is the difference (if any) between first-hand reports and proxy reports in assessing the QOL of individuals using AAC?
- How do changes in QOL relate to other outcome indicators such as self-determination, participation, membership, and happiness?
- How can existing measures be made more accessible to individuals using AAC?
     What is the iconicity of pictographic differentials used in existing QOL instruments?
     Are other graphic symbols used in AAC more iconic?
     Do graphic symbols in a person's existing repertoire lend themselves better to use as pictographic differentials than the symbols used in the existing instruments?
     Can existing AAC technologies for teaching symbol–referent relations be used for those people who fail the pretesting?
     What is the validity of alternate response formats (e.g., partner-assisted scanning) in completing QOL questionnaires?

CONCLUSION

The AAC field needs to devote a concerted effort to studying the outcomes of everyday interventions and services. Although there is a sense of urgency given the climate of accountability, there is merit in the careful conceptualization and design of outcomes research in AAC. A multidimensional approach to outcomes measurement, including the perspective of evaluation, the focus of evaluation, and the level of evaluation, was proposed toward that end. Relative to this model, the knowledge base is characterized by an inadequate representation of relevant stakeholder perspectives, a preoccupation with the validation of outcomes at the expense of other stages of service delivery, and an underrepresentation of studies focused on the outcomes of AAC interventions in terms of activity limitation and participation restriction. Nonetheless, the multidimensional model is intended as a conceptual framework that could drive (at least to some degree) how we tackle the study of AAC outcomes. Having taken a back seat as a field in outcomes measurement bears a myriad of problems—no one would argue with that. Sometimes, however, it affords the unique opportunity to avoid some of the "mistakes" made by the leading fields in outcomes measurement.

Communication is not really the point of all that is desired from interventions and services. Rather, changes in communication are intended to improve participation and membership of individuals using AAC. Even though researchers are only at the beginning of understanding the role of AAC interventions for participation, the AAC field has the tools (i.e., the Activity Standards Inventory), definitions (e.g., barriers), and processes (e.g., selecting a comparison standard) to serve as leader in providing specific meaning to the ICF construct of activity and participation.

REFERENCES

Asher, S., & Taylor, A. (1981). Social outcomes of mainstreaming: Sociometric assessment and beyond. *Exceptional Education Quarterly, 1,* 13–40.

Bailey, D., & Simeonsson, R. (1988). Investigation of use of goal attainment scaling to evaluate individual progress of clients with severe and profound mental retardation. *Mental Retardation, 26,* 289–295.

Beukelman, D.R., & Mirenda, P. (1998). *Augmentative and alternative communication: Management of severe communication disorders in children and adults* (2nd ed.). Baltimore: Paul H. Brookes Publishing Co.

Billingsley, F.F., White, O.R., & Munson, R. (1980). Procedural reliability: A rationale and an example. *Behavioral Assessment, 2,* 229–241.

Blackstone, S. (1995). Outcomes in AAC. *Augmentative Communication News, 7,* 1–8.

Burgee, M.L. (1996). A case study analysis of the intervention effect of goal attainment scaling in consultation. *Dissertation Abstract International Section A: Humanities and Social Sciences, 56*(8–A), 3053.

Calculator, S.N. (1991). Evaluating the efficacy of AAC intervention for children with severe disabilities. In J. Brodin & E. Björck-Åkesson (Eds.), *Methodological issues in research in augmentative and alternative communication: Proceedings from the First ISAAC Research Symposium* (pp. 22–31). Stockholm: The Swedish Handicap Institute.

Calculator, S.N. (1994). Communicative interventions as a means to successful inclusion. In S.N. Calculator & C.M. Jorgensen (Eds.), *Including students with severe disabilities in schools* (pp. 183–214). San Diego: Singular Publishing Group.

Calculator, S.N. (1999). AAC outcomes for children and youths with severe disabilities: When seeing is believing. *Augmentative and Alternative Communication, 15,* 4–12.

Carrow-Woolfolk, E. (1985). *Test for Auditory Comprehension of Language, Revised Edition.* Austin, TX: PRO-ED.

Cummins, R.A. (1993). *Comprehensive Quality of Life Scale–Intellectual Disability* (4th ed.). Melbourne: Deakin University.

Cummins, R.A. (1997). *Comprehensive Quality of Life Scale–Intellectual/Cognitive Disability* (5th ed.). Melbourne: Deakin University.

Cummins, R.A., McCabe, M.P., Romeo, Y., Reid, S., & Waters, L. (1997). An initial evaluation of the Comprehensive Quality of Life Scale–Intellectual Disability. *International Journal of Disability, Development and Education, 44,* 7–19.

Cytrynbaum, S., Birdwell, G.Y., Birdwell, J., & Brandt, L. (1979). Goal attainment scaling: A critical review. *Evaluation Quarterly, 3,* 5–40.

Dunn, L.M., & Dunn, L.M. (1981). *Peabody Picture Vocabulary Test–Revised.* Circle Pines, MN: American Guidance Service.

Fawcett, S.B. (1991). Social validity: A note on methodology. *Journal of Applied Behavior Analysis, 24,* 235–239.

Ferguson (1994). Is communication really the point? Some thoughts on interventions and membership. *Mental Retardation, 32,* 7–18.

Frattali, C.M. (1999). Outcome measurement: Definitions, dimensions and perspective. In C. Frattali (Ed.), *Measuring outcomes in speech-language pathology* (pp. 1–27). New York: Thieme.

Frattali, C.M., Thompson, C.K., Holland, A.L., Wohl, C.B., & Ferketic, M.M. (1995). *Functional Assessment of Communication Skills for Adults.* Rockville, MD: American Speech-Language-Hearing Association.

Fuqua, R.W., & Schwade, J. (1986). Social validation of applied behavioral research: A selective review and critique. In A.D. Poling & R.W. Fuqua (Eds.), *Research methods in applied behavior analysis* (pp. 265–292). New York: Plenum Publishers.

Giangreco, M.F., Cloninger, C.J., & Iverson, V.S. (1998). *Choosing outcomes and accommodations for children (COACH): A guide to planning for students with disabilities* (2nd ed.). Baltimore: Paul H. Brookes Publishing Co.

Goode, D. (1994). *Quality of life for persons with disabilities: International perspectives and issues.* Cambridge, MA: Brookline Books.

Granlund, M., & Blackstone, S. (1999). Outcomes measurement in AAC. In F. Loncke, J. Clibbens, H.H. Arvidson, & L.L. Lloyd (Eds.), *AAC: New directions in research and practice* (pp. 207–227). London: Whurr Publishers.

Granlund, M., & Steénson, A.-L. (1998). Team över tid [A longitudinal study of teams]. In M. Granlund (Ed.), *Barn med Flera Funktionsnedättingar i Särskolan* (pp. 265–382). Stockholm: Stifelsen ALA.

Hass, U., Anderson, A., Brodin, H., & Persson, J. (1997). Assessment of computer-aided assistive technology: Analysis of outcomes and costs. *Augmentative and Alternative Communication, 13,* 125–135.

Heal, L.W., & Sigelman, C.K. (1990). Methodological issues in measuring the quality of life of individuals with mental retardation. In R.L. Schalock (Ed.), *Quality of life:*

Perspectives and issues (pp. 161–176). Washington, DC: American Association on Mental Retardation.

Johnson, R. (1992). *The Picture Communication Symbols–Book III.* Solana Beach: Mayer–Johnson Co.

Jorgensen, C.M. (1994). Developing individualized inclusive educational programs. In S.N. Calculator & C.M. Jorgensen (Eds.), *Including students with severe disabilities in schools: Fostering communication, interaction, and participation* (pp. 27–74). San Diego: Singular Publishing Co.

Kangas, K., & Lloyd, L.L. (1998). Alternative and augmentative communication. In G.H. Shames, E.H. Wiig, & W.A. Secord (Eds.), *Human communication disorders: An introduction* (pp. 510–551). Needham Heignts, MA: Allyn & Bacon.

Kazdin, A.E. (1980). Acceptability of alternative treatments for deviant child behavior. *Journal of Applied Behavior Analysis, 13,* 259–273.

Kendall, P., & Norton-Ford, J. (1982). Therapy outcome research methods. In P. Kendall, & J. Butcher, (Eds.), *Handbook of research methods in clinical psychology* (pp. 429–460). New York: John Wiley & Sons.

Kind, P., Rosser, R., & Williams, A. (1982). A valuation of quality of life: Some psychometric evidence. In M.W. Jones-Lee (Ed.), *The value of life and safety* (pp. 159–170). Amsterdam: Elsevier North Holland.

Kiresuk, T., & Sherman, R. (1968). Goal attainment scaling: A general method for evaluating comprehensive mental health programmes. *Community Mental Health Journal, 4,* 443–453.

Kiresuk, T., Smith, A., & Cardillo, J. (1994). *Goal attainment scaling: Applications, theory, and measurement.* London: Lawrence Erlbaum Associates.

Lass, N., Ruscello, D., & Lakawicz, J. (1988). Listeners' perceptions of nonspeech characteristics of normal and dysarthric children. *Journal of Communication Disorders, 21,* 385–391.

Lewis, A.B., Spencer, J.H., Jr., Haas, G.L., & DiVittis, A. (1987). Goal attainment scaling: Relevance and replicability in follow-up of inpatients. *Journal of Nervous and Mental Disease, 175,* 408–418.

Light, J. (1989). Toward a definition of communicative competence for individuals using augmentative and alternative communication systems. *Augmentative and Alternative Communication, 5,* 137–144.

Light, J.C., & Binger, C. (1998). *Building communicative competence with individuals who use augmentative and alternative communication.* Baltimore: Paul H. Brookes Publishing Co.

Light, J., Collier, B., & Parnes, P. (1985a). Communication interaction between young nonspeaking physically disabled children and their primary caregivers: Part I. Discourse patterns. *Augmentative and Alternative Communication, 1,* 74–83.

Light, J., Collier, B., & Parnes, P. (1985b). Communication interaction between young nonspeaking physically disabled children and their primary caregivers: Part II. Communicative functions. *Augmentative and Alternative Communication, 1,* 98–107.

Light, J., Collier, B., & Parnes, P. (1985c). Communication interaction between young nonspeaking physically disabled children and their primary caregivers: Part III. Modes of communication. *Augmentative and Alternative Communication, 1,* 125–133.

Light, J.C., & Schlosser, R.W. (2003). *Outcomes research in augmentative and alternative communication: A multidimensional approach.* Manuscript in preparation.

Lund, S., & Light, J. (2001). *Fifteen years later: An investigation of long-term outcomes of augmentative and alternative interventions: Final grant report.* University Park: The Pennsylvania State University. (ERIC Document No. ED458727)

Lund, S., Light, J., & Schlosser, R.W. (2000, August). *Fifteen years later: Long-term outcomes of AAC interventions.* Paper presented at the Biennial Conference of the International Society for Augmentative and Alternative Communication (ISAAC), Washington, DC.

MacKay, G., Somerville, W., & Lundie, J. (1996). Reflections on goal attainment scaling (GAS): Cautionary notes and proposals for development. *Educational Research, 38,* 161–172.

Mount, B. (1987). *Personal futures planning: Finding directions for change.* Ann Arbor: University of Michigan Dissertation Information Service.

Office of Technology Assessment. (1978). *Assessing the efficacy and safety of medical technologies* (OTA-H-75). Washington, DC: U.S. Government Printing Office.

Olswang, L.B. (1990). Treatment efficacy: The breadth of research. In L.B. Olswang, C.K. Thompson, S.F. Warren, & N.J. Minghetti (Eds.), *Treatment efficacy research in communication disorders: Proceedings of the American Speech-Language-Hearing Foundation's National Conference on Treatment Efficacy* (pp. 99–103). San Antonio, TX: American Speech-Language-Hearing Association.

Ottenbacher, K.J., & Cusick, A. (1993). Discriminative versus evaluative assessment: Some observations on goal attainment scaling. *American Journal of Occupational Therapy, 47,* 349–354.

Ouelette-Kuntz, H. (1989). *A pilot study in the use of quality of life interview schedule with emphasis on the intra- and inter-rater agreement.* Unpublished master's thesis, Queens University, Kingston, Ontario.

Ouelette-Kuntz, H. (1990). A pilot study in the use of quality of life interview schedule. *Social Indicators Research, 23,* 283–298.

Ouellette-Kuntz, H., & McCreary, B. (1995). Quality of life assessment for persons with severe developmental disabilities. In R. Renwick, I. Brown, & M. Nagler (Eds.), *Quality of life in health promotion and rehabilitation: Conceptual approaches, issues, and applications* (pp. 268–278). Thousand Oaks, CA: Sage Publications.

Parilis, G.M. (1996). The effects of goal attainment scaling on perceived self-efficacy, motivation, and academic achievement. *Dissertation Abstracts International Section A: Humanities and Social Sciences, 56*(7-A), 2615.

Raphael, D., Brown, I., Renwick, R., & Rootman, I. (1996). Assessing the quality of life of persons with developmental disabilities: Description of a new model, measuring instruments, and initial findings. *International Journal of Disability, Development, and Education, 43,* 25–24.

Renwick, R., Brown, I., & Nagler, M. (Eds.). (1995). *Quality of life in health promotion and rehabilitation: Conceptual approaches, issues, and applications.* Thousand Oaks, CA: Sage Publications.

Renwick, R., Brown, I., & Raphael, D. (1998). *The Quality of Life Profile: People with physical and sensory disabilities.* Toronto: University of Toronto, Centre for Health Promotion.

Robey, R.R., & Schultz, M.C. (1998). A model for conducting clinical-outcome research: an adaptation of the standard protocol for use in aphasiology. *Aphasiology, 12,* 787–810.

Rockwood, K., Joyce, B., & Stolee, P. (1993). Use of goal attainment in measuring clinically important change in cognitive rehabilitation patients. *Journal of Clinical Epidemiology, 50,* 581–588.

Rockwood, K., & Stolee, P. (1993). Use of goal attainment scaling in measuring clinically important change in the frail elderly. *Journal of Clinical Epidemiology, 46,* 1113–1118.

Schalock, R.L. (1990). *Quality of life: Perspectives and issues.* Washington, DC: American Association on Mental Retardation.

Schalock, R.L. (1991). *The concept of quality of life in the lives of persons with mental retardation.* (ERIC Document Reproduction Service No. ED337924)

Schalock, R.L. (1994). Quality of life, quality enhancement, and quality assurance: Implications for program planning and evaluation in the field of mental retardation and developmental disabilities. *Evaluation and Program Planning, 17,* 121–131.

Schalock, R.L., & Keith, K.D. (1994). *Quality of life questionnaire.* Worthington, OH: IDS Publishing Corporation.

Schalock, R.L., Keith, K.D., & Hoffman, K. (1990). *Quality of Life standardization manual.* Hastings, NE: Mid-Nebraska Mental Retardation Services.

Schlosser, R.W. (1999). Social validation of interventions in augmentative and alternative communication. *Augmentative and Alternative Communication, 15,* 234–247.

Schlosser, R.W. (2002). On the importance of being earnest about treatment integrity. *Augmentative and Alternative Communication, 18,* 36–44.

Schlosser, R.W. (2003a). *The efficacy of augmentative and alternative communication: Toward evidence-based practice.* San Diego: Academic Press.

Schlosser, R.W. (2003b). *Measuring outcomes in speech-language pathology through goal attainment scaling.* Manuscript under review.

Schlosser, R.W., & Braun, U. (1994). Efficacy of AAC interventions: Methodologic issues in evaluating behavior change, generalization, and effects. *Augmentative and Alternative Communication, 10,* 207–223.

Schlosser, R.W., & Kovach, T. (2002). *Using goal attainment scaling to measure outcomes in augmentative and alternative communication.* Research in progress.

Schlosser, R.W., McGhie-Richmond, D., Blackstien-Adler, S., Mirenda, P., Antonius, K., & Janzen, P. (2000). Training a school team to integrate technology meaningfully into the curriculum: Effects on student participation. *Journal of Special Education Technology, 15,* 31–44.

Schwartz, I.S., & Baer, D.M. (1991). Social validity assessments: Is current practice state of the art? *Journal of Applied Behavior Analysis, 24,* 189–204.

Segalman, B. (2001). *Telephone service for people with speech disabilities is available nationally.* Paper submitted to the Biennial Conference of ISAAC 2002.

Siegel, S. (1956). *Nonparametric statistics for the behavioral sciences.* New York: McGraw-Hill.

Sigelman, C.K., Schoenrock, C.J., Budd, E.C., Winer, J.L., Spanhel, C.L., Martin, P.W., Hromas, S., & Bensberg, G.J. (1983). *Communicating with mentally retarded persons: Asking questions and getting answers.* Lubbock: Research and Training Center in Mental Retardation, Texas Tech University.

Simeonsson, R.J., Bailey, D.B., Huntington, G.S., & Brandon, L. (1991). Scaling and attainment of goals in family-focused early intervention. *Community Mental Health Journal, 27,* 77–83.

Slesaransky-Poe, G. (1997). *Outcomes in AAC: Communicative effectiveness and quality of life.* Paper presented at the Annual Meeting of the American Association on Mental Retardation, New York.

Smith, A. (1994). Introduction and overview. In T. Kiresuk, A. Smith, & J. Cardillo (Eds.), *Goal attainment scaling: Applications, theory, and measurement* (pp. 1–14). London: Lawrence Erlbaum Associates.

Stephens, T.E., & Haley, S.M. (1991). Comparison of two methods for determining change in motorically-handicapped children. *Journal of Physical and Occupational Therapy in Pediatrics, 11,* 1–17.

Stolee, P., Rockwood, K., Fox, R.A., & Streiner, D.L. (1992). The use of goal attainment scaling in a geriatric care setting. *Journal of the American Geriatric Society, 40,* 574–578.

Stolee, P., Stadnyk, K., Myers, A.M., & Rockwood, K. (1999). An individualized approach to outcome measurement in geriatric rehabilitation. *Journals of Gerontology: Series A: Biological Sciences and Medical Sciences, 54A*(12), M641–M647.

Tashakkori, A., & Teddlie, C. (1998). *Applied Social Research Methods Series: Vol. 46. Mixed methodology: Combining qualitative and quantitative approaches.* Thousand Oaks, CA: Sage Publications.

Tolley, K., Leese, B., Wright, K., Hennessy, S., Rowley, C., Stowe, J., & Chamberlain, A. (1995). Communication aids for the speech impaired. Cost and quality-of-life outcomes of assessment programs provided by specialist Communication Aids Centers in the United Kingdom. *International Journal of Technology Assessment in Health Care, 11,* 196–213.

Vandercook, T., York, J., & Forest, M. (1989). The McGill action planning system (M. A. P. S.): A strategy for building a vision. *Journal of the Association for Persons with Severe Handicaps, 14,* 205–215.

Wehmeyer, M.L., & Kelchner, K. (1995). *The Arc's Self-Determination Scale.* Arlington, TX: The Arc National Headquarters.

Wiederholt, J.L., & Blalock, G. (2000). *Gray Silent Reading Test.* Austin, TX: PRO-ED.

Wolf, M.M. (1978). Social validity: The case for subjective measurement, or how applied behavior analysis is finding its heart. *Journal of Applied Behavior Analysis, 11,* 203–214.

Woodend, A.K., Nair, R.C., & Tang, S-L. (1997). Definition of life quality from a patient versus health care professional perspective. *International Journal of Rehabilitation Research, 20,* 71–80.

World Health Organization. (1980). *International classification of impairments, disabilities, and handicaps.* Geneva: Author.

World Health Organization. (2001). *International classification of functioning, disability, and health.* Madrid: Author.

Index

Page numbers followed by *f* indicate figures; those followed by *t* indicate tables.

515